Handbook of Tuberculosis

Handbook of Tuberculosis

Edited by Megan Durham

hayle medical
New York

Hayle Medical,
750 Third Avenue, 9th Floor,
New York, NY 10017, USA

Visit us on the World Wide Web at:
www.haylemedical.com

ISBN: 978-1-63241-648-3

The publisher's policy is to use permanent paper from mills that operate a sustainable forestry policy. Furthermore, the publisher ensures that the text paper and cover boards used have met acceptable environmental accreditation standards.

Printed in China.

Cataloging-in-Publication Data

Handbook of tuberculosis / edited by Megan Durham.
p. cm.
Includes bibliographical references and index.
ISBN 978-1-63241-648-3
1. Tuberculosis. 2. Chest--Diseases. 3. Lungs--Diseases. 4. Mycobacterium diseases.
I. Durham, Megan.
RC311 .H36 2019
616.99--dc23

Table of Contents

Preface

The main aim of this book is to educate learners and enhance their research focus by presenting diverse topics covering this vast field. This is an advanced book which compiles significant studies by distinguished experts in the area of analysis. This book addresses successive solutions to the challenges arising in the area of application, along with it; the book provides scope for future developments.

The infectious disease caused by mycobacterium tuberculosis is known as tuberculosis (TB). Some common symptoms of this disease are cough characterized by blood-containing sputum, along with night sweats, weight loss and fever. It can be diagnosed by chest X-rays, tuberculin skin test, culture and microscopic examination of body fluids. Tuberculosis majorly affects the lungs. The tuberculosis that does not affect the lungs is known as extra-pulmonary tuberculosis. BCG vaccine is a commonly used vaccine for preventing TB. It has certain limitations due to which constant research is ongoing to develop better vaccinations along with medications to treat multi-drug resistant TB. This book includes some of the vital pieces of work being conducted across the world, on various topics related to the diagnosis, prevention and management of tuberculosis. This book, with its detailed analyses and data, will prove immensely beneficial to practicing doctors and medical students.

It was a great honour to edit this book, though there were challenges, as it involved a lot of communication and networking between me and the editorial team. However, the end result was this all-inclusive book covering diverse themes in the field.

Finally, it is important to acknowledge the efforts of the contributors for their excellent chapters, through which a wide variety of issues have been addressed. I would also like to thank my colleagues for their valuable feedback during the making of this book.

Editor

The Application of GeneXpert MTB/RIF for Smear-Negative TB Diagnosis as a Fee-Paying Service at a South Asian General Hospital

Poojan Shrestha,[1] Amit Arjyal,[1] Maxine Caws,[2,3] Krishna Govinda Prajapati,[4] Abhilasha Karkey,[1] Sabina Dongol,[1] Saruna Pathak,[1] Shanti Prajapati,[1] and Buddha Basnyat[1]

[1]*Oxford University Clinical Research Unit, Patan Hospital, Patan Academy of Health Sciences, P.O. Box 252, Kathmandu, Nepal*
[2]*Department of Clinical Sciences, Liverpool School of Tropical Medicine, Pembroke Place, Liverpool L3 5QA, UK*
[3]*Oxford University Clinical Research Unit, Hospital for Tropical Diseases, Wellcome Trust Major Overseas Programme, 764 Vo Van Kiet, District 5, Ho Chi Minh City, Vietnam*
[4]*Department of Microbiology and Immunology, Patan Hospital, Patan Academy of Health Sciences, P.O. Box 252, Kathmandu, Nepal*

Correspondence should be addressed to Buddha Basnyat; buddhabasnyat@gmail.com

Academic Editor: Vincent Jarlier

The GeneXpert MTB/RIF assay (Xpert) is a novel automated diagnostic tool for tuberculosis but its optimal placement in the healthcare system has not been determined. The objective of this study was to determine the possibility of additional case detection for pulmonary tuberculosis (PTB) by offering Xpert to smear-negative patients in a low-HIV burden setting with no *Mycobacterium tuberculosis* (*M.tb.*) culture facilities. Patients routinely presenting with symptoms suggestive of PTB with negative smears were offered single Xpert test on a fee-paying basis. Data were retrospectively reviewed to determine case detection in patients tested from February to December 2013. Symptoms associated with a positive test were analysed to determine if refinement of clinical criteria would reduce unnecessary testing. 258 smear-negative patients were included and *M.tb.* was detected in 55 (21.32%, $n = 55/258$). Using standard clinical assessment for selection, testing 5 patients detected one case of smear-negative PTB. These results demonstrate that fee-paying Xpert service in low-income setting can increase TB case confirmation substantially and further systematic studies of health economic implications should be conducted to determine optimal implementation models to increase access to Xpert in low- and middle-income countries.

1. Introduction

Tuberculosis (TB) continues to be a major public health problem, with 8 million cases and 1.3 million deaths each year [1]. One of the key challenges for TB control is to increase case detection and early treatment, thereby interrupting transmission chains and reducing individual morbidity. The most widely used test for TB, sputum smear microscopy, has a sensitivity of only 50% of active cases which contributes to delayed diagnosis resulting in continued transmission [2, 3]. In an advanced diagnostic setting, facilities such as culture, drug susceptibility testing (DST), and commercial molecular diagnostics may be available, but these facilities are lacking in most hospitals in high burden countries. Sputum smears with chest X-ray (CXR), where available, are the tests routinely applied for TB diagnosis. It is crucial to implement improved diagnostics in these endemic settings if we are to reach the targets of case detection, reduction in mortality, and prevalence of the disease [4, 5].

Derivations from case burden estimates suggest that only around 70% of active TB cases are diagnosed using current strategies [1]. The development and implementation of the Xpert assay (Cepheid, Sunnyvale, CA, USA), which has high sensitivity in detection of smear-negative TB, has raised hopes of increased case detection in low- and middle-income countries (LMICs). Xpert is the only fully automated real-time DNA-based test which can detect both TB and rifampicin resistance (RR) [6, 7]. The test is based on a heminested PCR test which detects the presence of *Mycobacterium tuberculosis* complex bacilli [8]. The PCR target, an 81-base-pair region of the *rpoB* gene, is the rifampicin resistance determining region (RRDR) [6, 9]. The reactions take place in a single-use cartridge making it easy to operate, without cross contamination, and giving a result in as little as 2 hours and thus potentially decreasing default due to delayed diagnosis [7, 10].

In the most recent meta-analysis, Xpert as an initial replacement for smear microscopy showed a pooled sensitivity of 89% (95% credible interval CrI 85% to 92%) and pooled specificity of 99% (95% CrI 98% to 99%), and as an add-on test following a negative smear microscopy, pooled sensitivity and specificity were 67% (95% CrI 60% to 74%) and 99% (95% CrI 98% to 99%), respectively [11]. For RR detection, it achieved a pooled sensitivity of 95% (95% CrI 90% to 97%) and a pooled specificity of 98% (95% CrI 97% to 99%) [11]. The test was first endorsed by WHO in 2010 [11, 12] and revised recommendations in 2013 included a recommendation that Xpert be used in all suspected TB cases, with the acknowledgement that this has substantial resource limitations [13].

However, despite a substantial negotiated price reduction on the test for LMICs, the 10 USD per cartridge remains expensive for low-income countries which often have per capita healthcare expenditure of <30 USD [14]. There have been limited reports of Xpert implementation on a fee-paying basis in such settings, with the majority of projects implementing free at point of care, a model which is dependent on sustained aid funding. Although the test cost is high to the patient, a confirmed diagnosis can avert often lengthy differential investigations and exploratory treatment which may cost substantially more. We therefore examined the impact on case detection of implementing Xpert as an optional fee-paying service to patients with suspected smear-negative TB.

In Nepal, the estimated incidence of TB is 163 per 100,000 with a prevalence rate of 241 per 100,000 population. In 2012-13, the Nepal Tuberculosis Programme (NTP) registered 17,788 sputum smear-positive cases and 8,367 sputum smear-negative cases [15]. In common with many LMICs, many pulmonary TB cases treated in the private sector go unreported and therefore there is likely to be discrepancy between official figures and the true numbers being diagnosed and treated. Although multidrug resistant tuberculosis (MDR TB) rates remain relatively low, at 2.2% in new and 17.2% among retreatment cases, only 262, one-quarter of the estimated MDR cases, were treated via the national programme in 2012-13 [15]. The positive predictive value of rifampicin resistance detection using Xpert in an unselected patient population will be low and confirmation of MDR is necessary before MDR treatment is initiated.

A recent Cochrane study concluded that more research would be helpful in evaluating the use of Xpert in TB programmes in high TB burden settings [11].

We report here the experience of implementing Xpert at a general hospital in Kathmandu, Nepal, and determine the number needed to test in order to detect one active case of smear-negative TB.

2. Materials and Methods

Patan Hospital is a 450-bed government general hospital providing emergency and elective outpatient and inpatient services, located in the Lalitpur area of the Kathmandu valley. The laboratory services are limited with acid-fast bacilli smear available but no provision for *M.tb.* culture.

From February 18, 2013, an Xpert machine was made available for testing. Clinical practitioners both from within and outside the hospital were invited to refer patients with symptoms consistent with TB and three negative sputum smears to testing by Xpert. Patients offered the test were informed about the test evaluation and asked for consent to collect baseline data on demographics and symptoms at presentation. This study was approved by the Institutional Review Board of Patan Hospital.

Patients with 3 negative Ziehl-Neelsen (ZN) sputum smears were referred for Xpert testing at the treating clinician's discretion. A new sputum sample was collected for Xpert testing. Data was collected on history of persistent cough (≥2 weeks), fever, drenching night sweats, weight loss (>1.5 kg in a month), loss of appetite, malaise, and shortness of breath or chest pain.

CXR reports were collected where available. For further analysis, CXR features were classified by the study investigators according to radiologist's report as upper lobe infiltrates, pleural effusion, diffuse infiltrates, cavitary lesions, other infiltrates, consolidation, other abnormalities, and normal. CXR reported as patchy infiltrates, bilateral infiltrates, and infiltrates without a specified location was classified as "other infiltrates." "Other abnormalities" comprised of pneumothorax, hyperinflation, lung abscess, mediastinal opacity, nodular opacity, mass lesion, and pleural thickening.

At Patan Hospital, the acid-fast bacilli microscopy is performed by experienced laboratory personnel following the guidelines set by the NTP and is monitored by the NTP external quality assessment (EQA) scheme. The sputum sample for the Xpert was processed according to manufacturer's guidelines. The patients were charged NPR 2000 (~20 USD) per test. This cost included freight charges (~$3 per cartridge), staffing, annual machine calibration ($450 per year), and annual maintenance charge (~$2,700 per year). The HIV status was reported by the patient but no confirmatory HIV testing was performed. Data on the treatment outcome was not collected.

We further examined whether restricting the tested population would miss cases of TB or improve efficiency of testing and reduce unnecessary patient charges. We determined the number needed to test if the tested population was restricted to (1) those with 2 or more symptoms consistent with TB (fever, night sweats, persistent cough (≥2 weeks), weight loss (≥1.5 kg in a month), malaise, shortness of breath, or chest pain) or (2) those with CXR abnormalities and 2 or more symptoms or (3) those with only the CXR abnormalities found in the Xpert positive group.

Categorical variables were compared between patient groups testing positive and negative by Xpert using Fisher's exact test with a P value of ≤ 0.05 considered as significant.

3. Results

Between February 18, 2013, and December 30, 2013, 258 smear-negative patients were tested by Xpert on sputum. Eighty-nine patients were referred from other hospitals throughout the Kathmandu valley, while 169 were from Patan Hospital clinics. Data were not systematically collected on patients who were smear-negative but not offered the test during the study period but no patients declined the test when offered at Patan Hospital. No patient declined consent for data collection and we therefore included all Xpert tested patients in the analysis.

During the study period, there were 2,222 new patients tested by smear microscopy at Patan Hospital. Of these, 1,070 had 3 negative sputum smears and 196 had at least one positive sputum smear. The remaining 956 patients did not complete 3 sputum smears. Therefore, 169/1070 (15.8%) of diagnostic subjects were offered an Xpert test. In the majority of cases, this was due to an alternative diagnosis being reached or symptom resolution/improvement during the smear and CXR diagnostic process, but this was not systematically evaluated.

Xpert was positive for *M.tb.* in 55 (n = 55/258, 21.3%) patients. Therefore, 4.7 patients needed to be tested to detect one active TB case. All patients with a positive Xpert test were referred for free treatment in the appropriate NTP DOTS facility.

A third of patients (n = 93/258, 37.98%) was female and the median age was 52 (interquartile range IQR 33–68). Four children were included (13, 15, and two 17 years of age). There were 2 patients (n = 2/258, 0.8%) with a positive result for rifampicin resistant TB by the Xpert test. The first patient was referred for sputum culture and phenotypic drug susceptibility testing at a tertiary centre (GENETUP, Nepal). The second rifampicin resistant patient was untraceable for follow-up by the phone number provided. No patient reported known HIV infection.

Table 1 shows the clinical features of the patients. The only clinical feature to show a statistically significant difference between the groups was shortness of breath, which was more common among Xpert negative patients (56.6 versus 72.2%, P = 0.04). As this finding nevertheless occurred in half of Xpert positive patients, it was not appropriate for refining the group of patients tested.

CXR was available for 187 patients (Table 2). Thirteen patients (n = 13/187, 6.9%) had no abnormality detected on CXR. Upper lobe infiltrates (P = 0.03) and cavitary lesions (P = 0.03) were more common among the Xpert positive group. Consolidation (P = 0.04) was not evident among the Xpert positive group while it was reported in 9.4% of Xpert negative patients.

Table 1: Comparison of clinical features of 251 patients with suspected smear negative TB testing positive and negative by Xpert.

Clinical features	Xpert positive	Xpert negative	P value
Cough	38 (71.7)	143 (72.2)	1
Fever	28 (52.8)	90 (45.5)	0.36
Night sweats	23 (43.4)	61 (30.8)	0.10
Loss of appetite	39 (73.6)	140 (70.7)	0.74
Weight loss	31 (58.5)	106 (53.5)	0.54
Malaise	42 (79.3)	164 (82.8)	0.55
Shortness of breath/chest pain	30 (56.6)	143 (72.2)	0.04
Total	53 (100)	198 (100)	

*Clinical questionnaire was not available for 7 patients.
kg = kilogram.

Table 2: Comparison of chest X-ray features of 187 patients testing positive or negative by Xpert.

Chest X-ray findings	Xpert positive	Xpert negative	P value
Upper lobe infiltrates	12 (31.57)	22 (14.86)	0.03
Cavitary lesions	5 (10.52)	5 (4.05)	0.03
Pleural effusion	9 (29.68)	27 (18.24)	0.49
Diffuse infiltration	7 (18.42)	26 (17.56)	1
Consolidation	0	14 (9.45)	0.04
Others	0	11 (6.75)	0.12
Normal	1 (2.6)	12 (8.10)	0.30
Other infiltrates	6 (13.15)	24 (16.89)	1
Infiltrates not in upper lobes	5 (13.15)	21 (14.18)	1
Total	39 (100)	148 (100)	

*Sum of the categories is greater than the total number of patients as one patient may be in more than one category.

No clinical questionnaire was available for 7 patients, leaving 251 patients in the symptom analysis (Table 3). If the Xpert testing was restricted to patients with 2 or more symptoms, the number needed to test was not altered and remained at 4.6 (n = 50/232, 21.6% positive). Three cases of TB would have been missed.

187 patients had an available questionnaire and CXR report. If CXR abnormalities and 2 clinical symptoms were required for Xpert testing, the number needed to test was 4.5 (n = 36/163, 22.1%). Three cases of TB would have been missed.

187 patients had CXR available. If testing were restricted to only those with an abnormal CXR showing at least one of the four characteristics, upper lobe infiltrates, cavitary lesions, pleural effusion, or infiltrates, then the number needed to test was 4 (n = 38/152 = 25%). 1 case would have been missed.

4. Discussion

This report demonstrates that application of Xpert testing as a fee-paying service in a general hospital can substantially

Table 3: Number of patients detected as positive by GeneXpert using different inclusion criteria for testing.

Patients	Number of patients with information n (%)	Number of patients tested	Numbers of Xpert positive n (%)	Number needed to test	Numbers of patients not meeting the criteria	Xpert positive in group not meeting criteria n (%)
At least 2 symptoms*	251 (93.7)	232	50 (21.6)	4.6	19	3 (15.8)
At least 2 symptoms + CXR**	187 (72.5)	163	36 (22.1)	4.5	24	3 (12.5)
At least the 4 listed CXR abnormalities	187 (72.5)	152	38 (25.0)	4.0	35	1 (2.9)

*7 patients had no available information of symptoms and were therefore excluded.
**71 patients did not have information of CXR report and were therefore excluded.

increase the yield of confirmed TB cases. Five patients need to be tested to detect one TB case by applying simple routine criteria to select smear-negative TB suspects. During the same time period, there were 196 smear-positive TB cases at Patan Hospital and the implementation of Xpert therefore resulted in a 28.1% ($n = 55/196$) increase in confirmed TB cases.

We assumed that the specificity of Xpert is high, as every study performed to date and meta-analysis has indicated consistently high specificity of 99% [10, 11, 16]. Therefore, although there is no culture confirmation for comparison, this was not an evaluation of diagnostic accuracy, which has been comprehensively reported elsewhere and it can be reasonably assumed that these cases are genuine, and the rate of false positive diagnosis is unlikely to exceed that of culture.

In areas of high TB prevalence such as Nepal, the majority of suspected TB cases are assessed by sputum smear microscopy and, where available, by CXR. Patients are often placed onto TB treatment on the basis of persistent cough or abnormal CXR alone. Modelling studies have indicated that Xpert scale-up may not increase the overall number of cases initiated on treatment due to these pragmatic empirical treatment practices. Instead, Xpert will divert treatment away from "false cases" to "true" smear-negative TB cases, thereby increasing the accuracy of treatment and cost-effectiveness, while reducing the burdens of toxicity and opportunity cost of treatment in patients who do not in fact have TB [17, 18]. The ability of Xpert to rapidly confirm TB in smear-negative cases offers the possibility of improving early TB case detection, but due to costs, recommendations for high burden, low-resource settings have so far focused on applying Xpert to HIV-infected individuals (where the sensitivity of smear is especially low and the complications of missed diagnosis are more severe) and patients with risk factors for MDR TB. Although WHO recommends applying the test to all smear-negative cases, the recommendation comes with the caveat that this is not financially feasible in most settings [13]. The low positive predictive value of Xpert for rifampicin resistance in a low MDR prevalence test population must also be considered. There has been considerable debate around the possibility of providing Xpert on a fee-paying basis to patients in low-income, high burden settings [19]. This study demonstrates that both uptake and case detection can be high in a targeted approach but further studies should be performed to determine the health economic impacts of such application, both on the individual patients including the opportunity costs of alternative health investigations and on household finances of testing costs and on hospital resource allocation.

The impact of delayed TB detection is threefold: firstly, morbidity to the individual is increased and in many cases will persist beyond the disease episode in severe permanent lung damage; secondly, undetected smear-negative TB will become progressively more infectious and transmit within the community; and finally the economic impact on the household is magnified by repeated visits to healthcare facilities, differential diagnostic testing and treatments, and loss of earnings due to healthcare seeking and morbidity.

The Xpert assay has also increased early detection of MDR-TB, particularly when applied to high-risk groups in accordance with WHO recommendations. Prior to application of this assay, patients at high risk for MDR TB would have to be referred to a tertiary setting and wait 6 to 8 weeks for results of phenotypic drug susceptibility testing resulting in high loss to follow-up and delays in treatment initiation. The line probe assays for MDR diagnosis have also largely been limited to tertiary centres in LMICs. In an unselected patient group without MDR risk factors and a low background prevalence of MDR TB, the positive predictive value of Xpert for rifampicin resistance is low and the result should be confirmed by a second test. However, early identification of possible MDR cases is key to reducing community transmission and reducing the incidence of MDR TB. The first patient positive for rifampicin resistant TB by Xpert in this study was referred to a tertiary centre for confirmatory testing by phenotypic DST according to the national guidelines. The phenotypic DST showed the patient was infected with TB resistant to isoniazid, rifampicin, streptomycin, and ethambutol. Without Xpert testing, this patient would have received a first line treatment regimen for a minimum of 5 months before being tested by phenotypic DST. The loss to follow-up of the second case despite the use of a rapid test demonstrates the problems associated with TB control beyond the need for accurate tests. This case could not be confirmed as a true positive for MDR and may not have received any TB treatment.

It is not clear how many of the patients testing positive for *M.tb.* by Xpert in this study would have been started on TB treatment based on the judgement of the treating clinician if Xpert testing was not available [20]. In the previous year (2011-2012) at Patan Hospital, 21 patients were empirically treated for TB, approximately one-third of those detected by Xpert during the study period (1.75/months versus 5.65/months, resp.). It is possible that the availability of Xpert increased the recognition of TB symptoms, although we can claim that in this endemic setting TB awareness is consistently high among clinicians. Conversely, it is possible that a negative Xpert test may have discouraged treatment in some cases which would otherwise have been treated, although clinicians were informed that a negative Xpert test does not exclude a TB diagnosis. Patients with a strong possibility of pulmonary TB despite a negative Xpert test were referred for further investigations including culture at a tertiary centre. The rate of smear positivity at Patan is 9.28% which is consistent with the results in other areas of similar endemicity; it is therefore unlikely that the Xpert diagnosis was inflated due to low smear microscopy confirmation [21–23].

The cost to the patients of the assay was 20 USD (which is equivalent to the price of eight CXRs in our hospital), including the full cost to the hospital of performing the assay and maintaining the service. Despite this, no clinician reported patients refusing the test for financial reasons, although this was not systematically evaluated. Studies of the patient acceptability of testing should be performed to determine the relative cost benefits for the patients of receiving a fee-paying Xpert test versus the traditional diagnostic route.

Scale-up of Xpert testing is underway in Nepal but funding is not available to provide Xpert testing free to all patients with suspected smear-negative TB and is unlikely to be so in the near to medium term. This is also true in other LMICs. In India, it was calculated that providing Xpert to all smear-negative TB suspects would consume the entire national healthcare budget [17].

Our study is consistent with other studies which have suggested the benefit of Xpert in smear-negative patients in developing countries [11, 24, 25]. The majority of these studies have been carried out in Africa where there is a substantially higher HIV burden than in South Asia. Three studies have been reported from low-HIV prevalence regions, including Peru and two hospitals (Hinduja Hospital and Christian Medical College Hospital) in India [8, 18, 25].

We examined the clinical features of groups testing positive and negative by Xpert to determine if further refinement of eligibility for testing criteria could guide the application of Xpert and reduce unnecessary testing and thereby costs to the patient. The number needed to test was reduced to 4 by restricting patients tested to only those with specific CXR criteria consistent with TB, while only a single case was missed. This strategy should be evaluated in a larger multicentre study to determine the optimal referral algorithm for Xpert testing in the general hospital setting.

By using only the classical broad definition of TB symptoms and CXR interpretation, the number needed to test for a single confirmed case of active TB is as low as five in this general hospital. Although smear microscopy, due to its simplicity, speed, and low cost, is used widely in low-resource settings, the low sensitivity precludes it from being an ideal test. The requirement for a rapid, simple TB diagnostic is evidenced by the widespread application of commercial serological tests which are inaccurate. These tests are widely provided at a cost to the patient and used to determine medical treatment. The government of India has recently banned the use of these tests following systematic evaluation by WHO [26]. Although the Xpert has several limitations, including requirement for stable electricity supply, limited temperature range, availability of maintenance, and bulky consumables, wider availability of the accurate Xpert assay may counter the use of these serological tests by providing a viable alternative to the patient and healthcare provider.

It is highly probable that a small number of cases of TB were missed in this study as Xpert does not have as high sensitivity as culture. There is a danger that clinicians will "exclude" a TB diagnosis on the basis of a negative Xpert test and it is important that education is carried out to ensure clinicians are aware of the test limitations prior to the test being implemented. However, it is not sustainable to implement TB culture facilities at general hospitals in South Asia and the long turnaround of results means loss to follow-up in the diagnostic pathway is high. This study was not an assessment of Xpert sensitivity and specificity, as this has been comprehensively evaluated in comparison with culture by others.

5. Conclusion

Our study has shown that by applying Xpert to test for smear-negative TB on a fee-paying basis in a general hospital in Nepal, five patients need to be tested to detect one case of active TB. Restriction of criteria for testing using CXR features can reduce the number needed to 4. Further research is needed evaluating the cost effectiveness, patient acceptability and impact on overall out-of-pocket expenditure of Xpert testing provided at a direct cost to the patient, to determine the optimal sustainable use of this technology while maximizing equality of access.

Authors' Contribution

Buddha Basnyat, Abhilasha Karkey, and Poojan Shrestha designed the study. Krishna Govinda Prajapati conducted the assays. Poojan Shrestha, Saruna Pathak, and Shanti Prajapati collected the data. Poojan Shrestha, Amit Arjyal, and Maxine Caws analyzed the data. Poojan Shrestha, Amit Arjyal, Maxine Caws, and Buddha Basnyat wrote the paper with additional inputs from Abhilasha Karkey, Sabina Dongol, and Krishna Govinda Prajapati. All the authors reviewed and approved the paper.

Acknowledgments

The authors would like to sincerely thank Dr. Raju Pangeni for his valuable suggestions. The authors thank their laboratory staff Jagyadeo Prasad Yadav, Srijana Shrestha, and Direndra Prasad Yadav and research nurses Niva Joshi and Manisha Risal, along with their community medical auxiliary workers—Balmukunda Neupane, Bijaya Karanjit, Nabin Adhikari, Nabraj Regmi, Rajendra Shrestha, and Surendra Shrestha for their invaluable technical assistance. Finally, the authors are indebted to all the patients who agreed to participate in the study.

References

[1] World Health Organization, *Global Tuberculosis Report*, WHO/HTM/TB/2013.11, World Health Organization, Geneva, Switzerland, 2013, http://www.who.int/tb/publications/global_report/en/.

[2] D. B. Young, M. D. Perkins, K. Duncan, and C. E. Barry III, "Confronting the scientific obstacles to global control of tuberculosis," *The Journal of Clinical Investigation*, vol. 118, no. 4, pp. 1255–1265, 2008.

[3] M. D. Perkins and J. Cunningham, "Facing the crisis: improving the diagnosis of tuberculosis in the HIV era," *Journal of Infectious Diseases*, vol. 196, supplement 1, pp. S15–S27, 2007.

[4] L. M. Parsons, Á. Somoskövi, C. Gutierrez et al., "Laboratory diagnosis of tuberculosis in resource-poor countries: challenges and opportunities," *Clinical Microbiology Reviews*, vol. 24, no. 2, pp. 314–350, 2011.

[5] M. Urdea, L. A. Penny, S. S. Olmsted et al., "Requirements for high impact diagnostics in the developing world," *Nature*, vol. 444, supplement 1, pp. 73–79, 2006.

[6] D. Helb, M. Jones, E. Story et al., "Rapid detection of *Mycobacterium tuberculosis* and rifampin resistance by use of on-demand, near-patient technology," *Journal of Clinical Microbiology*, vol. 48, no. 1, pp. 229–237, 2010.

[7] P. P. Banada, S. K. Sivasubramani, R. Blakemore et al., "Containment of bioaerosol infection risk by the Xpert MTB/RIF assay and its applicability to point-of-care settings," *Journal of Clinical Microbiology*, vol. 48, no. 10, pp. 3551–3557, 2010.

[8] C. C. Boehme, P. Nabeta, D. Hillemann et al., "Rapid molecular detection of tuberculosis and rifampin resistance," *The New England Journal of Medicine*, vol. 363, no. 11, pp. 1005–1015, 2010.

[9] H. H. El-Hajj, S. A. E. Marras, S. Tyagi, F. R. Kramer, and D. Alland, "Detection of rifampin resistance in *Mycobacterium tuberculosis* in a single tube with molecular beacons," *Journal of Clinical Microbiology*, vol. 39, no. 11, pp. 4131–4137, 2001.

[10] S. D. Lawn and M. P. Nicol, "Xpert MTB/RIF assay: development, evaluation and implementation of a new rapid molecular diagnostic for tuberculosis and rifampicin resistance," *Future Microbiology*, vol. 6, no. 9, pp. 1067–1082, 2011.

[11] K. R. Steingart, H. Sohn, I. Schiller et al., "Xpert MTB/RIF assay for pulmonary tuberculosis and rifampicin resistance in adults," *The Cochrane Database of Systematic Reviews*, vol. 1, Article ID CD009593, 2014.

[12] World Health Organization, *Automated Real-Time Nucleic Acid Amplification Technology for Rapid and Simultaneous Detection of Tuberculosis and Rifampicin Resistance: Xpert MTB/RIF System—Policy Statement*, World Health Organization, Geneva, Switzerland, 2011.

[13] World Health Organization, *Automated Real-Time Nucleic Acid Amplification Technology for Rapid and Simultaneous Detection of Tuberculosis and Rifampicin Resistance: Xpert MTB/RIF Assay for the Diagnosis of Pulmonary and Extrapulmonary TB in Adults and Children. Policy Update*, World Health Organization, Geneva, Switzerland, 2013.

[14] World Health Organization, *Global Health Observatory Data Repository*, World Health Organization, 2012, http://apps.who.int/gho/data/view.main.1920ALL?lang=en.

[15] National Tuberculosis Programme Nepal, *Annual Report 2012/13*, 2014, http://nepalntp.gov.np/index.php?view=publication.

[16] S. D. Lawn, P. Mwaba, M. Bates et al., "Advances in tuberculosis diagnostics: the Xpert MTB/RIF assay and future prospects for a point-of-care test," *The Lancet Infectious Diseases*, vol. 13, no. 4, pp. 349–361, 2013.

[17] D. W. Dowdy, A. Cattamanchi, K. R. Steingart, and M. Pai, "Is scale-up worth it? Challenges in economic analysis of diagnostic tests for tuberculosis," *PLoS Medicine*, vol. 8, no. 7, Article ID e1001063, 2011.

[18] A. Vassall, S. van Kampen, H. Sohn et al., "Rapid diagnosis of tuberculosis with the Xpert MTB/RIF assay in high burden countries: a cost-effectiveness analysis," *PLoS Medicine*, vol. 8, no. 11, Article ID e1001120, 2011.

[19] N. A. Baloch and M. Pai, "Tuberculosis control: business models for the private sector," *The Lancet Infectious Diseases*, vol. 12, no. 8, pp. 579–580, 2012.

[20] G. Theron, J. Peter, D. Dowdy, I. Langley, S. B. Squire, and K. Dheda, "Do high rates of empirical treatment undermine the potential effect of new diagnostic tests for tuberculosis in high-burden settings?" *The Lancet Infectious Diseases*, vol. 14, no. 6, pp. 527–532, 2014.

[21] International Union against Tuberculosis and Lung Diseases Paris, *Technical Guide: Sputum Examination for Tuberculosis by Direct Microscopy in Low Income Countries*, International Union against Tuberculosis and Lung Diseases Paris, 5th edition, 2000.

[22] S. Saleem, I. Shabbir, R. Iqbal, and S. U. Khan, "Value of three sputum smears microscopy in diagnosis of pulmonary tuberculosis," *Pakistan Journal of Medical Research*, vol. 46, no. 4, pp. 1–5, 2007.

[23] J. Seni, B. R. Kidenya, E. Obassy et al., "Low sputum smear positive tuberculosis among pulmonary tuberculosis suspects in a tertiary hospital in Mwanza, Tanzania," *Tanzania Journal of Health Research*, vol. 14, no. 2, pp. 1–9, 2012.

[24] A. Rachow, A. Zumla, N. Heinrich et al., "Rapid and accurate detection of *Mycobacterium tuberculosis* in sputum samples by Cepheid Xpert MTB/RIF assay—a clinical validation study," *PLoS ONE*, vol. 6, no. 6, Article ID e20458, 2011.

[25] C. C. Boehme, M. P. Nicol, P. Nabeta et al., "Feasibility, diagnostic accuracy, and effectiveness of decentralised use of the Xpert MTB/RIF test for diagnosis of tuberculosis and multidrug resistance: a multicentre implementation study," *The Lancet*, vol. 377, no. 9776, pp. 1495–1505, 2011.

[26] K. R. Steingart, A. Ramsay, D. W. Dowdy, and M. Pai, "Serological tests for the diagnosis of active tuberculosis: relevance for India," *Indian Journal of Medical Research*, vol. 135, no. 5, pp. 695–702, 2012.

2

Isoniazid Toxicity among an Older Veteran Population: A Retrospective Cohort Study

Christopher Vinnard,[1] Anand Gopal,[2] Darren R. Linkin,[3,4,5] and Joel Maslow[6]

[1] *Division of Infectious Diseases and HIV Medicine, College of Medicine, Drexel University, 245 N. 15th Street MS 461, New College Building 6314, Philadelphia, PA 19102, USA*
[2] *College of Arts and Sciences, University of Pennsylvania, Philadelphia, PA 19104, USA*
[3] *Division of Infectious Diseases, Department of Medicine, Perelman School of Medicine, University of Pennsylvania, Philadelphia, PA 19104, USA*
[4] *Department of Medicine, Philadelphia VA Medical Center, Philadelphia, PA 19104, USA*
[5] *Center for Clinical Epidemiology and Biostatistics, Perelman School of Medicine, University of Pennsylvania, Philadelphia, PA 19104, USA*
[6] *Division of Infectious Diseases, Morristown Medical Center, Morristown, NJ 07962, USA*

Correspondence should be addressed to Christopher Vinnard; christopher.vinnard@drexelmed.edu

Academic Editor: T. Ottenhoff

Background: our objective was to determine the incidence of toxicity among veterans initiating isoniazid therapy for latent tuberculosis infection (LTBI) and determine whether advancing age was a risk factor for toxicity. *Methods*: we performed a retrospective cohort study among all adults initiating isoniazid treatment for LTBI at a Veterans Medical Center from 1999 to 2005. We collected data on patient demographics, co-morbidities, site of initiation, and treatment outcome. *Results*: 219 patients initiated isoniazid therapy for LTBI during the period of observation, and the completion of therapy was confirmed in 100 patients (46%). Among 18/219 patients (8%) that discontinued therapy due to a documented suspected toxicity, the median time to onset was 3 months (IQR 1–5 months). In an adjusted Cox regression model, there was no association between discontinuation due to suspected toxicity and advancing age (HR 1.03, 95% CI 0.99, 1.07). In contrast, hepatitis C infection was a significant predictor of cessation due to toxicity in the adjusted analysis (HR 3.03, 95% CI 1.08, 8.52). *Conclusions*: cessation of isoniazid therapy due to suspected toxicity was infrequently observed among a veteran population and was not associated with advancing age. Alternative LTBI treatment approaches should be further examined in the veteran population.

1. Introduction

According to World Health Organization estimates, one-third of the world's population is latently infected with *M. tuberculosis*, and 10% of immunocompetent individuals will progress from latent to active tuberculosis infection within their lifetimes [1]. Detection and treatment of latent tuberculosis infection (LTBI) remain a cornerstone of the strategy to reduce the incidence of active tuberculosis in the United States. Daily isoniazid therapy for six to 12 months has been shown to significantly reduce the risk of progression from latent to active tuberculosis infection [2].

In the 1970's, several cases of fatal hepatotoxicity during isoniazid therapy for LTBI raised concerns regarding widespread isoniazid use and led to a reconsideration of its safety in older adults [3]. Subsequent studies of isoniazid toxicity have compared the risk of hepatotoxicity between adults less than and greater than 35 years of age [4–10], and a meta-analysis of these studies demonstrated a small but statistically significant increased risk of hepatotoxicity among adults greater than age 35 [11]. Because of these concerns, providers may be more reluctant to initiate isoniazid therapy in older patients with LTBI, particularly in the presence of comorbid illnesses [12].

Less is known about the relationship of advancing age and isoniazid toxicity among adults in later decades of life, particularly when used in clinical practice outside of tuberculosis control programs or public health clinics. Furthermore, although isoniazid treatment is recommended for use in long-term care facilities as a component of infection control programs [13], prior epidemiologic studies of isoniazid toxicity have been limited to outpatient settings.

Veterans are a unique population for LTBI-screening efforts, given their additional risk of tuberculosis exposure related to service deployments [14]. We sought to describe the incidence of toxicities among veterans initiating daily isoniazid treatment of LTBI and determine whether advancing age was associated with isoniazid discontinuation due to suspected toxicity.

2. Methods

We performed a retrospective cohort study of LTBI treatment with isoniazid at a single medical center. The Philadelphia Veterans Affairs (VA) Medical Center is a federal health care facility comprising an outpatient clinical facility, a 145-bed acute care hospital, and an adjoining 240-bed long-term care facility. We queried pharmacy records to identify all individuals prescribed isoniazid between January 1, 2000, and December 31, 2005. Among these patients, we limited study inclusion to individuals receiving isoniazid alone for the treatment of LTBI.

We reviewed clinical charts to extract demographic and comorbidity data, including HIV infection, hepatitis C infection, past or current alcohol abuse, and past or current intravenous drug use (IDU). Laboratory records were reviewed for baseline serum transaminase levels (defined as levels obtained within 6 months prior to initiation of isoniazid therapy), along with peak serum transaminase levels during treatment.

We classified treatment outcomes as completion of therapy, discontinuation due to a suspected toxicity, or discontinuation for unknown reasons (if completion could not be documented either by review of the clinical chart or the pharmacy records). We calculated the 95% confidence interval (CI) for the incidence of toxicities using the binomial test. We performed Cox regression analysis to determine the adjusted association of advancing age with treatment discontinuation due to suspected toxicity, which allowed us to account for differences in observation time. Stata v11.0 (College Station, TX, USA) was used for statistical analysis, and significance was declared for P values less than 0.05.

3. Results

Overall, 219 veterans initiated isoniazid therapy for LTBI, with a median age of 53 years (range 22–90). There were 18 patients (8%) with therapy discontinued due to suspected toxicity, 100 patients (46%) with successful completion of therapy, and 101 patients (46%) with therapy discontinued for unknown reasons. Isoniazid completion rates were higher among residents of the long-term care facility compared with nonresidents (64% versus 44%, $P = 0.07$), with similar rates of discontinuation for suspected toxicity between these two groups (9% versus 8%, $P = 0.88$). Among patients initiating treatment in the outpatient setting, there was no difference in completion rates for patients initiating treatment in the primary care clinics (40%) compared with the infectious disease clinic (49%, $P = 0.22$).

Baseline alanine transaminase (ALT) levels were obtained in 184 of 219 patients (84%). During isoniazid therapy, followup ALT levels were obtained in 156 of 219 patients (71%) overall, including 15 of 18 patients (83%) with subsequent cessation due to suspected toxicity (15/18, 83%) compared to 141 of 201 patients (70%) without treatment cessation due to suspected toxicity.

Discontinuation for suspected toxicity occurred in 18 patients (8%) after a median of 3 months (IQR 1–5 months). Hepatotoxicity was cited by the clinician as the reason for discontinuing therapy in 7 patients (3%, 95% CI 1–6%). Other suspected toxicities that led to early treatment cessation included 3 patients with rash (1%, 95% CI 0–4%) and 2 patients with nausea (1%, 95% CI 0–3%). Additional 5 patients had other types of clinical events attributed to isoniazid (malaise, back pain, thrombocytopenia, angioedema, and fever).

Characteristics of patients with and without isoniazid discontinuation due to suspected toxicity are shown in Table 1. The median age of patients that completed therapy was 53.4 years (IQR 45.8–66.1), and the median age of patients that discontinued therapy due to suspected toxicity was 54.5 years (IQR 50.5–61.5). Only hepatitis C infection was associated with discontinuation due to suspected toxicity ($P = 0.01$). There were two patients (1%, 95% CI 0–3%) with biochemically confirmed hepatotoxicity that met the definition of ATS/CDC treatment guidelines [2]. One 50-year-old patient with a history of alcohol abuse had an ALT rise from a baseline of 80 to a peak of 329 after 104 days of treatment, and a second 80-year-old patient without identifiable risk factors had an ALT rise from a baseline of 57 to a peak of 438 after 27 days of treatment. In both of these instances there was complete resolution of hepatotoxicity with cessation of isoniazid therapy.

In a proportional hazards model that included age, hepatitis C infection, and a history of alcohol use, age was not associated with treatment discontinuation due to suspected toxicity (HR 1.03, 95% CI 0.99, 1.07). In contrast, the relationship between hepatitis C infection and isoniazid discontinuation due to suspected toxicity remained significant even after adjusting for age and alcohol use (HR 3.03, 95% CI 1.08, 8.52).

4. Discussion

Daily isoniazid therapy remains the cornerstone of a targeted testing and treatment approach for LTBI [2]. In an older cohort of veterans initiating isoniazid treatment for LTBI, we found a high rate of discontinuation due to suspected toxicity. In contrast, the rate of biochemically confirmed hepatotoxicity was much lower and similar to previous

TABLE 1: Characteristics of veterans with and without isoniazid discontinuation due to suspected toxicity.

Characteristic	Treatment completion (%) (n = 100)	Discontinuation due to suspected toxicity (%) (n = 18)	P value
Age category			0.64
<35	5 (5)	0 (0)	
35–55	49 (49)	10 (56)	
56–75	35 (35)	5 (28)	
>75	11 (11)	3 (17)	
Sex			0.39
Male	98 (98)	17 (94)	
Female	2 (2)	1 (6)	
Comorbidities			
HIV	9 (9)	1 (6)	0.63
Hepatitis C	17 (17)	8 (44)	0.01
Alcohol use	33 (33)	8 (44)	0.35
IDU	11 (11)	5 (28)	0.06
Initiation setting			0.18
Outpatient			
Primary care clinic	33 (33)	7 (39)	
Infectious disease clinic	47 (47)	6 (33)	
Emergency department	3 (3)	0 (0)	
Inpatient			
Long-term care facility	14 (14)	2 (11)	
Acute care facility	3 (3)	3 (16)	

reports. We found that overall completion rates were lower than previous reports from public health clinics [15, 16].

Cessation of isoniazid therapy due to suspected toxicity was not associated with advancing age. Our work adds to prior studies of age-related isoniazid toxicity risk by enrolling a significant number of patients in later decades of life. The median age of participants in our study (53 years) is greater than any previous study of isoniazid therapy for LTBI. Treatment guidelines' use of 35 years of age has been called an "arbitrary" cutoff to define the risk of isoniazid-related toxicity [11], given that many other therapeutic drugs display significant changes in toxicity risk with advancing age. We found that isoniazid can be safely administered to older veterans provided that there is an appropriate clinical followup, consistent with current recommendations for the treatment of LTBI [2].

In contrast, we found that hepatitis C infection was associated with cessation of therapy due to concerns for toxicity. Our findings differ from a study of intravenous drug users in Spain that did not find a relationship between hepatitis C infection and hepatotoxicity [10]. One possible explanation for this difference is that providers in the VA were more cautious with discontinuation of therapy with minor elevations of transaminases that may not have resulted in biochemically confirmed hepatotoxicity. However, it is also possible that a biological interaction between age and hepatitis C led to our findings, given that our cohort was much older than the Spanish study (mean age 31 years). Further work is needed to characterize the complex relationship between hepatitis C and the risk of isoniazid-associated hepatotoxicity.

Interestingly, patients initiating isoniazid treatment in the long-term care facility, despite their older age and greater comorbidities, had higher rates of treatment completion compared with patients in all other settings. While isoniazid is recommended for the treatment of LTBI in long-term care facilities, there have not been specific investigations to evaluate its safety in this setting [12]. Our findings support the safety of current practices regarding LTBI screening and treatment in long-term care facilities.

Our retrospective cohort study had several limitations. Among patients lost to followup, we could not determine whether the development of side effects (such as gastrointestinal intolerance) contributed to their discontinuation of care. Furthermore, there was tremendous variability in clinical practices, with regards to testing for comorbidities (HIV or hepatitis C), number of isoniazid tablets provided per prescription, and frequency of followup visits. Our approach to ascertainment of comorbidities such as HIV or hepatiits C identified only those patients with a positive test, and the proportion of patients in the cohort without testing performed was not determined. Typical of a veteran population, women were underrepresented in this study. However, one strength of our approach was the ability to link centralized pharmacy records with clinical charts.

In summary, nine months of daily isoniazid therapy for the treatment of LTBI in an older veteran population were associated with low rates of treatment completion overall. Rates of treatment discontinuation due to suspected toxicities were similar to previous reports, and not associated with advancing age. Alternative LTBI treatment approaches should be further examined in the older veteran population.

Acknowledgment

This study was supported in part by the CDC Prevention Epicenters Program (U54 CK000163).

References

[1] C. Dye, S. Scheele, P. Dolin, V. Pathania, and M. C. Raviglione, "Global burden of tuberculosis: estimated incidence, prevalence, and mortality by country. WHO global surveillance and monitoring project," *Journal of the American Medical Association*, vol. 282, no. 7, pp. 677–686, 1999.

[2] American Thoracic Society and Centers for Disease Control and Prevention, "Targeted tuberculin testing and treatment of latent tuberculosis infection," *American Journal of Respiratory and Critical Care Medicine*, vol. 161, no. S221, S247 pages, 2000.

[3] D. E. Kopanoff, D. E. Snider, and G. J. Caras, "Isoniazid-related hepatitis: a U.S. Public Health Service cooperative surveillance study," *American Review of Respiratory Disease*, vol. 117, no. 6, pp. 991–1001, 1978.

[4] P. A. LoBue and K. S. Moser, "Use of isoniazid for latent tuberculosis infection in a public health clinic," *American Journal of Respiratory and Critical Care Medicine*, vol. 168, no. 4, pp. 443–447, 2003.

[5] H. Aziz, M. Shubair, V. A. DeBari, M. Ismail, and M. A. Khan, "Assessment of age-related isoniazid hepatotoxicity during treatment of latent tuberculosis infection," *Current Medical Research and Opinion*, vol. 22, no. 1, article no. 3148, pp. 217–221, 2006.

[6] F. F. Fountain, E. Tolley, C. R. Chrisman, and T. H. Self, "Isoniazid hepatotoxicity associated with treatment of latent tuberculosis infection: a 7-year evaluation from a public health tuberculosis clinic," *Chest*, vol. 128, no. 1, pp. 116–123, 2005.

[7] R. Van Hest, H. Baars, S. Kik et al., "Hepatotoxicity of rifampin-pyrazinamide and isoniazid preventive therapy and tuberculosis treatment," *Clinical Infectious Diseases*, vol. 39, no. 4, pp. 488–496, 2004.

[8] C. M. Nolan, S. V. Goldberg, and S. E. Buskin, "Hepatotoxicity associated with isoniazid preventive therapy: a 7-year survey from a public health tuberculosis clinic," *Journal of the American Medical Association*, vol. 281, no. 11, pp. 1014–1018, 1999.

[9] S. A. Gilroy, M. A. M. Rogers, and D. C. Blair, "Treatment of latent tuberculosis infection in patients aged ≥35 years," *Clinical Infectious Diseases*, vol. 31, no. 3, pp. 826–829, 2000.

[10] A. Fernandez-Villar, B. Sopena, R. Vazquez et al., "Isoniazid hepatotoxicity among drug users: the role of hepatitis C," *Clinical Infectious Diseases*, vol. 36, pp. 293–298, 2003.

[11] H. Kunst and K. S. Khan, "Age-related risk of hepatotoxicity in the treatment of latent tuberculosis infection: a systematic review," *International Journal of Tuberculosis and Lung Disease*, vol. 14, no. 11, pp. 1374–1381, 2010.

[12] D. J. Sorresso, J. B. Mehta, L. M. Harvill, and S. Bentley, "Underutilization of isoniazid chemoprophylaxis in tuberculosis contacts 50 years of age and older: a prospective analysis," *Chest*, vol. 108, no. 3, pp. 706–711, 1995.

[13] L. Thrupp, S. Bradley, P. Smith et al., "Tuberculosis prevention and control in long-term-care facilities for older adults," *Infection Control and Hospital Epidemiology*, vol. 25, no. 12, pp. 1097–1108, 2004.

[14] J. D. Mancuso and L. W. Keep, "Deployment-related testing and treatment for latent tuberculosis infection, part II," *Military Medicine*, vol. 176, pp. 1088–1092, 2011.

[15] K. R. Page, F. Sifakis, R. Montes De Oca et al., "Improved adherence and less toxicity with rifampin vs isoniazid for treatment of latent tuberculosis: a retrospective study," *Archives of Internal Medicine*, vol. 166, no. 17, pp. 1863–1870, 2006.

[16] R. M. Jasmer, J. J. Saukkonen, H. M. Blumberg et al., "Short-course rifampin and pyrazinamide compared with isoniazid for latent tuberculosis infection: a multicenter clinical trial," *Annals of Internal Medicine*, vol. 137, no. 8, pp. 640–647, 2002.

3

Initial Antituberculous Regimen with Better Drug Penetration into Cerebrospinal Fluid Reduces Mortality in HIV Infected Patients with Tuberculous Meningitis: Data from an HIV Observational Cohort Study

Gerardo Alvarez-Uria, Manoranjan Midde, Raghavakalyan Pakam, and Praveen Kumar Naik

Department of Infectious Diseases, Bathalapalli Rural Development Trust Hospital, Kadiri Road, Anantapur District, Bathalapalli 515661, Andhra Pradesh, India

Correspondence should be addressed to Gerardo Alvarez-Uria; gerardouria@gmail.com

Academic Editor: Luis E Cuevas

Tuberculous meningitis (TM) is the deadliest form of tuberculosis. Nearly two-thirds of HIV infected patients with TM die, and most deaths occur within one month. Current treatment of TM involves the use of drugs with poor penetration into the cerebrospinal fluid (CSF). In this study, we present the mortality before and after implementing a new antituberculous regimen (ATR) with a higher drug penetration in CSF than the standard ATR during the initial treatment of TM in an HIV cohort study. The new ATR included levofloxacin, ethionamide, pyrazinamide, and a double dose of rifampicin and isoniazid and was given for a median of 7 days (interquartile range 6–9). The new ATR was associated with an absolute 21.5% (95% confidence interval (CI), 7.3–35.7) reduction in mortality at 12 months. In multivariable analysis, independent factors associated with mortality were the use of the standard ATR versus the new ATR (hazard ratio 2.05; 95% CI, 1.2–3.5), not being on antiretroviral therapy, low CD4 lymphocyte counts, and low serum albumin levels. Our findings suggest that an intensified initial ATR, which likely results in higher concentrations of active drugs in CSF, has a beneficial effect on the survival of HIV-related TM.

1. Introduction

In 2011, there were 8.7 million incident cases of tuberculosis (13% of them in HIV infected patients) and 1.4 million deaths from tuberculosis (30% of them in HIV infected patients) [1]. With 25% mortality in non-HIV infected patients and 67% in HIV infected patients, tuberculous meningitis has the highest mortality among all forms of tuberculosis [2]. Moreover, tuberculous meningitis is more common in HIV infected patients and can comprise up to 19% of all cases of HIV-related tuberculosis [3, 4].

Currently, treatment of tuberculous meningitis involves the same drugs and doses as other forms of tuberculosis [5–7]. While isoniazid and pyrazinamide have good cerebrospinal fluid (CSF) penetration, rifampicin concentration in CSF may not reach the minimal inhibitory concentration for tuberculosis, and ethambutol and streptomycin have poor CSF penetration [2, 8]. Among second line drugs, levofloxacin, ethionamide and cycloserine have good penetration in CSF [8–10]. In a phase 2 randomized controlled trial investigating the safety of moxifloxacin and a higher intravenous dose of rifampicin during the first two weeks of treatment of tuberculous meningitis, the use of a higher dose of rifampicin was associated with a survival benefit [11]. These data suggest that increasing the CSF penetration of the initial treatment of tuberculous meningitis could potentially reduce its mortality.

The majority of deaths due to tuberculous meningitis occur within one month [4, 12]. Therefore, interventions to reduce mortality should be performed during the early stages of treatment. In this study, we present the mortality before and after implementing a new antituberculous regimen (ATR) with a higher drug penetration in CSF than the standard regimen during the initial treatment of HIV-related tuberculous meningitis.

2. Patients and Methods

2.1. Setting. This study was performed in the district of Anantapur, India. Rural Development Trust (RDT) is a nongovernmental organization that provides free medical care to HIV infected patients. The Vicente Ferrer HIV Cohort Study (VFHCS) is an open cohort study of all HIV infected patients who have attended RDT hospitals [13, 14]. Since September 2009, clinical information of the patients has been collected prospectively.

For this study, we selected all cases of tuberculous meningitis diagnosed from 6 June 2010 to 1 April 2013 in HIV infected adults living in Anantapur who were admitted to RDT Hospital Bathalapalli. The selection of patients from the database was executed on 27 May 2013. Patients who did not meet the proposed criteria for definite, probable, or possible tuberculous meningitis were excluded from the analysis [15]. Bacterial culture and cryptococcus antigen tests were performed on CSF to rule out other causes of meningitis.

2.2. Treatment. All patients were admitted to the hospital. Before 29 January 2012, patients were treated with the standard oral once daily ATR, that is, isoniazid 300 mg, rifampicin 450 mg, ethambutol 800 mg, and pyrazinamide 1500 mg. After 29 January 2012, patients received a new oral once daily ATR, including isoniazid 600 mg, rifampicin 900 mg, pyrazinamide 1500 mg, levofloxacin 750 mg, and ethionamide 750 mg. Therefore, we doubled the dose of rifampicin and isoniazid, and ethambutol, a drug with poor CSF penetration, was substituted by levofloxacin and ethionamide, which have better CSF penetration [16]. Although isoniazid has good CSF penetration, its dosage was increased due to its bactericidal effect during the first days of treatment [17]. The new ATR was given only during the admission, so once a clinical improvement was observed, patients who received the new ATR were discharged with the standard ATR. After discharge, patients from both groups were treated for at least nine months according to the Indian guidelines for tuberculosis [18]. All patients received pyridoxine 50 mg daily during the whole course antituberculous treatment.

Prophylaxis of deep vein thrombosis with subcutaneous sodium heparin (5000 IU every 12 hours) was given during the hospital admission to all patients. Intravenous dexamethasone was given the first day along with the ATR and was rapidly tapered if a clinical improvement was observed. The typical regimen was dexamethasone 16 mg IV every 6 hours for 3-4 days, dexamethasone 8 mg IV every 8 hours for 3-4 days, and then oral prednisolone 40 mg once daily before hospital discharge. After discharge, prednisolone was reduced 10 mg every two weeks, so corticosteroids were stopped after 8 weeks of hospital discharge. Patients with seizures were treated with a loading oral dose of 800 mg of valproate acid and then 600 mg every 8 hours. If seizures were

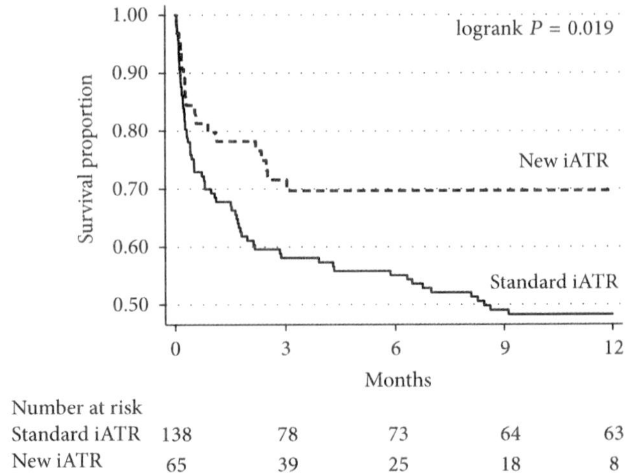

FIGURE 1: Kaplan-Meier survival estimates by the initial antituberculous regimen of 203 HIV patients with tuberculous meningitis. iATR, initial antituberculous regimen.

controlled, a further reduction to 400 mg every 8 hours was performed before hospital discharge.

2.3. Definitions. Designation of patients' community was performed by self-identification of the patients. Scheduled caste community is marginalized in the traditional Hindu caste hierarchy and, therefore, suffers social and economic exclusion and disadvantage. Scheduled tribe community is generally geographically isolated with limited economic and social contact with the rest of the population. Scheduled castes and scheduled tribes are considered socially disadvantaged communities and are supported by positive discrimination schemes operated by the Government of India [19]. Depressed level of consciousness was defined in patients with confusion, disorientation, or coma, but the Glasgow coma scale was not calculated.

2.4. Statistical Analysis and Ethics Statement. Statistical analysis was performed using Stata Statistical Software (Stata Corporation Release 11 College Station, TX, USA). The primary endpoint of the study was to evaluate the mortality in patients receiving the standard ATR versus the new ATR, so time-to-event methods were used. Time was measured from ATR initiation to death. Patients who did not die during the study period were censored at their last visit date. Crude and multivariable analyses were performed with Cox regression proportional hazard models. The proportional hazard assumption was assessed performing log-log survival curves based on Schoenfeld residuals [20]. CD4 cell count, sodium, haemoglobin, and albumin were not available in 12, 14, 8, and 10 cases, respectively. To include these patients in the multivariable analysis, missing values were imputed using multiple imputations by chained equation assuming missing at random [21]. In a sensitivity analysis, we also performed a multivariable analysis using only those cases with complete information. The study was approved by the ethical committee of the RDT Institutional Review Board.

TABLE 1: Baseline characteristics and differences between patients who received the standard antituberculous regimen and those who received a new antituberculous regimen with better cerebrospinal fluid penetration.

	Overall $N = 203$	Standard iATR $N = 138$	New iATR $N = 65$	P-value
Continuous variables	Median (IQR)	Median (IQR)	Median (IQR)	Wilcoxon rank-sum test
Age (years)	36.1 (30.3–43.4)	36.5 (30.9–45)	36 (30–42)	0.421
CD4 count (cells/μL)	107 (52–173)	108 (51.5–186)	107 (52–163)	0.744
Haemoglobin (g/dL)	10.3 (8.5–12)	10.5 (8.6–12.1)	9.7 (8.1–11.3)	0.182
Albumin (g/dL)	3.4 (2.7–4)	3.5 (2.8–3.9)	3.3 (2.6–4)	0.347
Sodium (mEq/L)	132 (126.8–136)	132.9 (126.9–136.7)	131.6 (126.8–134.9)	0.386
Categorical variables	N (%)	N (%)	N (%)	Chi^2 test
Gender				0.69
Female	60 (29.56)	42 (30.66)	18 (27.69)	
Male	143 (70.44)	95 (69.34)	47 (72.31)	
Disadvantaged community				0.703
No	140 (68.97)	94 (68.12)	46 (70.77)	
Yes	63 (31.03)	44 (31.88)	19 (29.23)	
Homeless				0.579
No	193 (95.07)	132 (95.65)	61 (93.85)	
Yes	10 (4.93)	6 (4.35)	4 (6.15)	
Illiterate				0.75
No	97 (47.78)	67 (48.55)	30 (46.15)	
Yes	106 (52.22)	71 (51.45)	35 (53.85)	
Depressed consciousness				0.172
No	114 (56.16)	82 (59.42)	32 (49.23)	
Yes	89 (43.84)	56 (40.58)	33 (50.77)	
Previous tuberculosis				0.407
No	163 (80.3)	113 (81.88)	50 (76.92)	
Yes	40 (19.7)	25 (18.12)	15 (23.08)	
Months on ART				0.755
>6 months	37 (18.23)	27 (19.57)	10 (15.38)	
<6 months	47 (22.15)	32 (23.19)	15 (23.08)	
No ART	119 (58.62)	79 (57.25)	40 (61.54)	

ART: antiretroviral therapy; iATR: initial antituberculous regimen; IQR: interquartile range.

3. Results

We identified 213 patients with diagnosis of tuberculous meningitis in the VFHCS database. After reviewing all cases, 10 patients were excluded for not meeting the criteria for tuberculous meningitis [15]. Of the 203 patients included in the analysis, 138 received the standard initial ATR and 65 received the new ATR. Baseline characteristics of the patients are presented in Table 1. Median age was 36 years and near one-third were women. One-third of patients belonged to disadvantaged communities, 5% were homeless, and over half were illiterate. 41% had started HIV antiretroviral therapy before the diagnosis of tuberculous meningitis and 20% had a previous episode of tuberculosis. 44% presented to the hospital with depressed consciousness, and the median CD4 lymphocyte count was 107 cells/μL. At presentation, the median sodium, haemoglobin, and albumin were 132 mEq/L, 10.3 g/dL, and 3.4 g/dL, respectively. We did not find statistically significant differences between patients who received the standard ATR and the new ATR (Table 1). Among patients who received the new ATR and did not die during the first admission, the median duration of the new ATR was 7 days (interquartile range (IQR), 6 to 9; range 3 to 24). Weight was measured in 102 patients who received the standard ATR and in 50 patients who received the new ATR, and the median weight was 43 kg (IQR 38–48) and 44 kg (IQR 40–50), respectively. Therefore, in patients who had their weight measured, the median dose of isoniazid and rifampicin was 7 mg/kg (IQR 6.3–7.9) and 10.5 mg/kg (IQR 9.4–11.8), respectively, for the group who received the standard ATR and 13.6 mg/kg (IQR 12–15) and 20.5 mg/kg (IQR 18–22.5), respectively, for the group who received the new ATR. In the group who received the standard ATR, the median followup was 7.5 months (IQR 0.4–23.5) and, during the first 12 months after the initiation of the ATR, 70 (51%) patients died, 5 (4%) were lost to followup, and 63 (46%) patients were alive. The group who received the new ATR had a smaller follow-up period, median 4.2 months (IQR 1.9–9.3), because the

TABLE 2: Crude and multivariable Cox regression analyses of factors associated with mortality in HIV patients with tuberculous meningitis.

	Crude analysis		Complete case MA $N = 176$		Multiple imputation MA $N = 203$	
	HR	95% CI	aHR	95% CI	aHR	95% CI
iATR						
New	1		1		1	
Standard	1.82*	(1.095–3.020)	1.88*	(1.081–3.261)	2.05*	(1.209–3.462)
Age (years)						
<35	1.06	(0.711–1.573)	1.16	(0.695–1.922)	1.09	(0.692–1.729)
>35	1		1		1	
Gender						
Female	1.05	(0.683–1.601)	0.93	(0.538–1.594)	0.85	(0.514–1.405)
Male	1		1		1	
Disadvantaged community						
No	1		1		1	
Yes	1.59*	(1.052–2.399)	1.19	(0.717–1.963)	1.27	(0.811–1.974)
Homeless						
No	1		1		1	
Yes	0.89	(0.361–2.201)	1.05	(0.382–2.874)	1.02	(0.378–2.766)
Illiterate						
No	1		1		1	
Yes	1.31	(0.877–1.954)	1.12	(0.662–1.889)	1.18	(0.736–1.881)
Depressed consciousness						
No	1		1		1	
Yes	1.36	(0.913–2.021)	1.21	(0.751–1.939)	1.30	(0.852–1.987)
Previous tuberculosis						
No	1		1		1	
Yes	1.09	(0.657–1.792)	1.54	(0.795–2.966)	1.50	(0.845–2.678)
Months on ART						
>6 months	0.63	(0.367–1.098)	0.82	(0.403–1.678)	0.76	(0.399–1.439)
<6 months	0.50*	(0.291–0.852)	0.59	(0.310–1.142)	0.56*	(0.311–0.995)
No ART	1		1		1	
CD4 count (cells/μL)						
≤50	3.04*	(1.885–4.901)	1.93*	(1.086–3.427)	1.95*	(1.132–3.372)
51–100	1.34	(0.766–2.346)	1.24	(0.665–2.322)	1.27	(0.707–2.279)
>100	1		1		1	
Sodium (mEq/L)						
≤135	1		1		1	
>135	0.58*	(0.358–0.956)	0.66	(0.379–1.133)	0.70	(0.410–1.181)
Albumin (g/dL)						
≤2.5	3.95*	(2.163–7.231)	3.66*	(1.490–9.008)	3.14*	(1.433–6.898)
2.6–3.8	1.92*	(1.139–3.227)	1.95*	(1.029–3.691)	1.92*	(1.093–3.380)
>3.8	1		1		1	
Haemoglobin (g/dL)						
≤9	1.48	(0.973–2.239)	0.78	(0.421–1.428)	0.76	(0.434–1.330)
>9	1		1		1	

* P value < 0.05; aHR, adjusted hazard ratio; ART: antiretroviral therapy; iATR: initial antituberculous regimen; HR: hazard ratio; MA: multivariable analysis.

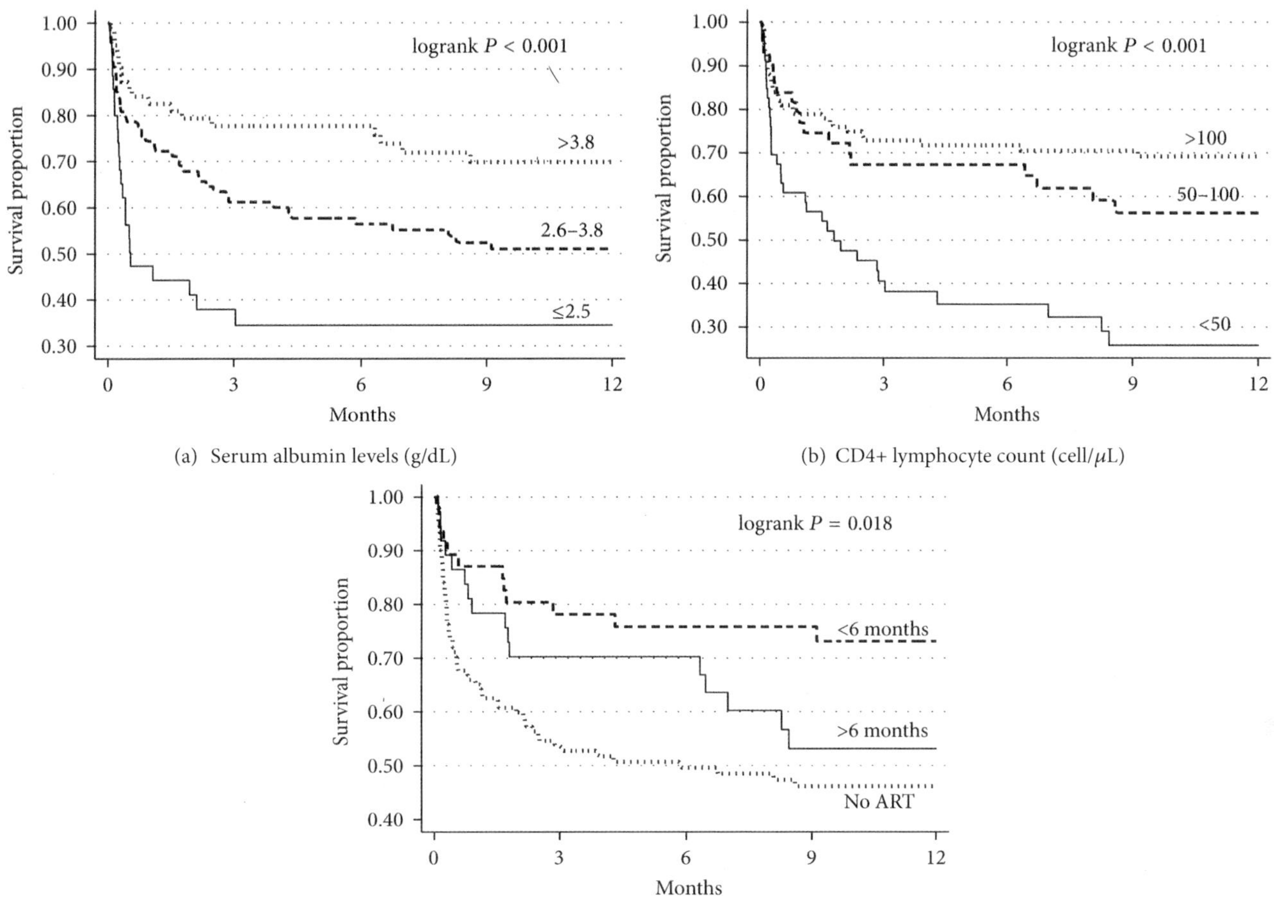

(a) Serum albumin levels (g/dL)

(b) CD4+ lymphocyte count (cell/μL)

(c) Duration of ART before TB meningitis

Figure 2: Kaplan-Meier survival estimates by baseline serum albumin levels (a), CD4 lymphocyte count (b), and duration of antiretroviral therapy (ART) of 203 HIV patients with tuberculous meningitis (c). ART, antiretroviral therapy; TB, tuberculous.

treatment was implemented in the hospital more recently. During the study period, 19 (29%) patients died, 43 (66%) attended the hospital within three months before the end of the study period, and 3 (5%) did not attend the hospital within three months before the end of the study period.

Figure 1 presents the Kaplan-Meier survival estimates by initial ATR. The study involved 2070.4 person-months. Patients who received the new ATR had a significant lower mortality than patients who received the standard ATR (P value = 0.019). The estimated absolute mortality reduction of the new ATR at 1, 3, 6, and 12 months was 10.5% (95% CI, −2 to 23), 13.5% (95% CI, −0.005 to 27.4), 14.6% (95% CI, 4.6 to 28.8), and 21.5% (95% CI, 7.3 to 35.7), respectively.

Crude and multivariable analyses of factors associated with mortality are presented in Table 2. Compared to the new ATR, the standard ATR had an adjusted hazard risk of mortality of 2.05 (95% CI, 1.21–3.42). In a sensitivity analysis including only those patients who had no missing values, the association between mortality and the standard ATR was also statistically significant. Other factors found to be associated with mortality were not being on antiretroviral therapy versus being on antiretroviral therapy <6 months, having a CD4 lymphocyte count <50 cells/μL and having a serum albumin <3.8 g/dL. Kaplan-Meier survival estimates by serum albumin levels, CD4 lymphocyte count, and duration of antiretroviral therapy before tuberculous meningitis are presented in Figure 2.

4. Discussion

In this study performed in a "real-life" resource-limited setting, the use of an initial ATR with better CSF drug penetration was associated with an estimated absolute mortality reduction at 12 months of 21.5%, and after adjusting by other variables, patients who received the standard ATR had two times higher risk of mortality than patients who received the new ATR. If these findings are confirmed by other studies, the result of this study could change the initial management of tuberculous meningitis in HIV infected patients.

The results of this study also add to the literature by showing new prognostic factors in HIV-related tuberculous meningitis that can be used in resource-limited settings. Patients who were on antiretroviral therapy at the time of tuberculous meningitis had a significant lower mortality than patients who had not started antiretroviral therapy. This may be explained by the fact that patients who were on antiretroviral therapy might have been asymptomatic at the moment of initiating HIV treatment. In these cases, tuberculous meningitis might have been unmasked after the immunological recovery due to antiretroviral therapy [22], suggesting that these patients had a less advanced form of tuberculous meningitis than those who were not on HIV treatment. In accordance with previous studies [23], patients with low CD4 counts were at a higher risk of mortality. But perhaps what is more interesting for resource-limited setting is that having low levels of serum albumin was strongly associated with mortality. Having low serum albumin levels has been associated with a higher risk of death in HIV-related tuberculosis and in patients initiating antiretroviral therapy [24, 25]. The present study shows that serum albumin can be used as a low-cost prognostic factor in HIV-related tuberculous meningitis.

The study has some limitations. Unlike clinical trials, observational studies can be biased due to unknown confounders. This is a retrospective study reflecting the routine clinical practice in a resource limited setting. Although we used the definition of possible tuberculous meningitis as the minimum criteria for patients to be included in the analysis [9, 15], the study was not designed to correctly classify cases as possible, probable, or definite tuberculous meningitis. We did not perform mycobacterial culture and drug sensitivity testing, so we do not know the proportion of patients who had drug resistant tuberculosis in each group. The Glasgow coma scale of patients was not calculated. Thus, we do not know whether patients who received the standard ATR had a more depressed level of consciousness than patients who received the new ATR. However, although not statistically significant, the proportion of patients with depressed consciousness was higher in the new ATR group (50.8% versus 40.6, P value = 0.17). The new ATR was well tolerated and we did not observe any severe adverse drug reaction. However, the study was not designed to detect adverse drug reactions, so the safety of the new ATR must be evaluated in further studies. The follow-up period of the group who received the new ATR was smaller than the one of the group who received the standard ATR because the new ATR was implemented more recently in our hospital. However, right censoring was corrected in multivariable analysis using Cox proportional hazard models. In summary, our findings must be interpreted with caution, and new studies, preferably randomized clinical trials, may be needed before adopting this new ATR into the clinical practice.

5. Conclusions

The results of this study indicate that improving the CSF drug penetration of the initial treatment of tuberculous meningitis can have a beneficial effect on survival in HIV infected patients. If these findings are confirmed by other studies, the result of this study could change the clinical management of tuberculous meningitis in HIV infected patients.

Disclosure

No external funding was received for this study.

Conflict of Interests

The authors declare that they have no conflict interests.

References

[1] World Health Organization, "Global tuberculosis control," 2012, http://apps.who.int/iris/bitstream/10665/75938/1/9789241564502_eng.pdf.

[2] F. Brancusi, J. Farrar, and D. Heemskerk, "Tuberculous meningitis in adults: a review of a decade of developments focusing on prognostic factors for outcome," *Future Microbiol*, vol. 7, pp. 1101–1116, 2012.

[3] C. Schutz, G. Meintjes, F. Almajid, R. J. Wilkinson, and A. Pozniak, "Clinical management of tuberculosis and HIV-1 co-infection," *European Respiratory Journal*, vol. 36, no. 6, pp. 1460–1481, 2010.

[4] G. Alvarez-Uria, P. K. Naik, R. Pakam, and L. Bachu, "Natural history and factors associated with early and delayed mortality in HIV infected patients treated of tuberculosis under directly observed treatment short course (DOTS) strategy: a prospective cohort study in India," *Interdisciplinary Perspectives on Infectious Diseases*, vol. 2012, Article ID 502012, 9 pages, 2012.

[5] G. Thwaites, M. Fisher, C. Hemingway, G. Scott, T. Solomon, and J. Innes, "British Infection Society guidelines for the diagnosis and treatment of tuberculosis of the central nervous system in adults and children," *Journal of Infection*, vol. 59, no. 3, pp. 167–187, 2009.

[6] World Health Organization, *Treatment of Tuberculosis: Guidelines for National Programmes*, 4th edition, 2009, http://www.who.int/tb/publications/tb_treatmentguidelines/en/.

[7] Centers for Disease Control and Prevention, "National Institutes of Health, HIV Medicine Association of the Infectious Diseases Society of America," Guidelines for the Prevention and treatment of Opportunistic Infections in HIV-Infected Adults and Adolescents, 2013, http://aidsinfo.nih.gov/Guidelines/HTML/4/adult-and-adolescent-oi-prevention-and-treatment-guidelines/0.

[8] P. R. Donald, "Cerebrospinal fluid concentrations of antituberculosis agents in adults and children," *Tuberculosis*, vol. 90, pp. 279–292, 2010.

[9] D. Heemskerk, J. Day, T. T. H. Chau et al., "Intensified treatment with high dose Rifampicin and Levofloxacin compared to standard treatment for adult patients with Tuberculous Meningitis (TBM-IT): protocol for a randomized controlled trial," *Trials*, vol. 12, article 25, 2011.

[10] G. E. Thwaites, S. M. Bhavnani, T. T. H. Chau et al., "Randomized pharmacokinetic and pharmacodynamic comparison of fluoroquinolones for tuberculous meningitis," *Antimicrob Agents Chemother*, vol. 55, pp. 3244–3253, 2011.

[11] R. Ruslami, A. R. Ganiem, S. Dian et al., "Intensified regimen containing rifampicin and moxifloxacin for tuberculous meningitis: an open-label, randomised controlled phase 2 trial," *The Lancet Infectious Diseases*, vol. 13, pp. 27–35, 2013.

[12] M. E. Torok, T. T. H. Chau, P. P. Mai et al., "Clinical and microbiological features of HIV-associated tuberculous meningitis in Vietnamese adults," *PLoS ONE*, vol. 3, no. 3, article e1772, 2008.

[13] G. Alvarez-Uria, M. Midde, R. Pakam, and P. K. Naik, "Gender differences, routes of transmission, socio-demographic characteristics and prevalence of HIV related infections of adults and children in an HIV cohort from a rural district of India," *Infectious Disease Reports*, vol. 4, article e19, 2012.

[14] G. Alvarez-Uria, M. Midde, R. Pakam et al., "Factors associated with late presentation of HIV and estimation of antiretroviral treatment need according to CD4 lymphocyte count in a resource-limited setting: data from an HIV Cohort Study in India," *Interdisciplinary Perspectives on Infectious Diseases*, vol. 2012, Article ID 293795, 7 pages, 2012.

[15] S. Marais, G. Thwaites, J. F. Schoeman et al., "Tuberculous meningitis: a uniform case definition for use in clinical research," *The Lancet Infectious Diseases*, vol. 10, pp. 803–812, 2010.

[16] G. E. Marx and E. D. Chan, "Tuberculous meningitis: diagnosis and treatment overview," *Tuberculosis Research and Treatment*, vol. 2011, Article ID 798764, 9 pages, 2011.

[17] P. R. Donald and A. H. Diacon, "The early bactericidal activity of anti-tuberculosis drugs: a literature review," *Tuberculosis*, vol. 88, supplement 1, pp. S75–S83, 2008.

[18] WHO, *Treatment of Tuberculosis: Guidelines for National Programmes*, 3rd edition, 2003, WHO/CDS/TB/2003.313, http://whqlibdoc.who.int/hq/2003/WHO_CDS_TB_2003.313_eng.pdf.

[19] G. Alvarez-Uria, M. Midde, and P. K. Naik, "Socio-demographic risk factors associated with HIV infection in patients seeking medical advice in a rural hospital of India," *Journal of Public Health Research*, vol. 1, article e14, 2012.

[20] D. G. Kleinbaum and M. Klein, *Survival Analysis, A Self-Learning Text*, Springer, 2nd edition, 2005.

[21] P. Royston, "Multiple imputation of missing values: further update of ice, with an emphasis on categorical variables," *Stata Journal*, vol. 9, no. 3, pp. 466–477, 2009.

[22] D. J. Pepper, S. Marais, G. Maartens et al., "Neurologic manifestations of paradoxical tuberculosis-associated immune reconstitution inflammatory syndrome: a case series," *Clinical Infectious Diseases*, vol. 48, no. 11, pp. e96–e107, 2009.

[23] D. Cecchini, J. Ambrosioni, C. Brezzo et al., "Tuberculous meningitis in HIV-infected patients: drug susceptibility and clinical outcome," *AIDS*, vol. 21, no. 3, pp. 373–374, 2007.

[24] C. R. Sudfeld, S. Isanaka, S. Aboud et al., "Association of serum albumin concentration with mortality, morbidity, CD4 T-cell reconstitution among tanzanians initiating antiretroviral therapy," *The Journal of Infectious Diseases*, vol. 207, pp. 1370–1378, 2013.

[25] P. Tabarsi, E. Chitsaz, A. Moradi et al., "Treatment outcome, mortality and their predictors among HIV-associated tuberculosis patients," *International Journal of STD & AIDS*, vol. 23, pp. e1–e4, 2012.

4

Awareness of the Warning Signs, Risk Factors, and Treatment for Tuberculosis among Urban Nigerians

Olufemi O. Desalu,[1] Adekunle O. Adeoti,[2] Abayomi Fadeyi,[3] Alakija K. Salami,[1] Ademola E. Fawibe,[1] and Olanrewaju O. Oyedepo[4]

[1] *Department of Medicine, University of Ilorin Teaching Hospital, PMB 1459, Ilorin 240001, Nigeria*
[2] *Department of Medicine, Ekiti State University Teaching Hospital, PMB 5355, Ado-Ekiti, Nigeria*
[3] *Department of Medical Microbiology, University of Ilorin Teaching Hospital, PMB 1459, Ilorin 240001, Nigeria*
[4] *Department of Anaesthesia, University of Ilorin Teaching Hospital, PMB 1459, Ilorin 240001, Nigeria*

Correspondence should be addressed to Olufemi O. Desalu, femuy1967@yahoo.co.uk

Academic Editor: José R. Lapa e Silva

Objectives. To determine the awareness of the warning signs, risk factors, and treatment of tuberculosis among urban Nigerians. *Methods.* This was a cross-sectional survey among 574 adults in Ilorin, Nigeria. Semistructured questionnaire was administered by trained interviewers to obtain information about awareness of tuberculosis warning signs, risk factors, and treatment. *Results.* Majority of the subjects (71.4%) were aware of at least one warning sign of tuberculosis. Cough (66.2%), weight loss (38.0%), and haemoptysis (30.7%) were the most identified warning signs. The predictors of awareness of warning sign were increasing age (r + 0.12), higher family income (r + 0.10), higher level of education (r + 0.10), and belonging to Christian faith (r + 0.11). Awareness of risk factors for tuberculosis was higher for tobacco smokers (77.0%) and history of contact with a case of TB (76.0%). Less than half were aware of HIV infection (49.8%), alcohol consumption (42.5%), chronic kidney disease (40.4%), extremes of ages (39.4%), cancers (36.9%), and diabetes mellitus (27.5%) as risk factors for TB. Tuberculosis was reported to be curable by 74.6% of the subjects and 67.9% knew that there are medications for treatment of tuberculosis, while 11.5% knew the duration of treatment. *Conclusion.* This study has revealed that the awareness of HIV and noncommunicable diseases as risk factors for TB is poor. This study has therefore demonstrated the need for health education programs that will emphasize recognition, identification, and modification of risk factor for TB.

1. Introduction

Tuberculosis (TB) is a chronic infectious disease caused by a bacterium called *Mycobacterium tuberculosis*. It usually affects the lungs in 80% of cases with warning signs of cough, haemoptysis, and chest pain, shortness of breath, fever, weight loss, and drenching night sweat [1]. TB is spread mainly through the air inform of droplets. When infectious people cough, sneeze, talk, laugh or spit, droplets containing *Mycobacterium tuberculosis* are sprayed into the air. People nearby may inhale the bacteria and become infected. *Mycobacterium tuberculosis* can remain viable as airborne droplet suspended in the air for a long time or as part of house dust for weeks. However, transmission usually occurs only after substantial exposure to someone with active TB [1, 2]. A person can be infected by *Mycobacterium tuberculosis* for many years without getting sick or spreading the organism to other people. If the immune system is weakened by immunosuppressive disease like HIV infection, diabetes mellitus, malignancy, chronic kidney disease, extremes of ages, and immunosuppressive agent, latent TB infection can develop into active disease [1, 2]. If a person with active disease is left untreated, he or she will infect on the average between 10 and 15 people every year [3]. TB accounts for 2.5% of the global burden of disease and is the commonest cause of death in young women, killing more women than all causes of maternal mortality combined [4–6]. Ninety-five per cent of all cases and 99% of deaths occur in developing countries, with the greatest burden in sub-Saharan Africa and South East Asia [7]. It currently holds the seventh place in the global ranking of causes of death. Unless intensive efforts are made, it is likely to maintain that position through to 2020, despite a substantial projected decline in disease burden from other infectious diseases [5, 6]. TB causes a significant socioeconomic burden: as three quarter of cases are within the economically productive age group of 15–54 years [8]. Tuberculosis is a serious public health problem in Nigeria with an estimated prevalence of nearly 900,000 TB cases and with the second highest TB disease burden in Africa and ranks 5th among the 22 high TB burden countries in the world [4]. In Nigeria, there were 90,447 TB cases notified in 2010 with 41, 416 (58%) cases as new smear positives, and a case detection rate of 40%. Ilorin city is the capital of Kwara State, a state that has one of the least TB notification rate (900 per annum) when compared with other states in the country like Lagos (8200 per annum) and Oyo (6000 per annum) that have the higher TB notification rate [9]. The outcome of TB control is determined by the clinical and social factors like delayed presentation and health care utilization which depend on the knowledge and awareness of TB symptoms among the population [10, 11]. For us to meet the Millennium Development Goal (MDG), the Global Plan to Stop TB and reverse the incidence of TB by 2015, we need to determine the level of awareness of the warning signs, risk factors, and treatment of tuberculosis among the population as modifiable factors in the TB control program. Therefore the objectives of our study were to determine the awareness of the warning signs, risk factors, and treatment of tuberculosis among urban residents in Ilorin, Nigeria.

2. Materials and Methods

This was a cross-sectional survey among subjects aged ≥18 years who reside in Ilorin West and East local government area Kwara state, Nigeria that was conducted between July 2011 and August 2011. The subjects were recruited by multi-stage stratified sampling method. A minimum sample size of 384 was arrived at using the Cochran formula $N = Z2pq/d2$, where N was the required sample size; p was (50%) [5]; q, ($1-p$); Z, an SD of 1.96 (which corresponds to a 95% confidence interval); and d is the degree of accuracy desired (0.05 for an acceptable error margin of 5%). The design effect of 1.0 which was derived from the homogeneity of the two council areas was used to adjust the minimum sample size. The local government areas consist of electoral wards that were divided into clusters and a sample frame containing the list of clusters was constructed by the investigators. The households in each cluster were randomly selected. The adults in each household were informed about the study by our trained interviewers and a maximum of two persons per household were selected in order to have normal spread and true representation of the study population. We then recruited individuals who met the inclusion criteria (age of 18–45 years, resided in Ilorin for at least 1 year, and willingness to participate in the study) from the selected households. Those who participated in the pretesting of the questionnaire and those with a past history of TB were excluded from the study as it was assumed that the former group would have been primed to seek for information on warning signs and risk factors for TB while the latter category would have a better knowledge of the warning signs having previously suffered from the disease.

A pretested semistructured questionnaire was administered face to face by trained interviewers in their place of residence or work. The questionnaire was in English, which is the official language of communication in Nigeria and translated to Yoruba language for few respondents who could not communicate in English. The questionnaire was used to obtain sociodemographic information, awareness of the warning sign of tuberculosis, the predisposing risk factors, and TB medication, cure and treatment duration. The question on awareness of the disease was based mostly on nonpersonal experience (individual level of enlightenment and public health education).

3. Data Analysis

The data were analyzed using SPSS version 15, Chicago Inc., IL, USA. Frequency statistics was performed for sociodemographic variables warning sign and risk factor for TB in the study population. The warning symptoms were analyzed according to gender using 2×2 cross tab, and chi square was calculated to determine the level of significance. $P < 0.05$ was considered to be statistically significant. Spearman correlation coefficient was used to determine the predictors of warning sign of TB. The confounding variables were identified by stratification of variables and they were used in adjusting the spearman correlation coefficient.

4. Results

A total of 574 subjects participated in the study; their median age was 30 with an interquartile range of (23–40). Of the 574, 308 (53.7%) were males and majority were unskilled workers and they earned below fifty thousand naira per month (three hundred and twelve dollars per month).

Majorities (459; 80%) were aware of TB as a disease. Four hundred and ten (71.4%) subjects were aware of at least one TB warning sign (Table 1). Of the 410 that were aware of the TB warning sign, 228 (55.6%) were males and 182 (44.4) were females. Majority of the subjects (66.2%) were aware of cough as TB warning sign, 218 (38.0%) were aware of weight loss, and 176 (30.7%) were aware of haemoptysis. Chronic cough was commonly reported as a warning sign by men (56; 18.2%) compared with women (18; 11.3%). Similarly, fever was commonly recognized by men (40; 13.0% versus 14; 5.3%) compared with women (Table 2).

The predictors of awareness of TB warning sign were increasing age ($r + 0.12$), higher family income ($r + 0.10$), higher level of education ($r+0.10$), and belonging to Christian faith ($r + 0.11$) (Table 3).

In this study, 442 (77.0%) subjects reported active tobacco smoking as a risk factor for TB, 436 (76.0%) reported history of contact with an index case of TB or chronic cough, while 342 (59.6%) cited health care related occupation as a risk

Table 1: General characteristics of the study subjects.

Characteristics	n (%)
Age	30 (23–40)*
Sex	
Male	308 (53.7)
Female	266 (46.6)
Education	
Primary/none	150 (26.1)
Secondary	148 (25.8)
Tertiary	276 (48.1)
Income (N)**	
<10,000	244 (42.5)
≤50,000	206 (39.5)
≤100,000	72 (12.5)
≤200,000	26 (4.5)
>N200,000	22 (3.8)
Occupational class	
Professional/administrators	21 (3.7)
Skilled	32 (5.6)
Unskilled	100 (17.4)
Others	421 (73.3)
Marital status	
Married	252 (43.9)
Others	322 (56.1)
Religion	
Islam	336 (58.5)
Christianity	236 (41.1)
Others	2 (0.3)
Aware of TB as a disease	
Aware	459 (80.0)
Unaware	115 (20.0)
Awareness of TB sign	
Aware	410 (71.4)
Unaware	164 (28.6)

*Median (interquartile range).
**4 missing.

Table 2: Identified TB warning sign according to gender.

Warning sign	Male (%) $N = 308$	Female (%) $N = 266$	Total (%) $N = 574$
Cough	212 (68.8)	168 (63.2)	380 (66.2)
Weight loss	126 (40.9)	92 (34.6)	218 (38.0)
Heamoptysis	104 (33.8)	72 (27.1)	176 (30.7)
Chronic cough	56 (18.2)	30 (11.3)	86 (15.0)*
Breathlessness	44 (14.3)	34 (12.8)	78 (13.6)
Chest pain	32 (10.4)	28 (10.5)	60 (10.5)
Fever	40 (13.0)	14 (5.3)	54 (9.4)*
Fatigue	16 (5.2)	20 (7.5)	36 (6.3)
Night sweat	20 (6.5)	10 (3.8)	30 (5.2)

*$P < 0.05$.

factor for TB. Three hundred and forty-four (59.0%) were aware of overcrowding and likewise environmental tobacco smoking as risk factor for TB, respectively. The use of biomass fuel as source of cooking energy was also reported by 326 (56.8%). Less than half of the subjects were aware of HIV infection (49.8%), alcohol consumption (42.5%), CKD/CRF (40.4%), extremes of ages (39.4%), and cancer (36.9%) as risk factors for TB. One hundred and fifty-eight subjects (27.5%) were aware of diabetes mellitus as risk factor for TB (Table 4).

In the treatment of TB, 428 (74.6%) reported that TB is curable, 390 (67.9%) were aware that there are drugs for treatment of tuberculosis, and only 66 (11.5%) knew the duration of treatment.

Table 3: Predictors of warning signs of TB.

Predictors	Crude r^2	Adjusted r^2
Age	+0.13*	+0.12*
Sex	+0.07	+0.06
Higher level of education	+0.06	+0.10*
Unskilled workers	+0.02	+0.03
Marriage	+0.04	+0.04
Higher family income	+0.18*	+0.10*
Christianity	+0.20*	+0.11*
Having a medical disease	+0.01	−0.04

Adjusted for age, sex, religion, and sociodemographic variables.
*$P < 0.05$.

Table 4: Awareness of the risk factors for TB in the subjects.

Reported risk factor	n (%)
Tobacco smoking	
-Active	442 (77.0)
-ETS	344 (59.0)
History of contact	436 (76.0)
Health care job	342 (59.6)
Overcrowding	344 (59.0)
Use of biomass fuel	326 (56.8)
Work-related pollution	322 (56.1)
Low income	312 (54.4)
HIV infection	286 (49.8)
Alcohol intake	244 (42.5)
CKD/CRF	232 (40.4)
Extremes ages	226 (39.4)
Cancer	212 (36.9)
Diabetes mellitus	158 (27.5)

5. Discussion

This present study was undertaken to determine the public awareness of warning symptoms, risk factors, and treatment of TB in Ilorin, Nigeria. Few studies on the awareness of TB exist in north-central Nigeria [12]. We defined TB warning sign as something perceived that informs or serves to warn a person about the presence or a future occurrence of tuberculosis.

In this study, about 71% of the subjects were aware of at least one warning sign of tuberculosis and about 29% could not mention a warning sign of TB. This result of this study is closer to the one by Vukovic et al. [13], among 1129 adults in Serbia where they found that almost a third of the subjects could not identify any sign of TB. Further analysis by gender showed that more men were aware of TB warning sign than the women. This pattern of observation may be explained by the result of Nigerian demographic health survey of 2008 which noted that in the same study region about 81% of men have heard of TB compared with 52% of women [12].

We also found that the most commonly identified TB warning sign was cough followed by weight loss and haemoptysis. Similar studies in Asia have also noted cough and haemoptysis as the common warning signs or symptoms of tuberculosis [14–18]. The most common warning sign in this study is cough and it is in contrast to what was reported in the Malaysian study where the respondents noted haemoptysis as the most common sign of TB [14]. Geographical variation in the awareness of TB warning sign may be attributed to the discrepancy in the burden of the disease in both these two countries, prior knowledge of TB, personal experience with a close friend, and family members affected by the disease. It also depends on sources of public health information.

The significant predictors of awareness of TB warning sign were increasing age, being a Christian, higher family income, and education. The association of increasing age with awareness of TB sign may be attributed to increasing knowledge of TB and lifetime experiences of close relative who had the disease. We also discovered that those who belong to Christian faith were more likely to be aware of TB sign than others after adjusting for confounding variable like age, sex, income, and level of education. Further subanalysis by stratification of the religion, was suffice to explain the religious predisposition as 0.8% of the Christians were uneducated compared with the Muslims that had 20.8% uneducated subjects in this study.

The association of higher family income and education with awareness of TB signs may be attributed to higher literacy. Higher level of educational attainment is often a factor for better family income. Families that have high income are able to purchase household assets like television, radio and Hi fi internet, and other communication appliances that increase their knowledge of health-related matters which are of public concern. Similar studies have also supported our observation that literates were more likely to be aware than the illiterates of signs and symptoms of TB [13, 16, 17, 19, 20]. A recent study in Pakistan also noted the association of higher monthly income with the knowledge of TB [21].

Our result also revealed that more than half of the subjects were aware of tobacco smoking (active and secondhand), history of contact, health care job, household overcrowding, use of biomass fuel as a source of cooking energy, work-related pollution, and low family income as a risk factor for TB. More than 50% were unaware of noncommunicable diseases (NCDs) like diabetes mellitus, cancers, chronic kidney disease, and behavioural factors like alcohol as risk factors for TB. Surprisingly half of the subjects did not report HIV which has a higher burden in sub-Saharan Africa as risk factor for TB. The NCDs are expected to increase by 2030 and as the impact of NCDs increases, and as population's age, annual NCD deaths are projected to continue to rise worldwide, and the greatest increase is expected to be seen in low- and middle-income regions. An extreme age of life was also cited by less than half of the subjects [22, 23]. Studies in Morocco [24] and Pakistan [17] have reported that significant percentages of the respondents in their study were unable to identify this as risk factor for TB. With regards to tuberculosis therapy, approximately 75% of the subjects reported that TB is curable, 67.9% were aware that there are drugs for treatment of tuberculosis, and only 11.5% knew the 6–8 months duration of treatment. Respondents in several studies have also noted TB as a curable disease [13, 21, 24, 25]. Singh et al. in 2002 [26] also reported that only 12.6% of their subjects in India knew the duration of TB therapy which is in agreement with 11.6% obtained in our study.

This study has determined the awareness of the warning sign, risk factor, and treatment for tuberculosis; however we have not explored the sociocultural belief and misconception of tuberculosis in the era of directly observed therapy which is not part of the objective of this study. This might be important direction in terms of research.

The study is limited by the small size of the population and power of the study, and nonvalidation of the study questionnaire in local language. The extent to which the translated items in questionnaire measure what it was intended to measure has not been statistically validated.

6. Conclusion

This study has shown the high level of awareness of TB warning sign and TB as a curable disease among the studied population. HIV, non communicable diseases like DM, alcohol consumption, and cancers were poorly reported as risk factors for TB.

Acknowledgment

The authors hereby thank the medical students of University of Ilorin 2011–2014 set for their assistance during the data collection.

References

[1] V. Kumar, A. K. Abbas, N. Fausto, and R. N. Mitchell, *Robbins Basic Pathology*, Saunders Elsevier, Philadelphia, Pa, USA, 8th edition, 2007.

[2] WHO Global Tuberculosis Programme WHO Fact sheet no.104, 2010, http://www.who.int/mediacentre/factsheets/fs-104/en/index.html.

[3] C. Dye, C. J. Watt, D. M. Bleed, S. M. Hosseini, and M. C. Raviglione, "Evolution of tuberculosis control and prospects for reducing tuberculosis incidence, prevalence, and deaths globally," *Journal of the American Medical Association*, vol. 293, no. 22, pp. 2767–2775, 2005.

[4] "Global tuberculosis control: surveillance, planning, financing," WHO Report WHO/HTM/TB/2008.393, World Health Organization, Geneva, Switzerland, 2008.

[5] C. Dye, S. Scheele, P. Dolin, V. Pathania, and M. C. Raviglione, "Global burden of tuberculosis: estimated incidence, prevalence, and mortality by country," *Journal of the American Medical Association*, vol. 282, no. 7, pp. 677–686, 1999.

[6] I. Smith, "What is the health, social, and economic burden of tuberculosis," in *Toman's Tuberculosis Case Detection, Treatment, and Monitoring: Questions and Answers*, T. Frieden, Ed., pp. 233–237, World Health Organization, Geneva, Switzerland, 2nd edition, 2004, WHO/HTM/TB/2004.334.

[7] C. Dye, "Global epidemiology of tuberculosis," *The Lancet*, vol. 367, no. 9514, pp. 938–940, 2006.

[8] World Health Organization, "Global tuberculosis control: surveillance, planning and financing," Tech. Rep. WHO/HTM /TB/2006. 362, WHO, Geneva, Switzerland, 2006.

[9] Nigeria Tuberculosis Fact Sheet. United States Embassy in Nigeria, http://photos.state.gov/libraries/nigeria/487468/pdfs/JanuaryTuberculosisFactSheet.pdf.

[10] L. V. Sacks and S. Pendle, "Factors related to in-hospital deaths in patients with tuberculosis," *Archives of Internal Medicine*, vol. 158, no. 17, pp. 1916–1922, 1998.

[11] T. A. Mathew, T. N. Ovsyanikova, S. S. Shin et al., "Causes of death during tuberculosis treatment in Tomsk Oblast, Russia," *International Journal of Tuberculosis and Lung Disease*, vol. 10, no. 8, pp. 857–863, 2006.

[12] National Population Commission (NPC) and ICF Macro, *Nigeria Demographic and Health Survey 2008*, National Population Commission and ICF Macro, Abuja, Nigeria, 2009, http://www.measuredhs.com/pubs/pdf/SR173/SR173.pdf.

[13] D. Vukovic, L. Nagorni-Obradovic, and V. Bjegovic, "Knowledge and misconceptions of tuberculosis in the general population in Serbia," *European Journal of Clinical Microbiology and Infectious Diseases*, vol. 27, no. 9, pp. 761–767, 2008.

[14] T. K. Koay, "Knowledge and attitudes towards tuberculosis among the people living in Kudat district, Sabah," *Medical Journal of Malaysia*, vol. 59, no. 4, pp. 502–511, 2004.

[15] M. U. Mushtaq, U. Shahid, H. M. Abdullah et al., "Urban-rural inequities in knowledge, attitudes and practices regarding tuberculosis in two districts of Pakistan's Punjab province," *International Journal for Equity in Health*, vol. 10, article 8, 2011.

[16] R. Malhotra, D. K. Taneja, V. K. Dhingra, S. Rajpal, and M. Mehra, "Awareness regarding tuburculosis in a rural population of Delhi," *Indian Journal of Community Medicine*, vol. 27, pp. 62–68, 2002.

[17] S. S. Ali, F. Rabbani, U. N. Siddiqui et al., "Tuberculosis: do we know enough? A study of patients and their families in an out-patient hospital setting in Karachi, Pakistan," *International Journal of Tuberculosis and Lung Disease*, vol. 7, no. 11, pp. 1052–1058, 2003.

[18] R. P. Croft and R. A. Croft, "Knowledge, attitude and practice regarding leprosy and tuberculosis in Bangladesh," *Leprosy Review*, vol. 70, no. 1, pp. 34–42, 1999.

[19] N. Sharma, R. Malhotra, D. K. Taneja, R. Saha, and G. K. Ingle, "Awareness and perception about tuberculosis in the general population of Delhi," *Asia-Pacific Journal of Public Health*, vol. 19, no. 2, pp. 10–15, 2007.

[20] S. P. Yadav, M. L. Mathur, and A. K. Dixit, "Knowledge and attitude towards tuberculosis among sandstone quarry workers in desert parts of Rajasthan," *Indian Journal of Tuberculosis*, vol. 53, pp. 187–195, 2006.

[21] S. I. Gilani and M. Khurram, "Perception of tuberculosis in Pakistan: findings of a nation-wide survey," *Journal of the Pakistan Medical Association*, vol. 62, no. 2, pp. 116–120, 2012.

[22] S. Wild, G. Roglic, A. Green, R. Sicree, and H. King, "Global prevalence of diabetes: estimates for the year 2000 and projections for 2030," *Diabetes Care*, vol. 27, no. 5, pp. 1047–1053, 2004.

[23] World Health Organization, *Global Status Report on Noncommunicable Diseases*, World Health Organization, Geneva, Switzerland, 2010.

[24] S. Ottmani, Z. Obermeyer, N. Bencheikh, and J. Mahjour, "Knowledge, attitudes and beliefs about tuberculosis in urban Morocco," *Eastern Mediterranean Health Journal*, vol. 14, no. 2, pp. 298–304, 2008.

[25] J. A. Khan, M. Irfan, A. Zaki, M. Beg, S. F. Hussain, and N. Rizvi, "Knowledge, attitude and misconceptions regarding tuberculosis in Pakistani patients," *Journal of the Pakistan Medical Association*, vol. 56, no. 5, pp. 211–214, 2006.

[26] M. M. Singh, T. Bano, D. Pagare, N. Sharma, R. Devi, and M. Mehra, "Knowledge and attitude towards tuberculosis in a slum community of Delhi," *Journal of Communicable Diseases*, vol. 34, no. 3, pp. 203–214, 2002.

5

Innovative Quality-Assurance Strategies for Tuberculosis Surveillance in the United States

Lilia Ponce Manangan, Cheryl Tryon, Elvin Magee, and Roque Miramontes

Division of Tuberculosis Elimination, National Center for HIV/AIDS, Viral Hepatitis, STD, and Tuberculosis Prevention, Centers for Disease Control and Prevention (CDC), Mailstop E-10, 1600 Clifton Road, Atlanta, GA 30033, USA

Correspondence should be addressed to Lilia Ponce Manangan, lpm2@cdc.gov

Academic Editor: Kashef Ijaz

Introduction. The Centers for Disease Control and Prevention (CDC)'s National Tuberculosis Surveillance System (NTSS) is the national repository of tuberculosis (TB) data in the United States. Jurisdictions report to NTSS through the Report of Verified Case of Tuberculosis (RVCT) form that transitioned to a web-based system in 2009. *Materials and Methods.* To improve RVCT data quality, CDC conducted a quality assurance (QA) needs assessment to develop QA strategies. These include QA components (case detection, data accuracy, completeness, timeliness, data security, and confidentiality); sample tools such as National TB Indicators Project (NTIP) to identify TB case reporting discrepancies; comprehensive training course; resource guide and toolkit. *Results and Discussion.* During July–September 2011, 73 staff from 34 (57%) of 60 reporting jurisdictions participated in QA training. Participants stated usefulness of sharing jurisdictions' QA methods; 66 (93%) wrote that the QA tools will be effective for their activities. Several jurisdictions reported implementation of QA tools pertinent to their programs. Data showed >8% increase in NTSS and NTIP enrollment through Secure Access Management Services, which monitors system usage, from August 2011–February 2012. *Conclusions.* Despite challenges imposed by web-based surveillance systems, QA strategies can be developed with innovation and collaboration. These strategies can also be used by other disease programs to ensure high data quality.

1. Introduction

In 2010, there were 8.8 million new cases of tuberculosis (TB) disease reported worldwide, with over 1 million TB deaths [1]. In the United States, 11,182 people were newly diagnosed with TB disease [2]. The mission of the Division of Tuberculosis Elimination (DTBE), Centers for Disease Control and Prevention (CDC) is to promote health and quality of life by preventing, controlling, and eventually eliminating TB from the United States, and by collaborating with other countries and international partners in controlling TB globally [3].

Tuberculosis surveillance is a core public health function. Ongoing and systematic collection, analysis, interpretation, and dissemination of surveillance data allow programs to target control interventions that provide the most impact in eliminating TB [4]. These surveillance data are essential in describing morbidity and mortality, monitoring trends in TB incidence and prevalence, detecting potential outbreaks, and defining high-risk groups. In addition, TB data are needed to evaluate TB control programs, identify deficiencies, and allocate resources. In order to perform these important functions, it is essential that surveillance data are collected and reported in an accurate, complete, and timely manner.

The CDC's National Tuberculosis Surveillance System (NTSS) is the national repository of TB surveillance data in the United States. CDC receives data on TB cases from reporting jurisdictions through a standardized data collection form, the Report of Verified Case of Tuberculosis (RVCT). NTSS has 60 reporting jurisdictions: all 50 US states, the District of Columbia, New York City, American Samoa, Federated States of Micronesia, Guam, Republic of the Marshall Islands, Commonwealth of the Northern Mariana Islands, Puerto Rico, Republic of Palau, and US Virgin Islands.

The RVCT was revised by a group of TB experts in 2009 and transitioned into a new web-based reporting system. An interdisciplinary CDC DTBE team collaborated with key national partners, state-based medical or health officers, and other local healthcare professionals to launch a national training program on the new RVCT [5, 6]. Extensive reviews of training materials enabled partners to provide feedback for improvements on the instructions for each of the 49 RVCT items [7]. The team also developed a self-study manual for participants that was used during facilitator-led trainings [8]. The manual can also be used as self-study for new TB staff and as a reference guide. In addition, a facilitator manual was developed and used during training-of-trainers courses to build RVCT training capacity throughout the reporting jurisdictions [9].

Quality assurance (QA) is a critical part of any successful surveillance system and is a continuous cycle of monitoring, evaluating, and improving data quality [10, 11]. Prior to 2009, jurisdictions depended on a CDC disk operating system (DOS) used for surveillance of TB data. This system provided a series of validation reports to jurisdictions for managing data. When CDC transitioned to a web-based system in 2009, there was a need for a standardized QA process that jurisdictions could adapt to their setting.

The team determined that a logical followup to the RVCT trainings was to enhance the QA knowledge and skills of TB surveillance staff. Furthermore, the RVCT training participants expressed concerns regarding the lack of data validation of some state systems and the inability of reporting areas to transmit all data electronically. DTBE staff began working individually with state public health partners to develop QA strategies. This paper describes these strategies to ensure the quality of TB data reported to the CDC's NTSS through the new web-based system.

2. Materials and Methods

The RVCT QA training team, in collaboration with key partners, developed innovative strategies to provide standardized methodologies, skills, and tools to enhance the capacity for conducting QA. Similar to the RVCT training course, the team used the systematic process for health education to develop these QA strategies [6, 12]. This process includes needs assessment, development, pilot testing, implementation, and outcome evaluation.

2.1. Quality Assurance Needs Assessment. During 2010-2011, the training team conducted a comprehensive needs assessment to determine strategies that could enhance QA for TB surveillance data. During the needs assessment, the team facilitated discussions of QA topics with prepared open-ended questions to jurisdictions and CDC staff.

The needs assessment included the following.

(i) meeting with TB program area staff from 11 reporting jurisdictions in either focus groups or individual interviews. Three incidence levels of TB-burden areas were represented including low (≤3.5 cases per 100,000 population in 2009), medium (3.6–3.8 cases per 100,000 population in 2009), and high TB incidence (>3.8 cases per 100,000 population in 2009). The staff described their surveillance system, and staff characteristics (training and expertise level), and shared their QA process and tools (i.e., tables, charts, graphs, processes, and templates). Staff suggested content topics and prioritized QA components that should be covered in the materials and a training course. In addition, they discussed successes and challenges experienced when conducting QA at their sites;

(ii) meeting with colleagues from DTBE who have a role in ensuring quality data including the subject matter experts in the laboratory, the Data Management and Statistics Branch, project officers for the National TB Indicators Project (NTIP), and the TB Genotyping Information Management System [13, 14]. These staff members collaborated to help develop and conduct a comprehensive training program and QA tools;

(iii) meeting with surveillance staff from other CDC divisions including the Division of STD Prevention, Division of Viral Hepatitis, and the Division of HIV/AIDS Prevention. Some of these colleagues indicated they conducted QA only after data arrived at CDC. None of the QA procedures or processes utilized by other divisions met the needs of DTBE;

(iv) conducting a review of available QA materials on surveillance data [15–38]. This review yielded information on various QA components and definitions (Table 1). However, the team did not find a comprehensive QA framework, practical step-by-step QA strategies for TB surveillance data, or practical models for a QA training course;

(v) reviewing the surveillance section of the Tuberculosis Elimination and Laboratory Cooperative Agreement, a portion of an agreement between DTBE and NTSS reporting jurisdictions that describes area surveillance activities [39]. This yielded QA components and a requirement to monitor data quality (Table 1).

2.2. Quality Assurance Strategies. The results of the needs assessment were used to develop 4 strategies for enhancing QA procedures in reporting jurisdictions. These include the following.

(1) Providing a QA Process That Includes Five Components and Categorizing Activities into Each of These Components. QA components include case detection, data accuracy, data completeness, data timeliness, and data security and confidentiality. These components provided logical steps for conducting QA activities and were designed to allow reporting areas to utilize those strategies that would benefit them.

(2) Providing QA Tools Including Guidance for a Written QA Protocol. The RVCT QA training team provided a template for a written QA protocol and other tools that jurisdictions can easily adapt and use to conduct QA. Staff from CDC and the various jurisdictions developed over 45 tools that were classified into each of the five QA components (Table 2). The

TABLE 1: Guidance* for developing a written protocol for quality assurance for tuberculosis surveillance data, United States, 2011.

(a) Case detection: Case detection is the discovery of the existence of a single instance of a specific disease or exposure, for example, tuberculosis (TB). This is a front-line surveillance activity and typically accomplished as a by-product of routine medical or veterinary care, laboratory work, or via an astute observer. The primary purpose is to find all patients with TB diagnosis to treat and prevent TB transmission and are reported to the TB surveillance system

Activities	Description	Data sources
Maintain a registry of TB cases.	Contains at a minimum the elements to produce data for the national TB case report, the revised Report of Verified Case of Tuberculosis (RVCT). All local jurisdictions should also have at least a log, if not a registry, that contains key demographic and clinical information on each reported TB suspect. Data on TB cases receiving diagnostic, treatment, or contact investigation services in the local jurisdiction, although not included in the annual morbidity total, should be included in the TB registry.	(i) TB suspect registries from all local jurisdictions.
Establish liaisons with appropriate reporting sources to enhance quality assurance (QA) of TB surveillance data.	Enhance identification, reporting, and followup of TB cases and suspects by establishing liaisons with appropriate reporting sources. Jurisdictions should provide a plan for case finding and how they will or have established appropriate liaisons. Thereafter, TB programs should provide periodic feedback and at minimum, an annual written report summarizing surveillance data to reporting sources.	(i) Hospitals. (ii) Clinics (e.g., TB and HIV/AIDS clinics). (iii) Laboratories performing tests for mycobacteria. (iv) Selected physicians (e.g., pulmonary and infectious disease subspecialists). (v) Correctional facilities. (vi) Community and migrant health centers. (vii) Pharmacies. (viii) Other public and private facilities providing care to populations with or at risk for TB.
Develop and implement active case detection activities.	At a minimum, ongoing active laboratory surveillance should be conducted by on-site visits in all areas to ensure complete reporting of all TB cases and suspects with positive acid-fast bacilli (AFB) smears and cultures for *M. tuberculosis*.	(i) Laboratory reports.
Evaluate the completeness of reporting of TB cases to the surveillance system.	Periodically (e.g., at least every two years) evaluate the completeness of reporting of TB cases to the surveillance system by identifying and investigating at least one population-based secondary data source to find potentially unreported TB cases.	Secondary data source, for example (i) statewide laboratory record review, (ii) pharmacy review, (iii) hospital discharge data review,
	Potential TB cases identified during the evaluation must be verified.	(i) medical records, (ii) physician, interviews, (iii) patient interviews.
	Reasons for nonreporting of TB cases should be determined and a plan for improvement developed and implemented.	

(b) Data accuracy: Data accuracy means that the data recorded match exactly what happens in a clinical encounter, whether or not it is clinically appropriate. The primary purpose is to identify and correct errors in the surveillance data

Activities	Description	Data sources
Evaluate accuracy/validity of RVCT data.	At least annually evaluate the accuracy/validity of RVCT data by comparing RVCT data and the jurisdiction's TB registry data to original data sources.	(i) RVCT data collection form. (ii) Patients' medical records. (iii) TB registry database.
Assess knowledge, skills, and abilities of staff and provide training if needed.	Assess the knowledge, skills, and abilities of all existing personnel and new hires whose duties involve the collection and reporting of registry and RVCT data. Provide training and evaluation. Training will focus on accurate and timely completion of the revised RVCT. All existing staff will be trained on the revised RVCT data collection, and new staff should be trained within 2 months of hire date.	(i) Personnel files. (ii) Staff interviews. (iii) Observations and evaluations of staff skills.

(c) Data completeness: Data completeness means that the information submitted contains the mandatory set of data items. The primary purpose is to capture all the relevant data on TB patients on the RVCT to support and improve the function of the TB surveillance system

Activities	Description	Data sources
Maintain completeness for all RVCT variables.	TB case data will be reported to CDC using the revised RVCT form via an electronic format that conforms to Public Health Information Network (PHIN) and/or National Electronic Disease Surveillance System (NEDSS) messaging standards.	(i) RVCT form via an electronic format.
	HIV status will be reported for at least 95 percent of all newly reported TB cases, age 25–44 years.	(i) HIV reports.
	A valid genotype accession number (generated by the CDC-sponsored genotyping laboratory) will be reported for at least 85 percent of all reported culture-positive cases.	(i) Genotyping reports.
	TB programs will maintain at least 95 percent reporting completeness for all variables existing on the pre-2009 RVCT.	(i) Pre-2009 RVCT form.
	By 2013, TB programs will achieve 95% completeness of all variables in the revised RVCT.	(i) Post-2009 RVCT form.
Match TB and AIDS registries.	Collaborate with the HIV/AIDS program to conduct at least annual TB and AIDS registry matches to ensure completeness of reporting of HIV and TB coinfected patients to both surveillance systems. Investigate and verify all TB cases reported to the HIV/AIDS program and not reported to the TB program. Update the TB registry and report to CDC as needed. At least annually assess reasons for incomplete HIV results on the RVCT for each verified case of TB.	(i) TB registries. (ii) HIV/AIDS registries.
	Determine if patients were not tested for HIV or were tested but results not reported to the TB program. Develop and implement plans for improvement in increasing HIV testing and reporting to patients and TB programs.	

(d) Data timeliness: Data timeliness is the speed between steps in the surveillance system. Data are current and available on time. The primary purpose is to ensure that data are available for TB program planning and for appropriate distribution of resources

Activities	Description	Data source
Report all newly diagnosed cases of TB to the CDC according to schedule.	Report all newly diagnosed cases of TB to the CDC according to a schedule agreed upon each year, generally monthly, and at least quarterly.	(i) RVCT reports.
Submit complete RVCT reports according to schedule.	The initial case reports should be submitted generally monthly and at least quarterly.	(i) RVCT report. (ii) Initial case report.
	Followup 1 report, which is only for TB cases with positive culture results, should be completed and submitted within 2 months after the initial RVCT was submitted, or when drug susceptibility results are available, whichever is later.	(i) RVCT reports. (ii) Followup 1 (Initial Drug Susceptibility Report).
	The followup 2 report, which should be submitted for all cases in which the patient was alive at diagnosis, should have data entered as it becomes available, and it should be complete when the case is closed to supervision. All followup 2 reports should be completed within two years of initial case reporting.	(i) RVCT reports. (ii) Followup 2 (Case Completion Report).
Analyze TB surveillance data at least quarterly.	At least quarterly, analyze TB surveillance data to monitor trends, detect potential outbreaks, and define high-risk groups. Produce and disseminate at least an annual report summarizing current data and trends.	(i) Surveillance data base.
Evaluate programmatic performance by using TB surveillance data at least annually.	At least annually, evaluate programmatic performance by using TB surveillance data to assist in compiling supporting evidence to determine the extent to which program objectives are being met and also to assist in developing strategies for improvement.	(i) National TB Indicators Project reports.

(e) Data security and confidentiality: Data security is the protection of public health data and information systems against unauthorized access. Data confidentiality is the protection of personal information collected by public health organizations. The primary purpose of security is to prevent unauthorized release of identifying information and accidental data loss or damage to the systems, while confidentiality is to ensure that personal information is not released without the consent of the person involved, except as necessary to protect public health

Activities	Description	Data sources
Ensure that TB surveillance data are kept confidentially and that all data files are secure.	Policies and procedures must be in place to protect the confidentiality of all surveillance case reports and files.	(i) Data security and confidentiality policies and procedures of the TB program. (ii) Surveillance case reports and files.
	Policies and procedures to protect HIV test results must conform to the confidentiality requirements of the state and local HIV/AIDS programs.	(i) Confidentiality requirements of the state and local HIV/AIDS programs. (ii) Observation of staff.
	Provide training on security and confidentiality of data.	

*Adopted from the 2011 cooperative agreement between the Division of Tuberculosis Elimination, Centers for Disease Control and Prevention and all 60 reporting jurisdictions of the National Tuberculosis Surveillance System.

tools include tables, charts, graphs, processes, and templates and are available in common electronic formats (e.g., Word, Excel, and PowerPoint). The team developed a main tool which is a template to help jurisdictions write a QA protocol required in the annual DTBE Cooperative Agreement (Table 2).

The National Tuberculosis Indicators Project (NTIP) is also an important QA tool [13]. During 2010, an NTIP module was developed to allow users to identify any TB case reporting discrepancies. This module has proven useful in recognizing data coding errors and data transmission problems, and highlighting the issue that errors are occurring more frequently than was previously recognized.

The reporting jurisdictions can access their NTIP and NTSS QA reports such as the missing and unknown (MUNK) reports through the Secure Access Management Services (SAMS). SAMS is a federal information technology system that gives authorized personnel secure, external access to nonpublic CDC applications.

(3) Developing and Conducting a QA Training Course. The training team developed and conducted a comprehensive QA training course to enhance the knowledge and skills needed by TB surveillance staff from the reporting jurisdictions for conducting QA. The results of the needs assessment and collaboration with subject matter experts were key to development of the QA course. The course focused on the QA process and five components, as well as other related topics to increase course participants' use of NTSS data for QA and program planning.

The course format included presentations from faculty (DTBE subject matter experts) with slides and handouts, exercises to apply the content to realistic situations, interactive discussions to share experiences and answer questions, and tools to use or adapt to their setting. Participants also described how they conducted QA at their sites and provided examples of QA challenges they encounter.

(4) Developing a Resource Guide and Toolkit. The training team is currently developing a resource guide and toolkit that can be used as a QA reference guide or a training manual. It will include many of the materials developed for the course such as handouts, exercises to apply the content, glossary, and examples of the tools (Table 2). A companion CD will provide the tools in easy-to-use formats (Word, Excel, and PowerPoint) so that jurisdictions can adapt them to their own setting. The guide and toolkit will be available in a print-based format with a companion CD that includes the tools. In addition, the materials will be downloadable from the CDC website.

3. Results and Discussion

3.1. Quality Assurance Training Evaluations. In July 2011, the team facilitated a pilot test of the 2-day QA training course with eleven TB surveillance experts from various state and local TB programs. The participants provided suggestions on how to improve the materials, the presentations, and the course schedule. The comprehensive course evaluation included written evaluations with qualitative and quantitative questions; discussions at the end of each of the five QA components; an end-of-course written evaluation; observations by course faculty. The team revised the materials and training course based on the analysis of the evaluation results (Table 3).

The team and other faculty members also conducted four 2-day trainings in Atlanta, GA, between August and September 2011. Course participants included 61 TB surveillance staff. Participants from the four trainings completed an end-of-course evaluation form consisting of qualitative and quantitative questions.

Results of the combined responses from the pilot course and four trainings evaluations (Table 3) indicated that participants learned about the QA process and benefited from sharing information on how other jurisdictions implement the QA components at their sites. The 73 participants (from the pilot course and four trainings) represented 34 (57%) of the 60 NTSS reporting jurisdictions. The 34 jurisdictions represent more than 80% of all TB cases reported to CDC each year.

Table 2: Master list of quality assurance tools for TB surveillance, United States, 2011.

(a) Quality assurance protocol tools

Tool number	Tool name	Description and how to use	Format
QA protocol-1	Cooperative agreement	The original version of the TB surveillance section of the cooperative agreement.	PDF
QA protocol-2	QA written protocol-requirements	A table that lists all of the cooperative agreement requirements for TB surveillance and sources for information.	Word
QA protocol-3	QA written protocol-guide	A guide to help jurisdictions write their own protocol.	Word

(b) Case detection tools

Tool number	Tool name	Description and how to use	Format
Case detection-1	TB program area module (TB PAM) flow chart	Flow chart to help with patient search. This flow chart was created initially to emphasize the importance of always searching for a patient within TB PAM so that duplicate patient records are not created. This flow chart also outlines the process for creating "Provider Verified" cases and addresses approval and rejection of notification.	Word
Case detection-2	Notification process	Flow chart that shows a tiered notification process for TB case notification. This flow chart identifies (1) what role each person (with a particular TB PAM right) has in the notification process and what happens when a notification is rejected or approved. Only TB program managers (a nurse within the TB program) creates a notification, and it must be approved by the TB Program Central Office Epidemiologist before it is sent to CDC for case counting.	Word
Case detection-3	TB suspects weekly report	This report is generated weekly for all suspects reported in TB PAM through Friday of the previous week. Suspects are classified as a case or not a case within 56 days from the date of report. There is a built-in calculation that calculates 56 days from the date of report (when the date of report is entered). All suspects that are past due (over 56 days) require a followup from one of the Central Office Nurse Consultants.	Excel
Case detection-4	Case verification and treatment status	Table that indicates case verification and treatment status. This spreadsheet is used to monitor treatment progress with the goal of completing treatment within 12 months. There are built-in calculations for 3, 6, 9, and 12 months from treatment start that are populated when the date therapy started is entered. Case verification is included to help identify how long treatment is anticipated for.	Excel
Case detection-5	Decline in reported tuberculosis cases survey	Sample survey to investigate decline in reported TB cases.	Word
Case detection-6	Counted tuberculosis case verification report	Form that indicates counted TB case verification.	PDF
Case detection-7	Investigation process for underreporting of TB	Table that provides a process for investigating underreporting of TB data.	Word
Case detection-8a	TB case closeout letter	Sample letter to accompany TB case close list (tool 8b) and TB case closeout form (tool 8c).	Word
Case detection-8b	TB case close list	List by jurisdiction indicating TB case closeout status.	Excel
Case detection-8c	TB case closeout form	Form for confirmation/signature of number of TB cases.	Word

(c) Accuracy tools

Tool number	Tool name	Description and how to use	Format
Accuracy-1a	Data accuracy checklist	A checklist for reviewing RVCT data for accuracy	Word
Accuracy-1b	Data accuracy checklist CDC SAS code	SAS code corresponding to the data accuracy checklist, accuracy tool-1a, and is based on CDC RVCT variable names.	Word
Accuracy-1c	CDC TB surveillance RVCT data dictionary	Data dictionary for interpreting the CDC RVCT variable names used in data accuracy checklist CDC SAS code, accuracy tool-1b	Excel
Accuracy-2	Options for prioritizing medical chart reviews when resources are limited	Various options to help prioritize medical chart reviews when resources are limited.	Word
Accuracy-3	RVCT surveillance database audit form	Checklist for checking the accuracy of RVCT.	Word
Accuracy-4	Accuracy checklist for sputum culture conversion	Table to indicate number of days for culture conversion by jurisdiction. This applies to cases that are sputum culture positive only. There are built-in calculations that calculate the date, that is, 30 and 60 days from treatment start (once the date therapy started is entered). There is also a built-in calculation for the number of days that it took for sputum culture conversion. This helps identify those patients who did not meet the National Tuberculosis Indicators Project (NTIP) Objective of converting their sputum culture within 60 days of treatment initiation.	Excel
Accuracy-5	Nucleic acid amplification test (NAAT) comparisons	Comparison of NAAT tests.	Excel
Accuracy-6	RVCT calculated variables	RVCT calculated variables algorithm for calculating vercrit.	Word
Accuracy-7	2009 RVCT form with public health information network (PHIN) variable identification	2009 RVCT form with PHIN variable identification by RVCT question number to use as a reference for report codes.	PDF

(d) Completeness tools

Tool number	Tool name	Description and how to use	Format
Completeness-1	Source list for locating RVCT data	Source document to locate information for each item on the RVCT.	Word
Completeness-2	Therapy status	Table to indicate therapy status by 12-month interval. This spreadsheet is used to monitor treatment progress with the goal of completing treatment within 12 months. There are built-in calculations for 3, 6, 9, and 12 months from treatment start that are populated when the date therapy started is entered. This tool targets the NTIP objective of treatment completion within 12 months.	Excel
Completeness-3	Culture and drug susceptibility status	Table to indicate culture and drug susceptibility status by jurisdiction. This report shows the susceptibility results for isoniazid, rifampin, pyrazinamide, and ethambutol. This shows those cases that are multidrug-resistant TB and also those who have an unknown or blank susceptibility report. This is for all culture-positive TB cases. This tool targets the NTIP objective of drug susceptibility reporting.	Excel
Completeness-4	TB Program area module (TB PAM)	Flow chart that shows the TB PAM process (initiation of RVCT through case closure). This flow chart was created for the TB PAM from initiating the RVCT to closing a case. This flow chart also identifies the responsible person(s) for the various steps.	Word
Completeness-5	Data abstraction instructions	Detailed procedures for RVCT quality control queries.	Word
Completeness-6a	RVCT variables used in NTIP	List of the RVCT variables used in the NTIP indicator calculation.	PDF
Completeness-6b	RVCT variables used in NTIP spreadsheet	Spreadsheet of the list of the RVCT variables used in the NTIP indicator calculation.	Excel

(e) Timeliness tools

Tool number	Tool name	Description and how to use	Format
Timeliness-1a	Building blocks—schedule for entering RVCT data	Timeline table. This is a building-block diagram addressing what RVCT variables should be entered and identifies the time frame when those variables should be entered. This helps field staff know when information should be available and when the state central office expects it to be entered.	Word
Timeliness-1b	Schedule for entering RVCT data	Timeline table similar to timeliness tool 1a. It is in a table format rather than the graphic of the building blocks.	Word
Timeliness-2	Quarterly case summary	Document that summarizes timeliness measures and objectives for a predetermined set of TB patients. Predefined case outcome objectives are presented for that particular set of TB patients.	Excel
Timeliness-3	Timeliness data dictionary	Description of the data used to calculate timeliness measures for analysis. These measures are used to determine completion of state objectives.	Word
Timeliness-4	2010 Final verbal case counts and data submissions	Spreadsheet for case count.	Excel
Timeliness-5	Timeline for reporting TB data to CDC	Timeline for reporting TB cases and final TB data transmissions to CDC.	PDF
Timeliness-6	Typical weekly data availability chart	Typical weekly data availability by day of the week.	PDF

(f) Data security and confidentiality tools

Tool number	Tool name	Description and how to use	Format
Data security and confidentiality-1	Standards for data security and confidentiality	List of minimum standards to facilitate data sharing and use of surveillance data for public health action.	Word
Data security and confidentiality-2	Initial assessment of TB program data security and confidentiality	Guide for the initial assessment of TB program's data security and confidentiality.	Word
Data security and confidentiality-3	Checklist for ongoing assessment of programs	Comprehensive checklist for assessing data security and confidentiality.	Word
Data security and confidentiality-4	Data security and QA checklist	A TB program's checklist for data security and QA.	Word

(g) Other tools

Tool number	Tool name	Description and How to Use	Format
Other-1	QA protocol example	Four-phase process for entering RVCT data, to conduct quality control, and ensure timeliness in reporting.	Word
Other-2	QA in surveillance literature sources	References for quality assurance of surveillance data.	Word
Other-3	2009 trending guidance	Mapping the old RVCT data to the new RVCT data and diagrams to illustrate the following three RVCT items: (i) 16—site of disease, (ii) 22A—X-ray, (iii) 46—type of health care provider. This document provides a visual explanation of the transition between old and revised RVCT variables. Mapping shows the user exactly how the definitions of previous variables match up with the new ones.	Word
Other-4	Cohort review preparation	Timeline for planning and conducting a cohort review session. Includes preparation timeline and job responsibilities. Determines when participants need to be notified of scheduled events leading up to the cohort review session.	Word
Other-5	TB case/suspect QA review form	A checklist to use when reviewing TB cases/suspects.	Word
Other-6	TB review and QA schedule	Quality assurance schedule for various reviews of TB cases/suspects.	Word

TABLE 3: Combined evaluation results of the quality assurance training courses, Centers for Disease Control and Prevention, July–September 2011.

Evaluation question	Combined responses from the pilot course and four trainings		
	Reponses $N = 73$		Participants' comments
Overall, how confident are you that the target audience can learn about QA after having attended this course?	Very confident/confident	99% (72)	"Great job! Please continue this class. It was very informative and I learned a lot." "Identified a number of good suggestions on how to improve my states level of accuracy with new tools provided by different topic speakers."
How effective will the QA process (as described in this course) help you conduct QA in your job?	Very effective/effective	100% (73)	"I learned a great deal from this pilot. This course will be valuable to the states and will lead to great discussions and changes in the way QA is performed. This will therefore lead to great improvement in the quality of the data."
How effective will the tools be in helping you conduct QA in your job?	Very effective/effective	93% (66)	"Very informative—lots of info I can actually use and apply to day-to-day activities (i.e., tools)"

Of the 73 participants, 66 (93%) stated that the QA tools will be effective in helping them conduct QA in their programs (Table 3). Participants stated that some of the most important things they learned were the five QA components and how they relate to the requirements in the cooperative agreement for a written QA TB surveillance protocol. Most of the participants appreciated the assessment of programmatic needs and the effort that went into implementing the course.

3.2. Quality Assurance Strategies with Limited Resources. In developing innovative strategies for QA of TB surveillance data, a key question for all programs is how best to maximize the use of limited resources to ensure data quality. The design and flexibility of the guide and toolkit enable health care staff to learn about the QA process in a self-study format or as part of a facilitator-led training course. Also, providing the materials in print-based format and the internet ensures accessibility to the materials without additional resources. Gaining knowledge and skills to conduct QA helps reporting jurisdictions remain vigilant in maintaining high quality of surveillance data despite limited resources.

3.3. Impact of Quality Assurance Strategies. This QA project represents a significant improvement to NTSS because it compiles for the first time guidelines, step-by-step process, and tools for monitoring and improving the quality of TB surveillance data. Additionally, CDC noticed an unprecedented timeliness and accuracy of all the required RVCT variables needed for publication on TB surveillance data in the Morbidity and Mortality Weekly Report issue for the World TB Day on March 24, 2012. The process to obtain data has been much easier than previous years because of improved understanding between CDC and jurisdictions fostered at the QA training.

Although the team conducted training on the QA strategies less than a year ago, CDC staff have also noticed better collaboration among NTSS reporting jurisdictions in sharing QA tools. Several jurisdictions sent letters to CDC shortly after the training stating that they have implemented QA tools that were pertinent to their programs.

In addition, SAMS portal reports indicated a 10% increase of NTSS enrollment from August 2011 to February 2012 and an 8% increase of NTIP enrollment for the same period. But it may be premature to attribute these results to the QA strategies.

The team also attempted to obtain MUNK reports of the jurisdictions represented during the QA training to examine any QA improvement, but this information was not readily available. This information can compare RVCT data and how missing or validation issues occur from the previous year. However, this may not be a reliable measurement of the impact of the QA strategies because the MUNK reports are influenced by changes in the number of TB cases, complexity of data-related issues, changes to state-based systems, or staff turnover.

The impact of the QA strategies to the quality of TB surveillance data can be better evaluated after the jurisdictions have fully implemented them. A survey of their QA practices may systematically evaluate the importance of these strategies.

Despite the limitations, these QA strategies support TB policies, laws, and regulations as they equip local jurisdictions with a systematic set of processes and tools that may be used to fulfill the requirements of the cooperative agreement to monitor data quality. Also, since reporting of a patient with TB disease to health authorities is mandated by state laws, the guidance on case detection, data accuracy, completeness, and timeliness helps reporting areas in complying with these laws.

In addition, these strategies are essential in collecting accurate and reliable TB surveillance data that are critical to making decisions to meet DTBE's priorities: interrupt transmission of *Mycobacterium tuberculosis,* reduce TB in foreign-born populations, reduce TB in racial/ethnic minority populations, mitigate/reduce impact of multidrug-resistant and extensively drug-resistant TB, and reduce HIV-associated TB.

Being vigilant in performing QA ensures high-quality data and ultimately helps accelerate progress toward elimination of TB in the United States.

4. Conclusions

Despite challenges imposed by various surveillance systems, economic constraints, and new diagnostic technologies, strategies for conducting QA can be developed with innovation and collaboration. Mobilizing the TB community to ensure high-quality data involves commitment, time, and energy of TB leaders and partners.

Guidelines, a step-by-step process, and tools for monitoring and improving the quality of TB surveillance data are essential for the TB community to effectively control TB. Future evaluation on the impact of these QA strategies will further demonstrate their importance in maintaining data quality.

Disclosure

This paper lists nonfederal resources in order to provide additional information to consumers. The views and content in these resources have not been formally approved by the U.S. Department of Health and Human Services (HHS). Listing these resources is not an endorsement by HHS or its components. The findings and conclusions in this paper are those of the authors and do not necessarily represent the views of CDC.

Acknowledgments

The authors would like to thank the TB program staff from various jurisdictions for participating in the needs assessment and those who submitted QA tools including Jason Cummins (TN), Sheanne Allen (WA), Jill Fournier (NH), Eyal Oren (Seattle/King County, WA), Janice Westenhouse (CA), and Gayle Wainwright (OR). They also thank the QA training course faculty for their hard work and commitment including Sandy Price and Stacey Parker (Data Flow and System QA Reports); Bob Pratt (Data Accuracy); Lori Armstrong (Data Validation Pilot Project); Carla Jeffries (Missing and Unknown Reports); Beverly Metchock and Angela Starks (Laboratory); Glenda Newell (Case Count Timeliness); Kai Young (National TB Indicators Project); Rachel Yelk-Woodruff (RVCT Completeness Study); Juliana Grant, Sandy Althomsons, and Brian Baker (TB Genotyping Information Management System). In addition, they would like to thank DTBE leadership for providing support for developing the QA project. Without their continued guidance, financial resources, and commitment to quality surveillance data, this project would not be possible. They also want to thank the dedication and hard work of all of the reporting jurisdictions that make TB surveillance successful.

References

[1] World Health Organization, *WHO Report, Global Tuberculosis Control*, 2011, http://www.who.int/tb/publications/global_report/2011/gtbr11_full.pdf.

[2] Centers for Disease Control and Prevention, *Reported tuberculosis in the United States*, Atlanta, Ga, USA, US Department of Health and Human Services, CDC, 2010, http://www.cdc.gov/tb/statistics/reports/2010/default.htm.

[3] Centers for Disease Control and Prevention. Division of Tuberculosis Mission Statement, 2012, http://www.cdc.gov/tb/about/mission.htm.

[4] Centers for Disease Control and Prevention, "Updated guidelines for evaluating public health surveillance systems," *Morbidity and Mortality Weekly Report*, vol. 50, no. 13, pp. 1–35, 2001.

[5] Centers for Disease Control and Prevention, DTBE's Comprehensive and Innovative Training Program on the Revised RVCT. TB Notes, no. 3, 2009, http://www.cdc.gov/tb/publications/newsletters/notes/TBN_3_09/rvct.htm.

[6] E. Magee, C. Tryon, A. Forbes, B. Heath, and L. Manangan, "The national tuberculosis surveillance system training program to ensure accuracy of tuberculosis surveillance data," *Journal of Public Health Management and Practice*, vol. 17, no. 5, pp. 427–430, 2011.

[7] Centers for Disease Control and Prevention, *Report of Verified Case of Tuberculosis (RVCT), Instruction Manual*, US Department of Health and Human Services, CDC, Atlanta, Ga, USA, 2009, http://www.cdc.gov/tb/programs/rvct/InstructionManual.pdf.

[8] Centers for Disease Control and Prevention, *Report of Verified Case of Tuberculosis (RVCT), Self-Study Modules, Participant Manual*, US Department of Health and Human Services, CDC, Atlanta, Ga, USA, 2009, http://www.cdc.gov/tb/programs/rvct/ParticipantManual.pdf.

[9] Centers for Disease Control and Prevention, *Report of Verified Case of Tuberculosis (RVCT), Self-Study Modules, Facilitator Manual*, US Department of Health and Human Services, CDC, Atlanta, Ga, USA, 2009.

[10] G. Krause, "From evaluation to continuous quality assurance of surveillance systems," *Eurosurveillance*, vol. 11, no. 11, p. 657, 2006.

[11] M. D. Decker, "Continuous quality improvement.," *Infection Control and Hospital Epidemiology*, vol. 13, no. 3, pp. 165–169, 1992.

[12] National Institutes of Health, *The Pink Book—Making Health Communication Programs Work*, National Cancer Institute; U.S. National Institutes of Health, 2012, http://www.cancer.gov/cancertopics/cancerlibrary/pinkbook/page1.

[13] CDC, National Tuberculosis Indicators Project Fact Sheet, 2012, http://www.cdc.gov/tb/publications/factsheets/statistics/NTIP.pdf.

[14] Centers for Disease Control and Prevention, Tuberculosis Genotyping Information Management System, 2012, http://www.cdc.gov/tb/programs/genotyping/tbgims/default.htm.

[15] American Immunization Registry Association (AIRA) Modeling of Immunization Registry Operations Workgroup, *Data Quality Assurance in Immunization Information Systems: Incoming Data*, AIRA, Atlanta, Ga, USA, 2008, http://www.immregistries.org/pdf/AIRA_MIROW_Chap3_DQA_0211-2008.pdf.

[16] M. W. Borgdorff, "New measurable indicator for tuberculosis case detection," *Emerging Infectious Diseases*, vol. 10, no. 9, pp. 1523–1528, 2004.

[17] Centers for Disease Control and Prevention, National Biosurveillance Strategy for Human Health, Version 2, 2010, http://www.cdc.gov/osels/pdf/NBSHH_V2_FINAL.PDF.

[18] Centers for Disease Control and Prevention, "Controlling tuberculosis in the United States," *Morbidity and Mortality Weekly Report*, vol. 54, no. 12, pp. 1–81, 2005.

[19] Centers for Disease Control and Prevention, "Decrease in reported tuberculosis cases—United States," *Morbidity and Mortality Weekly Report*, vol. 59, no. 10, pp. 289–294, 2010.

[20] Centers for Disease Control and Prevention, "Assessment of declines in reported tuberculosis cases—Georgia and Pennsylvania," *Morbidity and Mortality Weekly Report*, vol. 60, no. 11, pp. 338–342, 2011.

[21] Council of State and Territorial Epidemiologists Special Report: Public Health Surveillance Workshop, 2011, http://www.cste.org/webpdfs/SurveillanceWorkshopReportFINAL.pdf.

[22] A. B. Curtis, E. McCray, M. McKenna, and I. M. Onorato, "Completeness and timeliness of tuberculosis case reporting: a multistate study," *American Journal of Preventive Medicine*, vol. 20, no. 2, pp. 108–112, 2001.

[23] C. R. Driver, C. R. Braden, R. L. Nieves et al., "Completeness of tuberculosis case reporting, San Juan and Caguas Regions, Puerto Rico, 1992," *Public Health Reports*, vol. 111, no. 2, pp. 157–161, 1996.

[24] R. Dunbar, K. Lawrence, S. Verver et al., "Accuracy and completeness of recording of confirmed tuberculosis in two South African communities," *International Journal of Tuberculosis and Lung Disease*, vol. 15, no. 3, pp. 337–343, 2011.

[25] European Centre for Disease Prevention and Control, Tuberculosis Surveillance and Monitoring in Europe, 2012, http://www.ecdc.europa.eu.

[26] J. E. Golub, C. I. Mohan, G. W. Comstock, and R. E. Chaisson, "Active case finding of tuberculosis: historical perspective and future prospects," *International Journal of Tuberculosis and Lung Disease*, vol. 9, no. 11, pp. 1183–1203, 2005.

[27] N. B. Hoa, C. Wei, C. Sokun, J. M. Lauritsen, and H. L. Rieder, "Completeness and consistency in recording information in the tuberculosis case register, Cambodia, China and Viet Nam," *International Journal of Tuberculosis and Lung Disease*, vol. 14, no. 10, pp. 1303–1309, 2010.

[28] J. Hofferkamp, Ed., *Standards for Cancer Registries Volume III: Standards for Completeness, Quality Analysis, Management, Security and Confidentiality of Data*, North American Association of Central Cancer Registries, Springfield, Ill, USA, 2008, http://www.naaccr.org/LinkClick.aspx?fileticket=hvFzJKUcRM8%3d&tabid=134&mid=474.

[29] J. D. Mancuso, S. K. Tobler, A. A. Eick, and C. H. Olsen, "An evaluation of the completeness and accuracy of active tuberculosis reporting in the United States military," *International Journal of Tuberculosis and Lung Disease*, vol. 14, no. 10, pp. 1310–1315, 2010.

[30] D. McClish and L. Penberthy, "Using medicare data to estimate the number of cases missed by a cancer registry: a 3-source capture-recapture model," *Medical Care*, vol. 42, no. 11, pp. 1111–1116, 2004.

[31] H. L. Rieder and J. M. Lauritsen, "Quality assurance of data: ensuring that numbers reflect operational definitions and contain real measurements," *The International Journal of Tuberculosis and Lung Disease*, vol. 15, no. 3, pp. 296–304, 2011.

[32] J. E. Sprinson, E. S. Lawton, T. C. Proco, J. M. Flood, and J. L. Westenhouse, "Assessing the validity of tuberculosis surveillance data in California," *BMC Public Health*, vol. 6, article 217, 2006.

[33] M. J. Trepka, T. O. Beyer, M. E. Proctor, and J. P. Davis, "An evaluation of the completeness of tuberculosis case reporting using hospital billing and laboratory data; Wisconsin, 1995," *Annals of Epidemiology*, vol. 9, no. 7, pp. 419–423, 1999.

[34] United States Agency for International Development, *Data Quality Assurance Tool for Program-Level Indicators*, 2007, http://www.pepfar.gov/documents/organization/79628.pdf.

[35] J. T. Walkup, W. Wenhui, U. Sambamoorthi, and S. Crystal, "Sensitivity of an AIDS case-finding algorithm who are we missing?" *Medical Care*, vol. 42, no. 8, pp. 756–763, 2004.

[36] C. Weinbaum, D. Ruggiero, E. Schneider et al., "TB reporting," *Public Health Reports*, vol. 113, no. 4, p. 288, 1998.

[37] World Bank, *Public Health Surveillance Toolkit: A Guide for Busy Task Managers. World Bank*, 2002, http://siteresources.worldbank.org/INTPH/Resources/376086-1133371165476/PHSurveillanceToolkit.pdf.

[38] World Health Organization (WHO), WHO Statistical Information System. Tuberculosis Detection Rate Under DOTS, 2012, http://www.who.int/whosis/indicators/2007TBCasesDetectedDOTS/en/index.html.

[39] Centers for Disease Control and Prevention, Tuberculosis Elimination and Laboratory Cooperative Agreements: CDC-PS-10-1005. Continuation-Type 2, 2011.

Comparison of Overnight Pooled and Standard Sputum Collection Method for Patients with Suspected Pulmonary Tuberculosis in Northern Tanzania

Stellah G. Mpagama,[1,2] Charles Mtabho,[2] Solomon Mwaigwisya,[2] Liberate J. Mleoh,[1] I Marion Sumari-de Boer,[2] Scott K. Heysell,[3] Eric R. Houpt,[3] and Gibson S. Kibiki[2]

[1] *Kibong'oto National Tuberculosis Referral Hospital, P.O. Box 12, Kilimanjaro, Tanzania*
[2] *Kilimanjaro Clinical Research Institute and Kilimanjaro Christian Medical College, Kilimanjaro Moshi, Tanzania*
[3] *Division of Infectious Diseases and International Health, University of Virginia, Charlotteville, VA 22908, USA*

Correspondence should be addressed to Stellah G. Mpagama, s.mpagama@kcri.ac.tz

Academic Editor: Catharina Boehme

In Tanzania sputum culture for tuberculosis (TB) is resource intensive and available only at zonal facilities. In this study overnight pooled sputum collection technique was compared with standard spot morning collection among pulmonary TB suspects at Kibong'oto National TB Hospital in Tanzania. A spot sputum specimen performed at enrollment, an overnight pooled sputum, and single morning specimen were collected from 50 subjects and analyzed for quality, quantity, and time to detection in Bactec MGIT system. Forty-six (92%) subjects' overnight pooled specimens had a volume ≥ 5 mls compared to 37 (37%) for the combination of spot and single morning specimens ($P < 0.001$). Median time to detection was 96 hours (IQR 87–131) for the overnight pooled specimens compared to 110.5 hours (IQR is 137 right 137–180) for the combination of both spot and single morning specimens ($P = 0.001$). In our setting of limited TB culture capacity, we recommend a single pooled sputum to maximize yield and speed time to diagnosis.

1. Background

Tuberculosis (TB) and HIV are among the global leaders in infectious disease mortality [1]. Sub-Saharan Africa has one of the highest burdens of TB and HIV coinfection [2]. Prompt diagnosis of TB is critical to improve outcome, but diagnosis of TB is challenging in HIV-infected patients and especially in resource-limited settings [3]. HIV-infected patients have a higher rate of extrapulmonary TB, atypical chest radiographs and fewer pulmonary cavities [4–6]. As a consequence, HIV patients may be more likely to have a negative or paucibacillary sputum smear microscopy [7]. Subjects with paucibacillary specimens may be prone to being delayed in clinical diagnosis, either because acid-fast bacilli are not observed by microscopy or time to detection *Mycobacterium tuberculosis* (MTB) culture is prolonged [8]. Both poor quality and low quantity of sputum have a significant impact on TB detection rate [9, 10]. In settings reliant on smear microscopy as the only means of TB diagnosis, this may impact negatively the time to initiation of TB treatment. Ideal specimens should contain 5 mL or more of sputum without saliva. A previous study found that the quality and quantity of sputum were improved by pooling three versus a single "spot" collection [11]. However, collection on multiple days may unnecessarily burden health facilities and may be prone to contamination. In contrast, a single overnight pooled technique whereby a patient is given a sealable container in which to collect all expectorated sputum over the course of the night has been used in TB treatment trials and in assessment of early bactericidal activity of new TB medications [12, 13]. However it has not been examined in routine clinical practice.

At Kibong'oto National TB Hospital in Kilimanjaro, Tanzania, HIV co infection among TB suspects is common and it

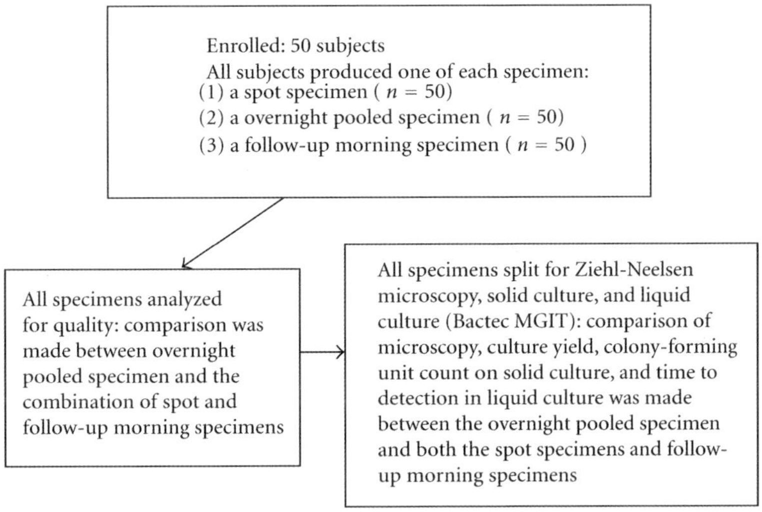

FIGURE 1: Study diagram of enrollment and specimen analysis.

TABLE 1: Demographic and clinical characteristics.

Variables ($N = 50$)	Measure
Sex	
Male	36 (72%)
Age (years) median (IQR)	38.5 (30–46)
Weight (kg) median (IQR)	51 (47–58)
HIV status	
Positive	8 (16%)
CD4 count (cells/μL) by HIV status in median (IQR)	
HIV positive	71 (30.5–158)
HIV negative	540 (409–614)
Chest X-ray findings	
Cavities	23 (46%)

has been observed that the minority of patients have cavitary chest radiographs. Furthermore it is a standard practice that each TB suspect is given a sealable mug to collect all sputum as an infection control measure. Thus, among a population at risk for lower bacillary yield, we sought to compare overnight pooled sputum in the sealable mugs to the standard spot technique for sputum quality, quantity, and time to MTB detection by culture in the Bactec MGIT system, a method which has correlated well with conventional colony counts [14, 15].

2. Methods

Subjects suspected of pulmonary TB at Kibong'oto National TB Hospital were recruited for enrollment. Subjects were eligible if they were 18 years and above and presenting with two weeks or more of cough. Each patient was asked to collect three sputum samples in calibrated wide mouthed container: (1) a spot specimen at the time of enrollment, (2) an overnight pooled specimen, and (3) a spot specimen on the morning after enrollment (Figure 1). Subjects were excluded if initiated on any antituberculosis medication prior to sample collection. Sputum samples were sent to Kilimanjaro Clinical Research Institute (KCRI) laboratory for processing. The specimens were assessed for volume collected, presence of blood, and color. Samples were analyzed for quality based on the following criteria: (1) volume equal to or more than 5 mls, (2) sputum color was white, yellow, green, or red, (3) presence of blood, and (4) thick consistency. Each sputum specimen was decontaminated with 4% NaOH and centrifuged at 1500 g for 10 minutes. The sediment was split equally for use in direct smear microscopy by Ziehl-Neelsen staining, MTB culture on solid agar with Lowenstein-Jensen slant and Middlebrook 7H11 media, and in liquid media using Bactec MGIT 960 machine (Becton Dickinson, USA). Positive culture growth was confirmed by secondary Ziehl-Neelsen stain. Colony-forming unit (CFU) count was performed on the Middlebrook 7H11 media.

Data were analyzed by Stata Version 11 statistical software (StataCorp, U.S.A). Values were presented as means with standard deviation (SD) or median with interquartile range (IQR) for data that was not normally distributed. Chi-square was used for dichotomous variables and Spearman's correlation coefficient for continuous variables to investigate the association with microscopy and culture yield. All tests were two sided with P values ≤ 0.05 regarded as statistically significant.

All subjects provided written informed consent. Ethical approval for the study was given by the IRB of the Kilimanjaro Christian Medical Center, Tumaini University and the National Ethical Review Board.

3. Results

Fifty pulmonary TB suspects were enrolled for the study, each produced three specimens, hence 150 samples were used for analysis. The median age of patients was 38.5 years (IQR 30–45) (Table 1). Thirty-six (72%) were male and 8 (16%)

Table 2: Comparison of overnight pooled and spot method of collection on quality and quantity of sputum.

Measure	Combination of spot and single morning specimen	Overnight pooled	P value
Quantity (≥5 mls)	37/100 (37%)	46/50 (92%)	$P < 0.001$
Color	92/100 (92%)	47/50 (94%)	$P = 0.79$
Thick consistency	66/100 (66%)	41/50 (82%)	$P = 0.12$
Presence of blood	11/100 (11%)	6/50 (12%)	$P > 0.99$

* P values are similar if pooled is compared with spot or single morning specimen, thus we combined spot and single for this table.

were HIV-1-infected patients. Among the HIV-infected subjects, the median CD4 count was 71 cells/μL (IQR 30.5–158). The median CD4 count for HIV-seronegative patients was 540 cell/μL (IQR 409–614). Twenty-three (46%) had cavitary disease (Table 1).

Overnight pooled sputum yielded a specimen of ≥5 mL in 46 (92%) of subjects compared to 37 (37%) for the combination of spot and single morning specimens ($P < 0.001$). Good quality of sputum specimen by color was observed in 47 (94%) of the patients for overnight pooled sputum—while combination of spot and single morning specimens was 92 (92%) ($P = 0.79$). Thick consistency was observed in 41 (82%) of patients for overnight pooled compared to combination of spot and single morning 66 (66%) ($P = 0.12$), and presence of blood was observed in 6 (12%) and 11 (11%), respectively ($P > 0.99$) (Table 2).

Overall 100 (67%) specimens were positive by smear microscopy. Thirty-four (68%) spot specimens were smear positive, compared to 31 (62%) single morning specimens, and 35 (70%) for overnight pooled ($P = 0.28$). Eighty-one (54%) culture-positive specimens were available for comparison of time to detection in the MGIT system from 27 subjects; 49 (33%) specimens were negative and bacterial contamination precluded analysis in 20 (13%). The MGIT contamination rate did not differ from that of Lowenstein-Jensen, found in 21 (14%) of all specimens. Furthermore, among MGIT specimens contamination did not vary by method of collection: spot (5.3%), single morning (3.3%) and overnight pooled (4.7%) ($P > 0.99$). However, the median time to detection was 96 hours (IQR 87–131) for the overnight pooled specimens which was significantly faster compared to 118 hours (IQR 98–167) for single morning specimen and 143 hours (IQR 108–194) for the spot specimens ($P < 0.005$) (Figure 2).

Only a limited number of pooled specimens were TB-culture positive on Middlebrook 7H11 to allow colony forming unit (CFU) count determination. The median CFU count among subjects with cavities on chest radiograph was 4.92 log/mL (IQR 4.3–6.28) compared to 3.95 log/mL (IQR 3.61–4.84) in patients without cavities ($P = 0.12$). Among the 8 HIV-infected subjects, only 2 (25%) had overnight pooled specimens available for CFU count. The median CFU count among HIV-infected subjects was 4.34 log/mL (IQR 3.9–4.72) compared to 4.84 log/mL (IQR 4.30–5.86) for the HIV-uninfected subjects ($P = 0.43$). There was no correlation between CD4 counts with CFU (Spearman's rho = −0.36) ($P = 0.16$).

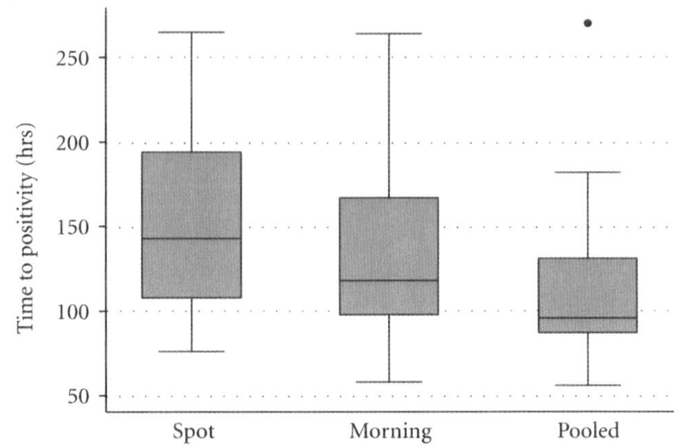

Figure 2: Median time-to-culture positivity among different collection method. * $P < 0.005$ comparing pooled to morning or spot.

4. Discussion

The major finding of this study was that in routine practice an overnight pooled sputum collection significantly improved the time to detection in the MGIT system among culture-positive samples. This is an important finding amidst the global scale-up of MTB culture.

Faster time to diagnosis in a TB suspect can speed drug susceptibility testing, hasten proper treatment, and potentially decrease transmission to the community and within the hospital. In settings with increasing rates of multidrug-resistant (MDR) TB, faster drug susceptibility results have been postulated to be one of the most important means of improving MDR TB outcome [16].

Sputum collection is the first and most critical step in laboratory diagnosis of pulmonary TB. In resource-limited settings such as ours, multiple specimen collection has been proposed to increase yield for rapid molecular probe diagnostics [17, 18]; however it can be overwhelming to the laboratory. Both microscopy and culture are time consuming and culture is costly. In Tanzania culture is recommended for smear-negative cases, for treatment failures and for monitoring MDR-TB patients. Currently there are few laboratories capable of culture and specimens must be sent long distances. In this setting, maximizing yield by sending the optimal specimen will conserve resources. We would strongly advocate sending pooled specimens in our context.

Our findings of increased culture yield with volumes of a minimum of 5 mls of adequate quality are consistent with previous studies that examined yield of microscopy [19, 20].

However, our microscopy yield did not approach the remarkable >95% rate of smear positivity reported by others when a 24-hour collection technique was used for diagnosis of selected subjects with pulmonary TB [21]. This is potentially contributed by the fact that we selected for pulmonary TB suspects and not confirmed cases. With an eye towards molecular diagnostics in the future, given the drop in sensitivity of the rapid molecular diagnostics in smear-negative sputum samples [17], we would expect that overnight pooled sputum collection would be equal to or improve upon molecular diagnostic yield compared with a spot specimen.

Our study has several limitations. For the CFU analysis on the overnight pooled specimens, fungal overgrowth limited examination of nine different plates. The contamination affected subjects with and without cavities so it is unlikely to have biased this finding; yet overall our total number of patients enrolled was small and may not have included enough HIV-infected patients to appreciate differences in this subgroup with regard to culture yield, CFU analysis, and time to detection. Bacterial contamination also limited evaluation of all samples in the MGIT, but the contamination was observed in all specimen collection techniques and has been reported in other evaluations of liquid culture in MGIT [22]. Furthermore, the culture yield for all techniques may have been diminished by splitting specimens for both solid and liquid culture.

In conclusion, we found that overnight pooled sputum collection improved the quantity of sputum without alteration in quality and led to faster time to detection. These findings can ultimately impact the decisions both of treatment and infection control. Overnight pooled sputum should be considered as an alternative to standard spot testing in resource-limited settings.

Acknowledgments

The authors would like to acknowledge the African Poverty Related-Infection Oriented Research Initiative (APRIORI) which supported grant of training in master degree of clinical research of which S. G. Mpagama is a recipient. S. G. Mpagama is also supported by the NIH Fogarty's Global Infectious Disease Research Training Program (D43 TW008270) which enabled final drafting of the paper.

References

[1] D. Maher, A. Harries, and H. Getahun, "Tuberculosis and HIV interaction in sub-Saharan Africa: impact on patients and programmes; implications for policies," *Tropical Medicine and International Health*, vol. 10, no. 8, pp. 734–742, 2005.

[2] C. Dye, S. Scheele, P. Dolin, V. Pathania, M. C. Raviglione, and The WHO Global Surveillance and Monitoring Project, Global Burden of Tuberculosis, "Global burden of tuberculosis: es-] timated incidence, prevalence, and mortality by country," *Journal of the American Medical Association*, vol. 282, no. 7, pp. 677–686, 1999.

[3] M. J. Reid and N. S. Shah, "Approaches to tuberculosis screening and diagnosis in people with HIV in resource-limited settings," *The Lancet Infectious Diseases*, vol. 9, no. 3, pp. 173–184, 2009.

[4] S. Shenoi, S. Heysell, A. Moll, and G. Friedland, "Multidrug-resistant and extensively drug-resistant tuberculosis: consequences for the global HIV community," *Current Opinion in Infectious Diseases*, vol. 22, no. 1, pp. 11–17, 2009.

[5] A. M. Elliott, K. Namaambo, B. W. Allen et al., "Negative sputum smear results in HIV-positive patients with pulmonary tuberculosis in Lusaka, Zambia," *Tubercle and Lung Disease*, vol. 74, no. 3, pp. 191–194, 1993.

[6] D. C. Perlman, W. M. El-Sadr, E. T. Nelson et al., "Variation of chest radiographic patterns in pulmonary tuberculosis by degree of human immunodeficiency virus-related immunosuppression. The Terry Beirn Community Programs for Clinical Research on AIDS (CPCRA). The AIDS Clinical Trials Group (ACTG)," *Clinical Infectious Diseases*, vol. 25, no. 2, pp. 242–246, 1997.

[7] A. D. Harries, H. T. Banda, M. J. Boeree et al., "Management of pulmonary tuberculosis suspects with negative sputum smears and normal or minimally abnormal chest radiographs in resource-poor settings," *International Journal of Tuberculosis and Lung Disease*, vol. 2, no. 12, pp. 999–1004, 1998.

[8] G. S. Kibiki, B. Mulder, D. van Ven et al., "Laboratory diagnosis of pulmonary tuberculosis in TB and HIV endemic settings and the contribution of real time PCR for M. tuberculosis in bronchoalveolar lavage fluid," *Tropical Medicine and International Health*, vol. 12, no. 10, pp. 1210–1217, 2007.

[9] P. Daley, A. Latha, Suzana S. et al., "Risk factors associated with poor quality sputum submission in India," *International Journal of Antimicrobial Agents*, vol. 34, p. S17, 2009.

[10] M. S. Khan, O. Dar, C. Sismanidis, K. Shah, and P. Godfrey-Faussett, "Improvement of tuberculosis case detection and reduction of discrepancies between men and women by simple sputum-submission instructions: a pragmatic randomised controlled trial," *Lancet*, vol. 369, no. 9577, pp. 1955–1960, 2007.

[11] Y. Merid, M. A. Yassin, L. Yamuah, R. Kumar, H. Engers, and A. Aseffa, "Validation of bleach-treated smears for the diagnosis of pulmonary tuberculosis," *International Journal of Tuberculosis and Lung Disease*, vol. 13, no. 1, pp. 136–141, 2009.

[12] R. Brindle, J. Odhiambo, and D. Mitchison, "Serial counts of Mycobacterium tuberculosis in sputum as surrogate markers of the sterilising activity of rifampicin and pyrazinamide in treating pulmonary tuberculosis," *BMC Pulmonary Medicine*, vol. 1, article 2, 2001.

[13] A. Jindani, C. J. Doré, and D. A. Mitchison, "Bactericidal and sterilizing activities of antituberculosis drugs during the first 14 days," *American Journal of Respiratory and Critical Care Medicine*, vol. 167, no. 10, pp. 1348–1354, 2003.

[14] A. H. Diacon, J. S. Maritz, A. Venter et al., "Time to detection of the growth of Mycobacterium tuberculosis in MGIT 960 for determining the early bactericidal activity of antituberculosis agents," *European Journal of Clinical Microbiology and Infectious Diseases*, vol. 29, pp. 1561–1565, 2010.

[15] C. Pheiffer, N. M. Carroll, N. Beyers et al., "Time to detection of Mycobacterium tuberculosis in BACTEC systems as a viable alternative to colony counting," *International Journal of Tuberculosis and Lung Disease*, vol. 12, no. 7, pp. 792–798, 2008.

[16] N. R. Gandhi, N. S. Shah, J. R. Andrews et al., "HIV coinfection in multidrug- and extensively drug-resistant tuberculosis results in high early mortality," *American Journal of Respiratory and Critical Care Medicine*, vol. 181, no. 1, pp. 80–86, 2010.

[17] M. Barnard, H. Albert, G. Coetzee, R. O'Brien, and M. E. Bosman, "Rapid molecular screening for multidrug-resistant tuberculosis in a high-volume public health laboratory in South Africa," *American Journal of Respiratory and Critical Care Medicine*, vol. 177, no. 7, pp. 787–792, 2008.

[18] D. Helb, M. Jones, E. Story et al., "Rapid detection of Mycobacterium tuberculosis and rifampin resistance by use of on-demand, near-patient technology," *Journal of Clinical Microbiology*, vol. 48, no. 1, pp. 229–237, 2010.

[19] B. Alisjahbana, C. R. Van, H. Danusantoso et al., "Better patient instruction for sputum sampling can improve microscopic tuberculosis diagnosis," *International Journal of Tuberculosis and Lung Disease*, vol. 9, no. 7, pp. 814–817, 2005.

[20] J. R. Warren, M. O. N. D. Bhattacharya, K. N. F. de Almeida, K. A. T. H. Trakas, and L. R. Peterson, "A minimum 5.0 ml of sputum improves the sensitivity of acid-fast smear for Mycobacterium tuberculosis," *American Journal of Respiratory and Critical Care Medicine*, vol. 161, no. 5, pp. 1559–1562, 2000.

[21] D. Gothi and J. M. Joshi, "Clinical and laboratory observations of tuberculosis at a Mumbai (India) clinic," *Postgraduate Medical Journal*, vol. 80, no. 940, pp. 97–100, 2004.

[22] M. Muyoyeta, J. A. Schaap, H. P. De et al., "Comparison of four culture systems for Mycobacterium tuberculosis in the zambian national reference laboratory," *International Journal of Tuberculosis and Lung Disease*, vol. 13, no. 4, pp. 460–465, 2009.

7

Five-Year Assessment of Time of Sputum Smears Conversion and Outcome and Risk Factors of Tuberculosis Patients in Central Iran

Fatemah Behnaz,[1] Mahmoud Mohammadzadeh,[1] and Golnaz Mohammadzade[2]

[1] *Department of Infectious Diseases, Shahid Sadoughi University of Medical Sciences, Yazd, Iran*
[2] *Shahid Sadoughi University of Medical Sciences, Yazd, Iran*

Correspondence should be addressed to Mahmoud Mohammadzadeh; mahmoudmohammadzadeh@yahoo.com

Academic Editor: Jacques Grosset

Objective. To evaluate risk factors which influence sputum smear conversion, outcome, and trends of conversion of sputum smear during 5 years and compare outcomes in patients with different regimens. *Methods.* In a retrospective cohort study, all patients with sputum smear positive tuberculosis were evaluated for comorbidities and demographic, microbiological, and therapeutic data and outcome. Smear examinations were performed at the beginning, at 2 months for CAT I, at 3 months for CAT II, at the end of second month of maintenance phase, and at the end of treatment. *Results.* This study enrolled 211 sputum smear positive patients, but 189 patients who completed the intensive phase of treatment were evaluated. Sputum smear of 158 patients converted at the end of intensive phase (83.6). Univariate analysis indicated that the risk of a persistent positive smear at the end of intensive phase was greater in diabetic patients ((odds 4.038, 95% CI 1.123–14.516) $P = 0.033$), and also a 3+bacillary load had risk of 2.933-fold ((95% CI 1.278–6.732) $P = 0.011$). Overall rate of unfavorable outcome was 20.9%. Factors associated with unfavorable outcome were age (P value 0.000), male gender (P value 0.027), diabetes (P value 0.000), and delayed conversion of sputum at the end of intensive phase (P value 0.000). Outcome for different regimens was not different significantly. Two specimens were isoniazid resistant. *Conclusions.* We suggest supervised treatment and care for diabetic patients and those with higher bacillary load. Paying attention to early diagnosis of tuberculosis in the elderly to reduce poor outcome and further measures to prevent transfer-out could improve the success rate.

1. Introduction

Tuberculosis (TB) remains a global health problem. In 2011, there were an estimated 8.7 million new cases of TB (13% coinfected with HIV) and 1.4 million people died from TB. Between 1995 and 2011, 51 million people were successfully treated for TB in countries that had adopted the WHO strategy, saving 20 million lives [1]. Successful control of tuberculosis (TB) depends on early and effective control of the transmission of *Mycobacterium tuberculosis* from infectious patients. Sputum smear conversion at the end of the intensive phase of treatment is used as an important early predictor of treatment success [2–4]. WHO continues to recommend performing smear microscopy at this stage because a positive smear should trigger an assessment of the patient, as well as additional sputum monitoring [1]. The sputum conversion results are used both for management of patients and for monitoring programmed performance [5]. Several studies evaluated risk factors such as age, smear grading, gender, influence of directly observed therapy (DOT), and associated comorbid conditions like HIV infection and diabetes mellitus among tuberculosis patients [5–8]. However, interest in geographic differences in response to TB treatment dates back to 1956 when Fox et al. compared clinical, radiographic, and microbiological outcomes in patients from Britain and Uganda [9]. In recent years Tuberculosis Trials Consortium Study 28 found later sputum culture conversion and lower rates of conversion in liquid media in African patients compared to non-African patients [10]. So, we studied risk factors which influence smear conversion and evaluated trends of conversion of sputum smear during a period of 5 years and compared outcomes in patients with pulmonary TB who received different regimens.

2. Materials and Methods

2.1. Study Design and Population. In a retrospective cohort study, all patients with sputum smear positive pulmonary TB who were referred to the Yazd Health Center from March 2007 to March 2012 were considered eligible for inclusion in this study. Comorbidities and demographic, microbiological, and therapeutic data were collected from patients' medical record. Based on the National Plan against Tuberculosis, all new smear positive pulmonary tuberculosis patients were classified as category (CAT I) regimen and all patients who were retreated were classified as CAT II regimen. Ethical clearance was obtained from the University Ethics Committee. This study did not need ethical consent.

2.2. Mycobacterial Examinations: Sputum Smear and Culture. Based on the National Plan against Tuberculosis, smear examinations were performed at the beginning, at 2 months for CAT I, 3 months for CAT II, at the end of second month of maintenance phase, and at the end of treatment. Culture and antimicrobial susceptibility were performed only for patients who were smear positive after three months of initiation of treatment. Sputum smears were examined for AFB by microscopy and Ziehl-Neelsen staining and graded by standard criteria and equivalent: 1–9 AFB/100 fields (1+); 1–9 AFB/10 fields (2+); and 1–9 AFB/field (3+) [11].

Smear conversion was defined as 2 consecutive negative samples. Smear and culture conversion time was defined as duration from the beginning of treatment to the date of the first negative sample. Delayed smear conversion was defined as persistent smear positivity after 2 months of treatment for patients in CAT I and 3 months for CAT II.

2.3. Treatment and Monitoring. A 6-month standard treatment based on international consensus 1 consists of intensive phase isoniazid (H), rifampicin (R), pyrazinamide (Z), and ethambutol (E) daily in the first 2 months; if the smear were positive, the intensive phase is extended by one more month for that patient. Treatment is followed by continuous phase (4 months), daily H and R, and can be prolonged in patients with concomitant hepatic and/or renal diseases and in case adverse effects occur. All new pulmonary TB patients were treated with this regimen irrespective of associated comorbid conditions. DOTS strategy was done in the intensive phase of all patients. All recurrent pulmonary TB patients were treated with HRZES daily for 2 months, HRZE daily for 1 month (intensive phase), and HRE daily for 5 months (continuous phase). Patients who were treated as CAT II were completely supervised for the entire course of treatment by DOTS strategy.

Outcome was defined as follows: cure: a patient whose sputum smear or culture was positive at the beginning of the treatment but who was smear or culture negative in the last month of treatment and on at least one previous occasion.

2.3.1. Definitions

Treatment Failure. Treatment failure is defined as a patient whose sputum smear or culture is positive at 5 months or later during treatment. Also included in this definition are patients found to harbor a multidrug resistant (MDR) strain at any point of time during the treatment, whether they are smear negative or positive.

Died. "Died" was defined as a patient who dies from any cause during the course of treatment.

Transfer-Out. Transfer-out is a patient who has been transferred to another recording and reporting unit and whose treatment outcome is unknown [12].

2.4. Statistical Analysis. Statistical analysis was performed using the SPSS version 17.0 software. All probabilities were two-tailed and P values <0.05 were regarded as significant.

Data were described as mean with standard deviation. The Chi-square test or the Fisher exact test was used to compare categorical variables whenever appropriate. Delayed smear conversion was a dichotomous dependent variable. Variables that were statistically significant and biologically plausible in univariate analysis were entered into a logistic regression model with forward stepwise conditional in order to identify the factors independently associated with that outcome. The odds ratios (OR) and 95% confidence intervals (CI) were determined.

3. Results

All of the two hundred and eleven sputum smear positive patients who have been treated during the time of study were retrospectively enrolled. The patients' mean age was 52.93 ± 22.19 (range: 2–95 years), and 114 patients were male, 54%. Study population included 110 Iranian and 101 non-Iranian patients, most of whom were immigrants from Afghanistan. Frequency of diabetes mellitus among patients with pulmonary TB in this study was 9.5%, which was the most common underlying comorbidity. Table 1 shows demographic characteristics, grading of sputum smear positivity at the initiation of treatment, anti-TB treatment regimens, treatment category, and comorbidities of enrolled patients at baseline.

Of 211 patients who were enrolled into the study, 22 had no record of sputum conversion at the end of the intensive phase; reasons were as follows: 9 patients were transferred out and 13 patients deceased during intensive phase of treatment. Of 189 patients who completed the intensive phase of treatment, sputum smear of one hundred and fifty-eight patients converted at the end of intensive phase (83.6%). Conversion rates of patients in CAT I were 144/173 (83.23%) and of patients in CAT II were 14/16 (87.5%) and conversion rate was not associated with category of treatment (P value = 0.660). The higher smear grading was associated with delayed conversion time (1+: 11.2%, 2+: 12.5%, and 3+: 30% (P = 0.01)). Diabetes mellitus and other comorbidities were associated with delayed conversion time (P = 0.012), whereas there

TABLE 1: Comorbidities and demographic and bacteriological variables of sputum smear positive pulmonary tuberculosis patients in Yazd ($n = 211$).

Characteristic		Number %
Sex	Male	114 (54)
Age	≤50	86 (40.7)
	>50	125 (59.3)
Nationality	Iranian	110 (52.1)
	Non-Iranian	101 (47.9)
Initial sputum grading	1+	122 (57.8)
	2+	36 (17.1)
	3+	53 (25.1)
Accompanying disease	DM	20 (9.5)
	HIV	4 (1.9)
	Malignancy	1 (0.5)
	Transplant	2 (0.9)
	Others*	10 (4.7)
Treatment regimen	HRZE	185 (87.7)
	HRZES	18 (8.5)
	HRE	6 (2.8)
	HZE	2 (0.9)
Treatment category	CAT I	191 (90.5)
	CAT II	20 (9.5)

*Corticosteroid therapy (3), COPD (3), chronic renal failure (2), inherited cell mediated immunodeficiency (1), and cirrhosis (1). H: isoniazid; R: rifampicin; Z: pyrazinamide; E: ethambutol; S: streptomycin.

was no association between age, sex, nationality, treatment regimens, and category of treatment with delayed conversion time in the present study (Table 2). In nine patients who had positive sputum culture and antimicrobial susceptibility, only two specimens of sputum were isoniazid resistant.

The outcome at the end of treatment for 211 enrolled patients was as follows: cure was achieved for one hundred and sixty-seven patients (79.1%) and unfavorable outcome during this study was 20.9% including treatment failure for 9 patients (4.3%), eight of whom were new smear positive cases, and death for nineteen patients (9%) during period of their treatment some of them due to diseases such as myocardial infarction, cerebrovascular accident, respiratory failure due to asthma, and COPD. The mean age of patients who died was 64 ± 18.86. From 16 patients (7.6%) who were transferred out, 9 patients returned to Afghanistan and health services could not trace them to find their outcomes. Factors associated with unfavorable outcome included age (P value 0.000), sex (P value 0.027), accompanying disease (P value 0.000), and sputum conversion at the end of intensive phase ((P value 0.000), Table 3). As is shown in Table 3 there was not any association between nationality, treatment regimen, initial sputum grading, or category of treatment and outcome in the present study.

As is shown in Table 4, after omitting patients who deceased and were transferred out, factors associated with failure included initial sputum grade (P value 0.004), diabetes mellitus (P value 0.00), and sputum conversion at the end of intensive phase (P value 0.00).

Univariate analysis indicated that the risk of a persistent positive smear at the end of 2nd month was greater in diabetic patients ((odds 4.038, 95% CI 1.123–14.516) $P = 0.033$), and also a 3+bacillary load had risk of 2.93-fold ((95% CI 1.28–6.73) $P = 0.011$) (Table 5).

Figure 1 illustrates sputum conversion rates and Figure 2 shows outcome during years of study.

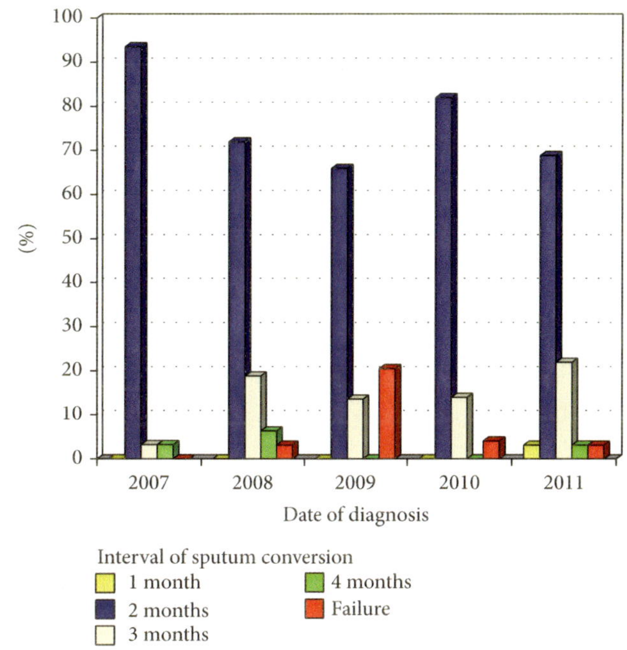

FIGURE 1: Time of sputum smear conversion of pulmonary tuberculosis regarding years of study.

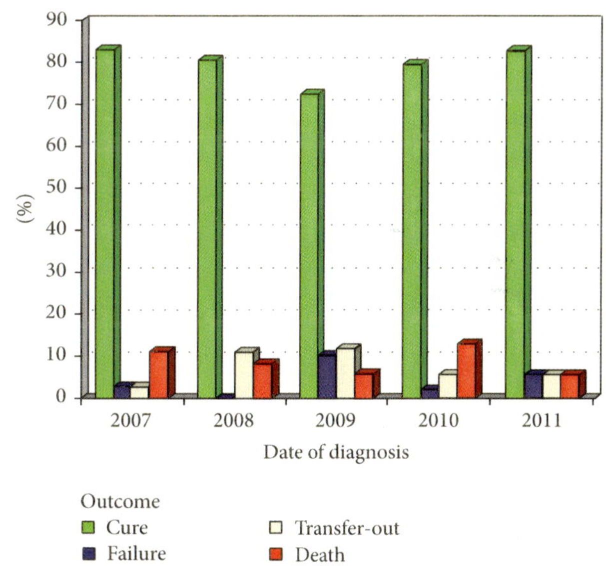

FIGURE 2: Outcome of pulmonary tuberculosis patients regarding years of study.

TABLE 2: Impact of comorbidities and demographic, microbiological, and therapeutic variables on sputum smear conversion at the end of the intensive phase ($N = 189$).

Characteristic		Sputum conversion status		P value
		Conversion number (%)	Nonconversion number (%)	
Sex	Male	83 (83.8)	16 (16.2)	0.925
	Female	75 (83.3)	15 (16.7)	
Age	≤50	60 (80)	15 (20)	0.279
	>50	98 (86)	16 (14)	
Nationality	Iranian	84 (85)	15 (15)	0.626
	Non-Iranian	74 (82.2)	16 (17.8)	
Initial sputum grading	≤2+	122 (88.4)	16 (11.6)	0.003
	3+	35 (70)	15 (30)	
Accompanying disease	DM	14 (70)	6 (30)	0.033
	Otherwise healthy (No comorbidity)	136 (87.8)	19 (12.2)	
Treatment regimen	HRZE	139 (83.7)	27 (16.3)	0.625
	HRZES*	13 (86.7)	2 (13.3)	
	HRE	4 (66.7)	2 (33.3)	
	HZE	2 (100)	0 (0)	
Treatment category	CAT I	144 (83.2)	29 (16.8)	0.660
	CAT II	14 (87.5)	2 (12.5)	

HRZES*: isoniazide, rifampicin, pyrazinamide, ethambutol, and streptomycin.

TABLE 3: Impact of comorbidities and demographic, microbiological, and therapeutic variables on outcome of patients ($N = 211$).

Characteristic		Outcome				P value
		Favorable	Unfavorable			
		Cure	Failure	Death	Transfer-out	
Sex	Male	83 (72.8)	6 (5.3)	11 (9.6)	14 (12.3)	0.027
	Female	84 (86.6)	3 (3.1)	8 (8.2)	2 (2.1)	
Age	≤50	65 (75.7)	2 (2.3)	4 (4.6)	15 (17.4)	0.000
	>50	102 (81.6)	7 (5.6)	15 (12)	1 (0.8)	
Nationality	Iranian	88 (80)	6 (5.5)	10 (9.1)	6 (5.5)	0.858
	Non-Iranian	79 (79)	3 (3)	9 (9)	9 (9)	
Initial sputum grading	≤2+	128 (81)	3 (1.9)	15 (9.5)	12 (7.6)	0.398
	3+	39 (75)	6 (11.5)	4 (7.7)	3 (5.8)	
Accompanying disease	DM	15 (75)	5 (25)	0 (0)	0 (0)	0.000
	Other comorbidities	10 (58.8)	0 (0)	6 (35.3)	1 (5.9)	
	No comorbidity	142 (81.6)	4 (2.3)	13 (7.5)	15 (8.6)	
Treatment regimen	HRZE	147 (80)	8 (4.3)	17 (9.2)	12 (6.5)	0.881
	HRZES*	13 (72.2)	1 (5.6)	1 (5.6)	3 (16.7)	
	HRE	59 (83.3)	0 (0)	1 (1.67)	0 (0)	
	HZE	2 (100)	0 (0)	0 (0)	0 (0)	
Treatment category	CAT I	153 (80.5)	8 (4.2)	17 (8.9)	12 (6.3)	0.53
	CAT II	14 (70)	1 (5)	2 (10)	3 (15)	
Sputum conversion	2 m for CAT I, 3 m for CAT II	146 (92.4)	2 (1.26)	4 (2.5)	6 (3.8)	0.000
	>2 m and >3	21 (67.8)	7 (28.6)	2 (6.4)	1 (3.2)	

*Isoniazide, rifampicin, pyrazinamide, ethambutol, and streptomycin.

4. Discussion

In pulmonary tuberculosis, the assessment of response to therapy is evaluated by disappearance of acid-fast bacilli (AFB) from sputum smear and the conversion of culture to negative [13]. Sputum smear of one hundred fifty-eight patients (83.6%) converted at the end of intensive phase in the present study. The conversion rate reported from India at the end of 2nd month was 84% [14].

Another study from Kuwait reported conversion rate of 88.5% in smokers and 94.2% in nonsmokers [15]. A study from Taiwan revealed that 11.1% of patients remained smear and culture positive after 2 months of treatment [16]. So the conversion rate in the present study is in the range of the mentioned studies. It has been known that the proportion of smear positive patients at the end of the intensive phase is a predictor of treatment success. So conversion rate of

TABLE 4: Impact of comorbidity and demographic, microbiological, and therapeutic variables on failure.

Characteristic		Outcome		P value
		Cure	Failure	
Sex	Female	84	3	0.32
	Male	83	6	
Age	≤50	65	2	0.31
	>50	102	7	
Nationality	Iranian	88	6	0.41
	Non-Iranian	79	3	
Initial sputum grading	≤2+	127	3	0.004
	3+	40	6	
Accompanying illness	Diabetic	15	5	0.00
	Otherwise healthy	152	4	
Treatment category	CAT I	153	8	0.775
	CAT II	14	1	
Sputum conversion	2 m for CAT I, 3 m for CAT II	146	2	0.00
	>2 m and >3	21	7	

TABLE 5: Risk estimate of nonconversion of sputum smear at the end of intensive phase.

Variable	Odds	95% CI	P
Age			
>50/≤50	0.694	0.291–1.658	0.412
Sex			
Female/male	1.048	0.462–2.377	0.910
Nationality			
Non-Iranian/Iranian	1.325	0.566–3.099	0.412
Initial sputum grading 3+/≤2+	2.933	1.278–6.732	0.011
Diabetic/other comorbidities			
No comorbidity	4.038	1.123–14.516	0.033

our patients is acceptable and indicates high compliance of patients, as well as the dosage and quality of TB medications.

The conversion rate was not different between Iranians and non-Iranians, most of whom were immigrants from Afghanistan and lived in Iran for a long time. We found higher initial smear grading which was associated with delayed conversion time ($P = 0.01$). This finding was observed in previous studies [7, 14, 15, 17].

Identification of risk factors for persistent smear positivity after 2 months of treatment which can predict treatment failure is very important [18].

Frequency of diabetes mellitus (DM) among patients with pulmonary TB in this study was 9.5% and was the most common underlying comorbidity. The data presented in this study showed that patients with DM and TB have more delayed sputum conversion and a higher probability of treatment failure. The risk of nonconversion of sputum at the end of intensive phase of treatment associated with DM in our study was 2.44-fold (95% CI 1.11–5.40). Treatment outcomes in patients with TB and DM have been a subject of debate. In a study performed in India smear conversion was similar in diabetic and nondiabetic patients [17], in contrast to another study conducted in México which identified diabetes as an independent risk of failure to treatment [19]. Defects in the immune system of patients with active TB and DM have been reported, including reductions in the activation of alveolar macrophages and the capacity to produce interleukin [20, 21], in addition to some degree of impaired limited numbers of diabetic patients' gastrointestinal drug absorption even in the absence of clinical gastroparesis [22]. This can explain delay of sputum smear conversion and higher unfavorable outcome in the present study. However, due to limited number of diabetic patients in this study, it could not be generalized.

Treatment outcome results serve as a tool to control the quality of TB treatment provided by the health care system. In our study, the outcome at the end of treatment was cure (79.1%). This is close to the WHO target of success rate of 85% of all smear positive cases. However, subgroups of patients contributing to unfavorable outcome should specifically be considered. In the present study 15 patients (7.1%) were transferred out; majority of them left this country to their own country (Afghanistan) while they were on treatment, so we have no information about their outcomes. This is a common problem in treatment of Afghani patients and efforts should be made to ensure the continuity of treatment for patients who move out of Iran for prevention of drug resistance. Six patients out of 15 transferred-out patients belonged to younger age group which explains poor outcome in this group. The death rate in our study was 9%; most patients who died were older than cured patients, and some of them also had other illnesses. It is difficult to know to what extent the death of patients whose only cause of death was TB could have been prevented. But because most of them happened during early phase of treatment, it might be due to delay in their diagnosis and treatment.

Nine patients had treatment failure (4.3%); most of them were new smear positive. Drug susceptibility at the beginning of treatment is not routine in our country, so this can be due to primary or secondary resistance. Limited culture and drug susceptibility have been done during this study, not indicating multiple drug resistance. However, failure also indicates problem in quality of TB treatment and must be considered in the program of TB control.

In our study men had more unfavorable outcome, because they had more transferred out and failure. Most of them returned to their initial country and we do not know their outcome and probably the rest of them did not have good adherence to treatment, so health care workers must give more information at the initiation of treatment about duration of therapy and importance of adherence to that. Efforts should be made to ensure the continuity of treatment for patients who move out of the country and, if possible, to allow them to complete their course of treatment, even if they have to leave the country later.

Time to sputum smear conversion was similar during the study and differences in outcome cannot be attributed to improved/worsening of TB treatment practices in our setting, because TB control program in our country did not change during the period in which the study subjects have been treated.

5. Conclusions

Our analysis showed that 16.4% of tuberculosis patients remained smear positive at the end of intensive phase. Risk factors for persistent positive smear at 2 months were diabetes and higher bacillary load at the beginning of treatment. The outcome at the end of treatment was cure of 79.1% of patients. Factors associated with unfavorable outcome included younger age, male gender, diabetes, and delayed conversion of sputum at the end of intensive phase. We conclude that intensified treatment and precautions for TB patients with mentioned risk factors, early diagnosis of TB in elderly patients to reduce the death rate, and further measures to prevent transfer-out could improve the success rate further.

Authors' Contribution

Fatemah Behnaz participated in concept and design of the study and prepared the paper. Mahmoud Mohammadzadeh contributed to analysis and interpretation of data and reviewed the paper critically for intellectual content. Golnaz Mohammadzade contributed to data collection and paper preparation.

Acknowledgment

This study was performed in Shahid Sadoughi University of Medical Sciences, Yazd, Iran.

References

[1] World Health Organization, *Global Tuberculosis Report 2012*, World Health Organization, 2012, http://who.int/tb/publications/global_report/en/.

[2] Z. Feng-zeng, M. H. Levy, and W. Sumin, "Sputum microscopy results at two and three months predict outcome of tuberculosis treatment," *International Journal of Tuberculosis and Lung Disease*, vol. 1, no. 6, pp. 570–572, 1997.

[3] S. Wen, Y. Su, and F. Zhang, "Analysis of short-term effects of short-course intermittent chemotherapies of the World Bank Loaned Project," *Chinese Journal of Tuberculosis and Respiratory Diseases*, vol. 19, no. 6, pp. 357–359, 1996.

[4] A. M. Chavez Pachas, R. Blank, M. C. Smith Fawzi, J. Bayona, M. C. Becerra, and C. D. Mitnick, "Identifying early treatment failure on Category I therapy for pulmonary tuberculosis in Lima Ciudad, Peru," *International Journal of Tuberculosis and Lung Disease*, vol. 8, no. 1, pp. 52–58, 2004.

[5] J. A. Kumaresan, A. K. M. Ahsan Ali, and L. M. Parkkali, "Tuberculosis control in Bangladesh: success of the DOTS strategy," *International Journal of Tuberculosis and Lung Disease*, vol. 2, no. 12, pp. 992–998, 1998.

[6] M. Senkoro, S. G. Mfinanga, and O. Mørkve, "Smear microscopy and culture conversion rates among smear positive pulmonary tuberculosis patients by HIV status in Dar es Salaam, Tanzania," *BMC Infectious Diseases*, vol. 10, article 210, 2010.

[7] V. V. Banu Rekha, R. Balasubramanian, S. Swaminathan et al., "Sputum conversion at the end of intensive phase of Category-1 regimen in the treatment of pulmonary tuberculosis patients with diabetes mellitus or HIV infection: an analysis of risk factors," *Indian Journal of Medical Research*, vol. 126, no. 5, pp. 452–458, 2007.

[8] S. Bawri, S. Ali, C. Phukan, B. Tayal, and P. Baruwa, "A study of sputum conversion in new smear positive pulmonary tuberculosis cases at the monthly intervals of 1st , 2nd & 3rd month under directly observed treatment, short course (dots) regimen," *Lung India journal*, vol. 25, no. 3, pp. 118–123, 2008.

[9] W. Fox, P. W. Hutton, I. Sutherland, and A. W. Williams, "A comparison of acute extensive pulmonary tuberculosis and its response to chemotherapy in Britain and Uganda," *Tubercle*, vol. 37, no. 6, pp. 435–450, 1956.

[10] W. R. M. Kenzie, C. M. Heilig, L. Bozeman et al., "Geographic differences in time to culture conversion in liquid media: tuberculosis trials Consortium Study 28. Culture conversion is delayed in Africa," *PLoS ONE*, vol. 6, no. 4, Article ID e18358, 2011.

[11] B. A. Forbes, D. F. Sahm, and A. S. Weissfeld, "Mycobacteria," in *Bailey & Scott's Diagnostic Microbiology*, p. 552, Mosby, St. Louis, Mo, USA, 11th edition, 2002.

[12] *Treatment of Tuberculosis: Guidelines*, WHO/HTM/TB/2009.420, 4th edition, 2009.

[13] J. B. Bass Jr., L. S. Farer, P. C. Hopewell et al., "Treatment of tuberculosis and tuberculosis infection in adults and children. American Thoracic Society and The Centers for Disease Control and Prevention," *American Journal of Respiratory and Critical Care Medicine*, vol. 149, no. 5, pp. 1359–1374, 1994.

[14] S. Bawri, S. Ali, C. Phukan, B. Tayal, and P. Baruwa, "A study of sputum conversion in new smear positive pulmonary tuberculosis cases at the monthly intervals of 1, 2 & 3 month under directly observed treatment, short course (dots) regimen," *Lung India*, vol. 25, no. 3, pp. 118–123, 2008.

[15] A. T. Abal, B. Jayakrishnan, S. Parwer, A. El Shamy, E. Abahussain, and P. N. Sharma, "Effect of cigarette smoking on sputum smear conversion in adults with active pulmonary tuberculosis," *Respiratory Medicine*, vol. 99, no. 4, pp. 415–420, 2005.

[16] J.-Y. Wang, L.-N. Lee, C.-J. Yu, Y.-J. Chien, and P.-C. Yang, "Factors influencing time to smear conversion in patients with smear-positive pulmonary tuberculosis," *Respirology*, vol. 14, no. 7, pp. 1012–1019, 2009.

[17] P. Caetano Mota, A. Carvalho, I. Valente, R. Braga, and R. Duarte, "Predictors of delayed sputum smear and culture conversion among a portuguese population with pulmonary tuberculosis," *Revista Portuguesa de Pneumologia*, vol. 18, no. 2, pp. 72–79, 2012.

[18] H. Ramarokoto, H. Randriamiharisoa, A. Rakotoarisaonina et al., "Bacteriological follow-up of tuberculosis treatment: a comparative study of smear microscopy and culture results at the second month of treatment," *International Journal of Tuberculosis and Lung Disease*, vol. 6, no. 10, pp. 909–912, 2002.

[19] R. N. Sanghani and Z. F. Udwadia, "The association of diabetes and tuberculosis: impact on treatment and post-treatment outcomes," *Thorax*, vol. 68, no. 3, pp. 202–203, 2013.

[20] C.-H. Wang, C.-T. Yu, H.-C. Lin, C.-Y. Liu, and H.-P. Kuo, "Hypodense alveolar macrophages in patients with diabetes mellitus and active pulmonary tuberculosis," *Tubercle and Lung Disease*, vol. 79, no. 4, pp. 235–242, 1999.

[21] N. Yaghini, M. Mahmoodi, G. R. Asadikaram, G. H. Hassanshahi, H. Khoramdelazad, and M. K. Arababadi, "Serum levels of interleukin 10 (IL-10) in patients with type 2 diabetes," *Iranian Red Crescent Medical Journal*, vol. 13, no. 10, pp. 751–752, 2011.

[22] M. Bashar, P. Alcabes, W. N. Rom, and R. Condos, "Increased incidence of multidrug-resistant tuberculosis in diabetic patients on the bellevue chest service, 1987 to 1997," *Chest*, vol. 120, no. 5, pp. 1514–1519, 2001.

8

Performance of Tuberculin Skin Test Measured against Interferon Gamma Release Assay as Reference Standard in Children

Michael Eisenhut[1] and Katy Fidler[2]

[1] *Paediatric Department, Luton & Dunstable University Hospital NHS Foundation Trust, Lewsey Road, Luton LU4 ODZ, UK*
[2] *Department of Infection and Immunology, Brighton & Sussex Medical School, University of Sussex, Brighton, East Sussex BN1 9PX, UK*

Correspondence should be addressed to Michael Eisenhut; michael_eisenhut@yahoo.com

Academic Editor: Carlo Garzelli

Objectives. International guidelines differ in the threshold of tuberculin skin test (TST) induration regarded as indicating *Mycobacterium (M.) tuberculosis* infection. Interferon gamma release assay (IGRA) results were used as reference to assess performance of TST induration thresholds for detection of *M. tuberculosis* infection in children. *Design.* Systematic review which included studies containing data on TST, IGRA, and Bacillus Calmette-Guérin (BCG) status in children. Data bases searched were PubMed, EMBASE, and the Cochrane library. Specificities and sensitivities were calculated for TST thresholds 5, 10, and 15 mm and correlated with age and geographical latitude. *Results.* Eleven studies with 2796 children were included. For BCG immunised children diameters of 5, 10, and 15 mm had median sensitivities of 87, 70, and 75% and specificities of 67, 93, and 90%, respectively. In non-BCG immunised children median sensitivities were 94, 95, and 83% and specificities 91, 95, and 97%. At the 10 mm threshold age correlated negatively with sensitivity of TST ($r = -0.65$, $P = 0.04$) and latitude correlated positively ($r = 0.71$, $P = 0.02$). *Conclusions.* For the 10 mm threshold the sensitivity of the TST is lower in BCG immunised children. Younger age and higher geographical latitude were associated with higher sensitivity of the TST.

1. Introduction

International guidelines differ in the threshold of tuberculin skin test (TST) induration regarded as indicating *Mycobacterium (M.) tuberculosis* infection in children with previous Bacillus Calmette-Guérin (BCG) immunisation. In the UK this is 15 mm and in the United States and Spain 10 mm [1]. The high risk posed by *M. tuberculosis* for children less than two years of age, with a risk of progression to disseminated tuberculosis and meningitis from 10 to 20% and tuberculosis in general of 50%, makes it essential to diagnose latent *M. tuberculosis* infection with maximum sensitivity. There is no gold standard test available to assess the sensitivity and specificity of tuberculin skin tests (TST) against in latent *M. tuberculosis* infection. Interferon gamma release assays (IGRA) have been shown to be more specific than TST particularly in BCG immunised persons [1] and may be more sensitive in children less than 2 years old and in low income countries where malnutrition and helminth and HIV infection are common [1–3]. Therefore the better performance characteristics of the IGRA compared to the TST make IGRA a suitable reference standard to determine the threshold of TST induration diameter used to define *M. tuberculosis* infection in children with and without BCG immunisation. This investigation adopted the methodology of a systematic review to address the following objectives:

(1) to define the TST induration diameter with the best sensitivity and specificity in diagnosing *M. tuberculosis* infection compared to IGRA in children with and without previous BCG immunisation;

(2) to determine the false negative rate of the TST with IGRA as reference standard for different TST induration thresholds;

(3) to assess the age dependency of sensitivity and specificity of TST;

(4) to assess the dependency of sensitivity and specificity of TST on geographical latitude.

2. Methods

2.1. Inclusion and Exclusion Criteria. Included were studies containing data on TST, IGRA, and BCG status of each participant in children (<16 years of age). Excluded were studies not allowing extraction of data on TST, IGRA, and BCG status in children or where results were only available for mixed adults and children groups. Excluded were data on patients with indeterminate IGRA.

2.2. Search Strategy. Data bases searched by the two authors independently were MEDLINE and Premedline (PubMed), EMBASE, and the Cochrane library using the key words: ELISPOT, QuantiFERON, interferon gamma release assay, IGRA, child, infant, newborn, neonate, and tuberculosis with a limit to: Human and English Language and Publication Year from 1993. Extracted were data on results for IGRA and TST and BCG immunisation, type of IGRA, procedure of TST, location of study, and proportion of children with active tuberculosis, comorbidities, and age. Documentation of the search strategy followed the PRISMA guidelines.

2.3. Data Analysis

2.3.1. Comparison of Sensitivities and Specificities for Different Tuberculin Skin Test Induration Thresholds. Sensitivities and specificities of TST induration thresholds measured against IGRA result as reference standard were calculated from individual patient data where it is possible using software MedCalc Statistical Software 11.5.0 (MedCalc Software bvba, Ostend, Belgium).

Medians for sensitivities and specificities across induration thresholds were compared by Kruskal-Wallis test to take into account multiple comparisons. The Mann-Whitney U test was used for comparison of specificities and sensitivities. Parameters in patients with and without BCG immunisation were compared by Fisher's exact test where original data were available. Because of the importance of not missing *M. tuberculosis* infection in children the proportions of negative TST with a positive IGRA were also calculated. For studies which contained data for different induration thresholds for the same population these were compared by Fisher's exact test.

2.3.2. Investigation of Inconsistency between Studies. Appropriate results were pooled in a meta-analysis to visualise and calculate heterogeneity with a summary statistic derived using the DerSimonian and Laird Random effects model where significant heterogeneity was detected using Meta-DISc 1.4 software (J. Zamora, V. Abraira, A. Muriel, KS. Khan, Coomarasamy A. Meta-DiSc: a software for meta-analysis of test accuracy data. BMC Medical Research Methodology 2006, 6:31). The I^2 statistic was used to quantify inconsistency (heterogeneity) of studies with $I^2 > 40\%$ representing moderate, >60% substantial, and >80% considerable inconsistency. Inconsistency (heterogeneity) of studies as documented in a meta-analysis was explored by investigation of an association of age, percentage of patients with active tuberculosis, and geographical latitude with sensitivities and specificities. Geographical latitude was investigated because BCG immunisation is known to have a lower impact on the immune response to tuberculin in areas closer to the equator. SPSS version 20 (SPSS Inc., Illinois, USA) was used to obtain correlations of age, latitude, and rates of active tuberculosis and specificities or sensitivities. Pearson's correlation coefficient and Spearman's rho were used for correlation analysis. Excel (Microsoft Office Excel (Microsoft Corporation, Seattle, WA, USA)) was used to generate graphic representations of sensitivities and specificities of different TST induration thresholds and the correlation of sensitivities and specificities and age or latitude. A P value of <0.05 was taken to indicate a statistically significant difference.

3. Results

3.1. Comparison of Sensitivities and Specificities for Different Tuberculin Skin Test Induration Thresholds. There were 245 records identified from PubMed, 196 in EMBASE, and 7 in the Cochrane library. 88 articles were retrieved for full text review and a total of 234 records were excluded (see Figure 1: PRISMA FLOW DIAGRAM). The 11 studies included had usable data on 2796 children (see Table 1). All studies investigated children as part of testing for *M. tuberculosis* infection. All but one study [4] used two tuberculin units of PPD RT 23 (Statens Serum Institute, Copenhagen, Denmark) for conduction of the tuberculin skin test. Eight studies used the QuantiFERON as IGRA, while three studies [1, 7, 13] used the ELISPOT version. Sensitivities, specificities, and percentages of false negative TST results for different TST induration thresholds were tabulated in Table 2.

In BCG immunised children 5, 10, and 15 mm induration thresholds had median (range) sensitivities of 87 (74.6 to 100.0), 70 (25 to 87), and 75 (60.9 to 83.6) %, respectively, and specificities of 67 (60.7 to 92.5), 93 (74.9 to 97.4), and 90 (70.7 to 97.0) %, respectively. In non-BCG immunised children median sensitivities were 94 (89 to 100), 95 (84 to 100), and 83.6% (one study only), respectively, and specificities were 91 (88.9 to 92.5), 95 (95 to 100), and 97% (one study only), respectively. There was no significant difference between sensitivities ($P = 0.43$) or specificities ($P = 0.13$) of induration thresholds with or without BCG immunisation (see Figures 4 and 5).

Comparison of sensitivities of induration thresholds 5, 10, and 15 mm with or without previous BCG immunisation is presented in Figure 4. There was no difference in sensitivities for a 5 or 15 mm induration threshold between patients

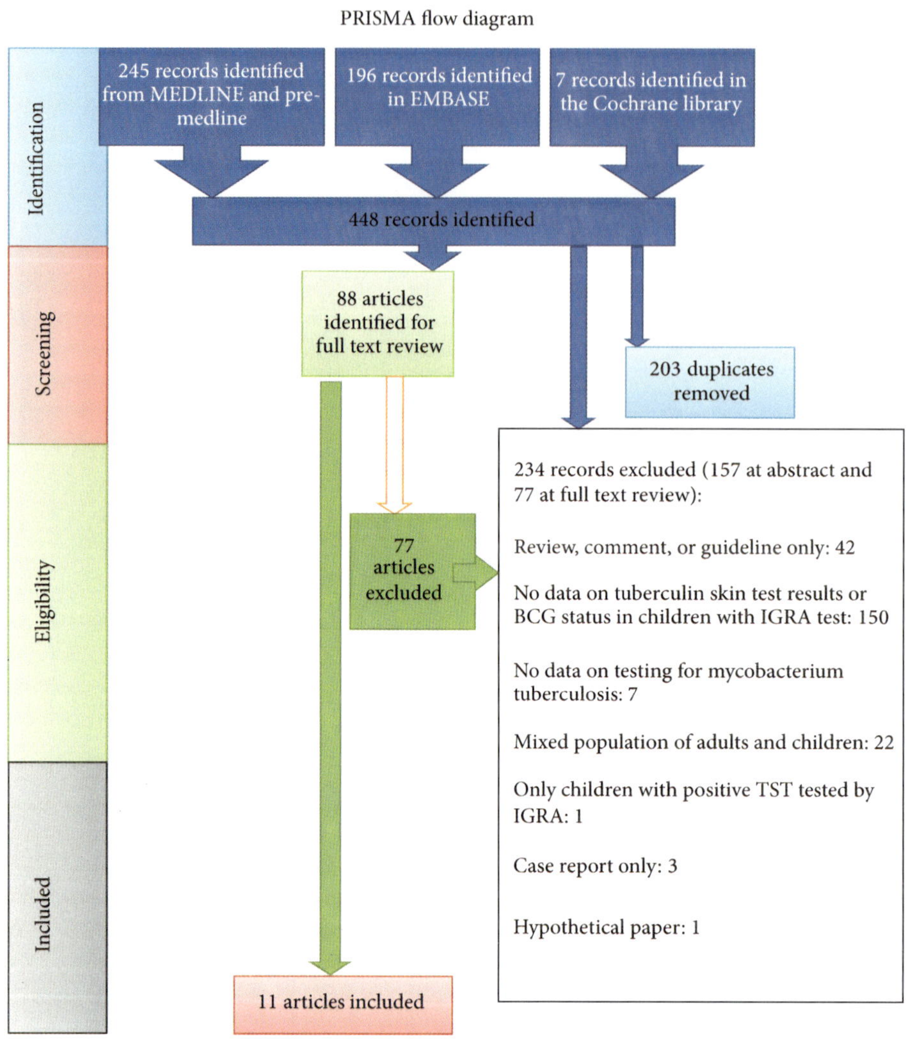

FIGURE 1: Study selection for systematic review—PRISMA flow diagram.

with and without BCG immunisation ($P = 0.26$ and $P = 0.50$, resp.). For the 10 mm induration threshold sensitivities were significantly lower and hence false negative TST's were significantly more common ($P = 0.014$) in children with BCG immunisation.

For this 10 mm induration threshold very low sensitivities were reported in one study from Uganda [13] (25%) and one from South Africa [9] (33.3%). Analysis of the Ugandan study's anthropometric data showed a low level of undernutrition, with prevalence of wasting being 5.4%. 13 (1.4%) of the participants were HIV infected, and the prevalence of other infections was as follows: asymptomatic malaria 4.0%, helminth infection 9.6%, and active tuberculosis 0.3%. In the South African study [9] all children had cancer: 61.8% haematological malignancies, 32.4% solid tumors, and 5.9% others.

One study with low specificity [1] (59.7%) was conducted in Istanbul, Turkey, with an ELISPOT, which was a precursor of the currently commercially available ELISPOT version. The other study showed a specificity of 60.8% [5] and was conducted in Seoul, South Korea, and 59.3% were clinically unwell with causes other than tuberculosis including pneumonia, chronic cough, fever of unknown origin, and lymphadenopathy.

3.2. Investigation of Inconsistency between Studies. For a 10 mm induration threshold in BCG immunised children a meta-analysis was employed to investigate for inconsistency (heterogeneity) between study results (see Figures 2 and 3). The studies Bakir 2009 and Mendez-Echevarria 2011 could not be included in the meta-analyses because the reports only allowed extraction of the sensitivities and specificities and not the raw data from which they were calculated. For other induration thresholds there were not enough studies available to allow for a meaningful meta-analysis to explore inconsistency between the majority of studies. The meta-analysis revealed considerable inconsistency (heterogeneity) of studies with regards to analysis of both sensitivities and specificities (see Figures 2 and 3).

TABLE 1: Characteristics of studies reporting on children with results on tuberculin skin test and interferon gamma release assay and information on BCG immunisation status (TB: tuberculosis).

Study reference	Country	Setting	Reason for testing	Age	Children with BCG immunisation	Children without BCG immunisation	Active TB (%)
Dogra et al. 2007 [4][a]	India	Rural Medical School	Suspect cases or contacts	Median: 6.0 years (range 1 to 12)	86	19	10.5
Chun et al. 2008 [5]	South Korea	Municipal Children's Hospital	Close and casual contacts and cases	Median 3.2 years (range 0–15.8)	145	—	3.0
Taylor et al. 2008 [6]	United Kingdom	Municipal Hospital	Contacts	Mean 10 years (range 4 to 16)	45	—	10.9 (suspected)
Nicol et al. 2009 [7]	South Africa	Semirural population	Suspected tuberculosis or contacts	Median 1.5 years (IQR 1.1 to 2)	214	—	26.8
Bakir et al. 2009 [1]	Turkey	Municipal clinics	Contacts	Median 7 years (IQR 3 to 11)	652	209	1.3
Soon et al. 2010 [8]	South Korea	Municipal Hospital	Contacts	Median 5 years	26	—	21.2
Stefan et al. 2010 [9]	South Africa	Municipal Hospital	Children newly diagnosed with cancer	Median 7 years (range 0.1 to 15)	29	—	2.9
Méndez-Echevarría et al. 2011 [10]	Spain	Municipal Hospitals	Immigrants from endemic areas, contacts, and cases	Mean age 4.73 (range 0.1 to 15)	213	246	14.8
Kasambira et al. 2011 [11]	South Africa	Rural clinics, District Hospital	Contacts	Median age 6 years (IQR 3 to 9)	236	—	19.0
Moyo et al. 2011 [12]	South Africa	Rural district	Contacts and suspected cases	Median 1.9 years (range 0.75 to 2.83)	376	—	13.1
Nkurunungi et al. 2012 [13]	Uganda	Municipal Hospital	Population based screening	5 years	300	—	0.3

[a]Numbers in brackets refer to the number of the reference in References of the paper.

We therefore explored potential sources of such inconsistency like presence of active tuberculosis, age, and geographical latitude.

The percentage of *M. tuberculosis* infected patients with features of active pulmonary tuberculosis did not correlate with sensitivity or specificity of the 10 mm threshold ($P > 0.10$).

Correlation analysis of sensitivity and age (Figure 6) or geographical latitude (Figure 7) was conducted for a subgroup of studies with data on an induration threshold of 10 mm and previous BCG immunisation. This subgroup was chosen as it was the only group with sufficient numbers to allow such an analysis.

Correlation of TST sensitivity with age (using an induration threshold of 10 mm) revealed a Spearman's rho correlation coefficient of −0.65 ($P = 0.04$) (Figure 6) indicating increased sensitivity of tuberculin skin testing relative to IGRA in younger children. Correlation of sensitivities with geographical latitude revealed a Pearson correlation coefficient of 0.71 ($P = 0.02$) indicating increased sensitivity of tuberculin skin testing with higher latitude (Figure 7).

Specificities for a threshold of 10 mm were equal or above 75% for all studies. There was no significant change in specificity at different ages or latitude.

3.3. Comparison of Sensitivity and Specificity of TST Induration Thresholds in BCG versus Not BCG Immunised Children.

Three studies contained original data or results of analyses on children both with and without BCG immunisation.

The first [4] allowed direct statistical comparison of sensitivities and specificities in BCG immunised versus not immunised children. For a 10 mm induration threshold sensitivity in BCG immunised children was 62.5% (95% CI 24.49 to 91.48) and in nonimmunised children 100.0% (95% CI 29.24 to 100.0) ($P = 0.49$). Specificity was also not significantly different between those immunised: 97.44% (95% CI 91.04 to 99.69) and those not immunised: 100% (95% CI 79.41 to 100.0) ($P = 0.90$).

The second study by Bakir et al. [1] demonstrated at a TST induration threshold of 10 mm a sensitivity of 81.8% (95% CI 76.5 to 86.4) in BCG immunised people similar to 84.5% (95%

TABLE 2: Sensitivities and specificities of tuberculin skin test thresholds and BCG immunisation status.

Study reference	BCG immunisation status (immunised +, not immunised −)	Sensitivity (95% confidence interval)	Specificity (95% confidence interval)	False negative rate as percentage (95% confidence interval) of people with negative tuberculin skin test amongst IGRA positive patients
TST induration threshold 5 mm				
Chun et al. 2008 [5][a]	+	86.7 (59.5 to 98.3)	60.8 (51.8 to 69.2)	13.3 (1.7 to 40.5)
Bakir et al. 2009 [1]	+	87.4 (82.6 to 91.2)	59.7 (54.7 to 64.5)	12.6 (8.8 to 17.4)
	−	89.1 (81.7 to 94.2)	88.9 (81.0 to 94.3)	10.9 (5.8 to 18.3)
Soon et al. 2010 [8]	+	100.0 (54.1 to 100.0)	75.00 (50.9 to 91.3)	0.0 (0.0 to 45.9)
Méndez-Echevarría et al. 2011 [10]	−	100.0 (95.0 to 100.0)	93.6 (88.7 to 96.5)	0.0 (0.0 to 5.0)
Kasambira et al. 2011 [11]	+	74.7 (63.3 to 84.0)	92.5 (87.3 to 96.1)	25.3 (16.0 to 36.7)
TST induration threshold 10 mm				
Dogra et al. 2007 [4]	+	62.5 (24.5 to 91.5)	97.4 (91.0 to 99.7)	37.5 (8.5 to 75.5)
	−	100.0 (29.2 to 100.0)	100.0 (79.4 to 100.0)	0.0 (0.0 to 70.8)
Chun et al. 2008 [5]	+	73.3 (44.9 to 92.2)	81.5 (73.8 to 87.8)	26.6 (7.8 to 55.1)
Bakir et al. 2009 [1]	+	81.8 (76.5 to 86.4)	74.9 (70.4 to 79.1)	18.2 (13.6 to 23.5)
	−	84.5 (76.4 to 90.7)	91.9 (84.7 to 96.4)	15.5 (9.3 to 23.6)
Nicol et al. 2009 [7]	+	87.0 (75.1 to 94.6)	77.5 (70.2 to 83.7)	13.0 (5.4 to 24.9)
Soon et al. 2010 [8]	+	66.7 (22.3 to 95.7)	95.0 (75.1 to 99.8)	33.3 (4.3 to 77.7)
Stefan et al. 2010 [9]	+	33.3 (0.008 to 90.6)	92.3 (74.9 to 99.0)	66.6 (9.4 to 99.2)
Kasambira et al. 2011 [11]	+	64.0 (52.1 to 74.8)	95.6 (91.2 to 98.2)	36.0 (25.2 to 47.9)
Méndez-Echevarría et al. 2011 [10]	+	82.6 (63.0 to 93.0)	86.0 (80.0 to 90.0)	17.4 (7.0 to 37.0)
	−	95.9 (88.6 to 98.6)	95.5 (91.1 to 97.8)	4.1 (1.4 to 11.4)
Moyo et al. 2011 [12]	+	83.8 (72.9 to 91.6)	95.8 (92.9 to 97.7)	16.1 (8.4 to 27.1)
Nkurunungi et al. 2012 [13]	+	25.0 (15.3 to 36.9)	97.4 (94.5 to 99.0)	75.0 (63.1 to 84.7)
TST induration threshold 15 mm				
Taylor et al. 2008 [6]	+	75.0 (19.4 to 99.4)	70.7 (54.5 to 83.9)	25.0 (0.6 to 80.6)
Bakir et al. 2009 [1]	+	75.5 (69.7 to 80.7)	90.5 (87.2 to 93.2)	24.5 (19.3 to 30.3)
	−	83.6 (75.4 to 90.0)	97.0 (91.4 to 99.4)	16.4 (10.0 to 24.6)
Méndez-Echevarría et al. 2011 [10]	+	60.9 (40.8 to 77.8)	97.0 (92.4 to 98.2)	39.1 (22.2 to 59.2)

[a]Numbers refer to the number of the reference in References of the paper.

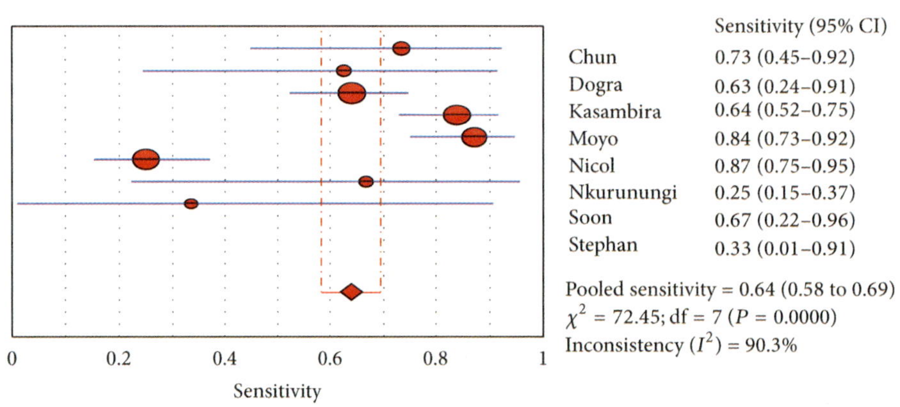

FIGURE 2: Meta-analysis of sensitivity of a 10 mm induration threshold of a tuberculin skin test in BCG immunised children (DerSimonian and Laird random effects model).

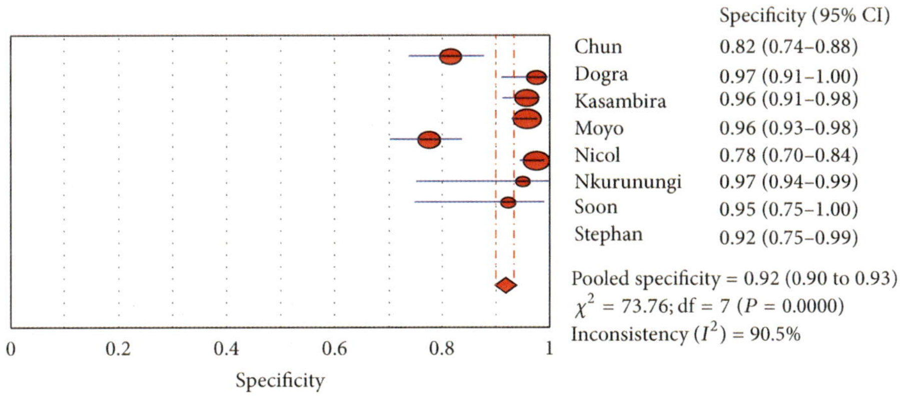

FIGURE 3: Meta-analysis of specificity of a 10 mm induration threshold of a tuberculin skin test in BCG immunized children (DerSimonian and Laird random effects model).

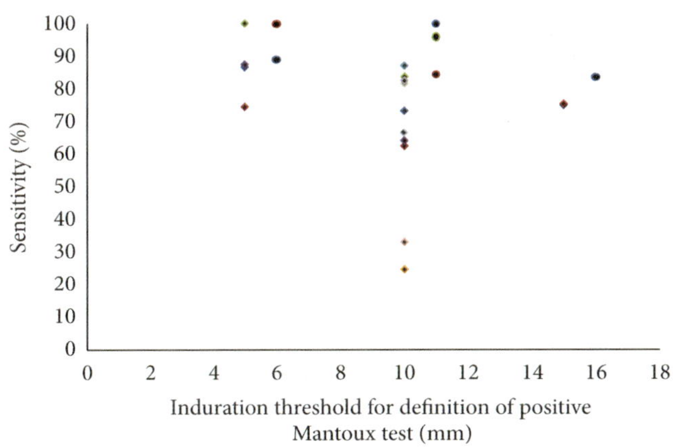

FIGURE 4: Sensitivity of different tuberculin skin test thresholds for detection of *M. tuberculosis* infection with (diamonds) and without (bullets) previous BCG immunisation with IGRA as a reference standard (each dot represents the result of one study).

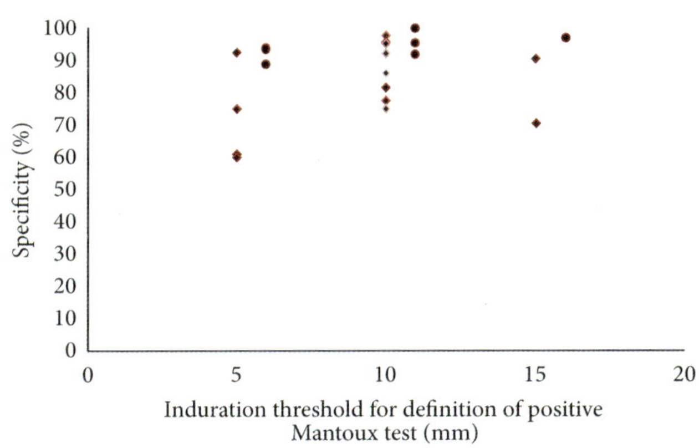

FIGURE 5: Specificity of different tuberculin skin test thresholds for detection of *M. tuberculosis* infection with (diamonds) and without (bullets) previous BCG immunisation with IGRA as a reference standard (each dots represents the result of one study).

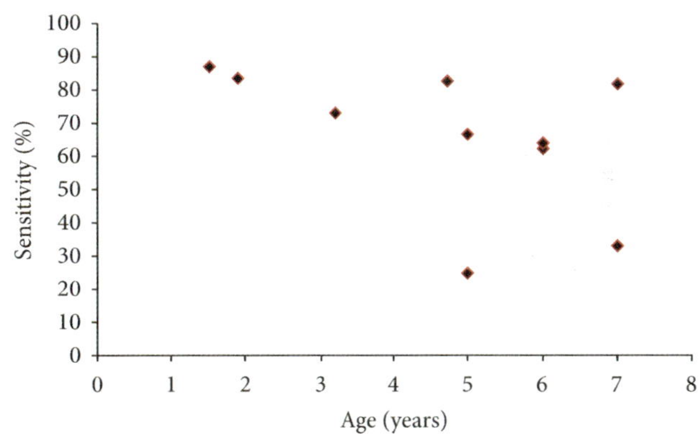

FIGURE 6: Sensitivity of a 10 mm threshold of induration of tuberculin skin test for detection of *M. tuberculosis* infection in relation to age in BCG immunised children using interferon gamma release assay as reference standard.

CI 76.4 to 90.7) in nonimmunised children. Specificity was significantly lower: 74.9% (95% CI 70.4 to 79.1) in immunised compared to nonimmunised children 91.9% (95% CI 84.7 to 96.4).

In the third study by Méndez-Echevarría et al. [10] sensitivity was 82.6% (95% CI 63 to 93) in BCG immunised people compared to 95.9% (95% CI 88.6 to 98.6) in non-immunised people and specificity was 86% (95% CI 80 to 90) in immunised people was significantly lower than in nonimmunised people with 95.5% (95% CI 91.1 to 97.8).

3.4. Comparison of False Negative TST Results with Different TST Induration Thresholds. In BCG immunised children 5, 10 and 15 mm induration thresholds had median (range) false negative rates of 13 (0.0 to 25.4), 30 (13 to 76), and 25 (16.4 to 39.1)%, respectively. In non-BCG immunised children median false negative rates were 6 (0.0 to 11), 5 (0.0 to 16), and 16.4%, respectively. There was no significant difference between false negative rates ($P = 0.43$) comparing different induration thresholds. The result was the same with or without BCG immunisation. For the 10 mm induration

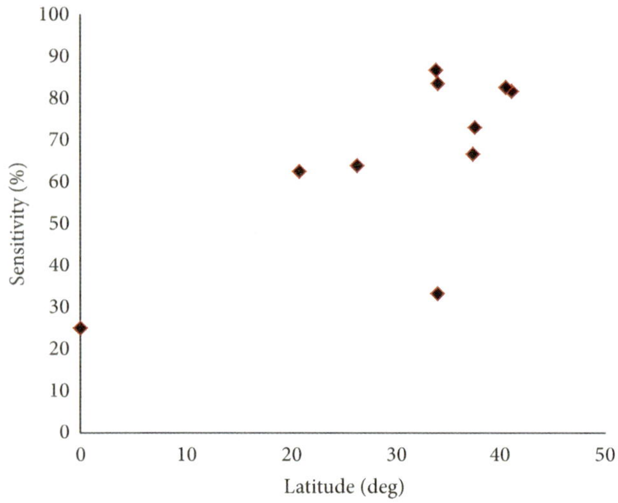

FIGURE 7: Correlation of sensitivity of a 10 mm tuberculin skin test induration threshold in BCG immunised children with geographical latitude of location where studies were conducted: each diamond shaped marker allocates a geographical latitude of the town where the study was located to the sensitivity of the 10 mm induration threshold for studies [1, 4, 5, 7–13].

threshold the false negative rate was significantly higher in BCG immunised versus non-BCG immunised children ($P = 0.014$).

Two studies [5, 11] allowed comparisons of sensitivities and the corresponding false negative TST rates (Table 2) within the same study. For Chun et al. [5] these were not significantly different between TST induration thresholds of 5 and 10 mm ($P = 0.65$). For the study by Kasambira et al. [11] there was also no significant difference in sensitivity and the corresponding false negative TST rates between these induration thresholds ($P = 0.21$).

4. Discussion

4.1. Comparing Parameters Determining Diagnostic Accuracy between Induration Thresholds. This investigation showed that there were no significant differences in sensitivities or specificities between TST induration thresholds of 5, 10, or 15 mm or children with and without BCG immunization, but the number of studies was too small and they were too heterogenous to exclude a clinically significant difference. For the 10 mm threshold BCG immunised children had a lower sensitivity of the TST compared to non-immunized children, which may be due to comorbidities in the South African study [9] (oncology patients) and coinfections in the Ugandan study [13] affecting the TST more than the IGRA. Future studies should investigate whether TST induration threshold should be lower in BCG immunised children to optimise sensitivity.

4.2. The Significance of a False Negative Tuberculin Skin Test. The better correlation of IGRA versus TST with exposure in previous contact investigations particularly in BCG immunised populations was reflection of a higher specificity of IGRA compared to TST. It is thus not the rate of negative IGRA results amongst positive TST results which is clinically relevant but the rate of negative TST results amongst patients with positive IGRA. This latter rate is not likely to represent false positive IGRA results but indicates lower sensitivity of the TST. In view of the increased risk of progression to potentially fatal tuberculous meningitis in children less than two years old the 13 and 16% false negative TST rates at a 10 mm induration in BCG immunised populations with a median age of less than two years of this review [7, 12] suggest that both TST and IGRA should be used simultaneously to investigate *M. tuberculosis* infection if this threshold is used to define TST positivity. A subgroup analysis contained in another of the included studies [1] which did not break down the results according to BCG vaccination status was derived from 32 less than 2-year-old children and found false negative rates for a 5 mm TST induration threshold of 21.9%, for a 10 mm threshold 34.4%, and for a 15 mm threshold 37.5%. Application of an induration threshold of 15 mm for definition of a positive TST in people with previous BCG immunisation was associated with an unacceptably high rate of false negative TST from 24 to 39% in the studies reviewed.

4.3. Investigation of Causes of Inconsistency. Higher geographical latitude was associated with higher sensitivity of the tuberculin skin test in BCG immunised children. This may be due to the fact that BCG immunisation is associated with a reduced effect on the Th1 response to tuberculin at lower latitudes [14, 15]. This may explain the low sensitivity in the Ugandan study. Causes for this observation may include a Th2 dominated immune response associated with helminth infections or concomitant malnutrition reducing a Th1 dominated delayed hypersensitivity reaction. Increased sensitivities of the 10 mm TST threshold with younger age with the highest between 80 and 90% in children between one and two years of age may indicate that there is no reduction of TST sensitivity in younger children.

4.4. Implications for Clinical Practice and Future Research. The use of 5 and 15 mm induration thresholds in TSTs in guidelines for testing of young children for *M. tuberculosis* infection is currently not evidence based. The literature search did not find studies exclusively conducted on infants. The studies available for this review did not contain data on a 5 mm or 15 mm induration threshold for less than two-year-old children but because of the high risk associated with missing *M. tuberculosis* infection an induration threshold of 15 mm should not be used in children <2 years of age. IGRA testing should not be reserved for confirmatory testing in children less than two years of age for any TST induration threshold.

Future studies need to assess sensitivities of TST thresholds for infants measured against IGRA results and need to investigate systematically the influence of systemic inflammatory response syndromes associated with nontuberculous infections and haematological malignancies on the sensitivity of TST compared to IGRA. The influence of BCG immunisation on TST specificity needs to be investigated for all induration thresholds to determine which threshold optimises specificity without compromising sensitivity for all age groups.

5. Conclusions

For the 10 mm threshold there was a lower sensitivity of the TST in BCG immunised children.

Younger age and higher latitude were associated with higher sensitivity of the tuberculin skin test.

Ethical Approval

Ethical or institutional approval and patients consent were not required for this systematic review, which only used anonymous data published in universally accessible journals.

Conflict of Interests

The authors have no conflict of interests and there was no funding involved in the conduct or writing up of the study.

Authors' Contribution

Michael Eisenhut devised the project, analysed the data, and wrote the paper. Katy Fidler and Michael Eisenhut devised the search strategy and independently conducted literature research. Katy Fidler critically revised the paper.

Acknowledgments

The authors thank Jill Fairclough, chief librarian at Brighton & Sussex Medical School, for support in performing a thorough literature search.

References

[1] M. Bakir, D. P. S. Dosanjh, J. J. Deeks et al., "Use of T cell-based diagnosis of tuberculosis infection to optimize interpretation of tuberculin skin testing for child tuberculosis contacts," *Clinical Infectious Diseases*, vol. 48, no. 3, pp. 302–312, 2009.

[2] D. A. Lewinsohn, M. L. Gennaro, L. Scholvinck, and D. M. Lewinsohn, "Tuberculosis immunology in children: diagnostic and therapeutic challenges and opportunities," *International Journal of Tuberculosis and Lung Disease*, vol. 8, no. 5, pp. 658–674, 2004.

[3] M. V. Rose, G. Kimaro, T. N. Nissen et al., "QuantiFERON-TB gold in-tube performance for diagnosing active tuberculosis in children and adults in a high burden setting," *PLoS ONE*, vol. 7, no. 7, Article ID e37851, 2012.

[4] S. Dogra, P. Narang, D. K. Mendiratta et al., "Comparison of a whole blood interferon-γ assay with tuberculin skin testing for the detection of tuberculosis infection in hospitalized children in rural India," *Journal of Infection*, vol. 54, no. 3, pp. 267–276, 2007.

[5] J.-K. Chun, C. K. Kim, H.-S. Kim et al., "The role of a whole blood interferon-γ assay for the detection of latent tuberculosis infection in Bacille Calmette-Guérin vaccinated children," *Diagnostic Microbiology and Infectious Disease*, vol. 62, no. 4, pp. 389–394, 2008.

[6] R. E. B. Taylor, A. J. Cant, and J. E. Clark, "Potential effect of NICE tuberculosis guidelines on paediatric tuberculosis screening," *Archives of Disease in Childhood*, vol. 93, no. 3, pp. 200–203, 2008.

[7] M. P. Nicol, M.-A. Davies, K. Wood et al., "Comparison of T-SPOT. TB assay and tuberculin skin test for the evaluation of young children at high risk for tuberculosis in a community setting," *Pediatrics*, vol. 123, no. 1, pp. 38–43, 2009.

[8] E.-G. Soon, B. K. Lim, H. M. Kim et al., "A tapping the usefulness of whole blood interferon-γ assay for diagnosing tuberculosis infection in children," *Tuberculosis and Respiratory Diseases*, vol. 68, no. 5, pp. 280–285, 2010.

[9] D. C. Stefan, A. Dippenaar, A. K. Detjen et al., "Interferon-gamma release assays for the detection of *Mycobacterium tuberculosis* infection in children with cancer," *International Journal of Tuberculosis and Lung Disease*, vol. 14, no. 6, pp. 689–694, 2010.

[10] A. Méndez-Echevarría, M. González-Muñoz, M. J. Mellado, F. Baquero-Artigao, R. Vecino, and E. Pérez, "Optimizing interpretation of the tuberculin test using an interferon-gamma release assay as a reference standard," *Pediatric Infectious Disease Journal*, vol. 30, no. 5, pp. 426–428, 2011.

[11] T. S. Kasambira, M. Shah, P. V. Adrian et al., "QuantiFERON-TB gold in-tube for the detection of *Mycobacterium tuberculosis* infection in children with household tuberculosis contact," *International Journal of Tuberculosis and Lung Disease*, vol. 15, no. 5, pp. 628–634, 2011.

[12] S. Moyo, F. Isaacs, S. Gelderbloem et al., "Tuberculin skin test and QuantiFERON assay in young children investigated for tuberculosis in South Africa," *International Journal of Tuberculosis and Lung Disease*, vol. 15, no. 9, pp. 1176–1181, 2011.

[13] G. Nkurunungi, J. E. Lutangira, S. A. Lule et al., "Determining *Mycobacterium tuberculosis* infection among BCG-immunised Ugandan children by T-SPOT.TB and tuberculin skin testing," *PLoS ONE*, vol. 7, Article ID e47340, 2012.

[14] M. E. Wilson, H. V. Fineberg, and G. A. Colditz, "Geographic latitude and the efficacy of bacillus Calmette-Guerin vaccine," *Clinical Infectious Diseases*, vol. 20, no. 4, pp. 982–991, 1995.

[15] G. A. W. Rook, K. Dheda, and A. Zumla, "Immune systems in developed and developing countries; implications for the design of vaccines that will work where BCG does not," *Tuberculosis*, vol. 86, no. 3-4, pp. 152–162, 2006.

9

Design of Thymidine Analogues Targeting Thymidilate Kinase of *Mycobacterium tuberculosis*

Luc Calvin Owono Owono,[1,2,3] Melalie Keita,[3,4] Eugene Megnassan,[3,4] Vladimir Frecer,[3,5,6,7] and Stanislav Miertus[3,7,8]

[1] *Laboratory for Simulations and Biomolecular Physics, Advanced Teachers Training College, University of Yaoundé I, P.O. Box 47, Yaoundé, Cameroon*
[2] *Centre for Atomic Molecular Physics and Quantum Optics (CEPAMOQ), University of Douala, P.O. Box 8580, Douala, Cameroon*
[3] *International Centre for Science and High Technology, UNIDO, Area Science Park, Padriciano 99, 34012 Trieste, Italy*
[4] *Laboratoire de Physique Fondamentale et Appliquée, Université d'Abobo-Adjamé, 02 BP 801 Abidjan 02, Cote d'Ivoire*
[5] *Cancer Research Institute, Slovak Academy of Sciences, 83391 Bratislava, Slovakia*
[6] *Department of Physical Chemistry of Drugs, Faculty of Pharmacy, Comenius University, 83232 Bratislava, Slovakia*
[7] *International Centre for Applied Research and Sustainable Technology (ICARST), 81404 Bratislava, Slovakia*
[8] *Faculty of Natural Sciences, University of Ss. Cyril and Methodius, 91701 Trnava, Slovakia*

Correspondence should be addressed to Eugene Megnassan; megnase@yahoo.com

Academic Editor: José R. Lapa e Silva

We design here new nanomolar antituberculotics, inhibitors of *Mycobacterium tuberculosis* thymidine monophosphate kinase (TMPK*mt*), by means of structure-based molecular design. 3D models of TMPK*mt*-inhibitor complexes have been prepared from the crystal structure of TMPK*mt* cocrystallized with the natural substrate deoxythymidine monophosphate (dTMP) (1GSI) for a training set of 15 thymidine analogues (TMDs) with known activity to prepare a QSAR model of interaction establishing a correlation between the free energy of complexation and the biological activity. Subsequent validation of the predictability of the model has been performed with a 3D QSAR pharmacophore generation. The structural information derived from the model served to design new subnanomolar thymidine analogues. From molecular modeling investigations, the agreement between free energy of complexation ($\Delta\Delta G_{\text{com}}$) and K_i values explains 94% of the TMPK*mt* inhibition ($pK_i = -0.2924\Delta\Delta G_{\text{com}} + 3.234$; $R^2 = 0.94$) by variation of the computed $\Delta\Delta G_{\text{com}}$ and 92% for the pharmacophore (PH4) model ($pK_i = 1.0206 \times pK_i^{\text{pred}} - 0.0832$, $R^2 = 0.92$). The analysis of contributions from active site residues suggested substitution at the 5-position of pyrimidine ring and various groups at the 5′-position of the ribose. The best inhibitor reached a predicted K_i of 0.155 nM. The computational approach through the combined use of molecular modeling and PH4 pharmacophore is helpful in targeted drug design, providing valuable information for the synthesis and prediction of activity of novel antituberculotic agents.

1. Introduction

A substantial number of the influenza A subtype H1N1 death cases reported by WHO occurred in patients with chronic respiratory conditions shedding light on possible impact of influenza on active tuberculosis (TB) patients [1]. Tuberculosis kills more than 2 million people [2] and infects around 2 billion worldwide [3] with more than 9 million cases annually [4]. According to WHO in the second millennium decade (2020), over 1 billion people will be newly infected and 36 million will die from TB [5, 6] making it a leading cause of mortality as infectious disease. In this regard, the millennium development goal (MDG) to halve by 2015 TB mortality relative to the 1990 level is problematic [7]. First, mortality in comparison with the 1990 level is slightly decreasing but not in Africa [2]. Secondly, the increased occurrence of MDR and XDR-TB strains is disqualifying the current 40-year-old and long-term DOTS drugs: isoniazid, rifampicin, pyrazinamide, and ethambutol [2]. Accordingly the need of new low-cost and short-term anti-TB therapies is more than urgent regardless those currently in the preclinical or early clinical phase since most of them are improvements on existing antimicrobial compounds with nonnegligible susceptibility to resistance.

The development of new drugs is entirely subordinated to the fulfillment of a particular profile: potency and rapid action short-term DOTS efficiency against MDR-TB safer than existing treatment coadministrable with anti-retrovirals easy to use in the field-action against latent as well as active forms [8]. Another requirement is the increased efficacy on targets relevant to dormancy phase and preventing from "nonproliferation and back resuscitation into growth phase" [3].

In the forthcoming of the availability of appropriated new targets, attention is given to enzymes catalyzing vital processes such as NAD supply [9] or ATP-dependent phosphorylation [10]. TMPK*mt* is the last specific enzyme for the synthesis of dTTP catalyzing dTMP conversion into dTDP using ATP as phosphoryl donor making its inhibitors potential anti-TB drugs targeting DNA replication [11]. So far the most potent thymidine-like inhibitors reported are in low micromolar range (3.5–5 μM) activity. The lack of leads for TMPK*mt* inhibitors and the availability of X-ray crystals structure of the enzyme bound to substrate open the gate to the design of new antitubercular agents with this scaffold [12].

The high-resolution 3D structures of TMPK*mt*-dTMP complexes (K_i = 4.5 μM) have been released at 1.6 Å-1GSI [13] and 1.9 Å-1G3U [14]. The first one with the highest resolution is displayed as 2D interaction view in Figure 1 depicting the interactions of thymine pyrimidine ring: stacking with Phe70 (d = 3.7 Å) and cation-π with Arg95 (d = 5.6 Å). Hydrogen bonds with Arg74 and Asn100 keep the orientation of the pyrimidine ring while the ribose ring's hydroxyl is bonded to Asp9. The orientation of Arg95 is also kept by its HB to one of the phosphate oxygen atoms; this polar group interacts with Tyr39 and the Mg^{2+} ion.

On the basis of these interactions, dTMP analogues have been reported by removing the monophosphate counterpart and Br substitution on the pyrimidine ring resulted in keeping the potency of the substrate [15] opening an important gate since the polarity of the dTMP analogues degrades their ADME profile due to their inability to cross cell-membrane [16]. Focusing on nucleosides instead of nucleotides with a hydroxyl group in place of OPO_3^{2-} for dTMP resulted in a sixfold drop of activity but a simple bromine substitution in the 5-position of the pyrimidine ring kept the initial potency (TMD4, K_i = 5 μM) [15]. This position is not suitable for other halogens F-212 μM, Cl-10 μM, and I-33 μM neither for hydroxyls OH-270 μM, CH_2OH-820 μM nor alkyl chains CH_3CH_2-1140 μM as repulsion was expected in the case of groups larger than CH_3 [15]. No phenyl ring has been tried in that position for this nucleoside but a sevenfold decrease in potency is observed in the case of dTMP with a benzyl ($C_6H_5CH_2$-28 μM) [16]. The stabilizing feature at the 5-position of the pyrimidine ring is not purely hydrophobic, and an orientational part has to be considered. For this we explore here the possibility to design analogues with different small groups in place of the above cited groups bearing both requirements.

The $2'$ position on the ribose ring has been occupied by hydroxyl and halogens with no specific improvement of potency neither. Various substitutions in $3'$ did not improve the potency. Differently the $5'$-position is the second enriching one after that on the pyrimidine ring. Few substitutions have been made beside OH : N_3, $NHCOCH_3$, NH_2, and halogens usually to keep the interactions involving the phosphate group in dTMP analogues. More recently attempts to replace the ribose ring with a phenyl [17] with no real improvement followed by a bicyclic sugar derivatives [18] reaching 3.5 μM and later by a spacer ended by acyclic nucleoside analogues exploring edge to face interaction between the naphthyl group and Tyr39 has led to 0.27 μM potency [19]. A Computer-assisted combinatorial design of bicyclic thymidine analogs as inhibitors of TMPK*mt* by Frecer et al. [20] identified submicromolar concentration range inhibitors with favorable ADME profile.

In the study reported herein the thymidine scaffold is kept with substituted small size group at position 5 of the phenyl ring, $2'$, $3'$ on the ribose ring and finally at $5'$-position taking in to account the structure of the training set (TS). A QSAR model of interaction with TMPK*mt* was built from a TS of 15 TMDs starting from the above mentioned 1GSI.pdb 3D structure to compute the free energy of complexation taking into account the interaction energy, the solvation free energy, numeric solution of the Poisson-Boltzmann scheme and finally the conformational entropy variation of the inhibitor upon binding. The predictability of the model was further crossed with a PH4 3D QSAR one used to screen a library of thymidine analogues (TMAs) for subnanomolar range analogues. The identified hits from the complexation QSAR equation finally reach a predicted activity in the picomolar concentration range.

2. Material and Methods

2.1. Training and Validation Sets. The training and validation sets of thymidine analogues inhibitors of TMPK*mt* used in this study were selected from the literature [15–17]. The inhibitory potencies of these derivatives cover sufficiently broad range of activity to allow a reliable QSAR model to be built ($5 \leq K_i^{exp} \leq 1900$ μM).

2.2. Model Building. Molecular models of the enzyme-inhibitor complexes ($E : I$), free TMPK*mt* (E) and inhibitors (I) were prepared from high-resolution crystal structure of the reference complex containing the deoxythymidine monophosphate TMPK*mt* : dTMP [13] (Protein Data Bank [21] entry code 1GSI at a resolution of 1.6 Å) using Insight-II molecular modeling program [22]. The structures of the E and $E : I$ complexes were considered to be at a pH of 7 with neutral N- and C-terminal residues and all protonizable and ionizable residues charged. No crystallographic water molecule was included into the model. The inhibitors were built into the reference structure complex by *in situ* replacing

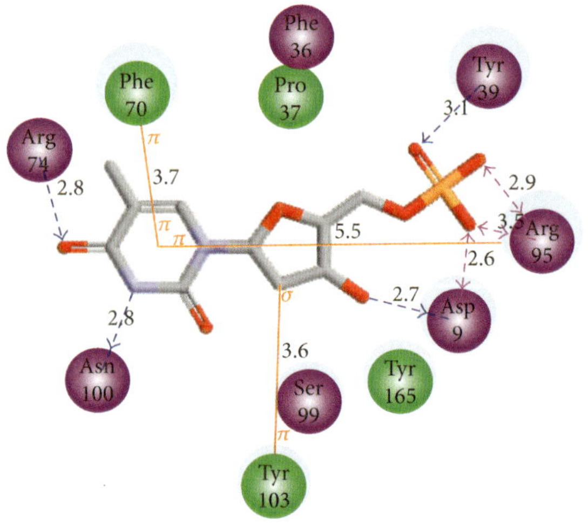

FIGURE 1: Interaction of dTMP with active site residues of TMPK*mt*.

of the derivatized R-group of the dTMP moiety (scaffold). An exhaustive conformational search over all rotatable bonds of the replacing function group, coupled with careful gradual energy minimization of the modified inhibitor and the TMPK*mt* active site residues located in the vicinity of the inhibitor (within 5 Å distance), was employed to identify the low-energy bound conformations of the modified inhibitor. The resulting low-energy structures of the $E : I$ complexes were then carefully refined by minimization of the whole complex. This procedure has been successfully used for model building of viral and protozoal protease-inhibitor complexes and design of peptidomimetic and hydroxynaphthoic inhibitors [23–27].

2.3. Molecular Mechanics. Simulations of the models of inhibitors, TMPK*mt,* and their complexes were carried out with all-atom representation using atomic and charge parameters of the class II consistent force field CFF91 [28]. A dielectric constant of 4 was used for all molecular mechanics (MM) calculations in order to take into account the dielectric shielding effect in proteins. Minimizations of the $E : I$ complexes, free E and I were carried out by relaxing the structures gradually, starting with added hydrogen atoms, continued with residue side chain heavy atoms and followed by the protein backbone relaxation. In all the geometry optimizations, a sufficient number of steepest descent and conjugate gradient iterative cycles were used with the convergence criterion for the average gradient set to 0.01 $\text{kcal}\cdot\text{mol}^{-1}\cdot\text{Å}^{-1}$.

2.4. Conformational Search. Free inhibitor conformations were derived from their bound conformations in the $E : I$ complexes by gradual relaxation to the nearest local energy minimum. Then a Monte Carlo search (with an upper limit of 50,000 iterations) for low-energy conformations over all rotatable bonds except those in the rings was carried out using Cerius^2 molecular modeling package [29]. Two hundred unique conformations were generated for each inhibitor by randomly varying torsion angles of the last accepted conformer by ±15° at 5000 K followed by subsequent energy minimization. During the minimization, a dielectric constant $\varepsilon = 80$ was used to account approximately for the dielectric screening effect of hydration upon the generated conformers. The conformer with the lowest total energy was selected and reminimized at $\varepsilon = 4$.

2.5. Solvation Gibbs Free Energies. The electrostatic component of solvation Gibbs free energy that incorporates also the effects of ionic strength through the solution of nonlinear Poisson-Boltzmann equation [30, 31] was computed by the DelPhi module in Discovery Studio [32]. The program treats the solvent as a continuous medium of high dielectric constant ($\varepsilon_o = 80$) and the solute as a cavity with low dielectric ($\varepsilon_i = 4$) with boundaries linked to the solute's molecular surface, which encloses the solute's atomic charges. The program uses a finite difference method to numerically solve for the molecular electrostatic potential and reaction field around the solute. DelPhi calculations were carried out on a (235×235×235) cubic lattice grid for the $E : I$ complexes and free E and (65 × 65 × 65) grid for the free I with full coulombic boundary conditions. Two subsequent focusing steps led in both cases to a similar final resolution of about 0.3 Å per grid unit at 70% filling of the grid by the solute. Physiological ionic strength of 0.145 $\text{mol}\cdot\text{dm}^{-3}$, atomic partial charges and radii defined in the CFF91 parameter set [28] and a probe sphere radius of 1.4 Å were used. The electrostatic component of the solvation Gibbs free energy was calculated as the reaction field energy [30, 33–35].

2.6. Entropic Term. The vibrational entropy change during the inhibitor binding to the E was calculated by normal mode analysis of the inhibitor vibrations using a simplified method of Fischer et al. [36, 37]. In this approach, vibrational analysis of the inhibitor bound at the active site of a "frozen" receptor (E) and of the low-energy conformer of the free inhibitor is computed for fully minimized structures using Discover [22] and $T\Delta S_{\text{vib}} = TS_{\text{vib}}\{I\}_E - TS_{\text{vib}}\{I\}$. It has been shown previously that for small and relatively stiff ligands this method gives a good approximation of the vibrational entropy change of the fully flexible system, that is, including the degrees of freedom of the protein receptor [36, 37]. The $TS_{\text{vib}}\{I\}$ term accounts for vibrational motions of the free inhibitor and represents an indicator of conformational flexibility of the molecule. Namely, low frequency vibrations, which correspond to collective motions of a number of atoms with larger amplitudes, that is, conformational changes, contribute most to this term. Relative values of $T\Delta\Delta S_{\text{vib}}$ with respect to a reference inhibitor were used to compensate partially for the restricted flexibility of E. Although enthalpic contribution to binding affinity is important, the enthalpy/entropy balance is acting more and more as descriptor of selectivity bringing drug optimization to a multidimensional approach [38].

2.7. Calculation of Binding Affinity. Inhibition constant (K_i) of a reversible inhibitor I is related to the standard Gibbs free energy (GFE) change of the formation of $E : I$ complex

(ΔG_{com}) in a solvent. The K_i value can thus be predicted from the complexation GFE $\Delta G_{\text{com}} = -\text{RT}\ln K_i$ assuming the following equilibrium:

$$\{E\}_{\text{aq}} + \{I\}_{\text{aq}} \longleftrightarrow \{E:I\}_{\text{aq}}, \quad (1)$$

where $\{\}_{\text{aq}}$ indicates solvated species. The standard GFE change of reaction (1) can be derived by molecular simulations of the complex and the free reactants:

$$\Delta G_{\text{com}} = G\{E:I\} - G\{E\} - G\{I\}. \quad (2)$$

In this work, we approximate the exact values of standard GFE for larger systems such as enzyme-inhibitor complexes by the expression [25, 26]:

$$G\{E:I\} \approx [E_{\text{MM}}\{E:I\} + \text{RT} - TS_{\text{trv}}\{E:I\}] + G_{\text{sol}}\{E:I\}, \quad (3)$$

where $E_{\text{MM}}\{E:I\}$ stands for the molecular mechanics total energy of the complex (including bonding and nonbonding contributions), and $G_{\text{sol}}\{E:I\}$ is the solvation GFE and $TS_{\text{trv}}\{E:I\}$ the entropic term:

$$TS_{\text{trv}}\{E:I\} = TS_{\text{tran}}\{E:I\} + TS_{\text{rot}}\{E:I\} + TS_{\text{vib}}\{E:I\} \quad (4)$$

composed of a sum of contributions arising from translational, rotational, and vibrational motions of $E:I$. Assuming that the trans and rot terms for the free E and the complex $E:I$ are approximately equal, we obtain

$$\begin{aligned}\Delta G_{\text{com}} \approx\ & [E_{\text{MM}}\{E:I\} - E_{\text{MM}}\{E\} - E_{\text{MM}}\{I\}] \\ & + [G_{\text{sol}}\{E:I\} - G_{\text{sol}}\{E\} - G_{\text{sol}}\{I\}] \\ & + TS_{\text{tran}}\{I\} + TS_{\text{rot}}\{I\} \\ & - [TS_{\text{vib}}\{E:I\} - TS_{\text{vib}}\{E\} - TS_{\text{vib}}\{I\}] \\ =\ & \Delta H_{\text{MM}} + TS_{\text{tran}}\{I\} + TS_{\text{rot}}\{I\} \\ & - \Delta TS_{\text{vib}} + \Delta G_{\text{sol}},\end{aligned} \quad (5)$$

where $TS_{\text{tran}}\{I\}$ and $TS_{\text{rot}}\{I\}$ describe the translational and rotational entropy terms of the free inhibitor, and ΔTS_{vib} represents the vibrational entropy change upon the complex formation.

Comparison between different inhibitors was done via relative changes in the complexation GFE with respect to a reference inhibitor, I_{ref}, assuming ideal gas behaviour for the rotational and translational motions of the inhibitors:

$$\begin{aligned}\Delta\Delta G_{\text{com}} &= \Delta G_{\text{com}}(I) - \Delta G_{\text{com}}(I_{\text{ref}}) \\ &= \Delta\Delta H_{\text{MM}} - \Delta\Delta TS_{\text{vib}} + \Delta\Delta G_{\text{sol}}.\end{aligned} \quad (6)$$

The evaluation of relative changes is preferable as it is expected to lead to partial cancellation of errors caused by the approximate nature of the molecular mechanics method as well as solvent and entropic effects description.

2.8. Interaction Energy. To calculate MM interaction energy (E_{int}) between enzyme residues and the inhibitor, a protocol available in Discovery Studio [32] that computes the nonbonded interactions (van der Waals and electrostatic terms) between defined sets of atoms was used. The calculations were performed using the CFF91 force field [28] with a dielectric constant of (5).

2.9. Pharmacophore Generation. Bound conformations of inhibitors taken from the models of $E:I$ complexes were used for building of 3D QSAR pharmacophore by means of Catalyst HypoGen algorithm [39] implemented in Discovery Studio [32]. The top scoring pharmacophore hypothesis was built up in three steps (constructive, subtractive, and optimization steps) from the set of most active inhibitors. Inactive molecules served for definition of the excluded volume. The maximum number of five features allowed by the HypoGen algorithm was selected based on the TMD scaffold and substituents during the pharmacophore generation, namely: hydrophobic aromatic (HYdAr), hydrophobic aliphatic (HYd), hydrogen bond donor, (HBD), hydrogen-bond acceptor (HBA), and ring aromatic (Ar). Adjustable parameters of the protocol were kept at their default values except the uncertainty on the activity, which was set to 1.5 instead of 3. This last choice to bring the uncertainty interval on experimental activity from the large $\langle K_i/3, 3 \times K_i\rangle$ to a relatively narrow $\langle 2 \times K_i/3, 3 \times K_i/2\rangle$ taking account in this way of the accuracy and homogeneity of the measured inhibitory activities since they are coming from the same work in the same laboratory. During the generation of 10 pharmacophores, the number of missing features was set to 0 and the best one was selected.

3. Results and Discussion

A training set of 15 TMDs and validation set of 6 TMVs were selected from 3 series of compounds with measured activities from the same laboratory [14–16]. They are listed in Table 1 and their experimental activity (5–1900 μM) covers a range sufficiently large to build a reliable QSAR model.

3.1. QSAR Models. The relative Gibbs free energy in (2) was computed for the complexes from *in situ* modification of dTMP as described in Material and Methods. Table 2 lists the Gibbs free energy and its components. The $\Delta\Delta G_{\text{comp}}$ reflects the mutual affinity between the enzyme and the inhibitor. Since it is computed from simulations in an approximate way, the consistency of the binding model is evaluated through a regression analysis leading to linear correlation with experimental activity K_i. The statistical data of these regressions are illustrated in Figure 3 and listed in Table 3. From the regression equation, the computed $\Delta\Delta G_{\text{comp}}$ for a novel compound similar to TMDs is used to predict its enzyme inhibitory activity K_i^{pred} provided they share the same binding mode. This process usually can narrow the filter to new lead compounds and save time compared with traditional synthesis approach. From the complexation model structures the computed breakdown of the contribution of

Table 1: Training and validation sets of TMD inhibitors for QSAR model.

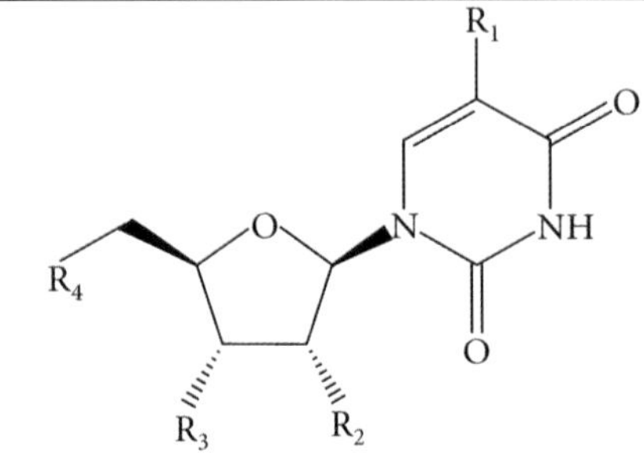

Training set	R_1	R_2	R_3	R_4	K_i^{exp} (μM)	Reference
TMD1	-------H	-------H	-------OH	-------OH	1020	[15]
TMD2	-------F	-------H	-------OH	-------OH	212	
TMD3	-------I	-------H	-------OH	-------OH	33	
TMD4	-------Br	-------H	-------OH	-------OH	5	
TMD5	-------CH_3	-------H	-------OH	-------N_3	7	[17]
TMD6	-------CH_3	-------OH^a	-------OH	-------OH	238	
TMD7	-------F	-------OH	-------OH	-------OH	521	
TMD8	-------CH_3	-------H	-------NH_2	-------OH	230	
TMD9	-------CH_3	-------OH	-------NH_2	-------H	1900	
TMD10	-------CH_3	-------H	-----/NH_2	-------OH	57	[16]
TMD11	-------CH_3	-------H	-------CH_2F	-------OH	45	
TMD12	-------CH_3	-------H	-------CH_2OH	-------OH	41	
TMD13	-------CH_3	-------OH	-----/NH_2	-------OH	393	
TMD14	-------CH_3	-------H	-----/‾‾‾OH	-------OH	156	
TMD15	-------CH_3	-------H	-------OH	-------OH	27	
Validation set	R_1	R_2	R_3	R_4	K_i^{exp} (μM)	Reference
TMV1	-------CH_3	-------H	-------OH	---HN–C(=O)–CH_3	90	[15–17]
TMV2	-------CH_3	-------OH	-------OH	-------OH	715	
TMV3	-------CH_2CH_3	-------H	-------OH	-------OH	1148	
TMV4	-------CH_3	-------H	-------F	-------OH	28	
TMV5	-------CH_2OH	-------H	-------OH	-------OH	820	
TMV6	-------OH	-------H	-------OH	-------OH	270	

[a]Hydroxyl in β position.

each TMPK*mt* active site residue to the interaction with TMD4 (K_i = 5 μM) E_{int}{TMPK*mt* : TMD4} is compared with the one of TMA12 (K_i^{pred} = 0.155 μM) E_{int}{TMPK*mt* : TMA12} in Figure 4. It comes out clearly from TMD4 to TMA12 that except Tyr39 all the residues involved in strong interaction with TMD4 remain in close contact with TMA12 (Figures 2 and 5(c)) with a noticeable increase of the contributions to E_{int} for Phe70, Pro37, Arg74, and Tyr165.

3.2. Binding Mode of Inhibitors. The binding modes of TMDs derived from the complexation model are illustrated in Figures 1 and 2. The main interactions at the active site formerly reported from the X-ray structure are conserved except the HBs involving the monophosphate moiety with Arg95, Tyr39, and ribose OH with Asp9 while additional HBs are established with Ala49 and Asp163. The stacking interaction pyrimidine ring, Phe70, is kept along with the

TABLE 2: Complexation energy and its components for the training set of TMPK*mt* inhibitors: TMD1–TMD15.

Training set[a]	M_w [b] ($g \cdot mol^{-1}$)	$\Delta\Delta H_{MM}$ [c] ($kcal \cdot mol^{-1}$)	$\Delta\Delta G_{sol}$ [d] ($kcal \cdot mol^{-1}$)	$\Delta\Delta TS_{vib}$ [e] ($kcal \cdot mol^{-1}$)	$\Delta\Delta G_{comp}$ [f] ($kcal \cdot mol^{-1}$)	K_i^{exp} [g] (μM)
TMD1	228	0	0	0	0	1020
TMD2	246	−3.942	3.537	−1.968	−2.373	212
TMD3	354	−4.695	1.873	−2.196	−5.017	33
TMD4	306	−1.631	−3.514	−1.742	−6.887	5
TMD5	333	−5.880	1.212	−2.238	−6.906	7
TMD6	258	−3.461	3.613	−1.371	−1.220	238
TMD7	262	−5.157	7.239	−1.510	0.571	521
TMD8	242	3.496	−4.720	0.378	−0.847	230
TMD9	242	1.916	−1.255	0.786	1.447	1900
TMD10	256	−0.110	−3.672	−0.390	−4.172	57
TMD11	258	−21.643	22.028	−3.572	−3.187	45
TMD12	256	−1.323	0.216	−2.213	−3.320	41
TMD13	272	3.727	−3.906	−2.715	−2.894	393
TMD14	270	−3.988	6.637	−3.934	−1.286	156
TMD15	242	−6.706	9.914	−5.140	−1.932	27
Validation set	M_w [$g \cdot mol^{-1}$]	$\Delta\Delta H_{MM}$ [$kcal \cdot mol^{-1}$]	$\Delta\Delta G_{sol}$ [$kcal \cdot mol^{-1}$]	$\Delta\Delta TS_{vib}$ [$kcal \cdot mol^{-1}$]	$\Delta\Delta G_{comp}$ [$kcal \cdot mol^{-1}$]	pK_i^{pred}/pK_i^{exp}
TMV1	283	−1.641	−0.724	−1.807	−4.172	1.100
TMV2	258	−4.852	6.608	−0.372	1.385	0.899
TMV3	256	−4.166	2.479	−0.282	−1.969	1.296
TMV4	244	2.350	−4.156	−1.145	−2.951	0.899
TMV5	258	−4.310	3.609	−0.527	−1.228	1.164
TMV6	244	−3.999	2.689	−1.471	−2.780	1.134

[a] For the chemical structures of the training set of inhibitors see Table 1.
[b] M_w is the molecular mass of the inhibitor.
[c] $\Delta\Delta H_{MM}$ is the relative enthalpic contribution to the Gibbs free energy change related to the protease-inhibitor complex formation derived by molecular mechanics (MM): $\Delta\Delta H_{MM} \cong [E_{MM}\{PR{:}TMDx\} - E_{MM}\{TMDx\}] - [E_{MM}\{PR{:}TMD1\} - E_{MM}\{TMD1\}]$, TMD1—is the reference inhibitor;
[d] $\Delta\Delta G_{solv}$ is the relative solvation Gibbs free energy contribution to the Gibbs free energy change related to protease-inhibitor complex formation: $\Delta\Delta G_{solv} = [G_{solv}\{PR{:}TMDx\} - G_{solv}\{TMDx\}] - [G_{sol}\{PR{:}TMD1\} - G_{sol}\{TMD1\}]$;
[e] $-\Delta\Delta TS_{vib}$ is the relative entropic contribution of the inhibitor to the Gibbs free energy related to protease-inhibitor complex formation: $\Delta\Delta TS_{vib} = [TS_{vib}\{TMDx\}_{PR} - TS_{vib}\{TMDx\}] - [TS_{vib}\{TMD1\}_{PR} - TS_{vib}\{TMD1\}]$;
[f] $\Delta\Delta G_{comp}$ is the relative Gibbs free energy change related to the enzyme-inhibitor complex formation: $\Delta\Delta G_{comp} \cong \Delta\Delta H_{MM} + \Delta\Delta G_{solv} - \Delta\Delta TS_{vib}$.
[g] K_i^{exp} is the experimental TMPK*mt* inhibition constant obtained from [15–17].
[h] Ratio of predicted and experimental inhibition constants $pK_i^{pre}/pK_i^{exp} \cdot K_i^{pre}$ was predicted from computed $\Delta\Delta G_{comp}$ using the regression equation for TMPK*mt* shown in Table 3.

TABLE 3: Statistical information on regression analysis of correlation for the training set between $\Delta\Delta G_{comp}$ and experimental activities (pK_i) respectively against TMPK*mt*.

$pK_i = -0.2924\,\Delta\Delta G_{comp} + 3.234$	
Statistical data of regression analysis	$\Delta\Delta G_{comp}$
Number of compounds n	15
Squared correlation coefficient of regression R^2	0.944
LOO cross-validated squared correlation coefficient R^2_{XV}	0.939
Standard error of the regression σ	0.184
Statistical significance of regression, Fisher F-test F	218.3
Level of statistical significance α	>95%
Range of activity of K_i (μM)	5–1900

cation-π interaction with Arg95. This last interaction is the main driving force of the substrate-like orientation of TMDs. The binding mode of dTMP scaffold as reported from X-ray structures is reproduced by our model based on thymidine scaffold making enrichment of interactions by new substitutions straightforward provided the accuracy of our predictive equation is sufficiently stable to cover the nanomolar range with the assumption that structurally similar ligands bind in a similar fashion. A quick analysis of the training set shows that halogen in the 5-position on pyrimidine ring is not the main feature for potency confirmed by the relatively low activity of TMD2-3. At the other ends in 5′-position only N3 bring substantial increase of potency. These two positions are of great importance for activity as indicated by the pharmacophore features in Figure 6. It is easy to appreciate the weight of each feature since CH3 in 5-position in a majority of inhibitors did not improve the inhibitory potency resulting in a 5-fold decrease in TMD15 (27 μM) compared with Br in TMD4 (5 μM). The cation-π

TABLE 4: Designed analogs with predicted activity.

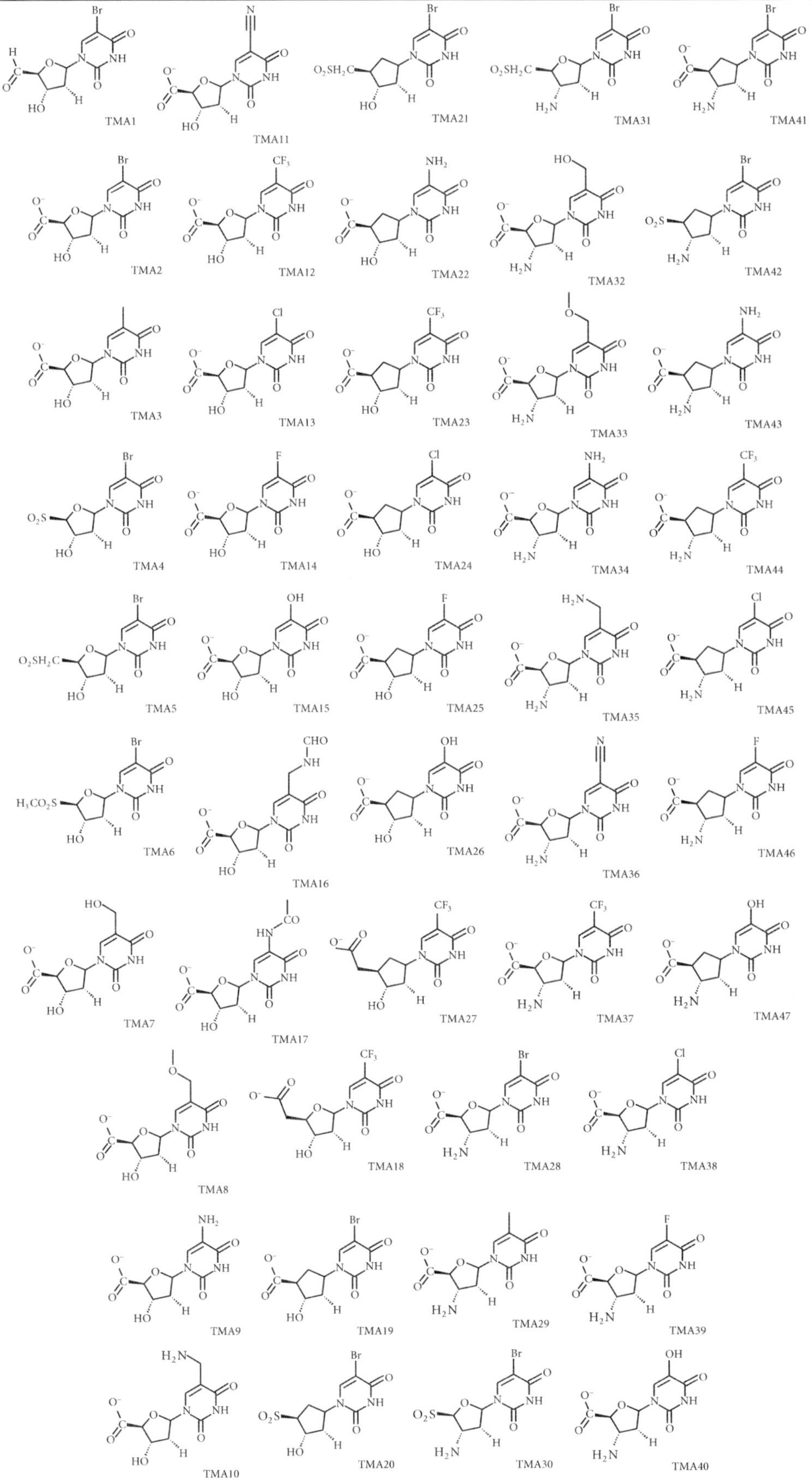

TABLE 4: Continued.

Analogue	M_w [b]	$\Delta\Delta H_{MM}$ [c]	$\Delta\Delta G_{sol}$ [d]	$\Delta\Delta TS_{vib}$ [e]	$\Delta\Delta G_{comp}$ [f]	K_i^{pre} (nM)
TMA1	305	−7.01	1.28	−1.52	−7.24	4457
TMA2	320	−16.01	3.67	−2.70	−15.03	24
TMA3	255	−14.98	3.25	−0.82	−12.55	125
TMA4	340	−7.76	−0.63	−4.21	−12.60	121
TMA5	354	−7.45	1.14	−5.05	−11.35	280
TMA6	355	−4.20	−2.90	−3.10	−10.21	606
TMA7	271	−18.39	4.66	−1.98	−15.71	15
TMA8	285	−17.68	6.85	−3.21	−14.03	46
TMA9	256	−14.51	4.59	−1.11	−11.03	348
TMA10	270	−14.88	3.32	−1.82	−13.38	72
TMA11	266	−14.67	4.31	−1.96	−12.32	146
TMA12	309	−21.47	3.47	−4.49	−22.49	0.155
TMA13	275	−15.99	3.31	−2.34	−15.02	24
TMA14	259	−14.85	2.97	−2.05	−13.93	49
TMA15	257	−16.21	3.82	−1.42	−13.82	53
TMA16	298	−20.08	3.41	−5.82	−22.50	0.155
TMA17	298	−19.78	3.14	−4.68	−21.32	0.341
TMA18	323	−21.50	18.09	−6.50	−9.91	741
TMA19	318	−15.10	3.43	−1.75	−13.42	69
TMA20	338	−5.13	−0.73	−2.60	−8.46	1962
TMA21	352	−6.36	0.77	−4.34	−9.92	733
TMA22	254	−13.68	4.05	−0.81	−10.44	518
TMA23	307	−21.15	15.85	−4.74	−10.04	676
TMA24	273	−15.14	2.31	−1.35	−14.18	42
TMA25	257	−14.61	3.02	−1.91	−13.50	66
TMA26	255	−15.25	2.97	−0.69	−12.97	94
TMA27	321	−19.66	19.04	−6.67	−7.29	4305
TMA28	319	−12.29	2.96	−2.17	−11.50	254
TMA29	254	−11.30	2.59	−0.77	−9.48	989
TMA30	339	−3.88	−1.82	−3.66	−9.36	1067
TMA31	353	−3.74	0.46	−5.27	−8.55	1849
TMA32	270	−14.46	3.17	−1.79	−13.08	87
TMA33	284	−13.86	6.19	−3.03	−10.71	431
TMA34	255	−10.78	3.93	−0.95	−7.80	3054
TMA35	269	−11.32	2.64	−1.73	−10.41	528
TMA36	265	−10.92	3.66	−1.45	−8.71	1658
TMA37	308	−17.88	2.81	−4.63	−19.70	1
TMA38	274	−12.24	2.62	−1.82	−11.44	265
TMA39	258	−11.05	2.26	−1.55	−10.34	554
TMA40	256	−12.45	3.23	−1.09	−10.31	564
TMA41	317	−12.78	2.85	−3.03	−12.96	95
TMA42	337	−2.27	−1.60	−3.68	−7.56	3606
TMA43	253	−11.28	3.32	−2.61	−10.57	474
TMA44	306	−17.31	15.03	−5.22	−7.50	3749
TMA45	272	−12.80	2.22	−2.69	−13.27	77
TMA46	256	−11.71	2.74	−2.29	−11.26	298
TMA47	254	−12.54	2.36	−1.30	−11.48	257

[a, b, c, d, e, f] See Table 2.

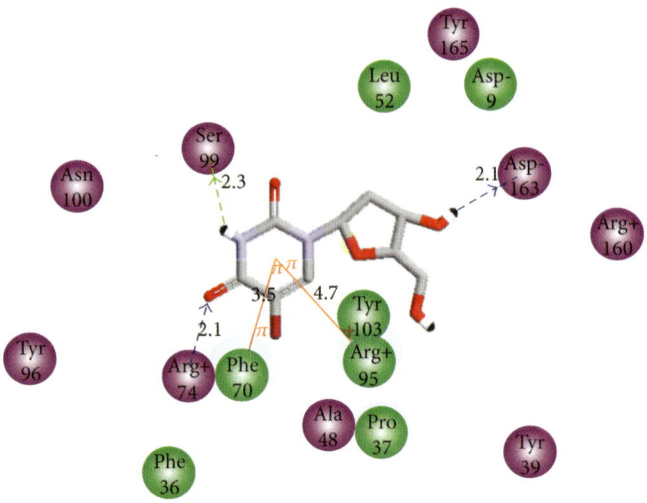

FIGURE 2: Interaction of TMD4 with active site residues of TMPK*mt*.

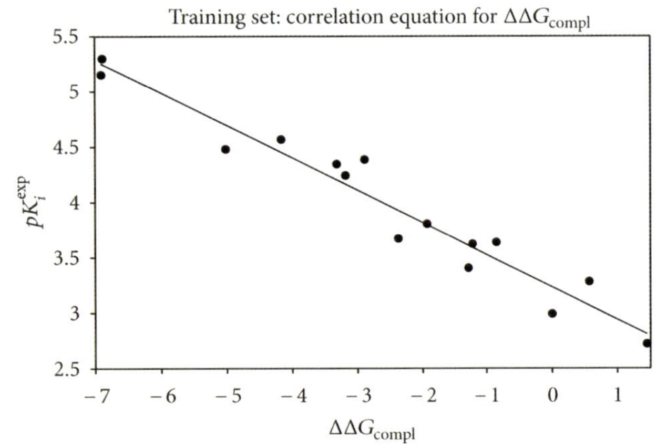

FIGURE 3: Plot of the correlation equation between pK_i^{exp} and relative complexation Gibbs free energy of the training set.

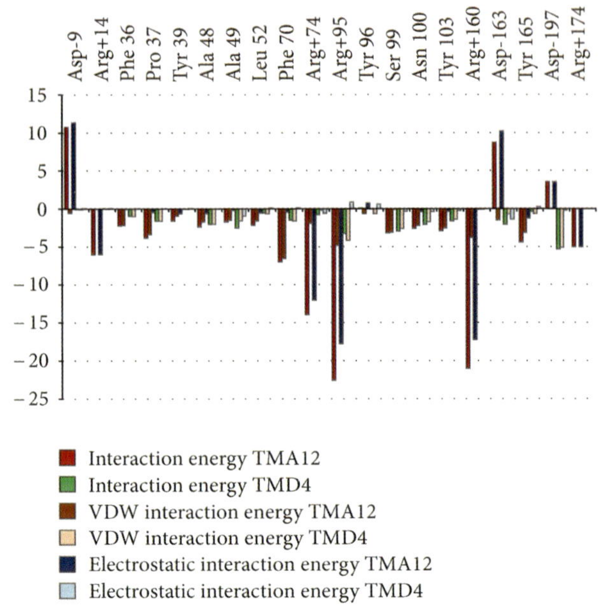

FIGURE 4: Interaction Energy breakdown comparison for the most active training set compound TMD4 and for the most active designed TMA12.

interaction between the pyrimidine ring and Agr95 (32% of E_{int}\{TMPK*mt* : TMA12\}) is conserved along with the π-π stacking involving Phe70 (10% of E_{int}\{TMPK*mt* : TMA12\}) as we can see in Figure 5(c).

3.3. Pharmacophore Model of Inhibitory Activity. The 3D QSAR PH4 generation process follows three main steps, the constructive, the subtractive, and the optimization steps. The constructive phase of HypoGen automatically selected as lead compounds ($5 \leq K_i \leq 7\,\mu$M) for which ($5 \times 1.5 - K_i/1.5 > 0$) TMD4 and TMD5 using these top two to generate all the starting PH4 features and retaining only those fitting the remaining leads. The subtractive phase in which inactive compounds ($\log(K_i) - \log(5) > 3.5$) are used to remove features that map more than 50% of them retained representatives of all the selected five features. In the optimization phase using the simulated annealing algorithm the highest scoring PH4s are retained according to their probability function-based cost. A total of 10 hypotheses were generated all displaying four features. The costs range from 55.1 (Hypo1) to 75.2 (Hypo10). This short gap supports the homogeneity of the hypotheses and the adequacy of the training set. The fixed cost (45.9) is lower than the null cost (157.4) by $\Delta = 111.5$. This difference is a major quality indicator of the PH4 predictability; $\Delta > 70$ corresponds to an excellent chance or a probability higher than 90% that the model represents a true correlation [32]. To be statistically significant the hypothesis has to be as closer as possible to the fixed and as further as possible from the null cost, for this set of 10 hypotheses $\Delta \geq 82.2$ attests the quality of the model. The standard indicators like the root-mean-square deviations (RMSD) and the correlation coefficients (R^2) range from 1.126 to 2.036 and from 0.96 to 0.88, respectively. Due to the closed values for the whole set of PH4s, the first hypothesis (Hypo1) has been retained for further analysis.

The data for the set of hypotheses (costs, RMSD, R) are listed in Table 5. The statistical data of Hypo1; $pK_i = 1.0206 \times K_i^{\text{pred}} - 0.0832$ ($n = 15$, $R^2 = 0.92$, $R^2_{\text{XV}} = 0.91$, $F = 132.1$, $\sigma = 0.231$ at a significance level >95%) are illustrated by the correlation plot in Figure 6 showing also the geometry of the pharmacophore and TMD4 and TMD5 mapping to it. To check the consistency of the model, we predicted the activity (pK_i) of the validation set (TMVs: TMV1-1.65; TMV2-1.16, TMV3-1.56, TMV4-1.26, TMV5-0.82, TMV6-1.02) all close to one except TMV1 and TMV3.

The randomization validation (Fisher method) of the PH4 model by CatScramble algorithm in Catalyst has been carried out from 49 random runs according to the 98% confidence level selected creating each time 10 valid hypotheses. Finally none of them was as predictive as the 10 lowest listed in Table 5, their costs ranged from 56 to 87 for the closest and from 116 to 135 for the highest; neither their

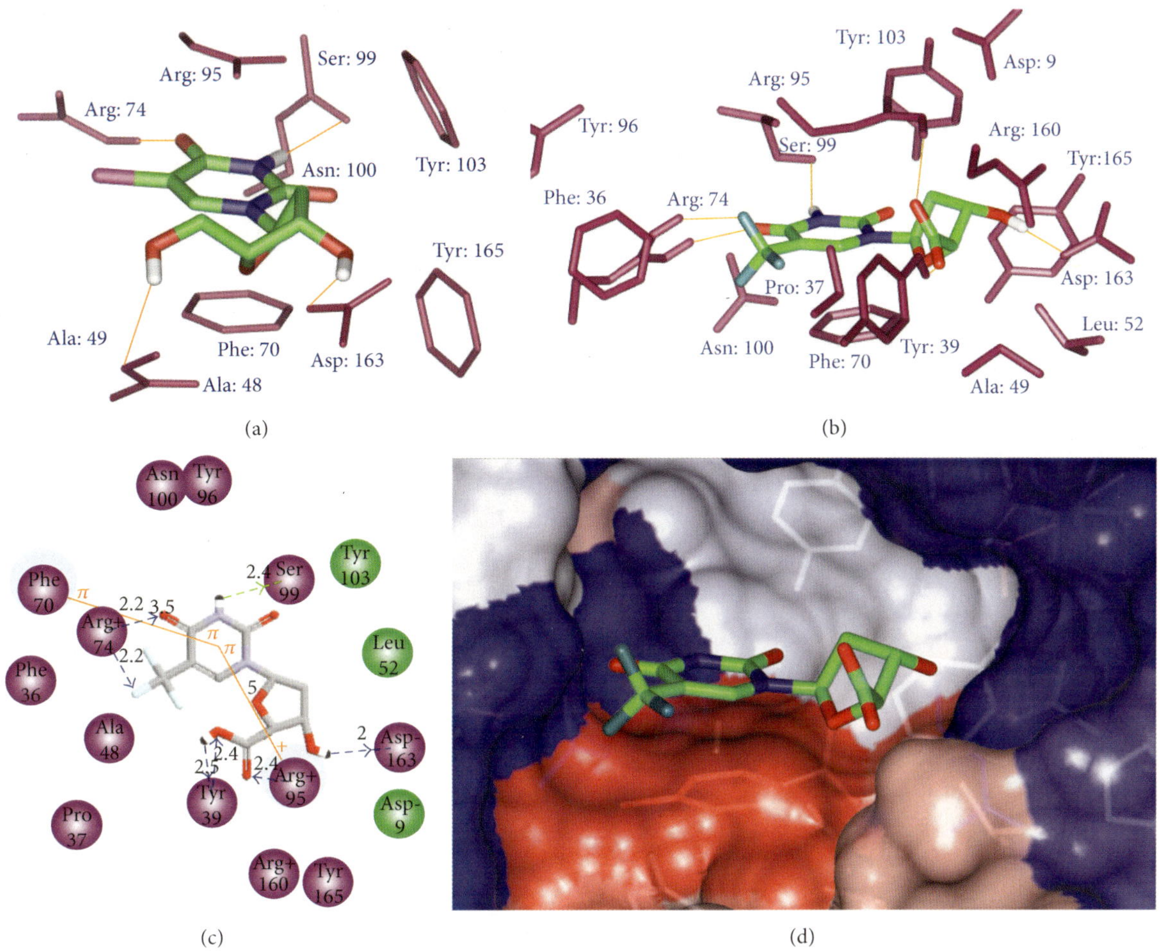

FIGURE 5: Close-up of TMD4 (a) and TMA12 (b) at the active site of TMPK*mt*. Hydrogen bonds are shown in orange color and the residues are in purple color. Interactions of inhibitor TMA12 at the active site in 2D depiction (c). Connolly surface of the same active site (d). The binding cleft surface is colored according to residue hydrophobicity: red-hydrophobic, blue-hydrophilic and white-intermediate residues.

TABLE 5: Output parameters of the 10 generated PH4 Hypotheses after CatScramble validation procedure for TMPK*mt* inhibitors listing RMSD, total cost and *R* correlation coefficient.

Hypothesis	RMSD	*R*	Total costs
Hypo1	1.126	0.964	55.1
Hypo2	1.207	0.958	57.1
Hypo3	1.477	0.936	61.1
Hypo4	1.802	0.904	68.7
Hypo5	1.831	0.901	69.7
Hypo6	1.941	0.888	72.3
Hypo7	1.975	0.883	73.7
Hypo8	2.016	0.878	74.4
Hypo9	2.023	0.877	75.2
Hypo10	2.036	0.876	75.2
Fixed cost	0	1.0	45.9
Null cost	4.213	0	157.4

correlation nor RMSD were better. To recapitulate there is 98% probability that the selected hypotheses provide a model at the same level of predictability as the complexation one for the biological activity of TMDs. The design of the new analogues of this work is based partially on the hydrophobic feature representing CH_3 group of the thymine ring. It was also the unique feature observed by Gopalakrishnan et al. [12] in a virtual screening approach for TMPK*mt* inhibitors. The difference between the null and the fixed cost in their case was 45 lower than the 70 threshold needed for a good predictability quality. Three HBA and one HBD features were added to the Hyd one in the model. The interfeature distances are different; in our model, the closest HBA to the Hyd is at 2.995 Å instead of 4.43 Å, 6.083 instead of 6.88 Å. It has to be indicated also that the HBD feature is related to the hydroxyl group of the ribose ring and accordingly the bound conformation being different from the free ligand one differences is expected from both pharmacophores and the nonavailability of the angle from their PH4 model makes a full comparison difficult.

The new inhibitors have been designed in respect to the PH4. A recent 3D pharmacophore study of substituted α-Thymidine Analogues inhibitors of TMPK*mt* using optimized receptor-independent (RI) 4D QSAR formalism [40]

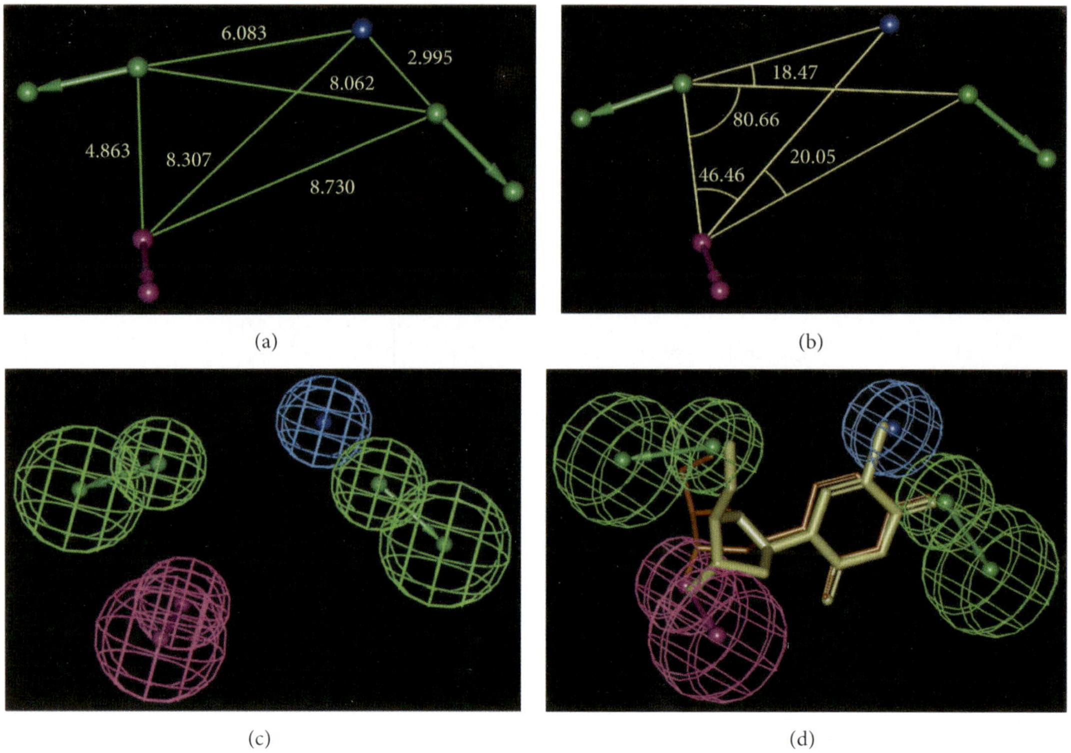

FIGURE 6: TMPK*mt* inhibition pharmacophore coordinates (a) and (b), features (c) and mapping (d) with TMD4 (purple) and TMD5 (yellow). The correlation plot of predicted versus experimental inhibitory activity is displayed in Figure 7.

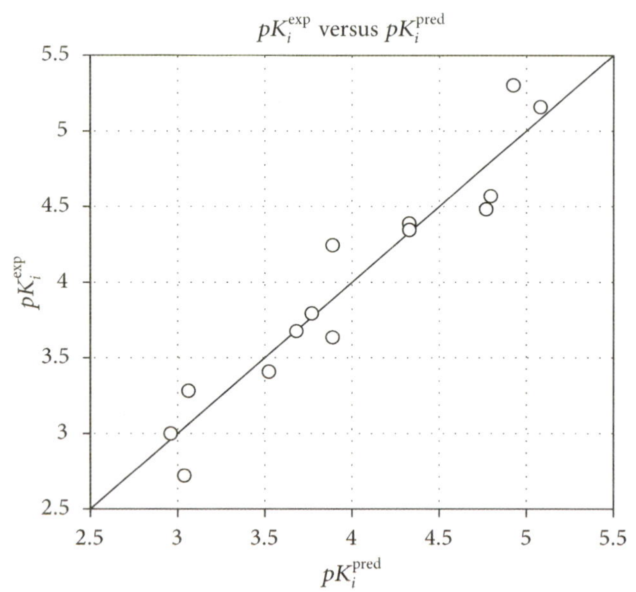

FIGURE 7: Plot of the correlation equation between pharmacophore (PH4) predicted and experimental inhibitory activity of the training set TMDs.

identified five Grid Cell Occupancy Descriptors (GCODs) for close interaction with Arg95 and Tyr103-Arg74-Asp163, Asp9 and Arg95-Ala35, Phe36, Pro37, and Arg160-Met66 and Phe70. One is inhibition-enhancing (close to the pyrimidine ring carbonyl in 4-position) and the other four inhibition diminishing. From this list only Ala35 and Met66 are missing in our QSAR model list of active site residues in close interaction with the inhibitors. The positions of the GCODs correspond globally with our generated PH4 model features.

3.4. New Inhibitors. The novel analogues are based mostly on the substitution in the 5-position on the pyrimidine ring, 2′ and 3′ of the ribose. More global replacement such as ribose → cyclopentane and a capping carboxylate at the 5′ end. They are listed in Table 4 (see also Figure 5), the most active ones reaching picomolar concentration range.

3.4.1. Substitution at the 5′ End (R_4). Keeping all the remaining moiety unchanged, the 5′ hydroxyl group in the training set has been replaced with various (TMA1-6, TMA18) polar groups among which the carboxylate COO^- performed the best but with a fivefold decrease of potency ($K_i = 24$ nM) from TMD4. As we can see from Figure 5(b), the carboxylate interacts through two HB with Arg95 and Tyr39 bringing substantial affinity towards TMPK*mt*. The former OH was not involved in any HB (Figure 2). About this additional HB with Tyr39 it is interesting to point out, among the few differences of the binding sites of TMPK*mt* and TMPK*h* (the human corresponding enzyme-PDB code 1E99) where Arg14, Tyr39 and Asn100 are replaced in the last one by Ser20, Arg45 and Gly102, respectively [41], the crucial opportunity to exploit this structural and functional difference (interaction with Tyr39) to design selective inhibitors for TMPK*mt*. Recent attempts of extension by replacement of the carboxylate COO^- with other groups resulting in 5′-modified thymidines are promising [42].

3.4.2. Substitution at the 5-Position of the Pyrimidine Ring (R_1). Keeping the carboxylate group and the ribose ring (R_2=H and R_3=OH) in place, replacement of bromine at the 5-position (TMA7-17) resulted in noticeable increase of potency for TMA12 $R_1=CF_3$-K_i = 0.155 nM, TMA16 $R_1=CH_2$–NH–CHO-K_i = 0.155 nM, and TMA17 R_1=NH–$COCH_3$-K_i = 0.341. The trifluoromethyl group is in a supplemental HB contact with Arg74 adding to the cation-π (Arg95) and π-π interaction (Phe70) of the pyrimidine ring (Figure 5(b)).

3.4.3. Substitution at the 3′ Position of the Ribose Ring (R_3). In order to improve the predicted potency for TMA12, 16 and 17 replacement of OH by NH_2 on the ribose ring does not result in any increase in predicted inhibitory activity, the best one TMA37 K_i = 1 nM being sixfold less potent than TMA12. Any other design modification, for example replacement of ribose by a cyclopentane, led to a decrease of potency (TMA19–27 and TMA41–47).

Figures 5(b) and 5(c) show the main interactions supporting the affinity of TMA12 in comparison with those coming out from our QSAR model for TMDs. The Connolly surface presented in Figure 5(d) suggests further design opportunities such as bicyclic 2′,3′-ring inhibitors of TMPK*mt* [20] and extension of the carboxylate end to derivatives carrying a naphtholactam or naphthosultam moiety at position 4 of a (Z)-butenyl chain [43]. The design of this class of inhibitors requires appropriate training set available (K_i: 0.42–0.75 μM). We are building the QSAR model and new analogues will be released in due course [44].

The contribution of the residues specific to TMPK*mt* to E_{int}{TMPK*mt* : TMA12} (Figure 4) globally 15% breakdown into Arg14 (9%), Tyr39 (2%) and Asn100 (4%) is encouraging compared with their value for E_{int}{TMPK*mt* : TMD4} globally 3.5% limited to Asn100 (3%) for the most active training set inhibitor.

4. Conclusions

The interaction model built based on complexation methodology and validated by a PH4 analysis provided structural information helpful in the design of new analogues. They are structurally close to reported dTMP analogues. Here a carboxylate in place of 5′-position hydroxyl increased their inhibitory potency reaching low to subnanomolar range (1–0.155 nM). One of the most potent new analogue TMA12 is HB bonded to the selective Tyr39 making the best of TMAs a promising set for synthesis and evaluation. A more systematic search through screening of combinatorial library and subsequent evaluation on enzymatic assay will lead to more potent analogues.

References

[1] P. Nunn and D. Falzon, "WHO information note on tuberculosis and pandemic influenza A, (H1N1)," 2009, http://www.who.int/tb/features_archive/h1n1_and_tuberculosis.pdf.

[2] E. L. Korenromp, A. L. Bierrenbach, B. G. Williams, and C. Dye, "The measurement and estimation of tuberculosis mortality," *International Journal of Tuberculosis and Lung Disease*, vol. 13, no. 3, pp. 283–303, 2009.

[3] D. J. Murphy and J. R. Brown, "Novel drug target strategies against *Mycobacterium tuberculosis*," *Current Opinion in Microbiology*, vol. 11, no. 5, pp. 422–427, 2008.

[4] "global tuberculosis control—surveillance, planning, financing," WHO Report, 2008, http://www.who.int/tb/publications/global_report/2008/en/index.html.

[5] M. D. Raviglione, D. E. Snider Jr., and A. Kochi, "Globa epidemiology of tuberculosis. Morbidity and mortality of a worldwide epidemic," *The Journal of the American Medical Association*, vol. 273, no. 3, pp. 220–226, 1995.

[6] WHO Global Tuberculosis Programme, "Tuberculosis," Fact sheet no. 104, 2002, http://www.who.int/mediacentre/factsheets/fs104/en/.

[7] C. Dye, D. Maher, D. Weil, M. Espinal, and M. Raviglione, "Targets for global tuberculosis control," *International Journal of Tuberculosis and Lung Disease*, vol. 10, no. 4, pp. 460–462, 2006.

[8] H. Lång, G. Quaglio, and O. F. Olesen, "Tuberculosis research in the European Union: past achievements and future challenges," *Tuberculosis*, vol. 90, no. 1, pp. 1–6, 2010.

[9] H. I. M. Boshoff, X. Xu, K. Tahlan et al., "Biosynthesis and recycling of nicotinamide cofactors in *Mycobacterium tuberculosis*: an essential role for NAD in nonreplicating bacilli," *Journal of Biological Chemistry*, vol. 283, no. 28, pp. 19329–19341, 2008.

[10] A. Lavie, N. Ostermann, R. Brundiers et al., "Structural basis for efficient phosphorylation of 3′-azidothymidine monophosphate by *Escherichia coli* thymidylate kinase," *Proceedings of the National Academy of Sciences of the United States of America*, vol. 95, no. 24, pp. 14045–14050, 1998.

[11] A. Haouz, V. Vanheusden, H. Munier-Lehmann et al., "Enzymatic and structural analysis of inhibitors designed against *Mycobacterium tuberculosis* thymidylate kinase: new insights into the phosphoryl transfer mechanism," *Journal of Biological Chemistry*, vol. 278, no. 7, pp. 4963–4971, 2003.

[12] B. Gopalakrishnan, V. Aparna, J. Jeevan, M. Ravi, and G. R. Desiraju, "A virtual screening approach for thymidine monophosphate kinase inhibitors as antitubercular agents based on docking and pharmacophore models," *Journal of Chemical Information and Modeling*, vol. 45, no. 4, pp. 1101–1108, 2005.

[13] T. Ursby, M. Weik, E. Fioravanti, M. Delarue, M. Goeldner, and D. Bourgeois, "Cryophotolysis of caged compounds: a technique for trapping intermediate states in protein crystals," *Acta Crystallographica Section D*, vol. 58, no. 4, pp. 607–614, 2002.

[14] I. Li De La Sierra, H. Munier-Lehmann, A. M. Gilles, O. Bârzu, and M. Delarue, "X-ray structure of TMP kinase from *Mycobacterium tuberculosis* complexed with TMP at 1.95 Å resolution," *Journal of Molecular Biology*, vol. 311, no. 1, pp. 87–100, 2001.

[15] S. Pochet, L. Dugué, G. Labesse, M. Delepierre, and H. Munier-Lehmann, "Comparative study of purine and pyrimidine nucleoside analogues acting on the thymidylate kinases of *Mycobacterium tuberculosis* and of humans," *ChemBioChem*, vol. 4, no. 8, pp. 742–747, 2003.

[16] V. Vanheusden, P. Van Rompaey, H. Munier-Lehmann, S. Pochet, P. Herdewijn, and S. Van Calenbergh, "Thymidine and thymidine-5′-O-monophosphate analogues as inhibitors of *Mycobacterium tuberculosis* thymidylate kinase," *Bioorganic and Medicinal Chemistry Letters*, vol. 13, no. 18, pp. 3045–3048, 2003.

[17] C. Gasse, D. Douguet, V. Huteau, G. Marchal, H. Munier-Lehmann, and S. Pochet, "Substituted benzyl-pyrimidines targeting thymidine monophosphate kinase of *Mycobacterium tuberculosis*: synthesis and in vitro anti-mycobacterial activity," *Bioorganic and Medicinal Chemistry*, vol. 16, no. 11, pp. 6075–6085, 2008.

[18] I. Van Daele, H. Munier-Lehmann, P. M. S. Hendrickx et al., "Synthesis and biological evaluation of bicyclic nucleosides as inhibitors of *M. tuberculosis* thymidylate kinase," *ChemMedChem*, vol. 1, no. 10, pp. 1081–1090, 2006.

[19] O. Familiar, H. Munier-Lehmann, A. Negri et al., "Exploring acyclic nucleoside analogues as inhibitors of *Mycobacterium tuberculosis* thymidylate kinase," *ChemMedChem*, vol. 3, no. 7, pp. 1083–1093, 2008.

[20] V. Frecer, P. Seneci, and S. Miertus, "Computer-assisted combinatorial design of bicyclic thymidine analogs as inhibitors of *Mycobacterium tuberculosis* thymidine monophosphate kinase," *Journal of Computer-Aided Molecular Design*, vol. 25, no. 1, pp. 31–49, 2011.

[21] H. M. Berman, J. Westbrook, Z. Feng et al., "The protein data bank," *Nucleic Acids Research*, vol. 28, no. 1, pp. 235–242, 2000.

[22] "Insight-II and discover molecular modeling and simulation package," version 2005, Accelrys, San Diego, Calif, USA, 2005.

[23] V. Frecer, M. Kabeláč, P. De Nardi, S. Pricl, and S. Miertuš, "Structure-based design of inhibitors of NS3 serine protease of hepatitis C virus," *Journal of Molecular Graphics and Modelling*, vol. 22, no. 3, pp. 209–220, 2004.

[24] V. Frecer, A. Jedinak, A. Tossi et al., "Structure based design of inhibitors of aspartic protease of HIV-1," *Letters in Drug Design and Discovery*, vol. 2, no. 8, pp. 638–646, 2005.

[25] V. Frecer, F. Berti, F. Benedetti, and S. Miertus, "Design of peptidomimetic inhibitors of aspartic protease of HIV-1 containing -PheΨPro- core and displaying favourable ADME-related properties," *Journal of Molecular Graphics and Modelling*, vol. 27, no. 3, pp. 376–387, 2008.

[26] B. Dali, M. Keita, E. Megnassan, V. Frecer, and S. Miertus, "Insight into selectivity of peptidomimetic Inhibitors with modified statine core for plasmepsin II of *Plasmodium falciparum* over human cathepsin D," *Chemical Biology and Drug Design*, vol. 79, no. 4, pp. 411–430, 2012.

[27] E. Megnassan, M. Keita, C. Bieri, A. Esmel, V. Frecer, and S. Miertus, "Design of novel dihydroxynaphthoic acid inhibitors of *Plasmodium falciparum* lactate dehydrogenase," *Medicinal Chemistry*, vol. 8, no. 5, pp. 970–984, 2012.

[28] J. R. Maple, M. J. Hwang, T. P. Stockfish et al., "Derivation of class II force fields. 1. Methodology and quantum force field for the alkyl functional group and alkane molecules," *Journal of Computational Chemistry*, vol. 15, no. 2, pp. 162–182, 1994.

[29] "Cerius2 life sciences molecular simulation software," version 4.6, Accelrys, San Diego, Calif, USA, 2002.

[30] M. K. Gilson and B. Honig, "The inclusion of electrostatic hydration energies in molecular mechanics calculations," *Journal of Computer-Aided Molecular Design*, vol. 5, no. 1, pp. 5–20, 1991.

[31] W. Rocchia, S. Sridharan, A. Nicholls, E. Alexov, A. Chiabrera, and B. Honig, "Rapid grid-based construction of the molecular surface and the use of induced surface charge to calculate reaction field energies: applications to the molecular systems and geometric objects," *Journal of Computational Chemistry*, vol. 23, no. 1, pp. 128–137, 2002.

[32] "Discovery studio molecular modeling and simulation program," version 2.5, Accelrys, San Diego, Calif, USA, 2009.

[33] C. J. F. Böttcher, *Theory of Electric Polarization*, Elsevier Press, Amsterdam, The Netherlands, 1973.

[34] S. Miertus, E. Scrocco, and J. Tomasi, "Electrostatic interaction of a solute with a continuum. A direct utilizaion of AB initio molecular potentials for the prevision of solvent effects," *Chemical Physics*, vol. 55, no. 1, pp. 117–129, 1981.

[35] V. Frecer and S. Miertus, "Polarizable continuum model of solvation for biopolymers," *International Journal of Quantum Chemistry*, vol. 42, no. 5, pp. 1449–1468, 1992.

[36] S. Fischer, J. C. Smith, and C. S. Verma, "Dissecting the vibrational entropy change on protein/ligand binding: Burial of a water molecule in bovine pancreatic trypsin inhibitor," *Journal of Physical Chemistry B*, vol. 105, no. 33, pp. 8050–8055, 2001.

[37] S. M. Schwarzl, T. B. Tschopp, J. C. Smith, and S. Fischer, "Can the calculation of ligand binding free energies be improved with continuum solvent electrostatics and an ideal-gas entropy correction?" *Journal of Computational Chemistry*, vol. 23, no. 12, pp. 1143–1149, 2002.

[38] E. Freire, "Do enthalpy and entropy distinguish first in class from best in class?" *Drug Discovery Today*, vol. 13, no. 19-20, pp. 869–874, 2008.

[39] H. Li, J. Sutter, and R. Hoffmann, "HypoGen: an automated system for generating 3D predictive pharmacophore models," in *Pharmacophore Perception, Development and Use in Drug Design*, O. F. Güner, Ed., pp. 171–189, International University Line, La Jolla, Calif, USA, 2000.

[40] C. H. Andrade, K. F. M. Pasqualoto, E. I. Ferreira, and A. J. Hopfmger, "Rational design and 3D-pharmacophore mapping of 5′-thiourea- substituted α-thymidine analogues as mycobacterial TMPK inhibitors," *Journal of Chemical Information and Modeling*, vol. 49, no. 4, pp. 1070–1078, 2009.

[41] N. Ostermann, A. Lavie, S. Padiyar et al., "Potentiating AZT activation: structures of wild-type and mutant human thymidylate kinase suggest reasons for the mutants' improved kinetics with the HIV prodrug metabolite AZTMP," *Journal of Molecular Biology*, vol. 304, no. 1, pp. 43–53, 2000.

[42] K. S. Toti, F. Verbeke, M. D. P. Risseeuw, V. Frecer, H. Munier-Lehmann, and S. Van Calenbergh, "Synthesis and evaluation of 5′-modified thymidines and 5-hydroxymethyl-2′-deoxyuridines as *Mycobacterium tuberculosis* thymidylate kinase inhibitors," *Bioorganic and Medicinal Chemistry*, vol. 21, no. 1, pp. 257–268, 2013.

[43] O. Familiar, H. Munier-Lehmann, A. Negri et al., "Exploring acyclic nucleoside analogues as inhibitors of *Mycobacterium tuberculosis* thymidylate kinase," *ChemMedChem*, vol. 3, no. 7, pp. 1083–1093, 2008.

[44] A. Kumar, E. Megnassan, I. Siddiqi, V. Frecer, and S. Miertus, "Rationa design of inhibitors of *Mycobacterium tuberculosis* Thymidine monophosphate kinase," In press.

10

Antimycobacterial Activities of Novel 5-(1H-1,2,3-Triazolyl)Methyl Oxazolidinones

Oludotun Adebayo Phillips,[1] Edet Ekpenyong Udo,[2] and Reny Varghese[1]

[1] *Department of Pharmaceutical Chemistry, Faculty of Pharmacy, Kuwait University, P.O. Box 24923, Safat 13110, Kuwait*
[2] *Department of Microbiology, Faculty of Medicine, Kuwait University, P.O. Box 24923, Safat 13110, Kuwait*

Correspondence should be addressed to Oludotun Adebayo Phillips, dphillips@hsc.edu.kw

Academic Editor: Zarir Farokh Udwadia

The antibacterial activities of a series of triazolyl oxazolidinones against *Mycobacterium tuberculosis* strain *in vitro* and *in vivo* in a mice model are presented. Most active compounds were noncytotoxic against VERO cells with acceptable selectivity indexes (SI) as measures of compound tolerability. Structure activity relationships (SARs) revealed that analogs with alkylcarbonyl (IC_{90}: < 0.2 to 0.422 μg/mL) and arylcarbonyl (IC_{90}: < 0.2 to 2.103 μg/mL) groups at the piperazine 4N-position-displayed potent antimycobacterium activities, comparable to the methanesulfonyl (IC_{90}: < 0.2 μg/mL) analog, linezolid (IC_{90}: < 0.2 μg/mL), and isoniazid (IC_{90}: < 0.034 μg/mL). The furanylcarbonyl derivative also displayed potent activity, while the arylsulfonyl analogs were inactive. Of the triazolyl oxazolidinones, the morpholino (PH-27) derivative with medium bioavailability in plasma was most active *in vivo*, but relatively less efficacious than isoniazid.

1. Introduction

Tuberculosis (TB) caused by *Mycobacterium tuberculosis*, a contagious and fatal disease, is considered a global epidemic and a major threat to public health. TB is becoming more prevalent in the world today than any other time in human history. It has been estimated that over a third of the world's population is infected with the TB bacilli, with 9.4 million new cases and nearly 1.7 million deaths in 2009 [1, 2]. Most infected people harbor latent TB infection (LTBI), and people with HIV/AIDS and compromised immune system are more likely to develop the disease. TB continues to be a leading cause of death in HIV/AIDS patients, forming a lethal combination.

A number of drugs, namely, isoniazid, rifampicin, ethambutol, and pyrazinamide are often administered over a prolonged period of time and may lead to the development of resistant strains due to patient-poor compliance among other factors. The development and spread of resistant *M. tuberculosis*, pose a vital challenge to the control of TB worldwide. In recent years, the emergence and spread of resistant *M. tuberculosis* strains has fuelled the TB epidemic by making it more difficult to treat. Multidrug-resistant (MDR) TB, which is resistant to the first line anti-TB agents, namely, isoniazid and rifampicin are increasing with >500,000/yr new cases of MDR-TB worldwide [3, 4]. Extensively drug-resistant (XDR) TB, resistant to first line anti-TB agents, namely, isoniazid, rifampicin, fluoroquinolones, and one of three injectable drugs, such as capreomycin, kanamycin, or amikacin is awfully difficult to treat and is considered a worldwide threat to TB control [3, 4]. These statistics serve as impetus for development of more effective and safer anti-TB drugs [5]. For more than 40 years, there has been a drought of new anti-TB drugs. However, more recently, there are increasing reports of newer agents demonstrating activity against drug-resistant *M. tuberculosis* strains [5–8]. Among these new agents are the oxazolidinones (linezolid—**LZD**; and **PNU-100480**; Figure 1), diarylquinoline (**TMC-207**; Figure 1), the nitroimidazole-oxazole (**OPC-67683**; Figure 1), the nitroimidazo-oxazine (**PA-824**, Figure 1), and some quinolone class of compounds. Linezolid (**LZD**; Figure 1), a prototypical oxazolidinone used in the clinic to treat gram-positive bacterial infections, the thiomorpholino derivative of **LZD** (**PNU-100480**; Figure 1), and others in

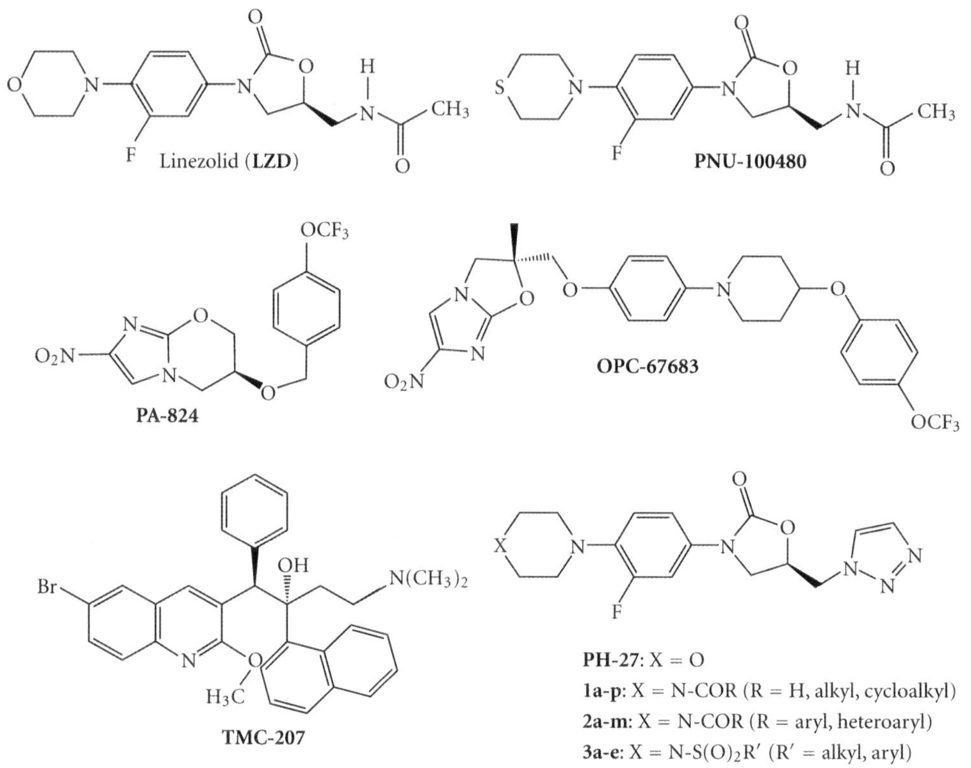

FIGURE 1: Chemical structure of oxazolidinone antibacterial agents and novel antimycobacterial agents.

this class, have demonstrated activity against susceptible and drug-resistant *M. tuberculosis.* Our laboratories have been interested in the synthesis of triazolylmethyl oxazolidinones of general structures **PH-27**, **1**, **2**, and **3** (Figure 1) with antibacterial activity [9–12]. Studies from other laboratories and ours have shown that the triazolyl oxazolidinones have potent activity against gram-positive bacterial species [9–14], comparable or superior to linezolid *in vitro*, thus affirming the bioisosteric replacement of the C5 acetamido functional group by the triazolyl moiety. On the basis of the potent antibacterial activities of the triazolyl oxazolidinones and the demonstrated antimycobacterium activities of representative oxazolidinones, namely, **LZD** and **PNU-100480**, we evaluated the anti*Mycobacterium tuberculosis* activity of selected novel triazolylmethyl oxazolidinones synthesized from our laboratories. Therefore, this study outlines the *in vitro* and *in vivo* antimycobacterial activity of selected triazolylmethyl oxazolidinones and to establish observable qualitative structure-activity relationships.

2. Materials and Methods

2.1. Synthesis of Compounds. The preparation of the compounds **1a-p**, **2a-m**, and **3a-e** has been described previously [9–12]. The reference antituberculosis agents isoniazid (**INH**) and linezolid (**LZD**) were provided by the Tuberculosis Antimicrobial Acquisition and Coordinating Facility (TAACF), Southern Research Institute, Birmingham, AL., USA.

2.2. Antituberculosis Susceptibility Testing. The *in vitro* antitubercular testing was determined according to the protocols of the Tuberculosis Antimicrobial Acquisition and Coordinating Facility (TAACF), USA [15, 16]. The activity of all compounds against replicating *M. tuberculosis* H37Rv (ATCC 27294, American Type Culture Collection, Rockville, MD, USA) was performed in BACTEC 12B medium using a fluorescence readout in the Microplate Alamar Blue Assay (MABA) according to the TAACF initial primary screen assays. Compounds were dissolved in 80% DMSO or 60% EtOH in water or H_2O and tested in ten 2-fold dilutions, ranging from 0.19 to 100 μg/mL; the IC_{90} (μg/mL) values defined as "inhibitory concentration" effecting a reduction in fluorescence of 90% relative to the controls. The values were determined from dose-response curves, and compounds with $IC_{90} \leq 10\,\mu$g/mL were considered active for antitubercular activity.

2.3. Mammalian VERO Cell Cytotoxicity (CC_{50}) Assay. The compounds were screened to assess toxicity to African green monkey kidney (VERO) cells using the Promage's Cell Titer Glo Luminescent Cell Viability assay by TAACF. The assay returns a CC_{50} value, which allows a selectivity index (SI: ratio of CC_{50}/IC_{90}) to be calculated. Compounds with SI value $\geq$ 10 are considered safe for further screening.

2.4. Preliminary In Vivo Bioavailability Testing (BioAssay). All *in vivo* assays/evaluations were determined according to

Table 1: *In vitro* antimycobacterium activity of 4N-acylpiperazinyl oxazolidinones against *M. tuberculosis* H37Rv.

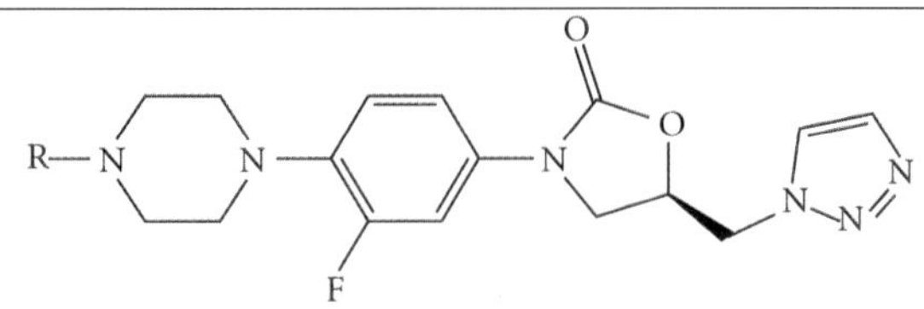

Compd.	–R	Clog *P* values	IC_{90} (μg/mL)	CC_{50} (μg/mL) VERO	SI
1a	HCO	−1.1502	<0.20	>37.43	>187.1
b	CH_3CO	−1.2042	<0.20	>41.64	>208.2
c	CF_3CO	−0.0952	0.281	>44.23	>156.8
d	$CHCl_2CO$	0.1218	<0.20	>45.72	>228.6
e	CH_3CH_2CO	−0.6752	0.334	>40.24	>120.4
f	CH_3CH_2OCO	0.9748	0.422	>41.84	>98.91
g	$(CH_3)_2CHCO$	−0.3662	0.283	>41.64	>146.6
h	$(CH_3)_3COCO$	1.6828	<0.20	>44.64	>223.2
i	$CH_3(CH_2)_4CO$	0.9118	<0.20	>44.45	>222.2
j	cyclohexanoyl	0.8268	2.095	>45.65	>21.79
k	$CH_3(CH_2)_5CO$	1.4408	<0.20	>45.85	>229.2
l	$CH_3(CH_2)_6CO$	1.9698	<0.20	>47.25	>236.2
m	$CH_3(CH_2)_7CO$	2.4988	<0.20	>48.65	>243.2
n	$CH_3(CH_2)_8CO$	3.0278	<0.20	>50.06	>250.3
o	$CH_3(CH_2)_9CO$	3.5568	<0.20	>51.46	>257.3
p	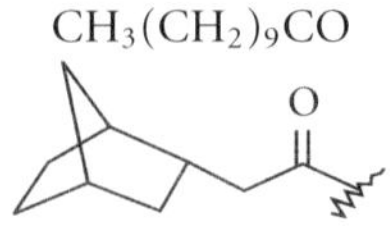	1.7208	<0.20	>48.25	>241.2
PH-27	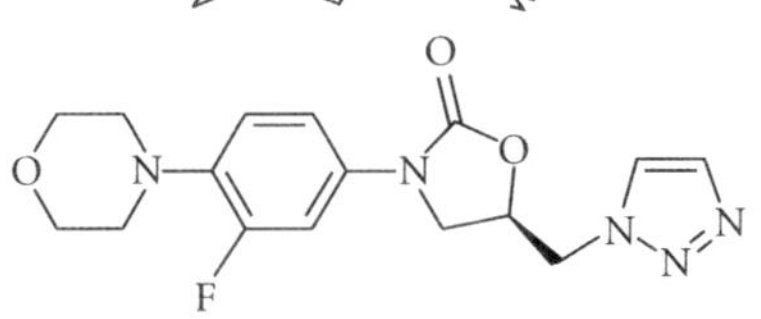	0.6308	0.466	>34.73	>74.53
LZD	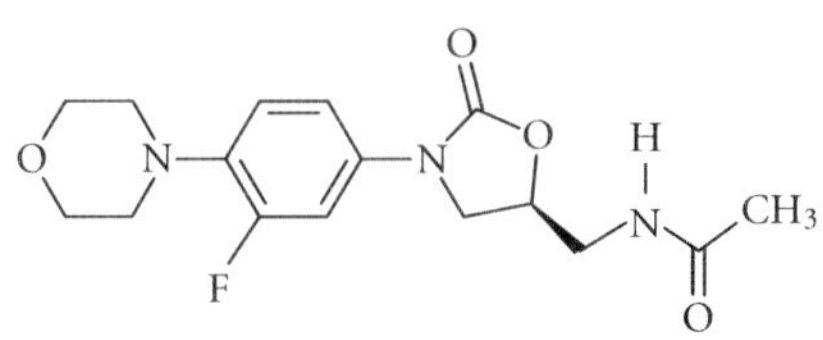	0.5321	<0.20	>33.73	>168.6
INH	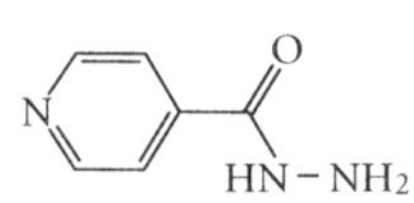	−0.668	0.034	>100	>2941

the TAACF protocols [15]. This assay was used to estimate drug levels in mice at specific time points after oral dosing, using the inhibition of growth of *M. tuberculosis* H37Rv as an indicator for drug activity. Selected compounds were orally dosed (300 mg/kg in 0.5% methyl cellulose) in three C57BL/6 mice and the animals were bled by nicking the lateral vein at 30 mins and 2.5 hrs, respectively, to collect blood samples. The blood samples were allowed to clot and centrifuged to collect serum, which were serially diluted and added to 96-well assay plates containing *M. tuberculosis* H37Rv (10^4 bacterial) on 100 μL 7H9 broth with 10% serum. Each assay also contains lanes of wells with drugs of known concentrations, with or without 10% mouse serum. Inhibition of bacterial growth was determined by optical density (λ = 600 nm) measurements every 3-4 days up to 14 days. The results were further confirmed by visual inspection at 10 days. Inhibition of bacterial growth in the assay (<50% of control without drugs) indicates sufficiently high concentration of compound in blood and hence an acceptable bioavailability.

2.5. In Vivo Efficacy Gamma Knock-Out (GKO) Mouse Model. Interferon gamma knockout female mice C57BL/6 IFN-KO ($n = 5$) unable to control an infection of *M. tuberculosis* were

Table 2: *In vitro* antimycobacterium activity of 4N-arylcarbonyl- and 4N-arylsulfonyl-piperazinyl oxazolidinones against *M. tuberculosis* H37Rv.

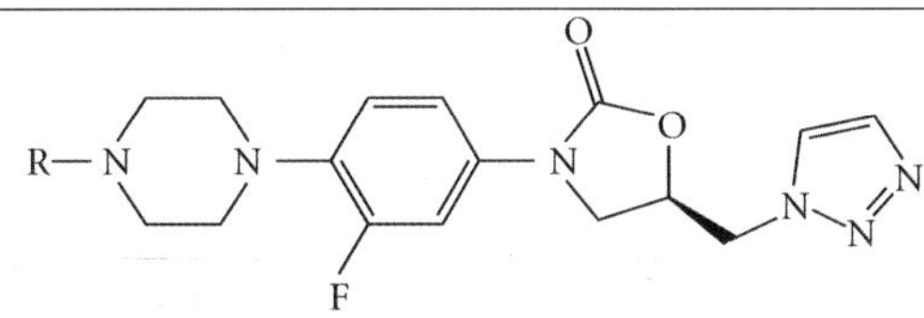

Compd.	–R	$C\log P$ values	IC_{90} (μg/mL)	CC_{50} (μg/mL) VERO	SI
2a	PhCO	0.6148	0.722	>45.04	>62.3
b	4-ClPhCO	1.4304	<0.20	>48.49	>242.4
c	3-NO_2PhCO	0.5198	0.759	>49.54	>65.27
d	2-CH_3PhCO	1.1138	3.375	>46.45	>13.76
e	3-CH_3PhCO	1.1138	0.422	>46.45	>110
f	4-CH_3PhCO	1.1138	2.103	>46.45	>22.08
g	2-CH_3OPhCO	0.8347	1.04	>48.05	>46.15
h	3-CH_3OPhCO	0.8347	0.829	>48.05	>57.89
i	4-CH_3OPhCO	0.8347	0.843	>48.05	>56.93
j	2-furylCO	−0.2092	<0.20	>44.04	>220.2
k	2-thienylCO	0.3913	0.209	>45.65	>217.3
l	3-pyridylCO	−0.4862	0.236	>45.14	>190.4
m	2-Cl 3-pyridylCO	0.2641	1.389	>48.59	>34.98
3a	CH_3SO_2	−0.6042	<0.20	>42.44	>212.2
b	2-furylSO_2	1.0658	>100 (0.419)[a]	n/d	n/d
c	PhSO_2	1.3448	5.469	>48.65	>8.896
d	3-CH_3PhSO_2	1.8438	>100 (1.024)[a]	n/d	n/d
e	4-CH_3PhSO_2	1.8438	>100[a]	n/d	n/d
PH-27	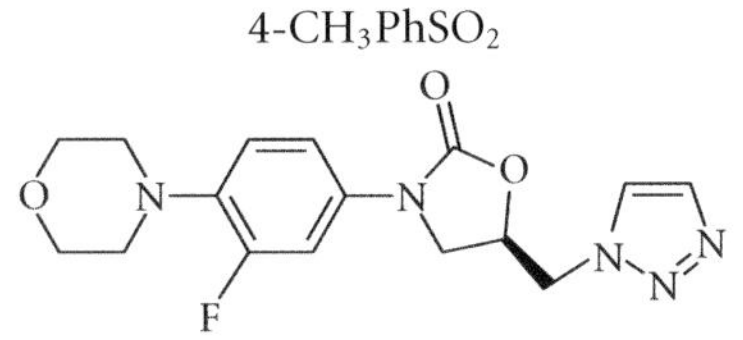	0.6308	0.466	>34.73	>74.53
LZD	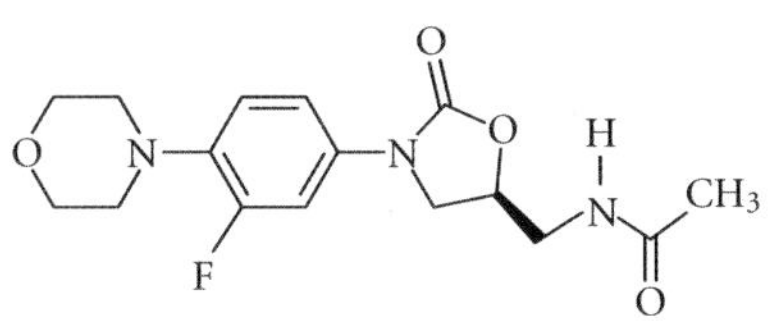	0.5321	<0.20	>33.73	>168.6
INH	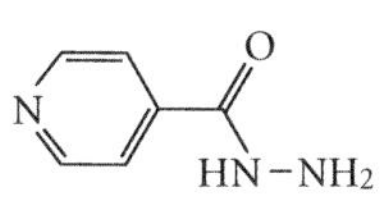	−0.668	0.034	>100	>2941

[a]Concentration that inhibited 50% growth of *M. tb.* (IC_{50}).

infected with *M. tuberculosis* ATCC 35801 (Erdman strain) by aerosol infection utilizing the Glass-Col Inhalation Exposure System. Treatment was started on day 13 after infection for 9 consecutive daily treatments until day 21. Test compounds were dissolved in 0.5% methyl cellulose and administered via oral gavage. An isoniazid (**INH**) control group, administered via oral gavage at 25 mg/Kg/day (H_2O), was included in each study. Mice were sacrificed on day 22 postinfection, and bacterial loads in the lungs and spleen were determined [15]. The Log10 CFU reduction values > 0.30 generally indicate activity.

3. Results and Discussion

The main goals of this study included evaluating the antimycobacterial activities of a series of triazolyl oxazolidinone derivatives **1a-p** and **2a-m** and **3a-e**, *in vitro* and *in vivo*, and explore recognizable structure-activity relationships (SARs) around the phenyloxazolidinone moiety. The synthesis of the compounds was described previously [9–12]. The results from the *in vitro* and *in vivo* (mice model) studies, presented in the Tables 1–5, were determined according to TAACF protocols [15, 16]. Data from *in vitro* antimycobacterium

TABLE 3: *In vivo* bioavailability of selected oxazolidinones.

Compd.	~ MIC (μg/mL) − serum	~ MIC (μg/mL) + serum	Dilution factor[a]	~ Compd in serum (μg/mL)	Bioavailability[b]
1g	1.1	3.3	1 : 20	22	low
1i	3.3	3.3	0	0	none
1o	0.37	3.3	0	0	none
2b	3.3	3.3	0	0	none
2j	1.1	1.1	0	0	none
2k	1.1	1.1	0	0	none
2l	1.1	0.37	1 : 10	11	low
3a	0.37	1.1	0	0	none
PH-27	1.1	0.37	1 : 80	88	medium
LZD	0.37	0.37	1 : 320	118.4	high
INH	0.014	0.041	1 : 320	4.48	high

[a]Dilution factor represents the last dilution step of the serum samples in which drug activity was still observed in the bioassay. (Drug levels in mouse serum are estimated by multiplying the dilution factor by the MIC value of the drug in absence of serum).
[b]Rating of bioavailability: low: activity of drug can be seen in 1 or 2 wells of the bioassay; medium: activity of drug can be seen in 3 or 4 wells of the bioassay; high: activity of drug can be seen in 5 or 6 wells.

TABLE 4: *In vivo* efficacy and observation at time of sacrifice.

Compd.	Lungs	Spleen	Other remarks
Control	+++	6 enlarged; 1 very large	2 with enlarged lymph nodes
INH	+	1 slightly enlarged; 4 normal	n/a
2l (306019)	++	1 enlarged; 4 slightly enlarged	Large intestine distended full of feces and air
1g (306027)	+	1 slightly enlarged; 4 normal	Large intestine distended full of feces and air
PH-27 (306006)	+	normal	Large intestine distended full of feces and air

+++; highly infected. ++/+; hardly any infected. n/a; not applicable.

and VERO cytoctoxicity assays are presented in Tables 1 and 2. From these data most of the compounds displayed potent to lack of activity against *M. tuberculosis* H37Rv strain with IC_{90} values in the range of <0.2 to >100 μg/mL, while the reference compounds linezolid (**LZD**) and isoniazid (**INH**) showed IC_{90} values of <0.2 and 0.034 μg/mL, respectively. The 4N-acylpiperazinyl derivatives displayed potent activity (IC_{90} range of >0.2–0.422 μg/mL, Table 1), in comparison to the 4N-aryl-carbonylpiperazinyl derivatives, which were relatively less active with IC_{90} in the range of <0.2–2.103 μg/mL. On the other hand, the 4N-arylsulfonyl derivatives were devoid of antimycobacterium activity (IC_{90} range of 5.469–100 μg/mL), while the methanesulfonylpiperazinyl derivative **3a** showed potent activity with IC_{90} value of <0.2 μg/mL. Although positive correlations between log *P* values and antimycobacterium activity have been demonstrated by previous other studies [17], however, such correlations could not be drawn in the present study since the MIC end-points were not determined. The *C* log *P* values of the compounds were estimated using ChemDraw Ultra 8.0.

In this study, interpretation of the *in vitro* assays (IC_{90} and VERO cell cytotoxicity: CC_{50}) data assisted in selection of compounds for further testing *in vivo*. Hence, data from the selectivity index (SI ratio = CC_{50}/IC_{90}, Tables 1 and 2) further indicated that most of the active compounds also displayed acceptable safety and therapeutic index profiles, represented by their SI ranges of >21 to >250. According to the TAACF criteria, compounds with SI value ≥ 10 are considered safe for further screening. In this regard, nine triazolyl oxazolidinones (**1g**, **1i**, **1o**, **2b**, **2j**, **2k**, **2l**, **3a**, and **PH-27**) along with **LZD** and **INH** as reference compounds were selected for preliminary bioavailability study. This bioassay was used to estimate the levels of the drug in mice at specific times after oral dosing. From the results presented in Table 3, the reference compounds **LZD** and **INH** displayed high concentrations (118.4 and 4.48 μg/mL) of the drugs in mice serum, suggesting high bioavailability of the drugs as demonstrated by the activity against *M. tuberculosis* H37Rv in 5 or 6 wells. While three of the triazolyl oxazolidinones, namely, **1g** (4N-isobutyryl), **2l** (4N-nicotinoyl), and **PH-27** (morpholino) displayed low to medium concentrations in mice, indicating low-to-medium bioavailability of drugs as demonstrated by activity in only 1 or 2 and 3 or 4 wells of the bioassay, respectively. In addition, the most lipophilic compound, the 4N-undecanoyl derivative **1o** (*C* log *P* = 3.5568) demonstrated 10 times higher MIC in the presence of serum suggesting that this compound probably has higher protein binding. Although all the other 5 compounds tested also showed relatively insignificant protein binding (Table 3), they also demonstrated no bioavailability similar to that of 4N-undecanoyl derivative **1o**. The probable reason(s) for this

Table 5: *In vivo* efficacy log10 CFU reduction in bacterial load in lungs and spleen.

Test group	Organ	Dose mg/Kg/dy	Mean ± SEM CFU	Log10 CFU reduction	Activity
Untreated **d13**	Lung	n/a	6.90 ± 0.11	n/a	n/a
	Spleen		4.75 ± 0.21		
Untreated **d22**	Lung	n/a	8.06 ± 0.11	n/a	n/a
	Spleen		6.38 ± 0.07		
INH	Lung	25	4.77 ± 0.12	3.29	Active
	Spleen		2.04 ± 0.38	4.34	Active
2l (306019)	Lung	150	7.67 ± 0.22	0.39	Inactive[a]
	Spleen		6.24 ± 0.06	0.14	Inactive[a]
1g (306027)	Lung	300	7.28 ± 0.14	0.78	Slightly active
	Spleen		5.95 ± 0.09	0.43	Inactive[a]
PH-27 (306006)	Lung	150	6.62 ± 0.08	1.44	Active
	Spleen		4.64 ± 0.21	1.74	Active

[a] 306027: slightly active in lung, but activity in spleen was not statistically significant.

lack of bioavailability of these other 5 compounds could be due to rapid metabolism and/or poor permeability of the compounds.

Finally, the *in vivo* antimycobacterial activities of the compounds that displayed bioavailability of low to high concentrations were evaluated against gamma knock-out (GKO) C57BL/6 female mice model, which are unable to control aerosol infection with the Erdman strains ATCC 35801. Treatment was initiated 13 days after infection by orally administering the drugs and treatment continued for 9 consecutive days until 21 days. The results of this *in vivo* study are presented in Tables 4 and 5 following sacrifice of the animals. As can be seen in Table 4, the triazolyl oxazolidinones **1g (306027)** and **PH-27 (306006)** demonstrated efficacy comparable to **INH** in mice lungs and spleen, while **2l (306019)** were less efficacious. Generally, the triazolyl compounds were more effective in lungs. Furthermore, mice treated with the triazolyl oxazolidinones presented with distended large intestine. The morpholino derivative **PH-27** was the most active of the triazolyl oxazolidinones tested providing 1.44 log CFU reduction in the lung and 1.74 log reduction in the spleen. While the 4N-isobutyryl derivative **1g** showed 0.78 log CFU reduction in the lungs, which was statistically significant, but no statistically significant activity was noted in the spleen. On the contrary, the 4N-nicotinoyl derivative **2l** did not show statistically significant log CFU reduction in either lung or spleen with 0.39 and 0.14 log CFU (Table 5), respectively. However, the reference compound **INH** provided 3.29 log and 4.34 log CFU reduction in lungs and spleen, respectively.

The main reason for the significant differences in the *in vivo* efficacy of these three derivatives 4N-isobutyryl **1g**, 4N-nicotinoyl **2l**, and morpholino **PH-27** is not clear, apart from the obvious differences in the preliminary bioavailability results. Although the bioavailability studies of the efficacious compounds are very preliminary in nature, the efficacy results seem to go well in hand with the reported oral exposure of the compounds. Previous studies from our laboratory have shown that these class of compounds are relatively stable in plasma at physiologic conditions and may bind to plasma protein [18]. In particular, the most probable reasons for lack of bioavailability of the six triazolyl oxazolidinones **1i**, **1o**, **2b**, **2j**, **2k**, and **3a** may be due to rapid *in vivo* metabolism and/or poor permeability upon oral administration. Further investigations on these class of compounds and other derivatives including their monoamine oxidase inhibitory activities are ongoing in our laboratories.

4. Conclusion

This study discloses the *in vitro* and *in vivo* antimycobacterium activity of a series of triazolyl oxazolidinones. Most of the compounds displayed potent *in vitro* activity against *M. tuberculosis* H37Rv, but this *in vitro* potency was not strongly reflected at the same level *in vivo*. This could be due to the low bioavailability of the compounds *in vivo*, however, the precise reason for this is unresolved. In conclusion, these derivatives may serve as templates for further modifications to attain more effective antimycobacterial compounds.

Acknowledgments

This work was supported by the Research Administration, Kuwait University Research Grant PC01/05 (OAP), and the Instrument Grants GS01/01, GS01/03, and GS01/05 awarded to the Science Analytical Facilities (SAF). Our gratitude to Tuberculosis Antimicrobial Acquisition and Coordinating Facility (TAACF), USA for performing biological screening assays.

References

[1] WHO, "The U.S government and global tuberculosis," *Fact Sheet*, March 2011.

[2] WHO, "The global tuberculosis epidemic," *Fact Sheet*, November 2010.

[3] A. Koul, E. Arnoult, N. Lounis, J. Guillemont, and K. Andries, "The challenge of new drug discovery for tuberculosis," *Nature*, vol. 469, no. 7331, pp. 483–490, 2011.

[4] WHO, "The global tuberculosis epidemic," *Fact Sheet*, no. 104, November 2010.

[5] A. Matteelli, A. C. C. Carvalho, K. E. Dooley, and A. Kritski, "TMC207: The first compound of a new class of potent anti-tuberculosis drugs," *Future Microbiology*, vol. 5, no. 6, pp. 849–858, 2010.

[6] G. F. Schecter, C. Scott, L. True, A. Raftery, J. Flood, and S. Mase, "Linezolid in the treatment of multidrug-resistant tuberculosis," *Clinical Infectious Diseases*, vol. 50, no. 1, pp. 49–55, 2010.

[7] E. C. Rivers and R. L. Mancera, "New anti-tuberculosis drugs in clinical trials with novel mechanisms of action," *Drug Discovery Today*, vol. 13, no. 23-24, pp. 1090–1098, 2008.

[8] W. W. Yew, M. Cynamon, and Y. Zhang, "Emerging drugs for the treatment of tuberculosis," *Expert Opinion on Emerging Drugs*, vol. 16, no. 1, pp. 1–21, 2011.

[9] O. A. Phillips, E. E. Udo, A. A. M. Ali, and N. Al-Hassawi, "Synthesis and antibacterial activity of 5-substituted oxazolidinones," *Bioorganic and Medicinal Chemistry*, vol. 11, no. 1, pp. 35–41, 2003.

[10] O. A. Phillips, E. E. Udo, A. A. M. Ali, and S. M. Samuel, "Synthesis and antibacterial activity of new N-linked 5-triazolylmethyl oxazolidinones," *Bioorganic and Medicinal Chemistry*, vol. 13, no. 12, pp. 4113–4123, 2005.

[11] O. A. Phillips, E. E. Udo, A. A. M. Ali, and S. M. Samuel, "Structure-antibacterial activity of arylcarbonyl- and arylsulfonyl-piperazine 5-triazolylmethyl oxazolidinones," *European Journal of Medicinal Chemistry*, vol. 42, no. 2, pp. 214–225, 2007.

[12] O. A. Phillips, E. E. Udo, and S. M. Samuel, "Synthesis and structure-antibacterial activity of triazolyl oxazolidinones containing long chain acyl moiety," *European Journal of Medicinal Chemistry*, vol. 43, no. 5, pp. 1095–1104, 2008.

[13] F. Reck, F. Zhou, M. Girardot et al., "Identification of 4-substituted 1,2,3-triazoles as novel oxazolidinone antibacterial agents with reduced activity against monoamine oxidase A," *Journal of Medicinal Chemistry*, vol. 48, no. 2, pp. 499–506, 2005.

[14] S. I. Hauck, C. Cederberg, A. Doucette et al., "New carbon-linked azole oxazolidinones with improved potency and pharmacokinetics," *Bioorganic and Medicinal Chemistry Letters*, vol. 17, no. 2, pp. 337–340, 2007.

[15] "Tuberculosis antimicrobial acquisition and coordinating facility (TAACF)," http://www.taacf.org/.

[16] L. A. Collins and S. G. Franzblau, "Microplate Alamar blue assay versus BACTEC 460 system for high- throughput screening of compounds against *Mycobacterium tuberculosis* and *Mycobacterium avium*," *Antimicrobial Agents and Chemotherapy*, vol. 41, no. 5, pp. 1004–1009, 1997.

[17] U. Das, S. Das, B. Bandy, J. P. Stables, and J. R. Dimmock, "N-Aroyl-3,5-bis(benzylidene)-4-piperidones: A novel class of antimycobacterial agents," *Bioorganic and Medicinal Chemistry*, vol. 16, no. 7, pp. 3602–3607, 2008.

[18] O. A. Phillips, L. H. Sharaf, M. E. Abdel-Hamid, and R. Varghese, "Assessment of the stability of novel antibacterial triazolyl oxazolidinones using a stability-indicating high-performance liquid chromatography method," *Medical Principles and Practice*, vol. 20, no. 1, pp. 51–59, 2011.

11

Evaluation of MGIT 960 System for the Second-Line Drugs Susceptibility Testing of *Mycobacterium tuberculosis*

Hyejin Kim,[1] Minji Seo,[2] Young Kil Park,[1] Jae-Il Yoo,[3] Yeong Seon Lee,[3] Gyung Tae Chung,[3] and Sungweon Ryoo[1]

[1] *Korean Institute of Tuberculosis, 168-5, Osong sangmyung 4 ro, Osong-eup, Cheongwon-gun, Chungbuk 363-954, Republic of Korea*
[2] *Novartis Korea LTD, CD&MA, Namdaemunro 5-ga, Joon-gu 100-753, Republic of Korea*
[3] *Centers for Infectious Diseases, National Institute of Health, Korea Centers for Disease Control and Prevention, 187 Osong sangmyung 2 ro, Osong-eup, Cheongwon-gun, Chungbuk 363-951, Republic of Korea*

Correspondence should be addressed to Sungweon Ryoo; scientist1@empal.com

Academic Editor: Alexander S. Apt

Many laboratories validate DST of the second-line drugs by BACTEC MGIT 960 system. The objective of this study is to evaluate the critical concentration and perform DST for the 2nd line drugs. We evaluated 193 clinical strains of *M. tuberculosis* isolated from patients in South Korea. Testing the critical concentration of six second-line drugs was performed by MGIT 960 and compared with L-J proportion method. The critical concentration was determined to establish the most one that gave the difference between drug resistance and susceptibility in MGIT960 system. Good agreement of the following concentrations was found: Concordance was 95% for 0.5 μg/mL of moxifloxacin; 93.6%, 1.0 μg/mL of levofloxacin; 97.5%, 2.5 μg/mL of kanamycin; 90.6%, 2.5 μg/mL of capreomycin; 86.2%, 5.0 μg/mL of ethionamide; and 90.8%, 2.0 μg/mL of ρ-aminosalicylic acid. The critical concentrations of the four drugs, moxifloxacin, levofloxacin, kanamycin, and capreomycin, were concordant and reliable for testing 2nd line drug resistance. Further study of ethionamide and ρ-aminosalicylic acid is required.

1. Introduction

Tuberculosis represents a major public health concern especially due to the increasing number of multidrug-resistant tuberculosis TB (MDR TB). Particularly in developing countries, extensively drug-resistant tuberculosis TB (XDR TB) continues to pose serious problem [1–5]. The increase in MDR/XDR TB rates prompts effective diagnostic methods so that appropriate treatments can be given to infected patients [6–8]. Many studies reported that MGIT 960 (Becton Dickinson Diagnostic System, Sparks, MD) provided reliable and rapid results in the detection and recovery of mycobacterium from clinical specimens and also the drug susceptibility testing (DST) of the TB isolates for the first line drugs isoniazid, rifampicin, ethambutol, streptomycin, and pyrazinamide [9, 10]. Recently, laboratories are facing great hindrances to provide DST for second-line drugs to ensure effective treatment of MDR/XDR TB by using MGIT 960 system [11–16]. However, in most of these studies, the tested numbers of second-line anti-TB drug were limited and the critical concentrations ranges of the second-line drugs were also discordant [11–13]. Despite the recommendation by WHO in 2008 for the use of liquid media for the second-line DST using MGIT 960, it is still unreliable due to the difficulty in determining the critical concentration [16]. It is not easy to calibrate newly developed DST methods using altered conditions. *In vitro* results of DST to second-line drugs were affected by criteria for measuring resistance such as the critical concentrations and critical proportions of drugs. For instance, DST with L-J solid media was established MICs that was defined as the drug concentration on which <20 colonies were found, while MIC in MGIT 960 was defined as the drug concentration at which the daily change in growth unit was less than that of the 1 : 100 control [17].

The Korean Institute of Tuberculosis (KIT) is a government operating research institute founded in 1970. KIT has been working as a main organization for conducting National TB program including diagnosis, basic research, and vaccine production. According to Korean Guidelines for Tuberculosis there are 5 practical tips for building treatment regimen for MDR-TB patients. Step 1 includes available 1st line drugs: pyrazinamide and ethambutol. Step 2 : choose one of the injectable drugs: kanamycin, amikacin, streptomycin, capreomycin. Step 3: choose one of the quinolone drugs: levofloxacin, moxifloxacin, ofloxacin. Step 4: choose available drugs among group IV: ρ-aminosalicylic acid, cycloserine, prothionamide. Step 5: if 4 drugs are not composed until step 4 group V drugs can be considered: amoxicillin/clavulanate, clarithromycin, high-dose isoniazid, clofazimine, linezolid, thioacetazone (not for HIV patients).

The L-J proportion method has been used for both first- and second-line DST for a long time in Korea, but recently, a switch to MGIT 960 method has been initiated for first-line DST. In this study, we tested the various critical concentrations published second-line TB drugs, moxifloxacin, levofloxacin, kanamycin, capreomycin, ethionamide, and ρ-aminosalicylic acid and used L-J proportion method as a reference for comparison with the MGIT 960 system.

2. Materials and Methods

2.1. Strains. Cultures submitted to the Korean Institute of Tuberculosis from the Public Health Center in Korea were evaluated. A total of 193 clinical strains of *M. tuberculosis*, including 134 pansusceptible strains and 59 resistant strains whose drug susceptibility results were previously determined by L-J, were tested. All isolates were analyzed by each patient category with treatment history (Table 1). All isolates were freshly subcultured on L-J medium before being used and tested by the MGIT 960.

Table 1: Clinical *M. tuberculosis* strains used in the study.

Test drugs	Number of strains	
	Susceptible	Resistant[a]
MXF		
New cases	37	4
Previously treated cases	3	15
LEV		
New cases	40	4
Previously treated cases	0	15
KM		
New cases	40	6
Previously treated cases	0	10
CPM		
New cases	39	5
Previously treated cases	1	6
ETH		
New cases	39	2
Previously treated cases	0	6
PAS		
New cases	40	6
Previously treated cases	0	11

[a]Treatment period of drug in resistant strains was >6 months.

2.2. Chemicals. All drugs were in chemically pure powder form. Levofloxacin (LEV), Capreomycin (CPM), Kanamycin (KM), Ethionamide (ETH), and ρ-aminosalicylic acid (PAS) were obtained from Sigma-Aldrich (St. Louis, MO), and Moxifloxacin (MXF) was obtained from Bayer (Bayer Health Care AG, Germany). The powders were stored at −20°C in desiccators as recommended by the manufacturer. LEV, CPM, KM, and PAS were dissolved in deionized water (DW), MXF in 0.1 N NaOH with subsequent dilutions in DW, and ETH solubilized in DMSO with subsequent dilutions in DW. All stock solutions were sterilized by membrane filtration through 0.22 μm-pore-size Millex-GS filter units (Millipore, Bedford, MA). All stock solutions were stored at −80°C in small aliquots. The frozen drug solutions were used immediately after thawing and the remaining was discarded and never stored in freezer again. Working solution was prepared freshly from the stock solution and the serial dilutions were carried out to achieve the desired concentrations.

2.3. Drug Susceptibility Test by the MGIT960 Method. MGIT DST was performed with strains grown from L-J slope, which were identified as *M. tuberculosis* with ZN staining. For the preparation of inoculums from L-J culture, 4 mL of Middlebrook 7H9 broth was added to a sterile tube with cap containing six to ten 2 mm glass beads. 1~2 colonies were extracted using a sterile loop from a growth culture that was not older than 14 days. The colonies were suspended in the Middlebrook 7H9 broth and vortexed for 2-3 minutes to break up the larger clumps. The suspension was left for 30 minutes to settle down the sediment to the bottom of the tube. Then, the supernatant fluid was transferred to another sterile tube and the suspension was left for another 15 min. Using 7H9 broth, the suspension was adjusted to a 0.5 McFarland standard. 1 mL of the adjusted suspension was diluted in 4 mL of sterile saline (1 : 5 dilutions). A 0.5 mL of the 1 : 5 dilutions was inoculated into tubes containing test drugs. In preparation of the second-line drug growth control tube, 0.1 mL of the previously mentioned suspension was pipetted into a total of 10 mL of sterile saline to prepare the 1 : 100 GC suspensions (1% growth control). The GC suspension was mixed thoroughly by gently inverting 3 to 4 times and then inoculated with 0.5 mL of the 1 : 100 GC suspensions into MGIT tubes. To interpret the results for 2nd drugs, the standard protocol recommended by the first-line drug manufacturers was followed for DST by the MGIT 960 method. When the growth unit (GU) of the growth control reaches 400 within 4–13 days, the GUs values of the drug-containing vials were evaluated. The GU of the drug-containing tubes were found 100 and >100; the result reported susceptible and resistant strains, respectively. Evaluated concentrations of each drug are listed in Table 2.

2.4. Drug Susceptibility Test by the L-J Proportion Method. L-J proportion method was the reference method for this study. All strains were previously tested on L-J medium by standard procedures at concentrations of MXF 2.0 μg/mL, LEV

TABLE 2: Drug concentrations tested in MGIT 960 and L-J proportion method.

Drug	Concentration evaluated (μg/mL) MGIT960	L-J
Moxifloxacin	0.25, 0.5, 1.0, 2.0, 4.0	2.0
Levofloxacin	0.25, 0.5, 1.0, 2.0, 4.0, 8.0	2.0
Kanamycin	0.625, 1.25, 2.5, 5.0, 6.0, 10.0	40.0
Capreomycin	0.625, 1.25, 2.5, 5.0	40.0
Ethionamide	0.625, 1.25, 2.5, 5.0	40.0
p-aminosalicylic acid	0.5, 1.0, 2.0, 4.0, 8.0, 16.0	1.0

2.0 μg/mL, KM 40 μg/mL, CPM 40 μg/mL, ETH 40 μg/mL, and PAS 1.0 μg/mL [18].

2.5. Genotypic Characterization. Strains that have shown discrepancy between the MGIT960 and L-J DST were retested in two methods. Also, we analyzed by DNA sequencing the key regions involved in the following genes; *gyrA* and *gyrB* for MXF and LEV, *rrs* for both KM and CPM, *tlyA* for CPM, and *inhA* promoter, *inhA*, *ethA*, and *ethR* for ETH.

3. Results and Discussion

A total of 193 strains including 134 pansusceptible strains and 59 resistant strains with various drug susceptibility profiles (19 isolates were resistant to MXF and LEV, 16 isolates were resistant to KM, 11 isolates were resistant to CPM, 8 isolates were resistant to ETH, and 17 isolates were resistant to PAS according to the L-J method) were tested for susceptibilities for the second-line drugs. To determine the minimal inhibitory antimicrobial test concentrations (MICs) for 6 drugs, we analyzed twelve references having DST data using MGIT 960 for second-line drugs. To determine the critical concentration, it is based on the basis of distinguishable susceptible and resistant strains. The DST results for each 6 drugs are presented in Table 3. On testing both susceptible and resistant strains, the critical concentrations were obtained: 0.5 μg/mL for MXF, 1.0 μg/mL for LEV, 2.5 μg/mL for KM, 2.5 μg/mL for CPM, 5.0 μg/mL for ETH, and 2.0 μg/mL for PAS. Good agreement of critical concentration between the MGIT 960 and L-J proportion method results was observed for MXF, LEV, KM, and CPM.

The MICs for MXF have been reported between 0.125 and 2.0 μg/mL and resistant strains for this drug are characterized by a higher MIC [12, 13, 19, 20]. For example, MIC of clinical isolates and pansusceptible strains was reported on the basis of the MGIT960 method [12]. Also, it was reported that MICs of *gyrA* mutant strains were higher than those for pansusceptible and resistant strains [21]. We evaluated extended concentrations among 0.25~4.0 μg/mL to determine MIC of resistant strain for MXF in this study (Table 2).

For moxifloxacin, the agreement was 95% concordant at 0.5 μg/mL. We found four strains with discordant result. One of those isolates was resistant at 1.0 μg/mL as false resistant when repeated using the MGIT960 method. Three strains were susceptible when tested by L-J method, but resistant (at <0.5 μg/mL) and susceptible (at ≥1.0 μg/mL) when tested by MGIT960 (Table 4). Historically, those isolates were from each patient in the followup. To elucidate isolates with reduced susceptibility to MXF, we analyzed the mutation associated with resistance to MXF. Although either *gyrA* or *gyrB* mutations was not detected, those strains possibly carry a mutation which is located outside the QRDRs, or the resistance may be caused by other mechanisms.

The MICs for LEV were recommended between 0.5 and 2.0 μg/mL in previous papers [22, 23]. According to Sanders's paper, they tested MICs with both pansusceptible and resistant strain. MICs of resistant strains (2.0 μg/mL) were higher than those for the pansusceptible strains (1.0 μg/mL), which showed bimodal pattern like MXF [24]. We evaluated concentrations among 0.25~8.0 μg/mL for LEV to determine MIC of resistant strains (Table 2). For levofloxacin, the agreement was 94% at 1.0 μg/mL. Applying the 1.0 μg/mL for the MGIT method, 18 of 19 resistant strains yielded resistant results and 37 of 40 susceptible strains yielded susceptible results (sensitivity 94.7%, specificity 92.5%). The three susceptible strains were susceptible at >1.0 μg/mL when tested using the MGIT960 method. For the three susceptible strains, we analyzed gene sequence in those discordant strains and did not harbor the *gyrA* and *gyrB* mutations (Table 4).

The MICs for KM were recommended 1.25~4.0 μg/mL in the previous reports [19, 20]. Critical concentration of this drug is commonly recommended between 2.5 and 5.0 μg/mL but it is greater than 20 μg/mL in the case of using KM-resistant strains [6, 11, 19]. Range of MIC was chosen 0.625~10 μg/mL to evaluate MICs of KM in our study (Table 2).

For kanamycin, the use of the 2.5 μg/mL critical concentration for the MGIT960 method led to yielding 97.5% concordance. 16 of 16 resistant strains yielded resistant results and 38 of 40 susceptible strains yielded susceptible results. The two discrepant strains did not harbor the *rrs* mutation (Table 4). We suggest the critical concentration for KM as a 2.5 μg/mL to yield the best discrimination between susceptible and resistant strains.

The MICs for CPM were reported 1.0~5.0 μg/mL [19, 23, 25]. We evaluated MICs of CPM among 0.625~5.0 μg/mL (Table 2). The concordance between both DST methods was 91% in capreomycin testing. Applying the 2.5 μg/mL for the MGIT method, 10 of 11 resistant strains yielded resistant results and 37 of 40 susceptible strains yielded susceptible results (sensitivity 90.9%, specificity 90.3%). Three discordant susceptible strains were susceptible at >2.5 μg/mL when tested using the MGIT960 method. Those strains were sequenced *rrs* and *tlyA* genes for genetic analysis but no mutations were detected in the two genes (Table 4). Resistant strain was found to be susceptible at >0.625 μg/mL by MGIT 960. This isolate was from XDR-TB patient in the 4th follow-up sample. This strain also proved susceptible at >0.625 μg/mL by MGIT 960 but resistant by L-J method. The resistance to fluoroquinolones was reported; aminoglycosides were developed during therapy [26]. Although it was isolated from patient during treatment, it seemed to obtain more susceptible results with the MGIT 960 instrumentation than with the comparative L-J method.

TABLE 3: Drug susceptibility testing results of each drug determined by use of the MGIT 960 system to be compared with L-J.

Drug	Conc. evaluated (μg/mL)	No. of strains with indicated results by L-J/MGIT 960				Sensitivity (%)	Specificity (%)
		R/R	*S/S*	*R/S*	*S/R*		
MXF	0.5	19	36	0	4	100	90.0
LEV	1.0	18	37	1	3	94.7	92.5
KM	2.5	16	38	0	2	100	95.0
CPM	2.5	10	37	1	3	90.9	90.3
ETH	5.0	6	38	2	1	75.0	97.4
PAS	2.0	16	35	1	5	94.1	87.5

TABLE 4: Drug susceptibility and genotypic characterization of isolates show discrepant results between L-J and Bactec MGIT 960.

Discordant isolates	Susceptibility at the following concentration (μg/mL)				KIT number	Genotypic characterization
MXF	0.25	0.5	1.0			
S/R	*R*	*R*	*S*		1176, 1503, 1574	*gyrA*, wt; *gyrB*, wt
	R	*R*	*R*		1575[a]	
LEV	0.5	1.0	2.0			
R/S	*R*	*S*	*S*		2933[b]	*gyrA*, wt; *gyrB*, wt
S/R	*R*	*R*	*S*		1147, 1155, 4900	
KM	1.25	2.5	5.0			
S/R	*R*	*R*	*R*		1562, 1565	*rrs*, wt
CPM	0.625	1.25	2.5	5.0		
R/S	*R*	*S*	*S*	*S*	4831	*rrs*, wt; *tlyA*, wt
S/R	*R*	*R*	*R*	*S*	1168, 1182, 2809	
ETH	1.25	2.5	5.0			
R/S	*R*	*S*	*S*		5189	*ethA*, *ethR*, *inhA*, wt
	R	*R*	*S*		5298[c]	*ethA*, S266R; *ethR*, *inhA*, wt
S/R	*R*	*R*	*R*		2934	*ethA*, *ethR*, *inhA*, *wt*
PAS	0.5	1.0	2.0	4.0		
R/S	*R*	*S*	*S*	*S*	4891	
S/R	*R*	*R*	*R*	*S*	1201, 1212, 1214, 1573	Not done
	R	R	R	R	4537	

[a]Determined as a false-resistant result.
[b]Treatment period of drug in this patient was 17 months.
[c]Determined as a false-susceptible result.

ETH was recommended among 0.5~2.5 μg/mL [19, 23, 25, 27]. We evaluated among 0.625~5.0 μg/mL for ETH (Table 2).

For ethionamide, we proposed 5.0 μg/mL critical concentrations in the MGIT960. Using a concentration of 5.0 μg/mL of ETH, one isolate with discordant results was to be false resistance, giving a sensitivity of 75%. This strain harbored an S266R of *ethA* mutation related to ETH resistance (Table 4). Based on the suggested concentration for ETH, MGIT960 test results compare poorly with those of the L-J method, at 86.2% concordance. Although the 86.2% agreement was found, this population with resistant is small. This discordance is not a novel observation, although its extent is larger than that observed in previous studies [12, 28]. Acute ETH DST has always been difficult to obtain because the drug is thermolabile [29]. ETH is an important drug for the treatment of MDR-TB and required for further DST testing and studies.

For PAS, an MIC of 4.0 μg/mL was reported [19]. PAS was tested among 0.5~16.0 μg/mL in this study (Table 2).

PAS, when applying the 2.0 μg/mL for the MGIT method, was 91% concordant (94.1% sensitivity, 87.5% specificity). One discrepant strain from new cases patients had low-level resistance (at 0.5 μg/mL) but susceptible at >1.0 μg/mL.

The agreement for ETH and PAS was low, since we were not able to decide the concentration at which 100% of the resistant strains grew in the presence of the drug and 100% of the susceptible strains were inhibited. Larger studies are needed to define the further susceptibility test.

In summary, MGIT960 and L-J proportion methods for second-line DST for *M. tuberculosis* were established for six drugs. The critical concentration for moxifloxacin was determined 0.5 μg/mL, for levofloxacin 1.0 μg/mL, for kanamycin 2.5 μg/mL, for capreomycin 2.5 μg/mL, for ethionamide 5.0 μg/mL, and ρ-aminosalicylic acid 2.0 μg/mL using MGIT 960. These critical concentrations were reliable for testing 2nd line drug resistance. The two drugs whose ETH and PAS were low with agreement are required for further DST testing and studies.

Acknowledgments

This study was supported by a research grant of the Korea Centers of Disease Control and Prevention (CDC), Republic of Korea (Grant no. 2009-E00479-00). Special thanks to Mr. Byungchul Ahn, Jangho Park, and Ms. Heekyung Yu for the preparation of the materials.

References

[1] M. A. Aziz, A. Wright, A. Laszlo et al., "Epidemiology of antituberculosis drug resistance (the Global Project on Anti-tuberculosis Drug Resistance Surveillance): an updated analysis," *Lancet*, vol. 368, no. 9553, pp. 2142–2154, 2006.

[2] R. Banerjee, G. F. Schecter, J. Flood, and T. C. Porco, "Extensively drug-resistant tuberculosis: new strains, new challenges," *Expert Review of Anti-Infective Therapy*, vol. 6, no. 5, pp. 713–724, 2008.

[3] N. R. Gandhi, A. Moll, A. W. Sturm et al., "Extensively drug-resistant tuberculosis as a cause of death in patients co-infected with tuberculosis and HIV in a rural area of South Africa," *Lancet*, vol. 368, no. 9547, pp. 1575–1580, 2006.

[4] M. C. Raviglione and I. M. Smith, "XDR tuberculosis—implications for Global Public Health," *New England Journal of Medicine*, vol. 356, no. 7, pp. 656–659, 2007.

[5] N. S. Shah, A. Wright, G. H. Bai et al., "Worldwide emergence of extensively drug-resistant tuberculosis," *Emerging Infectious Diseases*, vol. 13, no. 3, pp. 380–387, 2007.

[6] A. Martin, J. C. Palomino, and F. Portaels, "Rapid detection of ofloxacin resistance in *Mycobacterium tuberculosis* by two low-cost colorimetric methods: resazurin and nitrate reductase assays," *Journal of Clinical Microbiology*, vol. 43, no. 4, pp. 1612–1616, 2005.

[7] N. Morcillo, B. Di Giulio, B. Testani, M. Pontino, C. Chirico, and A. Dolmann, "A microplate indicator-based method for determining the susceptibility of multidrug-resistant *Mycobacterium tuberculosis* to antimicrobial agents," *International Journal of Tuberculosis and Lung Disease*, vol. 8, no. 2, pp. 253–259, 2004.

[8] T. Prammananan, W. Arjratanakool, A. Chaiprasert et al., "Second-line drug susceptibilities of Thai multidrug-resistant *Mycobacterium tuberculosis* isolates," *International Journal of Tuberculosis and Lung Disease*, vol. 9, no. 2, pp. 216–219, 2005.

[9] P. Bemer, T. Bodmer, J. Munzinger, M. Perrin, V. Vincent, and H. Drugeon, "Multicenter evaluation of the MB/BACT system for susceptibility Testing of *Mycobacterium tuberculosis*," *Journal of Clinical Microbiology*, vol. 42, no. 3, pp. 1030–1034, 2004.

[10] L. Heifets, T. Linder, T. Sanchez, D. Spencer, and J. Brennan, "Two liquid medium systems, mycobacteria growth indicator tube and MB redox tube, for *Mycobacterium tuberculosis* isolation from sputum specimens," *Journal of Clinical Microbiology*, vol. 38, no. 3, pp. 1227–1230, 2000.

[11] I. Bastian, L. Rigouts, J. C. Palomino, and F. Portaels, "Kanamycin susceptibility testing of *Mycobacterium tuberculosis* using Mycobacterium growth indicator tube and a colorimetric method," *Antimicrobial Agents and Chemotherapy*, vol. 45, no. 6, pp. 1934–1936, 2001.

[12] A. Krüüner, M. D. Yates, and F. A. Drobniewski, "Evaluation of MGIT 960-based antimicrobial testing and determination of critical concentrations of first- and second-line antimicrobial drugs with drug-resistant clinical strains of *Mycobacterium tuberculosis*," *Journal of Clinical Microbiology*, vol. 44, no. 3, pp. 811–818, 2006.

[13] M. Palaci, S. Y. M. Ueki, D. N. Sato, M. Alice da Silva Telles, M. Curcio, and E. A. M. Silva, "Evaluation of mycobacteria growth indicator tube for recovery and drug susceptibility testing of *Mycobacterium tuberculosis* isolates from respiratory specimens," *Journal of Clinical Microbiology*, vol. 34, no. 3, pp. 762–764, 1996.

[14] S. Rüsch-Gerdes, G. E. Pfyffer, M. Casal, M. Chadwick, and S. Siddiqi, "Multicenter laboratory validation of the BACTEC MGIT 960 technique for testing susceptibilities of *Mycobacterium tuberculosis* to classical second-line drugs and newer antimicrobials," *Journal of Clinical Microbiology*, vol. 44, no. 3, pp. 688–692, 2006.

[15] M. Sharma, L. Thibert, P. Chedore et al., "Canadian multicenter laboratory study for standardized second-line antimicrobial susceptibility testing of *Mycobacterium tuberculosis*," *Journal of Clinical Microbiology*, vol. 49, no. 12, pp. 4112–4116, 2011.

[16] World Health Organization, "Policy guidance on drug-susceptibility testing (DST) of 2nd antituberculosis drug," WHO/HTM/TB/2008.392. Geneva, Switzerland, 2008.

[17] K. M. Kam, A. Sloutsky, C. W. Yip et al., "Determination of critical concentrations of second-line anti-tuberculosis drugs with clinical and microbiological relevance," *International Journal of Tuberculosis and Lung Disease*, vol. 14, no. 3, pp. 282–288, 2010.

[18] G. Canetti, W. Fox, A. Khomenko et al., "Advances in techniques of testing mycobacterial drug sensitivity, and the use of sensitivity tests in tuberculosis control programmes," *Bulletin of the World Health Organization*, vol. 41, no. 1, pp. 21–43, 1969.

[19] C. Rodrigues, J. Jani, S. Shenai, P. Thakkar, S. Siddiqi, and A. Mehta, "Drug susceptibility testing of *Mycobacterium tuberculosis* against second-line drugs using the Bactec MGIT 960 System," *International Journal of Tuberculosis and Lung Disease*, vol. 12, no. 12, pp. 1449–1455, 2008.

[20] J. Van Ingen, S. Simons, R. De Zwaan et al., "Comparative study on genotypic and phenotypic second-line drug resistance testing of *Mycobacterium tuberculosis* complex isolates," *Journal of Clinical Microbiology*, vol. 48, no. 8, pp. 2749–2753, 2010.

[21] C. Piersimoni, C. Lacchini, V. Penati et al., "Validation of the agar proportion and 2 liquid systems for testing the susceptibility of *Mycobacterium tuberculosis* to moxifloxacin," *Diagnostic Microbiology and Infectious Disease*, vol. 57, no. 3, pp. 283–287, 2007.

[22] S. Y. G. Lin, E. Desmond, D. Bonato, W. Gross, and S. Siddiqi, "Multicenter evaluation of Bactec MGIT 960 system for second-line drug susceptibility testing of *Mycobacterium tuberculosis* complex," *Journal of Clinical Microbiology*, vol. 47, no. 11, pp. 3630–3634, 2009.

[23] C. A. Sanders, R. R. Nieda, and E. P. Desmond, "Validation of the use of middlebrook 7H10 agar, BACTEC MGIT 960, and

BACTEC 460 12B media for testing the susceptibility of *Mycobacterium tuberculosis* to levofloxacin," *Journal of Clinical Microbiology*, vol. 42, no. 11, pp. 5225–5228, 2004.

[24] F. Giannoni, E. Iona, F. Sementilli et al., "Evaluation of a new line probe assay for rapid identification of gyrA mutations in *Mycobacterium tuberculosis*," *Antimicrobial Agents and Chemotherapy*, vol. 49, no. 7, pp. 2928–2933, 2005.

[25] T. S. Huang, S. S. J. Lee, H. Z. Tu et al., "Use of MGIT 960 for rapid quantitative measurement of the susceptibility of *Mycobacterium tuberculosis* complex to ciprofloxacin and ethionamide," *Journal of Antimicrobial Chemotherapy*, vol. 53, no. 4, pp. 600–603, 2004.

[26] S. Feuerriegel, H. S. Cox, N. Zarkua et al., "Sequence analyses of just four genes to detect extensively drug-resistant *Mycobacterium tuberculosis* strains in multidrug-resistant tuberculosis patients undergoing treatment," *Antimicrobial Agents and Chemotherapy*, vol. 53, no. 8, pp. 3353–3356, 2009.

[27] B. Springer, K. Lucke, R. Calligaris-Maibach, C. Ritter, and E. C. Böttger, "Quantitative drug susceptibility testing of *Mycobacterium tuberculosis* by use of MGIT 960 and EpiCenter instrumentation," *Journal of Clinical Microbiology*, vol. 47, no. 6, pp. 1773–1780, 2009.

[28] M. J. Ruiz-Serrano, L. Alcala, L. Martinez et al., "In vitro activities of six fluoroquinolones against 250 clinical isolates of *Mycobacterium tuberculosis* susceptible or resistant to first-line antituberculosis drugs," *Antimicrobial Agents and Chemotherapy*, vol. 44, no. 9, pp. 2567–2568, 2000.

[29] D. A. Mitchison, "Drug resistance in tuberculosis," *European Respiratory Journal*, vol. 25, no. 2, pp. 376–379, 2005.

12

The Poor Survival among Pulmonary Tuberculosis Patients in Chiapas, Mexico: The Case of Los Altos Region

J. C. Nájera-Ortiz,[1,2] H. J. Sánchez-Pérez,[1,2] H. Ochoa-Díaz-López,[1] G. Leal-Fernández,[3] and A. Navarro-Giné[4]

[1] *Área Académica Sociedad, Cultura y Salud, El Colegio de la Frontera Sur (Ecosur), 29290 San Cristóbal de Las Casas, Chiapas, Mexico*
[2] *Grups de Recerca d'Amèrica i Àfrica Latines, GRAAL-Ecosur, San Cristóbal de Las Casas, Chiapas, Mexico*
[3] *Departamento de Atención a la Salud, Universidad Autónoma Metropolitana-Xochimilco, 04960 México, DF, Mexico*
[4] *Grups de Recerca d'Amèrica i Àfrica Latines (GRAAL), Unitat de Bioestadística, Facultat de Medicina, Universitat Autónoma de Barcelona (UAB), 08193 Barcelona, Spain*

Correspondence should be addressed to J. C. Nájera-Ortiz, jcnajerao@hotmail.com

Academic Editor: T. Ottenhoff

Objective. To analyse survival in patients with pulmonary tuberculosis (PTB) and factors associated with such survival. *Design.* Study of a cohort of patients aged over 14 years diagnosed with PTB from January 1, 1998 to July 31, 2005. During 2004–2006 a home visit was made to each patient and, during 2008-2009, they were visited again. During these visits a follow-up interview was administered; when the patient had died, a verbal autopsy was conducted with family members. Statistical analysis consisted of survival tests, Kaplan-Meier log-rank test and Cox regression. *Results.* Of 305 studied patients, 68 had died due to PTB by the time of the first evaluation, 237 were followed-up for a second evaluation, and 10 of them had died of PTB. According to the Cox regression, age (over 45 years) and treatment duration (under six months) were associated with a poorer survival. When treatment duration was excluded, the association between poorer survival with age persisted, whereas with having been treated via DOTS strategy, was barely significant. *Conclusions.* In the studied area it is necessary that patients receive a complete treatment scheme, and to give priority to patients aged over 45 years.

1. Introduction

Tuberculosis (TB) continues to be one of the leading causes of disease, disability, and death. Seventy-five percent of people with TB belong to the economically active age group (15–54 years) and 95% of the cases and 99% of deaths occur in developing countries [1].

The incidence rate of TB in Mexico in 2007 was 20/100,000 and the death rate was 2.4/100,000 [2]. Nevertheless, given the socioeconomic conditions in the country such as high rurality, high levels of poverty, and shortage of health resources in marginalized areas, both figures might be higher.

Chiapas is among the Mexican states with the highest indices of poverty [3]. This state shows one of the highest proportions of rural and indigenous population, has the lowest human development index of the whole country [3], has the lowest *per capita* availability of health resources [4, 5], and has the highest rates of prevalence and mortality due to TB [6].

This situation is even worse in rural indigenous populations of Chiapas, like Los Altos region, where in many communities access to basic services turns out to be more a privilege than a right. In such circumstances, control and anti-TB treatment of TB patients via the directly observed treatment short-course (DOTS) strategy is very difficult.

Therefore the results of this situation are high levels of underdiagnosis and of treatment defaulting, multidrug resistance, and deaths due to TB [7–9].

In Los Altos region of Chiapas, despite the well-known high underdiagnosis of cases [10], the recorded levels of morbimortality due to TB are very high. The poor living and health conditions of Chiapas together with a deficient population coverage and poor quality of the health care services and the high prevalence of diseases such as diabetes, HIV/AIDS, malnutrition, and alcoholism might be associated with the poor survival of TB patients [7].

The survival in patients with pulmonary tuberculosis (PTB) has not been analysed before in Chiapas. Therefore, the aim of the present study was to analyse survival among patients diagnosed with PTB during the period 1998–2005 in Los Altos region of Chiapas and to investigate socioeconomic, demographic, and anti-TB treatment-related factors associated with their survival.

2. Study Population and Methods

A longitudinal prospective study was carried out in a cohort of patients aged 15 years and over, diagnosed with PTB by the Health District of Los Altos Region (Ministry of Health) by acid fast smear or culture, between 1 January 1998 and 31 July 2005 in Los Altos region of Chiapas.

The study began in 2004-2005 with an initial phase which consisted of visiting the homes of those patients diagnosed between 1998 and 2002 ($n = 431$) [7]. Subsequently in 2006, a second visit was made to locate those patients diagnosed between 2003 and July 2005 ($n = 98$). All patients ($n = 529$) were evaluated in terms of their PTB status.

The disturbing findings of the first study (95 deaths—of which 68 were probably due to PTB—plus 237 located alive, and 197 not found) motivated a second study involving all patients located alive in the first study ($n = 237$). We undertook a follow-up visit to these patients during 2008-2009. Out of the 237 patients, 10 had died due to PTB, 175 were located alive, and 52 could not be located as they had moved.

In both studies, patients located alive were interviewed at home; when they had died, a verbal autopsy was carried out with their family, in which the date, place, and cause of death were investigated, among other aspects.

Survival time was defined as the number of days between the recorded date of PTB diagnosis and the date of death or, in the case of patients located alive, between diagnosis date and the date of their last interview.

Survival was analysed in terms of demographics (sex, age, type of community of residence, indigenous condition and whether they spoke Spanish or not), socioeconomic status (educational level, occupation, social security), treatment-related variables: treated under DOTS strategy or not, and duration of anti-TB treatment: complete or not (six months or less, resp.).

A patient treated under the DOTS strategy was defined as the one who is under the anti-TB drug intake program and he/she is directly and constantly supervised by either health staff or a trained relative.

The survival function was estimated using the Kaplan-Meier method [11], and survival curves were compared among different categories of a given variable using the Log-rank test [11]. Finally, for those variables found to be associated with survival time, two multivariate analyses (Cox regression) were carried out, one taking into account the duration of treatment and the other ignoring this duration due to the possibility of a correlation effect between duration of treatment and survival time, which could lead to overestimation of the true effect of treatment duration. For example, a patient who dies two months after he is diagnosed, might not have received more than two-month treatment.

In all statistical analyses a significance level of $\alpha = 0.05$ was assumed. The analyses were conducted using the statistical packages *SPSS* version 15 [12] and Stata version 11.1 [13].

3. Results

3.1. Demographic and Socioeconomic Indicators of the Patients Studied. Table 1 shows the main demographic, socioeconomic, and treatment-related indicators for the 305 patients studied, according to their alive or deceased condition.

Only 12.8% of the patients studied reported having received their anti-TB treatment under DOTS strategy, and one in five (22.3%) had less than six months of anti-TB treatment.

3.2. Survival. The average follow-up time per patient for the entire cohort was 2,032 days (median 2,137; range 0 to 4,089), for patients located alive was 2,464 days (median 2,601; range 382 to 4,089), and for patients who died (from the PTB diagnosis date to their date of death) was 774 days (median 670; range 0 to 3,185). The incidence of mortality by person-years of follow-up was 4.6 by 100 person-years.

Of the 78 deaths suffering from PTB, 25% died during the six months following diagnosis (i.e., during treatment), 38% by the end of the first year from the date of diagnosis, 53% had died by the end of the second year, 72% after three years, 86% after four years, and 92.3% after five years; only one of the 78 patients who had died survived for seven years and over.

3.3. Factors Related to Survival. No significant differences were found between survival curves in terms of the following variables: sex, indigenous condition, type of community of residence (rural-urban), occupation, or social security (yes or no). Statistically significant differences were observed for age (poorer survival in those aged over 45 years) (Figure 1), educational level (poorer survival in patients with under three years of schooling), whether treated via the DOTS strategy (poorer survival in those not treated under DOTS) (Figure 2), and duration of treatment (poorer survival in those not completing treatment) (Figure 3).

In the multivariate analysis performed, the only two variables which continued to show statistically significant

TABLE 1: Demographic, socioeconomic, and antituberculosis treatment-related indicators among the study patients.

Indicator (%)	Total $n = 305$	Alive $n = 227$	Deceased $n = 78$	Significance (x^2 Mantel-Cox)
		Demographic		
Sex				
Male	51.1	52.6	50.7	0.556
Female	48.9	47.4	49.3	
Age group (years)				
15–34	46.9	52.9	29.5	<0.001
35–44	18.4	18.9	16.7	
45 and over	34.8	28.2	53.8	
Type of community of residence				
Rural	69.8	69.2	71.8	0.493
Urban	30.2	30.8	28.2	
Speak Spanish				
Yes	69.2	70.5	65.4	0.328
No	30.8	29.5	34.6	
Indigenous				
Yes	85.6	85.9	84.6	0.903
No	14.4	14.1	15.4	
		Socioeconomic		
Educational level				
0–3 years of schooling	73.1	69.2	84.6	0.020
More than 3 years of schooling	26.9	30.8	15.4	
Occupation				
Agricultural	41.6	39.2	48.7	0.113
Non-agricultural	58.4	60.8	51.3	
With social security				
Yes	22.0	22.9	19.2	0.102
No	78.0	77.1	80.8	
		Antituberculosis treatment related		
DOTS strategy treatment				
Yes	12.8	15.0	6.4	0.041
No	87.2	85.0	93.6	
Duration of treatment (completion)				
Not	22.3	11.9	52.6	<0.001
Yes	77.7	88.1	47.4	

associations with survival were age and the duration of anti-TB treatment. Patients aged 45 years and over ($n = 106$) presented poorer survival than the younger patients (Table 2). The median survival time of those in this age group who died ($n = 42$) was 718 days (range 0 to 3,185). Of these 42 only 9.5% received anti-TB treatment via the DOTS strategy, and in 47.6% the duration of such treatment was not completed. The median survival time of those who died in the reference group consisting of patients aged 15–34 years (23/143) was 688 days (range 8–1,841).

With regard to the duration of anti-TB treatment, those patients with incomplete treatment presented poorer survival than those treated with complete treatment (Table 2). The median survival time of the 41 patients out of those with incomplete treatment was 261 days (range 0–1,658), whereas among those dying in the other group ($n = 37$) the median survival time was 1,137 days (range 202–3,185).

4. Discussion

This study represents one of the first attempts to measure survival among PTB patients in Chiapas, Mexico, an area of high socioeconomic deprivation and strong presence of indigenous population.

From the cohort of PTB patients diagnosed between 1998 and 2005, and followed up between 2004 and 2008, 15% of them had died from PTB. Chiapas is one of the Mexican states with higher levels of PTB mortality. For example,

Table 2: Deaths, incidence density, and hazard ratios according cox regression models.

Factor	Including variable "duration of treatment"[a]					
	Number of deaths	Incidence density*	HR	95% CI		P
Age						
15–34 ($n = 143$)	23	2.8	1			
35–44 ($n = 56$)	13	3.7	1.03	0.51	2.10	0.927
45 and over ($n = 106$)	42	8.1	2.10	1.22	3.61	0.007
Duration of treatment (completion)						
Yes ($n = 237$)	37	2.6	1			
Not ($n = 68$)	41	16.0	5.74	3.59	9.18	<0.001

*Expressed in terms of 100 person-years of follow-up.
[a]The following variables were not statistically significant: sex ($P = 0.234$), educational level ($P = 0.172$), and DOTS treament ($P = 0.145$).

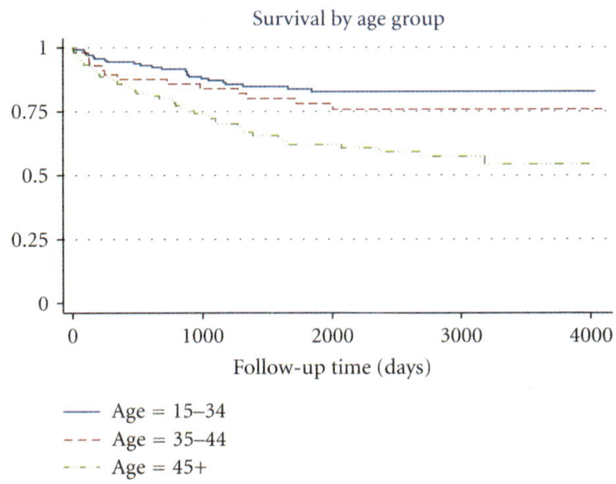

Figure 1: Survival functions for variable: Age.

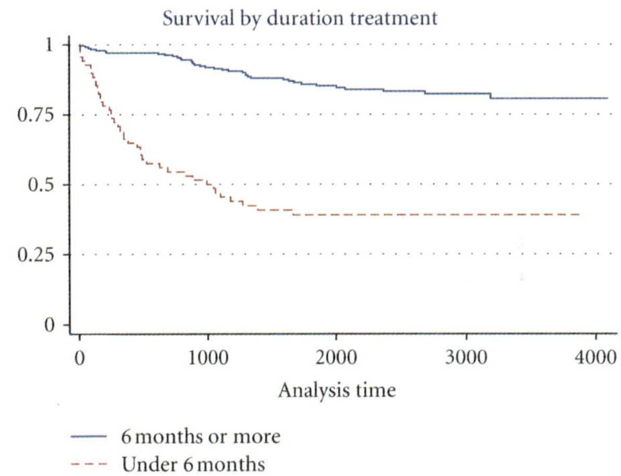

Figure 3: Survival functions for variable: duration of treatment.

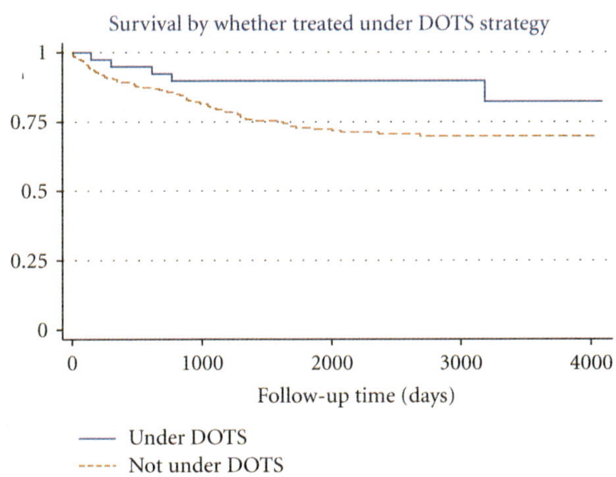

Figure 2: Survival functions for variable: treated under DOTS strategy.

in 2008 and 2009 the PTB mortality for the country was 1.8 and 1.7/100000, respectively, whereas in Chiapas the PTB mortality rate was 4.68 and 3.79 for the same years. Moreover, the studied region is one of the regions of Chiapas with the highest PTB morbidity and mortality rates. This is likely due to the fact that Los Altos region is one of the regions with the worst living conditions and highest level of poverty, with mainly rural population, a high proportion of indigenous communities, great problems of access to health services, and scarce opportunities to get a proper diagnosis [7].

Therefore, the results of this study are consistent with the situation described previously. The findings also provide evidence that in the study area, patients being aged 45 years and over, not having completed the established six months treatment, and not having been treated via the DOTS strategy are associated with an increased risk of dying from PTB.

The fact that patients aged 45 years and over have a lower chance of survival may be a reflection of the accumulation of unfavourable living conditions related to their poverty (lower education, higher levels of malnutrition during childhood, etc.) which probably made them more vulnerable to TB.

Regarding whether they completed six months of treatment or not, it should be mentioned that the study area is characterized by having a significant proportion of indigenous and peasant populations living in severe conditions of poverty and deprivation. Also, both access to and quality of health services are deficient. There is considerable evidence of the mistreatment of patients by the health services staff [14], deficient application of the DOTS strategy in anti-TB treatment (in the present study only 13% were treated under DOTS), and the frequent shortages of supply of anti-TB drugs [10]. All this contributes to have a high proportion of PTB patients who start anti-TB treatment but who do not complete it, leading to a higher mortality among these patients, as well as increasing their chances of becoming multidrug resistant cases [9].

Thus, the fact that the patients whose treatment duration was less than six months had a lower chance of survival is consistent with the documented evidence that points out that six-month treatment is the minimum time for a person to have a 96–98% chance of being cured (in new cases) [15]. Of those patients receiving anti-TB treatment of less than six-month duration ($n = 68$), 60% had died by the time of this study, whereas the proportion of deceased patients among those treated for six months or more was 15.6%.

The high proportion of deceased patients found by this study (26% of those patients with the required information to be included in the survival analyses) is much higher than that found in a similar study conducted in Peru [16], where only 4.5% had died. The differences in findings between these two studies may be the result from the following two aspects: in our study the median days of patient follow-up was 2,137 days, whereas in the Peruvian study it was 178 days. In the Peruvian study the main factor associated with survival time was HIV-TB coinfection; in our study no data were available to assess this association.

Regarding survival time, we would like to stress the following points.

(1) One quarter of deaths occurred in the first six months following their PTB diagnosis (during the time they were supposedly in treatment). It is also remarkable that two years after diagnosis slightly more than half of the deaths had already occurred. These two facts suggest, on the one hand, problems with the quality of health care services provided, such as delay in the diagnosis (at the moment when the health services made a PTB diagnosis, the patient might have already had a severe health condition). On the other hand, the living and health conditions of the patients under study are highly precarious, making them particularly vulnerable to PTB. However, it is noteworthy that another important proportion of deaths occurred between three and four years after diagnosis.

(2) According to the literature reviewed [17], mortality among nontreated PTB patients is 50% at five years after diagnosis. In the present study, in which all patients were diagnosed and received anti-TB treatment (according to current Mexican legislation, all patients diagnosed with PTB must be treated under DOTS), mortality was 23.6% at five years following diagnosis. The importance of our results lies in the fact that the patients were diagnosed and consequently received anti-TB treatment. Thus, a necessary question arises: what survival can be expected among patients not diagnosed or treated? This is an important issue to consider given that the socioeconomic conditions and degree of deprivation in the region are mostly unfavourable. Several studies conducted in the communities of Chiapas have shown the high levels of underdiagnosis, reaching 55–76% of prevalent PTB cases in rural areas [18].

Regarding the study constraints, the following issues are pointed out.

(i) First is the high attrition rate of follow-up patients. We think that this situation is due to population movements. The migration in this region is mainly due to economic factors (patients by themselves or accompanying a relative look for better job opportunities; some rural patients move to the urban areas looking for health care). These patients are registered by the health services as urban patients when in fact they are not. Once they finished their treatment, they go back to their rural communities or look for another place to live without notifying it to the health services. Therefore, it is not possible to follow up them after they have finished their treatment.

(ii) Among the group of 78 patients who died from PTB, only five were treated via DOTS. This did not make possible to undertake a multivariate analysis including the variable treatment via DOTS. The difference in the death proportion between those not treated via DOTS and those treated via DOTS was considerable (93.6% versus 6.4%, resp.).

5. Conclusions

The poor survival associated with age (45 years and over), with not having anti-TB treatment for six months, and not being treated via the DOTS strategy, may be considered as failures in the performance of the TB prevention and control programme in the study region. Thus, in the studied area, it is necessary to establish mechanisms to ensure that patients receive at least six months of anti-TB treatment and to pay special attention to patients aged 45 years and over.

Acknowledgment

The authors are grateful to Rosario García Miranda for her contributions in the revision of the final paper.

References

[1] World Health Organization, *An Expanded DOTS Framework for Effective Tuberculosis Control*, WHO/CDS/TB/2002.297, Geneva, Switzerland, 2002.

[2] World Health Organization, *Global Tuberculosis Control. Epidemiology, Strategy, Financing*, WHO/HTM/TB/2009.411, Ginebra, Switzerland, 2009.

[3] Gobierno de los Estados Unidos Mexicanos, Presidencia de la República, "Plan Nacional de Desarrollo 2007-2012," México, D.F., 2007.

[4] Organisation for Economic Co-operation and Development (OECD), *OECD Reviews of Health Systems: MEXICO*, OECD, Paris, France, 2005.

[5] Dirección General de Información en Salud, "Sistema de Cuentas Nacionales y Estatales de Salud (SICUENTAS), Secretaría de Salud, México. Estadísticas de recursos financieros públicos para la salud en México, 2003," *Salud Publica Mex*, vol. 47, pp. 90–98, 2005.

[6] E. González-Pier, C. Gutiérrez-Delgado, G. Stevens et al., "Definición de prioridades para las intervenciones de salud en el Sistema de Protección Social en Salud de México," *Salud Publica Mex*, vol. 49, pp. s27–s52, 2007.

[7] J. C. Nájera-Ortiz, H. J. Sánchez-Pérez, H. Ochoa-Díaz, M. Arana-cedeño, M. S. Lezama, and M. M. Mateo, "Demographic, health services and socio-economic factors associated with pulmonary tuberculosis mortality in Los Altos Region of Chiapas, Mexico," *International Journal of Epidemiology*, vol. 37, no. 4, pp. 786–795, 2008.

[8] I. Reyes-Guillén, H. J. Sánchez-Pérez, J. Cruz-Burguete, and M. Izaurieta-De-Juan, "Anti-tuberculosis treatment defaulting. An analysis of perceptions and interactions in Chiapas, Mexico," *Salud Publica de Mexico*, vol. 50, no. 3, pp. 251–257, 2008.

[9] H. J. Sánchez Pérez, A. Díaz-Vázquez, J. C. Nájera-Ortiz, S. Balandrano, and M. Martín-Mateo, "Multidrug-resistant pulmonary tuberculosis in Los Altos, Selva and Norte regions, Chiapas, Mexico," *International Journal of Tuberculosis and Lung Disease*, vol. 14, no. 1, pp. 34–39, 2010.

[10] M. Arana-Cedeño, "Dos padecimientos de la pobreza y la exclusión en Chiapas: la desnutrición y la tuberculosis," Pérez Arguelles Mariana (coord.) Cinco miradas sobre el derecho a la salud. Estudios de caso en México, El Salvador y Nicaragua. México, D.F., Fundar, Centro de Análisis e Investigación, A.C., pp: 177–230, 2010.

[11] P. Armitage, *Statistical Methods in Medical Research*, Blackwell Scientific, Oxford, Miss, USA, 1997.

[12] SPSS Inc, *SPSS for Windows Version 15.0*, SPSS Inc, Chicago, Ill, USA, 2006.

[13] "Stata SE/11.1," College Station: Stata Corp, 2010.

[14] E. Ticona, "Tuberculosis: Se agotó el enfoque biomédico," *Revista Peruana de Medicina Experimental y Salud Pública*, vol. 26, pp. 273–275, 2009.

[15] Secretaría de Salud, "Modificación a la Norma Oficial Mexicana NOM-006-SSA2-1993 para la Prevención y Control de la Tuberculosis en la Atención Primaria a la Salud," Diario Oficial de la Federación, México, D.F., Octubre 2000.

[16] A. Bernabé-Ortiz, "Factores asociados a supervivencia en pacientes con tuberculosis en Lima, Perú," *Revista Chilena de Infectología*, vol. 25, pp. 104–107, 2008.

[17] R. García-Ramos, F. L. Lado Lado, V. Tunez Bastida et al., "Tratamiento Actual de la Tuberculosis," *Anales de Medicina Interna*, vol. 20, pp. 91–100, 2003.

[18] H. J. Sánchez-Pérez, M. A. Hernán, S. Hernández-Díaz, J. M. Jansá, D. Halperin, and A. Ascherio, "Detection of pulmonary tuberculosis in Chiapas, Mexico," *Annals of Epidemiology*, vol. 12, no. 3, pp. 166–172, 2002.

13

Hair Analysis for Determination of Isoniazid Concentrations and Acetylator Phenotype during Antituberculous Treatment

Michael Eisenhut,[1] Detlef Thieme,[2] Dagmar Schmid,[3] Sybille Fieseler,[3] and Hans Sachs[2]

[1] *Paediatric Department, Luton & Dunstable University Hospital, NHS Foundation Trust, Luton LU40DZ, UK*
[2] *Forensisch Toxikologisches Centrum, Munich 80335, Germany*
[3] *Institut fur Rechtsmedizin, Ludwig-Maximilians Universität München, Munich 80336, Germany*

Correspondence should be addressed to Michael Eisenhut, michael_eisenhut@yahoo.com

Academic Editor: T. Ottenhoff

Background. Analysis of isoniazid (INH) uptake has been based on measurement of plasma concentrations providing a short-term and potentially biased view. *Objectives.* To establish hair analysis as a tool to measure long-term uptake of INH and to assess whether acetylator phenotype in hair reflects N-acetyltransferase-2 (NAT2) genotype. *Design and Methods.* INH and acetyl-INH concentrations in hair were determined in patients on INH treatment for *M. tuberculosis* infection using high pressure liquid chromatography/mass spectrometry. Acetyl-INH/INH ratios were correlated with NAT-2 genotype. *Results.* Hair concentrations of INH, determined in 40 patients, were not dependent on ethnic group or body mass index and were significantly higher in male compared to female patients (median (range) 2.37 ng/mg (0.76–4.9) versus 1.11 ng/mg (0.02–7.20) ($P = 0.02$). Acetyl-INH/INH ratios were a median of 15.2% (14.5 to 31.7) in homozygous rapid acetylator NAT-2 genotype and 37.3% (1.73 to 51.2) in the heterozygous rapid acetylator NAT-2 genotype and both significantly higher than in the slow acetylator NAT-2 genotype with 5.8% (0.53 to 14.4) ($P < 0.05$). *Conclusions.* Results of hair analysis for INH showed lower concentrations in females. Acetyl-INH/INH ratios were significantly lower in patients with slow acetylator versus rapid acetylator genotypes.

1. Introduction

The first application of hair analysis in monitoring of anti-infective treatment was the measurement of hair concentrations of indinavir, a protease inhibitor, in patients with HIV infection. Indinavir hair concentrations were significantly higher in responders compared to nonresponders [1]. Previous studies analysed antiepileptic drugs in segments of hair of patients on treatment for epilepsy and found that variability of hair drug concentrations, reflecting variable antiepileptic drug ingestion over time, was greater in epileptic patients with sudden unexplained death [2]. Hair analysis in patients on carbamazepine for treatment of epilepsy showed a significant linear relationship between the prescribed dose, hair concentration, and total plasma concentration [3].

Failure of tuberculosis treatment and relapse of tuberculosis, with selection of drug resistance mutations, have not been associated with low maximum concentrations of antituberculosis drugs such as isoniazid (INH). These conditions have been, however, associated with low areas under the concentration curve (AUC) in plasma, which is found in patients with intermittent noncompliance to treatment, widely spaced intermittent therapy, and chronically reduced absorption as found in HIV patients [4–6]. Other factors, which may contribute to subtherapeutic INH concentrations, are age below 5 years and high body mass index [7, 8]. A low AUC for INH has also been associated with the development of acquired rifamycin resistance despite directly observed therapy, leading to isolated rifamycin resistance and multidrug resistant tuberculosis by a lack of protection by INH against resistance development [9]. We introduce the development of hair analysis as a novel tool for quantification of long-term uptake and metabolism of INH. This may help to define the threshold of long-term presence of INH required for effective treatment. Hair analysis has several

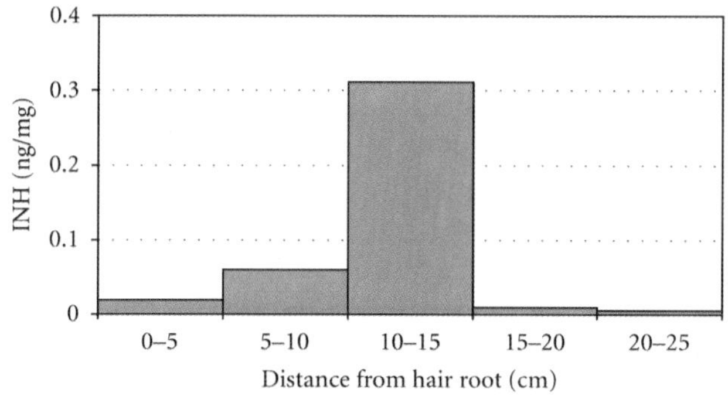

FIGURE 1: Isoniazid (INH) concentration in the hair shaft as function of distance from the scalp (cm) obtained 9 months after cessation of a 3-month course of treatment.

advantages compared to conventional monitoring of INH drug serum concentrations for generation of an AUC in serum. Hair sampling is painless and not distressing, which is particularly important when children are involved in a study or routine monitoring of INH uptake. INH is not stable in human serum at room temperature unlike in hair. In developing countries with resource limitations, the logistics and expense associated with repeated blood sampling and freezing and transport of blood samples are considerably more challenging compared to obtaining a hair sample with the possibility of storage at room temperature for months if necessary and ease of transport sealed in a plastic bag by ordinary mail to a reference centre where analysis can be performed. The aims of this study were to establish a method for quantification of long-term uptake of INH and the INH acetylator phenotype by measurement of the acetyl-INH/INH ratio in hair samples and to explore determinants of hair concentrations of INH.

2. Study Population and Methods

2.1. Study Population. Eligible for inclusion into the study were all adults and children commenced on INH treatment for *Mycobacterium tuberculosis* disease or latent infection. Excluded were patients who had received INH treatment prior to the current episode or those who decided to keep their hair very short.

Patients were consecutive patients recruited from adult and paediatric out-patient clinics as well as wards of the Luton & Dunstable University Hospital, NHS Foundation Trust, UK, between 2007 and 2009 and enrolled following informed, written consent by patients and/or parents/legal guardians as appropriate. The majority of patients were recruited from pupils of a school outbreak of *M. tuberculosis* infection described previously [10]. The study had ethical approval by the Hertfordshire Local Research Ethics Committee and approval and full support by the Department of Research and Development of the Luton & Dunstable University Hospital, NHS Foundation Trust.

Included were patients who agreed not to have their hair cut short for at least 3 months after commencement of treatment.

2.2. Hair Analysis for INH and Acetyl-INH. Hair sampling was done by cutting hair at the occipital hairline. A segment of hair grown during treatment, assuming a growth rate of 1 cm per month [11], was then cut off from the scalp end of the hair sample.

The hair sample was sent to the Forensic Toxicological Centre in Munich, Germany, and processed there for INH and acetyl-INH concentrations by high pressure liquid chromatography/mass spectrometry: Samples were decontaminated by 5 min agitation in a gas tight tube with 5 mL petroleum benzene (boiling range to 40°C, Merck, Germany), dried and cut into lengths of 1-2 mm. After adding ~50 ng of the internal standard (INH propionate) and 2 mL of formic acid (98–100%, technical grade, AppliChem, Germany), the samples were extracted and derivatised in gas tight tubes by 3 h ultrasonification at 55°C. Respective signals to noise ratios were for INH (as formyl-INH) = 17.2 and Acetyl-INH = 11.8. Similarly, the average signal intensity in 7 blank hair samples (from participants not exposed to isoniazid) corresponded to INH = 0.015 ng/mg and Ac-INH = 0.009 ng/mg.

The linearity of the calibration was confirmed for both analytes within the calibration range, that is, 0.05–1 ng/mg. Relevant correlation coefficients were formyl-INH = 0.975 and acetyl-INH = 0.989. To demonstrate the suitability of hair analysis for retrospective analysis of INH treatment, segments of the hair strand of one patient were analysed 9 months after a three-month course of treatment (see Figure 1). The isoniazid concentration in hair of this participant directly after treatment was 0.27 ng/mg. The maximum concentration in segments of a hair sample of the same patient obtained 9 months after treatment was 0.31 ng/mg. This supported a lack of leaching of isoniazid over time and its stability in hair. The fact that this concentration was even slightly higher may relate to desiccation of the hair shaft increasing drug concentrations in hair over time. This demonstrated the preservation of INH in hair for months after treatment and correlation of its presence with time of treatment.

2.3. Determination of NAT-2 Genotype. Mouth swabs to obtain cells from the buccal mucosa were obtained in duplicate for DNA analysis and sent to the Institut fur Rechtsmedizin, Ludwig-Maximilians Universität München, Munich, Germany, where samples were analysed by PCR for the arylamine N-acetyltransferase-2 (NAT-2) genotype.

Genomic DNA was isolated using BioRobot EZ1 system from QIAGEN (Hilden, Germany) [12]. For genotyping NAT2, a fragment of 769 bp was amplified with following primers [13]:

NAT2f 5′-GAG TTG GGC TTA GAG GCT ATT T-3′

NAT2fr 5′-TTG GGT GAT ACA TAC ACA AGG G-3′.

The PCR was carried out in a total volume of 25 μL in the presence of 1 ng of genomic DNA as template, 5 pmol of each primer, 10x Gold Buffer (Applied Biosystems, Foster City, CA, USA), 10x dNTP mix, 3 mM $MgCl_2$ and 1,25 U *Ampli Taq Gold* (Applied Biosystems, PE Corporation, Foster City,

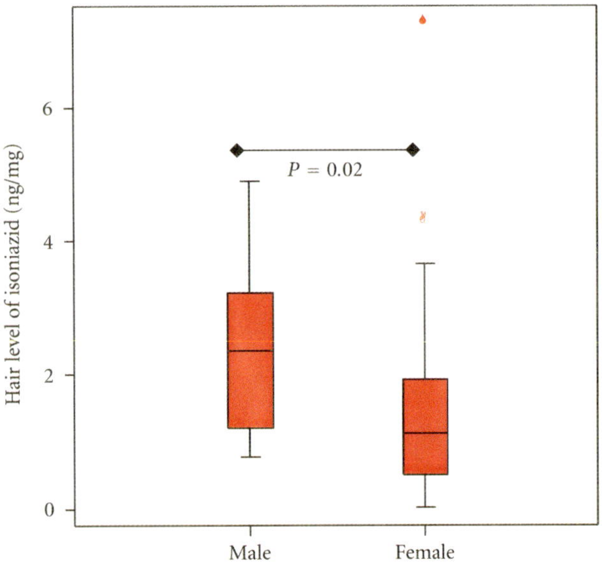

FIGURE 2: Isoniazid concentration in hair and gender.

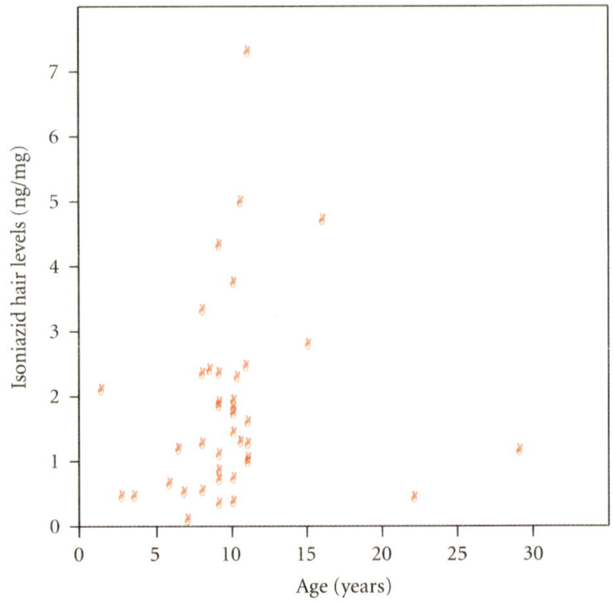

FIGURE 3: Correlation of isoniazid concentration in hair and age.

CA, USA). After initial denaturation at 94°C for 12 min, 35 cycles of 30 sec at 94°C, 45 sec at 63°C, and 1 min at 72°C were carried out. The final elongation step was at 72°C for 10 min.

Afterwards, the PCR products were sequenced by the BigDye Terminator v1.1 Cycle Sequencing Kit (Applied Biosystems, PE Corporation, Foster City, CA, USA) according to the manufacturer's instructions.

2.4. Statistical Analysis. Statistical analysis was by Mann-Whitney U-test for comparison of continuous data with nonparametric distribution and Pearson and Spearman's rank correlation coefficients were used in calculation of linear and nonlinear correlations as appropriate. Multiple comparisons of nonparametric data were performed by the Kruskal Wallis test and simultaneous multivariate linear regression analysis was conducted to determine which factor independently predicted INH hair concentrations. The software used was SPSS release 18.0. A P value of <0.05 was taken to indicate a statistically significant difference.

3. Results

3.1. Study Population. We recruited a total of 40 patients. 13 were treated for tuberculosis disease and 27 for latent *M. tuberculosis* infection. The mean age was 9.8 years (range: 1.3–29 years). Thirty-one female and nine male patients were recruited. There were 16 Caucasian patients, 14 Asian patients, 9 African or Afro-Caribbean patients, and 1 with unknown ethnic origin. All patients were on an equivalent of 5 mg/kg/day of INH. Treatment for active disease was with INH/rifampicin/pyrazinamide with or without ethambutol in the intensive (2 months) and INH and rifampicin in the continuation phase (4 months). Patients treated for latent *M. tuberculosis* infection were treated with three months of INH and rifampicin. In none of these patients was there any concern about compliance which was directly supervised and documented by the parents in the children (all but two participants) of this study.

3.2. Relation of INH Concentrations and Acetyl-INH/INH Ratios to Patient Characteristics. Investigation of the relationship of gender and INH concentrations and acetyl-INH/INH ratios revealed that INH concentrations were with a median of 2.37 ng/mg (range 0.76–4.9) significantly higher in male compared to female patients with 1.11 ng/mg (0.02–7.20) ($P = 0.02$) (see Figure 2). Acetyl-INH/INH ratios were not different between genders with a median of 11.5 (range 0.74–51.22) in male and 6.7 (0.48–47.5) in female patients ($P = 0.32$). Correlation of age with INH concentrations revealed a significant correlation with $r = 0.28$ (Spearman's rank correlation coefficient) (one-tailed $P = 0.04$) (see Figure 3) and weight with $r = 0.275$ (Pearson's correlation coefficient) (one-tailed $P = 0.043$) (see Figure 4).

Comparison of the predictive power of age and gender in determination of INH concentrations by simultaneous multiple linear regression analysis revealed that gender was with $t = -1.79$ ($P = 0.081$) a better predictor than age with a $t = 0.55$ ($P = 0.58$) but none of these patient characteristics was significantly associated in this analysis. There was no correlation of INH concentrations with BMI ($r = 0.213$, $P = 0.1$). There was also no correlation of acetyl-INH/INH ratio and weight or age, ($P = 0.356$ and 0.276, resp., by Spearman's rank correlation coefficient). Comparison of INH concentrations between African, Asian, and Caucasian ethnic groups revealed a median of 1.66 ng/mg (range 0.02–7.20) in African patients, 0.83 (0.27–2.72) in Asian, and 1.74 (0.3–4.23) in Caucasian patients and there was no significant difference between groups ($P = 0.130$). Comparison of INH hair concentrations in patients with active versus latent *M. tuberculosis* infection revealed that there was with a median

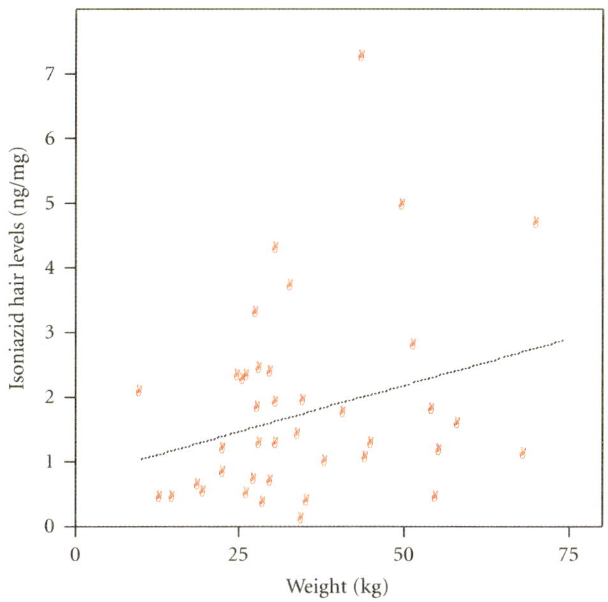

FIGURE 4: Correlation of isoniazid concentrations and body weight (regression line inserted).

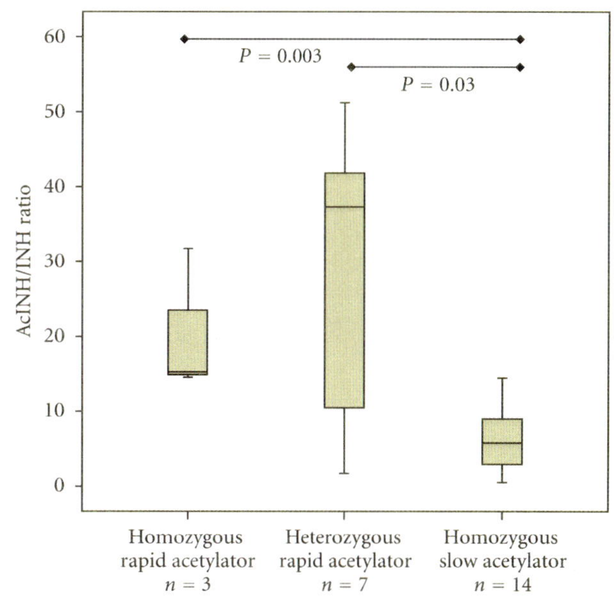

FIGURE 5: Acetylator phenotype represented as acetylisoniazid/isoniazid ratio (AcINH/INH ratio) and arylamine N-acetyltransferase 2 genotype ($n = 24$).

of 1.76 ng/mg (range 0.35–4.6) in patients with active tuberculosis no significant difference from hair concentrations of patients with latent *M. tuberculosis* infection of 1.19 (0.02–7.2) ($P = 0.66$).

3.3. Relationship of Acetylator Phenotype and Genotype. Acetylator phenotype represented as acetyl-INH/INH ratio was with a median of 15.2 ng/mg (range 14.5–31.7) in patients with a homozygous rapid acetylator genotype and with a median of 37.3 (1.73–51.2) in patients with heterozygous rapid acetylator genotype significantly higher than in patients with a slow acetylator genotype of 5.8 (0.53–14.49) ($P = 0.013$) (see Figure 5). The difference between homozygous rapid acetylator and heterozygous rapid acetylator genotype was not statistically significant ($P = 0.517$). There was no significant correlation between INH concentrations in all patients and acetyl-INH/INH ratio ($r = 0.1$, $P = 0.538$). INH concentrations in patients with homozygous rapid acetylator genotype had a median of 0.36 ng/mg (range 0.02–7.2), in patients with heterozygous rapid acetylator genotype 0.90 ng/mg (0.56–4.9) and in patients with slow acetylator genotype 1.91 ng/mg (0.27–3.23) and the difference between the groups was not significant ($P = 0.503$). There was no difference in age, gender, or weight in different acetylator genotypes.

4. Discussion

To our knowledge, we present the first data on hair concentrations of INH and its determinants. We demonstrated that hair analysis can be used to analyse INH uptake and acetylator phenotype. Results of this acetylator phenotype analysis were validated by analysis of the acetylator genotype. The wide variability of acetylator phenotypes within the heterozygous rapid acetylator genotype has been found previously on analysis of the acetyl-INH/INH ratios in peripheral blood [14]. We did not find a significant correlation of acetylator phenotype or genotype and INH hair concentrations. This may be due to the fact that group sizes were small. INH concentrations increased in ascending order from homozygous rapid over heterozygous rapid to slow acetylator genotype, but this was not significant. A previous study investigating areas under the concentration—time curve for INH during 12 hours after dosing—found a highly significant association with NAT-2 genotype [6]. The lack of association of age with acetylator phenotype in hair supported results of a previous study showing that the acetylator phenotype calculated from the acetyl-INH/INH ratio in plasma 3 hours after dosing is age dependent, that is increases with age up to the age of 4 years, but is not age-dependent after this age [15]. In our study, only 3 patients were younger than 5 years of age. We found that on univariate analysis gender was significantly associated with hair INH concentrations. A previous investigation demonstrated that the half-life of INH in serum was significantly longer in males compared to female patients [16]. This may provide a mechanism for increased accumulation of INH in hair of male patients over time found in our study. In a study conducted in India, more patients with low concentrations four and a half hours after administration were found in female compared to male patients independent of age and body weight [17]. In contrast to these results, a more recent investigation showed a significantly higher area under the INH concentration curve for female adults compared to male adults in the 8 hours after application of INH [18]. Another recent investigation showed no significant gender difference in INH concentrations in plasma one or four hours after INH application or in epithelial lining fluid or alveolar cells four hours after application [19].

With regards to age dependency of INH concentrations a previous cohort study in South African children found that each year increase in age was associated with increases in INH peak concentrations of 6% [20] but age was noncontributory to a multivariate analysis model describing the effects of genotype and dose in mg/m^2. AUCs for INH in children in another study showed, on within genotype regression, a significant increase with age [7]. In our study, the contribution of age was not statistically significant in a multivariate model.

The significantly faster elimination of INH by infants and younger children has been ascribed to the relatively greater mass of the liver in proportion to total body weight and it has been proposed that more optimal doses would be calculated on the basis of body surface area rather than body weight.

Body weight was not associated with INH hair concentrations on multivariate analysis. A previous investigation noted a positive correlation of body weight with plasma INH concentrations [21].

The fact that INH hair concentrations were not different in cases of active tuberculosis compared to latent *M. tuberculosis* infection indicates that active tuberculosis was not associated with malabsorption of INH, a phenomenon postulated for patients with active tuberculosis previously [22].

Previous studies noted an enhanced drug uptake of darker hair due to its higher melanin content [23]. Our study found no difference between ethnic groups making it unlikely that hair colour is a significant factor in hair concentrations of INH.

Hair analysis is uniquely placed to investigate the causes of treatment failure or relapse in and outside a trial setting. Hair analysis can offer identification of causes of disease relapse to establish whether it is due to a loss of pharmacological efficacy (drug resistant strain) or noncompliance. It also overcomes the limitations of plasma monitoring in identifying patients who, following periods of total noncompliance, comply with the prescribed dose a few days prior to clinical visits so as to achieve respectable steady state concentrations [3].

A low INH concentration in the hair of a patient with treatment failure could be interpreted as follows.

(i) By the analysis of segments of a hair shaft increased variability of INH concentrations between segments indicates poor compliance.

(ii) A decreased INH/acetyl-INH ratio indicates homo- or heterozygous rapid acetylator status.

(iii) A uniformly low INH concentration in all segments of a hair shaft in the absence of a low INH/acetylINH ratio, age, or weight could indicate malabsorption.

5. Conclusions

Results of hair analysis for INH showed lower concentrations in females. Acetyl-INH/INH ratios were significantly lower in patients with slow acetylator versus rapid acetylator genotypes.

References

[1] L. Bernard, A. Vuagnat, G. Peytavin et al., "Relationship between levels of indinavir in hair and virologic response to highly active antiretroviral therapy," *Annals of Internal Medicine*, vol. 137, no. 8, pp. 656–659, 2002.

[2] J. Williams, C. Lawthom, F. D. Dunstan et al., "Variability of antiepileptic meditation taking behaviour in sudden unexplained death in epilepsy: hair analysis at autopsy," *Journal of Neurology, Neurosurgery and Psychiatry*, vol. 77, no. 6, pp. 481–484, 2006.

[3] J. Williams, P. N. Patsalos, and J. F. Wilson, "Hair analysis as a potential index of therapeutic compliance in the treatment of epilepsy," *Forensic Science International*, vol. 84, no. 1–3, pp. 113–122, 1997.

[4] P. R. Donald, D. P. Parkin, H. I. Seifart et al., "The influence of dose and N-acetyltransferase-2 (NAT2) genotype and phenotype on the pharmacokinetics and pharmacodynamics of isoniazid," *European Journal of Clinical Pharmacology*, vol. 63, no. 7, pp. 633–639, 2007.

[5] P. Gurumurthy, G. Ramachandran, A. K. H. Kumar et al., "Decreased bioavailability of rifampin and other antituberculosis drugs in patients with advanced human immunodeficiency virus disease," *Antimicrobial Agents and Chemotherapy*, vol. 48, no. 11, pp. 4473–4475, 2004.

[6] M. Weiner, W. Burman, A. Vernon et al., "Low isoniazid concentrations and outcome of tuberculosis treatment with once-weekly isoniazid and rifapentine," *American Journal of Respiratory and Critical Care Medicine*, vol. 167, no. 10, pp. 1341–1347, 2003.

[7] H. S. Schaaf, D. P. Parkin, H. I. Seifart et al., "Isoniazid pharmacokinetics in children treated for respiratory tuberculosis," *Archives of Disease in Childhood*, vol. 90, no. 6, pp. 614–618, 2005.

[8] M. Kinzig-Schippers, D. Tomalik-Scharte, A. Jetter et al., "Should we use N-acetyltransferase type 2 genotyping to personalize isoniazid doses?" *Antimicrobial Agents and Chemotherapy*, vol. 49, no. 5, pp. 1733–1738, 2005.

[9] M. Weiner, D. Benator, W. Burman et al., "Association between acquired rifamycin resistance and the pharmacokinetics of rifabutin and isoniazid among patients with HIV and tuberculosis," *Clinical Infectious Diseases*, vol. 40, no. 10, pp. 1481–1491, 2005.

[10] S. Paranjothy, M. Eisenhut, M. Lilley et al., "Extensive transmission of Mycobacterium tuberculosis from 9 year old child with pulmonary tuberculosis and negative sputum smear," *British Medical Journal*, vol. 337, p. a1184, 2008.

[11] O. Braun-Falco and G. P. Heilgemeir, "The trichogram," *SEM for Dermatologists*, vol. 4, article 40, 1985.

[12] K. Anslinger, B. Bayer, B. Rolf, W. Keil, and W. Eisenmenger, "Application of the BioRobot EZ1 in a forensic laboratory," *Legal Medicine*, vol. 7, no. 3, pp. 164–168, 2005.

[13] A. Khedhaier, E. Hassen, N. Bouaouina, S. Gabbouj, S. B. Ahmed, and L. Chouchane, "Implication of Xenobiotic Metabolizing Enzyme gene (CYP2E1, CYP2C19, CYP2D6, mEH and NAT2) polymorphisms in breast carcinoma," *BMC Cancer*, vol. 8, article 109, 2008.

[14] K. Fukino, Y. Sasaki, S. Hirai et al., "Effects of N-acetyltransferase 2 (NAT2), CYP2E1 and glutathione-S-transferase (GST) genotypes on the serum concentrations of isoniazid and metabolites in tuberculosis patients," *Journal of Toxicological Sciences*, vol. 33, no. 5, pp. 187–195, 2008.

[15] A. Pariente-Khayat, E. Rey, D. Gendrel et al., "Isoniazid acetylation metabolic ratio during maturation in children," *Clini-*

cal Pharmacology and Therapeutics, vol. 62, no. 4, pp. 377–383, 1997.

[16] O. Paulsen and L. G. Nilsson, "Distribution of acetylator phenotype in relation to age and sex in Swedish patients. A retrospective study," *European Journal of Clinical Pharmacology*, vol. 28, no. 3, pp. 311–315, 1985.

[17] P. R. Gangadharam, A. L. Bhatia, S. Radhakrishna, and J. B. Selkon, "Rate of inactivation of isoniazid in South Indian patients with pulmonary tuberculosis," *Bulletin of the World Health Organization*, vol. 25, pp. 765–777, 1961.

[18] H. McIlleron, P. Wash, A. Burger, J. Norman, P. I. Folb, and P. Smith, "Determinants of rifampin, isoniazid, pyrazinamide, and ethambutol pharmacokinetics in a cohort of tuberculosis patients," *Antimicrobial Agents and Chemotherapy*, vol. 50, no. 4, pp. 1170–1177, 2006.

[19] J. E. Conte, J. A. Golden, M. McQuitty et al., "Effects of gender, AIDS, and acetylator status on intrapulmonary concentrations of isoniazid," *Antimicrobial Agents and Chemotherapy*, vol. 46, no. 8, pp. 2358–2364, 2002.

[20] H. McIlleron, M. Willemse, C. J. Werely et al., "Isoniazid plasma concentrations in a cohort of South African children with tuberculosis: implications for international pediatric dosing guidelines," *Clinical Infectious Diseases*, vol. 48, no. 11, pp. 1547–1553, 2009.

[21] D. A. Evans, P. B. Storey, and V. A. Mckusick, "Further observations on the determination of the isoniazid inactivator phenotype," *Bulletin of the Johns Hopkins Hospital*, vol. 108, pp. 60–66, 1961.

[22] V. G. F. Pinheiro, L. M. A. Ramos, H. A. S. Monteiro et al., "Intestinal permeability and malabsorption of rifamicin and INH in active pulmonary tuberculosis," *Brazilian Journal of Infectious Diseases*, vol. 10, pp. 374–379, 2006.

[23] M. Gandhi and R. M. Greenblatt, "Hair it is: the long and short of monitoring antiretroviral treatment," *Annals of Internal Medicine*, vol. 137, no. 8, pp. 696–697, 2002.

14

Treatment Outcome of Tuberculosis Patients Registered at DOTS Centre in Ogbomoso, Southwestern Nigeria: A 4-Year Retrospective Study

Olarewaju Sunday,[1] Olanrewaju Oladimeji,[2] Folorunso Ebenezer,[1] Babatunde Akintunde,[1] Temitayo-Oboh Abiola,[1] Abdulsalam Saliu,[1] and Oluwatoyin Abiodun[3]

[1] *Department of Community Medicine, Ladoke Akintola University Teaching Hospital, Ogbomoso, Nigeria*
[2] *Liverpool School of Tropical Medicine, Pembroke Place, Liverpool, UK*
[3] *Department of Medical Microbiology, Ladoke Akintola University of Technology, Ogbomoso, Oyo State, Nigeria*

Correspondence should be addressed to Olarewaju Sunday; biosunfoundation@yahoo.com

Academic Editor: Carlo Garzelli

Background Information. Monitoring outcome of tuberculosis treatment and understanding the specific reasons for unsuccessful treatment outcome are important in evaluating the effectiveness of tuberculosis control program. This study investigated tuberculosis treatment outcomes and predictors for unsuccessful treatment outcome in Ogbomoso town, Southwestern Nigeria. *Methodology.* Medical records of all tuberculosis patients registered from January 2008 to December 2011 in 5 Local Government areas, Ogbomoso, Southwestern Nigeria, were reviewed. Treatment outcome and tuberculosis type were categorized according to the national tuberculosis control guideline. Bivariate analysis was used to analyse the association between treatment outcome and potential predictor variables. *Results.* Out of the 965 total TB patients (579 males and 386 females) with mean age 42.4 ± 1.9 years, 866 (89.74%) were categorized as pulmonary tuberculosis and 109 (11.30%) as extrapulmonary tuberculosis. Treatment outcome among total 914 subjects was as follows: 304 (33.26%) patients got cured, 477 (52.19%) completed treatment, 87 (9.52%) died, 9 (0.98%) defaulted, and 1 (0.11%) failed treatment while 36 (3.94%) were transferred out. Higher treatment success rate was associated with those on Category 1 treatment ($P < 0.05$). *Conclusion.* The treatment success rate of tuberculosis patients was high (85.45%) compared to national target. However, certain proportion of patients died (9.52%) and defaulted (0.98%), which is a serious public health concern that needs to be addressed urgently.

1. Introduction

Tuberculosis (TB) has reemerged as a major global public health concern since the mid-1980s. Globally, tuberculosis accounted for 1.2–1.5 million deaths (including mortality due to tuberculosis as well as TB and HIV coinfection), with 85% of this occurring in developing countries and 26% in Africa. Possible causes of reemergence are due to rapid increase in poverty, poor living conditions with overcrowding, war, malnutrition, lack of drugs, the chronic problem of underfunding of National Tuberculosis Programmes (NTPs), and nonadherence to programme policies. These factors may contribute to increased transmission of mycobacterium tuberculosis in the community and/or to an increased risk of progression from latent to overt clinical TB [1]. Nigeria is a high burden for tuberculosis (TB). Although the exact burden of tuberculosis in Nigeria is not known, the WHO estimates an incidence rate for all forms of tuberculosis to be 311 per 100,000 populations, incidence of smear positive annually 131 per 100,000 population and prevalence of 546 per 100,000 populations [2]. These figures place Nigeria 4th among the 22 high burden countries in the world [2].

Early diagnosis and adequate treatment of infectious patients with pulmonary TB are necessary to reduce transmission of M. tuberculosis and ultimately to achieve elimination of TB. If TB is detected early and properly treated using a combination of medicines for 6 to 9 months, the patients quickly become noninfectious and are eventually cured. Important challenges for TB control are human immunodeficiency virus (HIV) coinfection and drug resistance [3, 4]. HIV coinfection is the strongest known risk factor for progression of latent TB infection to TB disease [5]. Although HIV coinfection has been shown not to affect the failure rate of TB treatment, high mortality has been reported among HIV-infected TB patients in sub-Saharan Africa [6].

In Nigeria, the National Tuberculosis Control Programme (NTBLCP) was well established body facilitating policy and human development, tertiary care, resource mobilization, and technical support to the state programs in the control of TB, leprosy, and Buruli ulcer while the LGA is the operational level of the program based on the primary health care (PHC) principle (the main thrust of health care in Nigeria). Directly Observed Treatment Short Course strategy based on 5 components, that is, political commitment, case detection by bacteriology, standardized treatment with supervision, effective drug supply, and treatment monitoring, recommended by World Health Organization (WHO) was adopted by NTBLCP to eliminate tuberculosis since 1993 [7]. Moreover, the standardized treatment as recommended by WHO consists of 2-month intensive phase, in which patients take drugs directly under the observation of health care providers, and 4-month continuation phase for new TB cases while the retreatment cases have 3-month intensive phase and 5-month continuation phase. The utility of DOTS has also been demonstrated by Ige et al. who reported 90% sputum conversion rate at second month among 97 patients in a 3-year short course chemotherapy among pulmonary tuberculosis in Ibadan, between April 3, 1995, and April 6, 1998, Ibadan with no relapse after 18 months follow-up while Erhabor et al. at Obafemi Awolowo University Teaching Hospital, Ile-Ife reported a cure rate of 86.1% and compliance rate of 93.8% [8, 9].

Monitoring the outcome of treatment using standardized approach is essential in order to evaluate the effectiveness of the intervention and for comparison. World Health Organization in conjunction with International Union Against Tuberculosis and Lung Disease (IUATLD) provided recommendations on how to evaluate treatment outcomes using standardized categories [10]. This would make it possible to recognize and amend system failures before the incidence and proportion of resistant isolates rise. However, treatment outcome of tuberculosis patients has not been assessed yet in Ogbomoso, Southwestern Nigeria. Therefore, this study aimed to assess treatment outcomes of all TB patients on treatment over 4-year period by reviewing register and case records which will enable us to ascertain the effectiveness or otherwise of this regimen and possible emergence of resistance to antituberculosis drugs in this environment.

2. Materials and Method

2.1. Study Area. This study was carried out in Ogbomoso, Southwestern Nigeria. It is a city in Oyo State, Southwestern Nigeria, founded in the mid-seventeenth century with a population approximately 645,000 as of 1991. The city is considered one of Nigeria's largest urban centers. The majority of the people are members of the Yoruba ethnic group. Yams, cassava, maize, and tobacco are some of the notable agricultural products of the region.

2.2. Study Design. A retrospective analysis of the profile and treatment outcome of all tuberculosis patients registered from January 2008 to December 2012 at DOTS Clinic was conducted. The registration documents reviewed contain basic information such as patient's age, sex, address, tuberculosis type, and treatment outcome. Institutional ethical clearance was obtained from the ethical committee, Lautech Teaching Hospital, Ogbomoso, Oyo State.

2.3. Definitions. According to the standard definitions of the National Tuberculosis and Leprosy Control Program guideline (NLCP) adopted from WHO 6, the following clinical case and treatment outcome definitions were used [11].

2.4. Pulmonary TB, Smear-Positive. A patient was with at least two sputum specimens which were positive for acid-fast bacilli (AFB) by microscopy.

2.5. Pulmonary TB, Smear-Negative. A patient was with symptoms suggestive of TB, with at least two sputum specimens which were negative for AFB by microscopy, and with chest radiographic abnormalities consistent with active pulmonary TB (including interstitial or miliary abnormal images).

2.6. Extrapulmonary TB (EPTB). This included tuberculosis of organs other than the lungs, such as lymph nodes, abdomen, genitourinary tract, skin, joints, bones, and meninges. Diagnosis of EPTB was based on fine needle aspiration cytology or biochemical analyses of cerebrospinal/pleural/ascitic fluid or histopathological examination or strong clinical evidence consistent with active extrapulmonary tuberculosis, followed by a decision of a clinician to treat with a full course of antituberculosis chemotherapy. In all the cases of EPTB, sputum examinations and chest radiographs were used to investigate the involvement of lung parenchyma.

2.7. Treatment Outcome. The treatment outcome was divided into seven categories according to NTLCP guideline. These categories were cured (finished treatment with negative bacteriology result at the end of treatment), completed treatment (finished treatment, but without bacteriology result at the end of treatment for those who are smear-positive), failure (remaining smear-positive at five months despite correct intake of medication), defaulted treatment (patients who interrupted their treatment for two consecutive months or more after registration), died (patients who died from any cause during the course of treatment), transferred out (patients whose treatment results are unknown due to transfer to another health facility), and successfully treated (a patient who was cured or completed treatment).

Table 1: Socio-demographic status of respondents.

Variable (N = 965)	Frequency	Percentage
Sex		
Male	579	60.0
Female	386	40.0
LGA		
Surulere	62	6.4
Ogbomoso N	471	48.8
Ogbomoso S	268	27.8
Orire	56	5.8
Ogo Oluwa	108	11.2
Age group		
0–9	39	4.0
10–29	51	5.3
20–29	154	16.0
30–39	185	19.2
40–49	180	18.7
>50	356	36.9

2.8. Statistical Analysis. Data collected was analyzed using SPSS statistical package after data cleaning and ensuring data validity through random checks and double entry of data. Frequency data were generated. Both bi- and logistic regression were done in addition to Chi squared testing to demonstrate association between variables of interest. P value was set at less than or equal to 0.05 for all inferential statistics having to do with significance tests.

2.9. Study Limitation. A large proportion of reported cases (i.e., 486 cases) with missing information were excluded from the study while information on other factors such as education, occupation, housing, and other sociocultural factors that could also affect the treatment outcome was not captured in the register.

3. Results

A total of 965 patients with complete documentation were analyzed, age range 1–90 years. Five hundred and seventy-nine (60.0%) were males while 386 (40.0%) were females giving a male to female ratio of 1.5 : 1. The total mean age group for male patients is 43 ± 19 years while that of the female group is 40 ± 17 years and the total mean age group is 42.0 ± 1.9 years (see Table 1).

Likewise, the disease was pulmonary in 854 (88.5%) and extrapulmonary in 111 (11.5%). Nine hundred and seventeen (95.1%) were registered as new cases and put on Category 1 treatment while 48 (4.9%) were registered as retreatment cases and put on Category 11 treatment (see Table 2).

Of the overall 965 patients seen, 477 (33.3%) were cured, 477 (52.2%) had completed treatment given an overall treatment success of 87.5%, 87 (9.52%) died, and 36 (3.94%) were transferred out while 1 (0.01%) failed treatment (see Table 3).

Table 2: Distribution of patients in relation to site of disease and treatment category.

Variable	Frequency	Percentage
Pulmonary	854	88.5
Extra-pulmonary	111	11.5
Total	**965**	**100.0**
Cat 1	917	95.1
Cat 11	48	4.9
Total	**965**	**100.0**

Table 3: Overall outcome of patients with tuberculosis treatment in Ogbomoso, Oyo State.

Variable	Frequency	Percentage
Cured	304	33.3
Treatment completed	477	52.2
Treatment failure	1	0.01
Dead	87	9.52
Defaulted	9	0.98
Transfer out	36	3.94

Table 4: Factors associated with favorable treatment outcome.

Variable	Odds ratio	Confidence interval	P value
Treatment Category 1	5.14	2.8–9.3	0.00
Local Government			
Surulere	0.033	0.013–0.80	0.00
Ogbomoso North	0.72	0.42–1.22	0.23
Ogbomoso South	4.77	2.4–9.6	0.00
Orire	5.49	1.23–24.9	0.026

The Local Government area (i.e., Surulere, Ogbomoso South, and Orire LGA) where the patient is taking treatment (P = 0.00) as well as treatment category (P = 0.00) had significantly associated with favourable treatment outcome (see Table 4).

4. Discussion

DOTS is a highly effective and efficient means of managing tuberculosis. The treatment success rate of all tuberculosis cases was 85.5% which is comparable with results from other regions of the world where DOTS strategy is currently being operated. In Cotonou, Benin Republic, 82% and 78% success rates were reported among new and retreatment cases with 1% and 3% failure rates, respectively [12]. In another study, 66.5% cure rate was reported after 7-month short course chemotherapy among smear-positive Rwandan and Burundian refugees [13]. Similarly, 77.2% and 68.3% cure rates, respectively, were reported among smear-positive and smear-negative tuberculosis patients in Sudan [14]. This may be due to full supervision of DOTS Strategy in the treatment centres for 2 months on Category 1 and 3 months for Category 2 during the intensive phase while patients are expected to collect their drugs on monthly basis during the continuation phase.

However, the study also documented unfavourable treatment outcome of 9.52% death, 3.94% transferring out, and 0.01% treatment failure. Other information on responsible factors highlighted from previous studies such as HIV status, occupation, educational status, and poor living conditions was not documented in the record used for this study.

A greater proportion of the TB patients registered within the period were males compared to females. Patients who were mostly affected were within the age range group 20–49 years which is in conformity with findings of Nwachokor et al. and Thomas et al., where predominantly patients below 40 years of age were infected with a peak in the 21 to 30 years of age range. The age groups most affected from this work also conform with global trend in which the middle age groups are most at risk of being infected with tuberculosis. Reasons deduced from this include drug abuse, alcoholism, smoking, and poor living conditions occasioned by unemployment and poverty thus portending grave danger to the society [15]. Also, as observed from the result, there were more than 88.5% and 11.5% cases of pulmonary and extrapulmonary tuberculosis, respectively. This goes to show that pulmonary tuberculosis remains to be the major type of tuberculosis in Ogbomoso by extension Nigeria. This finding is supported by another finding in Ibadan, Southwestern Nigeria, by Cadmus and Salami in Ilorin, North Central Nigeria [16, 17]. Although occurrence of tuberculosis was higher in males than females (1.5 : 1), there remains a great cause for concern on the growing impact of TB as a major cause of morbidity and mortality among women. However, those with favourable outcome had no significant association with gender, age group, type of TB lesion, and new or retreatment TB cases similar to the outcome of the study done by Egbewale et al. in a 4-year review of tuberculosis treatment outcome among 879 TB patients in State Hospital, Osogbo, Southwestern Nigeria [18]. It disagrees with other studies done by Salami and Oluboyo in Ilorin and Gninafon et al. at Cotonou, Benin Republic, where strong association exists with male gender and increasing age [12, 17]. Outcome in our study depends on compliance with therapy and level of monitoring by the community extension workers compared to type of lesion, age, and gender.

There were some limitations to this study: culture for tubercle bacilli was not done; therefore the smear-conversion rate may be underestimated since some bacilli present in the sputum smear may be dead. Also drug susceptibility tests were not done, so we could not assess the degree of resistance to anti-TB drugs. Also, other sociocultural factors and socioeconomic factors such as education, housing, and income that can affect the outcome of patients on treatment could not be retrieved from the register. DOTS is a highly effective and efficient means of managing TB. Efforts should be made to increase treatment centres so as to make them available to patients in developing countries that bear a large burden of the disease. Use of a comprehensive approach, which may include the provision of incentives, transportation, feeding, and others, will go a long way in enhancing DOTS.

References

[1] *Global Tuberculosis Control: Surveillance, Planning, Financing. WHO Report 2010*, World Health Organization, Geneva, Switzerland, 2010, (WHO/HTM/TB/2004.331); 2010 Contract No.: Document Number.

[2] WHO Global Tuberculosis Report 2009, 2009.

[3] E. L. Corbett, C. J. Watt, N. Walker et al., "The growing burden of tuberculosis: global trends and interactions with the HIV epidemic," *Archives of Internal Medicine*, vol. 163, no. 9, pp. 1009–1021, 2003.

[4] C. Dye, M. A. Espinal, C. J. Watt, C. Mbiaga, and B. G. Williams, "Worldwide incidence of multidrug-resistant tuberculosis," *Journal of Infectious Diseases*, vol. 185, no. 8, pp. 1197–1202, 2002.

[5] T. R. Frieden, T. R. Sterling, S. S. Munsiff, C. J. Watt, and C. Dye, "Tuberculosis," *The Lancet*, vol. 362, no. 9387, pp. 887–899, 2003.

[6] Y. D. Mukadi and A. Harries, "Tuberculosis case fatality rates in high HIV prevalence populations in sub-Saharan Africa," *AIDS*, vol. 15, no. 2, pp. 143–152, 2001.

[7] NTBLCP annualReport 2009.

[8] O. M. Ige, N. A. Bakare, and B. O. Onadeko, "Modified short-course chemotherapy of pulmonary tuberculosis in Ibadan, Nigeria—a preliminary report," *African Journal of Medicine and Medical Sciences*, vol. 29, no. 1, pp. 51–53, 2000.

[9] G. E. Erhabor, O. Adewole, A. O. Adisa, and O. A. Olajolo, "Directly observed short course therapy for tuberculosis—a preliminary report of a three-year experience in a teaching hospital," *Journal of the National Medical Association*, vol. 95, no. 11, pp. 1082–1088, 2003.

[10] J. Veen, M. Raviglione, H. L. Rieder et al., "Standardized tuberculosis treatment outcome monitoring in Europe," *European Respiratory Journal*, vol. 12, no. 2, pp. 505–510, 1998.

[11] Ministry of Health of Nigeria (MOH), *Tuberculosis and Leprosy and Control Programme Workers Manual.*

[12] M. Gninafon, L. Tawo, F. Kassa et al., "Outcome of tuberculosis retreatment in routine conditions in Cotonou, Benin," *International Journal of Tuberculosis and Lung Disease*, vol. 8, no. 10, pp. 1242–1247, 2004.

[13] E. Rutta, R. Kipingili, H. Lukonge, S. Assefa, E. Mitsilale, and S. Rwechungura, "Treatment outcome among Rwandan and Burundian refugees with sputum smear-positive tuberculosis in Ngara, Tanzania," *International Journal of Tuberculosis and Lung Disease*, vol. 5, no. 7, pp. 628–632, 2001.

[14] E.-S. Al Kah, D. A. Enarson, O. Baraka, S. A. Mustafa, and G. Bjune, "Treatment results of DOTS in 1797 sudanese tuberculosis patients wit h or without HIV co-infection," *International Journal of Tuberculosis and Lung Disease*, vol. 6, no. 12, pp. 1058–1066, 2002.

[15] A. Kochi, "The global tuberculosis situation and the new control strategy of the World Health Organization," *Tubercle*, vol. 72, no. 1, pp. 1–6, 1991.

[16] S. I. Cadmus, "Insight into the epidemiology of laboratory confirmed human tuberculosis in Ibadan, Nigeria," *African Journal of Medicine and Medical Sciences*, vol. 39, pp. 213–218, 2010.

[17] A. K. Salami and P. O. Oluboyo, "Hospital prevalence of pulmonary tuberculosis and co-infection with human immunodeficiency virus in Ilorin: a review of nine years (1991–1999)," *West African Journal of Medicine*, vol. 21, no. 1, pp. 24–27, 2002.

15

Application of Cox Proportional Hazards Model in Case of Tuberculosis Patients in Selected Addis Ababa Health Centres, Ethiopia

Kabtamu Tolosie and M. K. Sharma

Addis Ababa University, Addis Ababa, Ethiopia

Correspondence should be addressed to M. K. Sharma; mk_subash@yahoo.co.in

Academic Editor: Brian Eley

Introduction. Tuberculosis (TB) is a chronic infectious disease and mainly caused by mycobacterium tuberculosis (MTB). It has been one of the major causes of mortality in Ethiopia. The objective of the study was to identify factors that affect the survival of the patients with tuberculosis who started treatment for tuberculosis. *Methods*. This was a retrospective study in six randomly selected health centres in Addis Ababa, Ethiopia. The data were obtained from medical records of TB patients registered from September 2012 to August 2013 and treated under directly observed treatment surgery (DOTS) strategy. Kaplan Meier plots, logrank tests, and Wilcoxon tests were used to assess the survival pattern. Cox proportional hazards model for multivariable analysis was discussed. *Results*. Out of the total 826 registered TB patients, 105 (12.71%) died during the study period and 712 (87.29%) were censored. Based on Kaplan Meier survival curves, logrank test, and Wilcoxon test, it was found that the patients had statistically significant differences in survival experience with respect to age, body weight at initiation of treatment, TB patient category, and HIV status. Multivariable Cox hazards regression analysis revealed that the covariates age, TB patient category, HIV, and age by HIV interaction were significant risk factors associated with death status in TB patients. *Conclusion*. Deaths of individuals with diseases especially HIV coinfected and nonnew TB cases were high. Therefore, this needs to strengthen the follow-up of patients with TB treatment from the day of anti-TB treatment initiation to completion days.

1. Introduction

Tuberculosis (TB) is the leading cause of death from a single bacterial species among adults around the world. The World Health Organization (WHO) estimated that one-third of the world population is infected with *Mycobacterium tuberculosis*, with 9.4 million new cases and 1.3 million deaths in 2009 [1].

Reducing death, eliminating disease, and preventing the development of drug-resistant TB are the major goals of TB control [2]. TB-related death is often referred to as a TB control indicator [3].

Although the developed countries in Europe and North America have well-equipped treatment facilities and provide free and sufficient anti-TB drugs, treatment success rates there are still below WHO's goal of 85%, which may be because of the relatively high death rates. In those countries, TB cases are found in the relatively higher age group and are associated with comorbidities [4].

In previous studies, even in developed countries with good national TB control programs, more than 10% of cases died during the follow-up period. In high-resource settings, but not in most high TB-burden countries, most cases of death during TB treatment are often because of causes other than TB [5].

On March 24, 1882, Dr. Robert Koch announced the discovery of *Mycobacterium tuberculosis*, the bacteria that cause tuberculosis (TB). Dr. Koch's discovery was the most important step taken toward the control and elimination of this deadly disease. In 1982, a century after Dr. Koch's announcement, the first World TB Day was sponsored by the World Health Organization (WHO) and the International Union against Tuberculosis and Lung Disease (IUATLD). The event was intended to educate the public about the devastating health and economic consequences of TB, its effect on developing countries, and its continued tragic impact on global health [6].

Tuberculosis (TB) has been one of the major causes of morbidity and mortality in Ethiopia for long. Accordingly, the Ethiopian Ministry of Health and its stakeholders have put their unreserved and integrated efforts in this health problem. Among these efforts is the well developed Health Management Information System (HMIS) for Tuberculosis programs. However, the direction where Tuberculosis in Ethiopia is heading has not been well analyzed and unpackaged by epidemiologically relevant factors. So, what are the factors that affect the survival of TB patients? It might be gender, age, TB patients category, type of TB, smear result, HIV, and body weight at initiation of treatments of patients. Therefore, to fill this gap there is a need to study the factors that are affecting the survival of patients with tuberculosis. The objectives of this study are (i) to identify the factors that are affecting the survival of the patients with tuberculosis, (ii) to estimate survival time probabilities of the TB patients, (iii) to compare the survival probabilities of the TB patients with respect to different risk factors, and (iv) to identify the factors influencing death status of patient by using the Cox proportional hazards model.

2. Data and Methodology

2.1. The Data. The data was a retrospective cohort study based on TB patients that were registered in unit TB registers in the health facilities providing DOTS in six randomly selected Addis Ababa Governmental health centres, Addis Ababa, Ethiopia. In this study we used secondary data which was collected from patient follow-up records. Information for this study was extracted from documents of all TB cases registered from September 2012 to August 2013 in six DOTS clinics located in six randomly selected health centres.

2.2. Variables in the Study. The explanatory (independent) variables of interest in this study include demographic factors disease, and medicine related factors, and characteristics of the disease. The response (dependent) variable is continuous; it is length of time of treatment for tuberculosis patients.

2.3. The Response Variable. The dependent variable or response is the waiting time until the occurrence of an event (dead: 1, alive or censored: 0). Observations are censored, in the sense that, for some units, the event of interest has not occurred at the time the data are analyzed.

2.4. Predictor Variables. Predictors or explanatory variables which are called covariates are those whose effect on the waiting time we wish to assess. The predictor (covariate) variables which are assumed to influence the survival of TB patients included in the model are (i) age, (ii) gender, (iii) TB patients category, (iv) type of TB, (v) smear result, (vi) initial weight of patients, and (vii) HIV status.

3. Method of Data Analysis

3.1. Survival Analysis. The study focused on time to event (time to death by tuberculosis), so the appropriate method of this particular study was survival analysis. We have used Kaplan-Meir estimator and Cox proportional hazard model for the analysis and model building. We have also used logrank tests and Wilcoxon tests for comparison of survival functions. Kaplan Meier analysis was used to study survival pattern; the KM plot, which is a step function, gives some indications about the shape of the survival distribution. The figure in general shows if the pattern of one survivorship function lies above another which means the group defined by the upper curve lived longer, or had a more favourable survival experience, than the group defined by the lower curve.

3.2. The Proportional Hazards Model. It was used for multivariate analysis to identify factors associated with death from tuberculosis and Cox proportional hazards (PH) model given by

$$\lambda(t \mid z) = \lambda_0(t) e^{\mathbf{Z}^T \boldsymbol{\beta}}, \tag{1}$$

where $\mathbf{Z} = (Z_1, \ldots, Z_p)^T$ and $\boldsymbol{\beta} = (\beta_1, \ldots, \beta_p)^T$, $\mathbf{Z}$ is a $p \times 1$ vector of covariates such as treatment indicators and prognostic factors, and $\boldsymbol{\beta}$ is a $p \times 1$ vector of regression coefficient.

The parameter was estimated by using partial likelihood functions. We used three different tests to assess the significance of the coefficients in Cox proportional hazards model: the partial likelihood ratio test, the Wald test, and the score test.

3.3. Selection of Covariates. We used Hosmer and Lemeshow [7] and Collett [8] that recommended the procedure in variable selection, including all variables that are significant in the univariable analysis at the 20 to 25 percent level and also any other variables which are presumed to be clinically important to fit the initial multivariable model.

3.4. Overall Goodness of Fit. To assess the overall goodness of fit of a Cox proportional hazards regression model Arjas [9] suggests plotting the cumulative observed versus the cumulative expected number of events for subjects with observed (not censored) survival times. If the model fit is adequate, then the points should follow a 45-degree line beginning at the origin.

4. Results

The statistical packages SAS and STATA have been used to analyze the data.

4.1. Summary Statistics. Out of the total 826 registered TB patients 105 (53 male and 52 female) or 12.71% died during the study period and 712 (87.29%) were censored. The age group (≥45 years) showed the highest percentage (18.3%)

with respect to death proportions among the other two age groups. In TB patient category nonnew case had higher percentage (21.93%) of death. The percentages of death 10.4%, 13.99% and 12.99% occurred in the patients with pulmonary positive, pulmonary negative, and extrapulmonary types of TB, respectively, and the patients with positive smear result had lower death percentage. HIV-positive TB patients are the highest risk group for death, that is, 22.18%. Patients with body weight at initiation of treatment (≥35 kg's) had lower risk group for death (Table 1).

4.2. Descriptive Survival Analysis. Table 2 exhibits that out of 826 TB patients, 721 patients were censored (87.29%) and 105 patients died (12.71%). The median follow-up time was 168 days for patients that are censored (range from 15 to 284 days); 25% of the patients had 176 days of follow up (upper quartile). The median time of death was 52 days (range from 1 to 190 days). This shows that most of the events/deaths occurred in the earlier months of anti-TB treatment.

Figure 1 exhibits that there were differences among survivor curves of age category, initial weight, TB patient category, and HIV status for TB patients. However, there were not clear differences among survivor curves of gender, smear result, and type of TB.

Based on Table 3, we find that logrank test and Wilcoxon test are not significant in survival experience between the various categories of gender, smear result, and type of TB. But, they are significant in survival experience of the patients in different categories of age, body weight at initiation of treatment, TBC, and HIV status (at $\alpha = 5\%$).

4.3. Results of the Cox Proportional Hazards Model. We begin with a multivariable model that contains all variables which were significant in the univariate Cox proportional hazard model at the 20–25 percent level.

Table 4 exhibits the summary of seven covariate variables in the univariate analysis. The most appropriate subset of these predictors will be selected in the multivariable model based on their contribution to the maximized log partial likelihood of the model (−2LL). The highest reduction in $-2\text{LL}(\widehat{\beta})$ is observed for HIV status. This difference is 24.599 which is statistically significant (P value < 0.0001) and suggests that an improvement over the null model would be achieved by including HIV status. The reduction in $-2\text{LL}(\widehat{\beta})$ on adding TBC to the null model is 8.19, which is significant. The next reduction in $-2\text{LL}(\widehat{\beta})$ on adding age of patients to the null model is 6.728, which is also significant. By using the Wald chi-Square test, the variable age, smear result, TB category, and HIV status are significant at the 25-percent level and therefore they are candidates for inclusion in multivariable model. Age, TB Category, and HIV status have relatively strong associations with the death of TB patients. Omitting the predictors or covariates gender, initial weight, and type of TB from the model does not bring significant changes in the value of $-2\text{LL}(\widehat{\beta})$. Therefore, these predictors become the first to be removed from the multivariable models.

The next step is to fit the multivariable Cox proportional model that contains age, smear result, TBC, and HIV status. So, at this stage we have a multivariable model which includes the three main effect covariates age, TB category (TBC), and HIV status (HIV). These covariates are significant at 5% level of significance.

The other important step is considering variables that are nonsignificant at univariable analysis but may be confounders. The effect of adding each of the three variables gender, weight, and types of TB (TTB) in the model is shown in Table 5. In particular, when gender, initial weight, and TTB are added, the increase in $-2\text{LL}(\widehat{\beta})$ is nonsignificant values, that is, 0.228, 2.142, and 0.736, respectively.

The final step in the model building process is the consideration of interaction terms shown in Table 6. The Wald test was used to assess the significance of reasonable and possible interactions. The decision for rejection of the null hypothesis is $-2\text{LL}_2 - (-2\text{LL}_1) > \chi^2\ (\alpha = 0.05) = 3.84$. Table 6 shows that the interaction HIV × age was significant. And this is an indication that the interaction of HIV and the age of the patient affects the survival time of the patient.

The results shown in Table 6 ensure that the preliminary model of the study will contain three main effects and one interaction effect. Now, all covariates are significant at 5% level of significance (Table 7). The next step is to check the linearity of continuous covariates in the preliminary multivariable model.

4.4. Checking for Linearity of Continuous Covariates in the Model. It can be seen that the plots of martingale residuals in Figure 2 are random showing no systematic patterns or trends, and the LOESS smoothed curve appears to lie about a horizontal line through zero, supporting the inclusion of the untransformed covariates age and age and HIV interaction have a linear relationship with the survival time in Cox model.

After a preliminary model has been fitted to an observed set of survival data, our next step would be to assess the adequacy of the fitted model. The model will not be identified as the final model until its fit and adherence to model assumptions.

4.5. Diagnosis of the Mode

4.5.1. Assessment of the Proportional Hazards Assumption. The results of tests of all the time-dependent variables in Table 8 were not significant either individually or collectively, so we do not have enough evidence to reject proportionality assumption of all covariates at 5% level of significance.

The plots of the scaled Schoenfeld residuals and the lowness smooth curves shown in Figures 3(a)–3(d) support the assumption of proportional hazards for each of the four covariates. That is, each subplot in the figure is random, smooth and approximates a horizontal through zero or slope approximately equal to zero. This indicates that none of the four covariates had interaction with log of time; also the plots support the proportional hazards assumption.

4.5.2. Identification of Influential and Poorly Fit Data. The score residuals for age in Figure 4(a) display fan shape with the smallest distance near the mean age of 35 and increasing

TABLE 1: Characteristics of tuberculosis patient data under DOTS from six randomly selected governmental health centers in Addis Ababa, Ethiopia, from September 2011 to August 2012.

Patients characteristics	Summary of the number of death and censored values				
	Total	Death	Percent death	Censored	Percent censored
Gender					
Male	414	53	12.80	361	87.20
Female	412	52	12.62	360	87.38
Age categories					
0–24	284	22	7.75	262	92.25
25–44	389	55	14.14	334	85.86
≥45	153	28	18.30	125	81.70
TB patients cat.					
New	712	80	11.24	632	88.76
Nonnew	114	25	21.93	89	78.07
Type of TB					
Pul. positive	202	21	10.40	181	89.60
Pul. negative	293	41	13.99	252	86.01
Extra pulmonary	331	43	12.99	288	87.01
Smear result					
Positive	202	21	10.4	181	89.60
Negative	624	84	13.46	540	86.54
HIV status					
Positive	239	53	22.18	186	77.82
Negative	587	52	8.86	535	91.14
Initial weight					
<35	62	13	20.97	49	79.03
≥35	764	92	12.04	672	87.96

TABLE 2: Summary statistics of status of TB patients and days of follow-up time.

(a)

Status	Status of TB patients Frequency	Percent
Censored	721	87.29
Dead	105	12.71

(b)

Status of patients	N. Obs.	Mean	Std. Dev.	Median	Lower quartile	Upper quartile	Min.	Max.
Censored	721	170.791	18.291	168.000	168.000	176.000	15.000	284.000
Dead	105	63.867	47.012	52.000	29.000	88.000	1.000	190.000

TABLE 3: Results of the Logrank test, Wilcoxon test and −2log (LR) for the categorical variables of TB patients under DOTS in six randomly selected AA health centers.

Covariates	DF	Test of no difference in survival over strata					
		Logrank		Wilcoxon		−2log (LR)	
		Chi-Square	Pr > Chi-Square	Chi-Square	Pr > Chi-Square	Chi-Square	Pr > Chi-Square
Gender	1	0.0020	0.9641	0.0167	0.8973	0.0011	0.9740
Age	2	11.0320	0.0040	10.4640	0.0053	11.5554	0.0031
Weight	1	4.4974	0.0339	5.6019	0.0179	3.9437	0.0470
Smear res.	1	1.6355	0.2009	1.7743	0.1828	1.7244	0.1891
TBC	1	9.7252	0.0018	11.3382	0.0008	8.4141	0.0037
TTB	2	1.8631	0.3939	2.0941	0.3510	1.9208	0.3827
HIV	1	27.6614	<0.0001	28.9458	<0.0001	25.6999	<0.0001

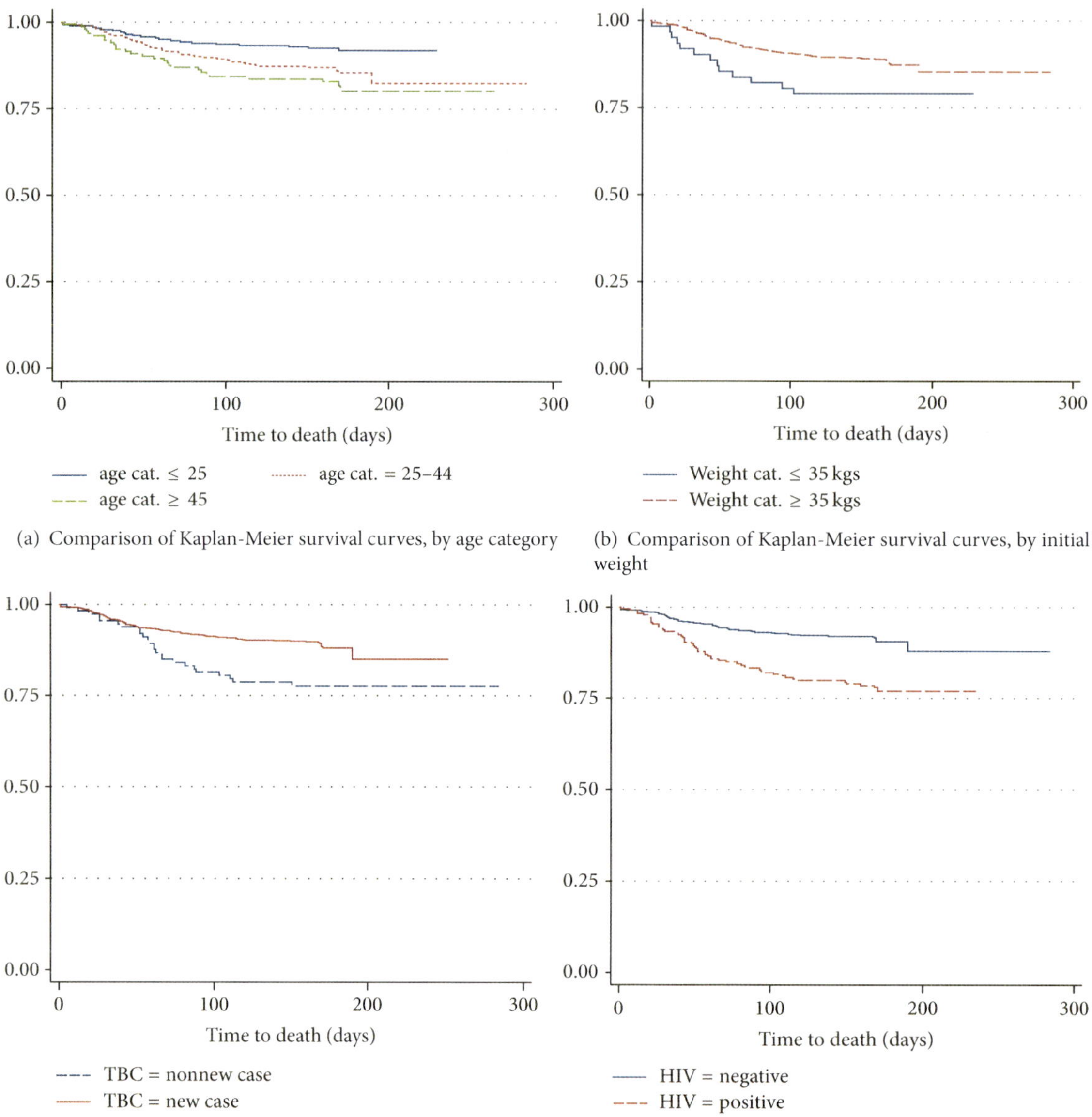

(a) Comparison of Kaplan-Meier survival curves, by age category

(b) Comparison of Kaplan-Meier survival curves, by initial weight

(c) Comparison of Kaplan-Meier survival curves by TB category

(d) Comparison of Kaplan-Meier survival curves by HIV status

Figure 1: The plot of the estimate of Kaplan-Meier survivor curves of TB patients under DOTS in AA health centers (a) age category, (b) initial weight of patients, (c) TB patient category, and (d) HIV status.

Table 4: Results of the univariable proportional hazards Cox regression model of TB patients DOTS in six randomly selected AA health centers.

Analysis of maximum likelihood estimates								
Covariates	DF	Parameter estimate	Standard error	−2LL	Lik. ratio P value	Score P value	Wald P value	Hazard ratio
Gender	1	−0.00878	0.19526	1382.970	0.9641	0.9641	0.9641	0.991
Age	1	0.01626	0.00608	1376.244	0.0095	0.0072	0.0074	1.016
Weight	1	−0.00859	0.00772	1381.761	0.2711	0.2665	0.2659	0.991
S. result	1	−0.31097	0.24441	1381.251	0.1896	0.2012	0.2033	0.733
TBC	1	−0.70235	0.22993	1374.782	0.0042	0.0018	0.0023	0.495
TTB cat. II	1	0.26331	0.26657	1381.039	0.3805	0.3944	0.3233	1.301
TTB cat. III	1	0.36374	0.26882				0.1760	1.439
HIV	1	0.98580	0.19524	1358.373	<0.0001	<0.0001	<0.0001	2.680
The value of −2LL for the null model is 1382.972								

Table 5: Result of partial likelihood ratio test for those variables not significant in the univariable analysis fitted by being included in the model containing those variables significant in multivariable analysis one at a time.

Variables	$-2LL(\hat{\beta})$	$-2LL(\hat{\beta})$ difference	DF	Pr > ChiSq
Age + TBC + HIV	1349.058			
Age + TBC + HIV + gender	1348.830	0.228	1	0.633
Age + TBC + HIV + weight	1346.916	2.142	1	0.143
Age + TBC + HIV + TTB	1348.302	0.736	2	0.692

Table 6: Result of partial likelihood ratio test for the contribution of the interaction effect.

	Model fit statistics			
Interactions	$-2LL_2$ with main effects only	$-2LL_1$ with main and interaction effects	$-2LL_2$- $(-2LL_1)$	Sig.
Age, TBC	1368.802	1368.189	0.613	Do not reject
Age, HIV	1353.644	1345.312	8.332	Reject
TBC, HIV	1353.368	1350.085	3.283	Do not reject

Table 7: Results of the multivariable proportional hazards Cox regression model containing the main and interaction effect.

(a)

	Testing global null hypothesis: bETA = 0		
Test	Chi-Square	DF	Pr > ChiSq
Likelihood ratio	42.6252	4	<0.0001
Score	45.1009	4	<0.0001
Wald	40.3081	4	<0.0001

(b)

			Analysis of maximum likelihood estimates					
Covariates	DF	Parameter estimate	Standard error	Chi-Square	Pr > ChiSq	Hazard ratio	95% HR Conf. limit	
Age	1	0.02745	0.00760	13.0603	0.0003	1.028	1.013	1.043
TBC	1	−0.54298	0.23231	5.4629	0.0194	0.581	0.369	0.916
HIV	1	2.29131	0.50215	20.8209	<0.0001	9.888	3.695	26.457
Age * HIV	1	−0.04028	0.01354	8.8468	0.0029	0.961	0.935	0.986
			The value of −2LL for the model is 1340.347					

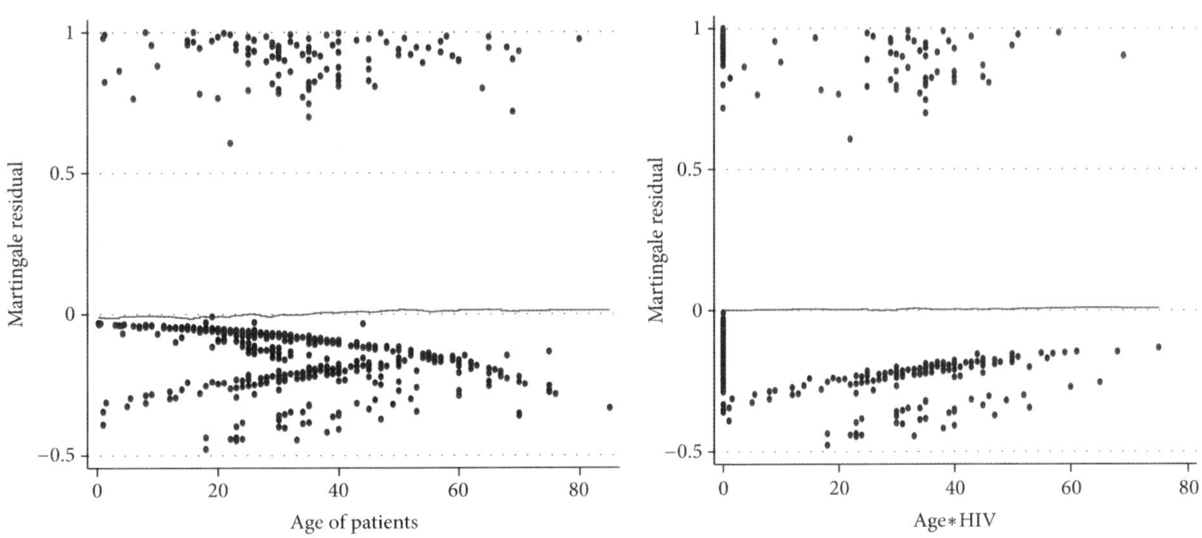

(a) Martingale residuals vs. age of patients

(b) Martingale residuals vs. age and HIV status interaction

Figure 2: Plots of Martingale residuals computed for continuous covariates of TB patients under DOTS in AA health centers (a) age and (b) age and HIV status interaction.

TABLE 8: Result of test of proportionality assumption containing the variables in Table 7 and their interaction with log time.

(a)

Analysis of maximum likelihood estimates						
Covariates	DF	Parameter estimate	Standard error	Chi-Square	Pr > ChiSq	Hazard ratio
Age	1	0.01919	0.02212	0.7526	0.3857	1.019
TBC	1	0.20274	0.95433	0.0451	0.8318	1.225
HIV	1	1.09680	1.13372	0.9359	0.3333	2.995
AgHIV	1	−0.02914	0.01722	2.8638	0.0906	0.971
Age ∗ log (time)	1	0.00223	0.00561	0.6904	0.6904	1.002
TBC ∗ log (time)	1	−0.19525	0.23829	0.6714	0.4126	0.823
HIV ∗ log (time)	1	0.31882	0.27050	1.3891	0.2385	1.375
agHIV ∗ log (time)	1	−0.0001785	0.0001725	1.0712	0.3007	1.000

(b)

Linear hypotheses testing results			
Label	Wald Chi-Square	DF	Pr > ChiSq
Test proportionality	2.1579	4	0.7067

in absolute value for ages increasingly older or younger than 35. The purpose of the plot is to see whether there are subjects whose ages yield unexpectedly large values. This would be seen in the graph as a point lying well away from the others in the plots. In the figure there is one point in the top right at age 80 that falls a bit away from the rest of the points. However, the distance between this point and the others is not striking. The oldest subject, age 85, has score residuals that are well within range of values. Thus, we conclude that there are no high leverage values for age of TB patients.

The score residuals for age × HIV interaction are plotted in Figure 4(b). The plots have one point in the top left corner that fall a bit away from the rest of the other points. But the distance between these points and the others is not striking. The two subsets, one in the top right and one in the bottom right, have score residuals that are well within range of values. Thus, we conclude that there are no high leverage values for age by HIV interaction. In general, the plots in Figure 5 have shown that there are no strikingly large score residuals.

The first six largest changes in parameter estimates are shown in Table 9. To begin with the largest difference for covariate age is observed for patient numbered 730. The result exhibits that the change in the parameter estimate, if the data for this patient is discarded, is 0.0023234. The standard error, of the parameter estimate for age in the full data set is 0.0076. That is, the percentage change in parameter estimate if the observation is removed is about 30.57% of the standard error that is, less than one standard error. Thus, removing this observation would not bring a significant change on age of patients. It is similar for covariates TBC, HIV, and age by HIV interaction. Therefore, it can be concluded that there was no aberrant observation in the data set that illegitimately inflated the estimates of the parameters of the covariates in the final model.

4.5.3. Checking for Overall Goodness of Fit. The cumulative hazard plot of the Cox-Snell residuals is shown in Figure 5. We see that the hazard function is reasonably straight line that has a unit slope and zero interception. It approximates the 45-degree line very closely except for very large values of time. Overall we would conclude that the final model fits the data very well. Therefore, the model with estimates as given in Table 7 is the final model.

4.5.4. Interpretation of the Results. The results of the fitted final model in Table 7 are interpreted in terms of hazard ratios (HR). The coefficient of the categorical covariates is interpreted as the logarithm of the ratio of the hazard of death to the baseline (reference group) hazard. That is, they are interpreted by comparing the reference group with others. Similarly, the coefficient for a continuous explanatory variable indicates the estimated change in the logarithm of the hazard ratio for a unit increase in the value of the respective covariate when the remaining covariates in the model are controlled.

Only the covariate TB patient category (TBC) has hazard ratio that is estimated by exponentiating its estimated coefficient. This is because the covariates age and HIV are involved in interaction. The estimated coefficient for a new case of TB was −0.54298, which decreases the hazards of experiencing death by a factor exp(−0.54289) = 0.581 (95% CI: 0.369–0.916); that is, the patients with a new case of TB have about 41.9% lower mortality rate than patients with nonnew case TB. The 95-percent confidence interval suggested that the rate could be as much as 63.1 percent lower to only 8.4 percent lower. The estimated hazard ratio pointed to a significant benefit for the new case of the two TB patient categories, controlling for all other model covariates.

Age and HIV status are present in the model, with both main effects and their interaction. Since HIV status is at two levels, we present hazard ratios for age at each HIV status rather than for HIV status at each age. For example, the estimate hazard ratios for an increase of 15 years of age at HIV-negative and HIV-positive were found to be 1.51, 0.82,

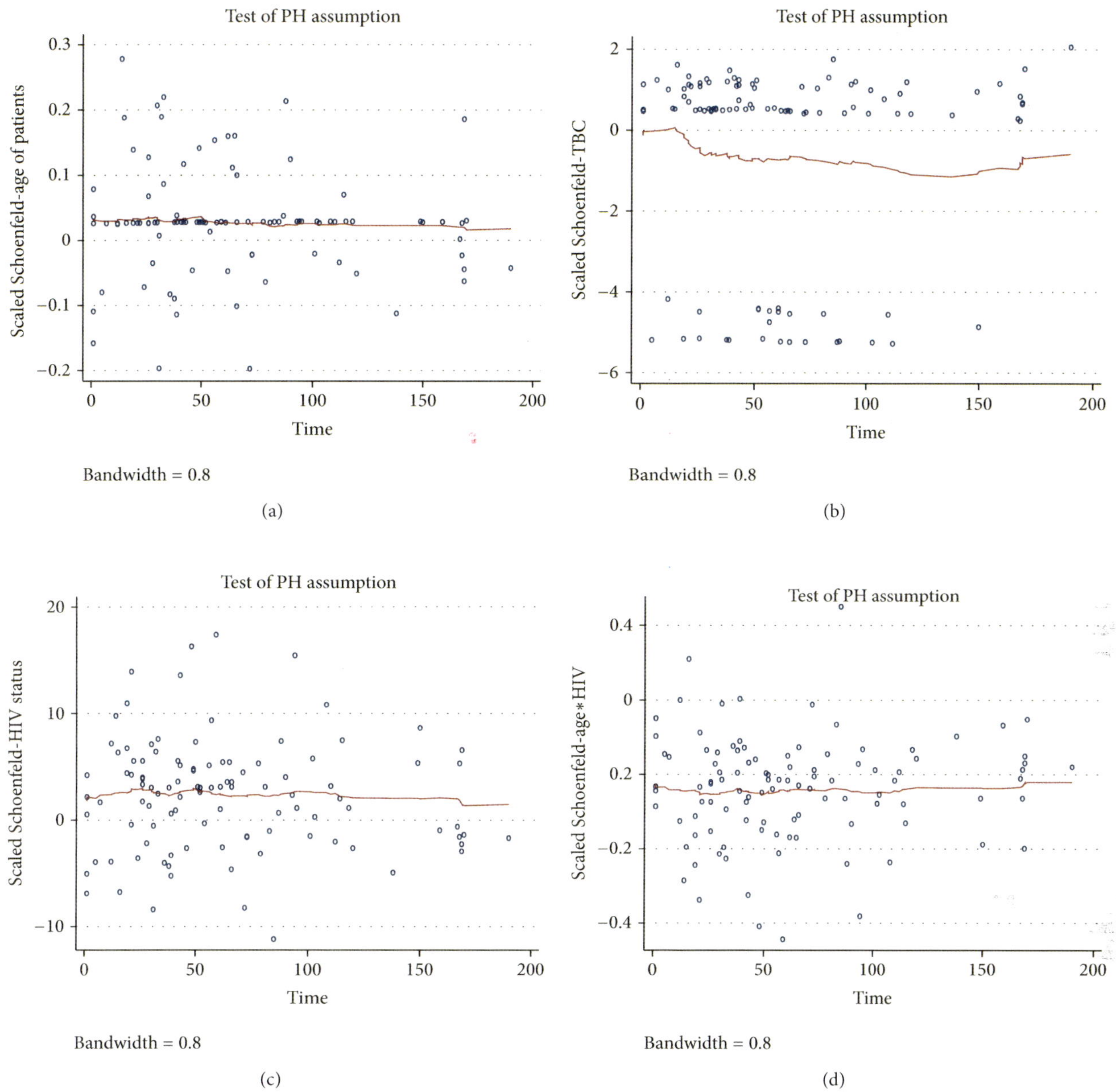

FIGURE 3: Graphs of the scaled Schoenfeld residuals and their LOESS smooth curves for the covariates: (a) age of patients, (b) TB patient category, (c) HIV status, and (d) age and HIV status interaction.

respectively. This means that being older by 15 years at HIV-negative increased the rate of death by about 51 percent and HIV-positive reduces the rate of death by about 18 percent.

5. Discussion

This study is an attempt to identify the factors that affect the survival of the patients with tuberculosis; we found that from the Kaplan-Meier survival estimates there was a significant difference in survival by the age, body weight at initiation of treatment, TB patient category, and HIV status. However, there were no differences among survival curves of gender, smear result, and type of TB patients. The logrank test also showed that there was no significant difference in survival experience between the various categories of gender, smear result, and type of TB (P value > 0.05). However, the test showed that the survival experience of patients in different categories of age (logrank statistic = 11.0320, P value = 0.0053), initial weight (logrank statistic = 4.4974, P value = 0.0179), TBC (logrank statistic = 9.7252, P value = 0.0008), and HIV status (logrank statistic = 27.6614, P value ≤ 0.0001) differ significantly. The multivariable Cox proportional hazards regression results analysis indicated that the three covariates age, TB patient category, HIV, and the interaction age by HIV were significantly associated with death among TB patients. Gender, body weight at initiation of treatment,

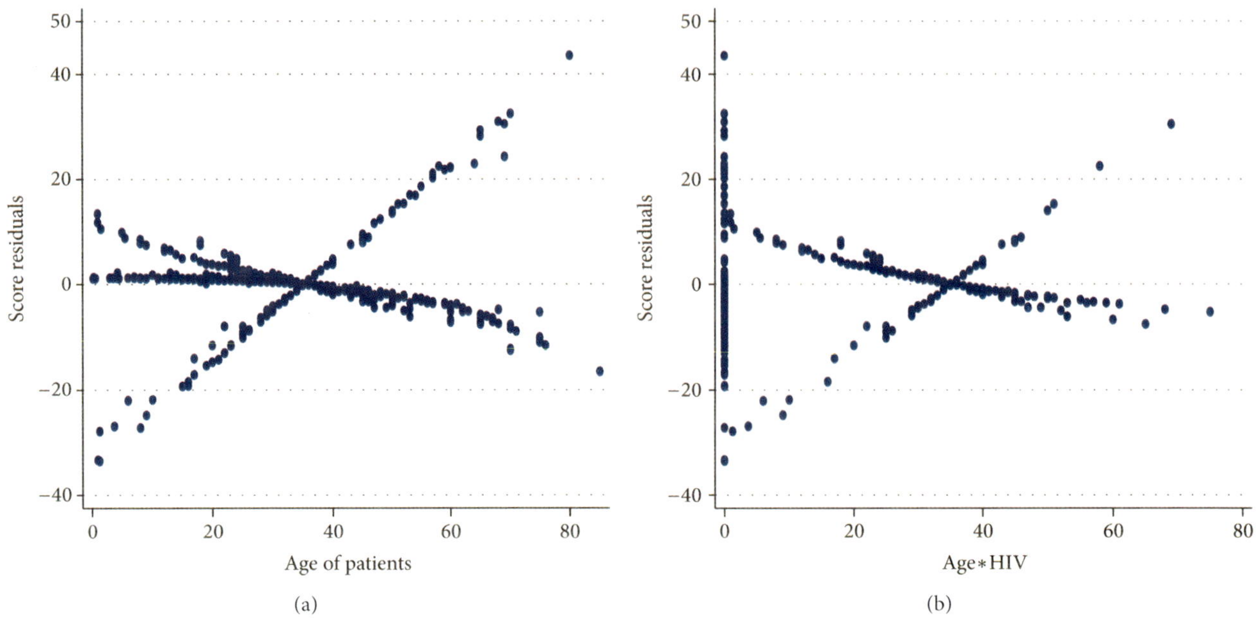

FIGURE 4: Graphs of the score residuals computed from the model in Table 7 for (a) age of TB patients and (b) age by HIV status interaction.

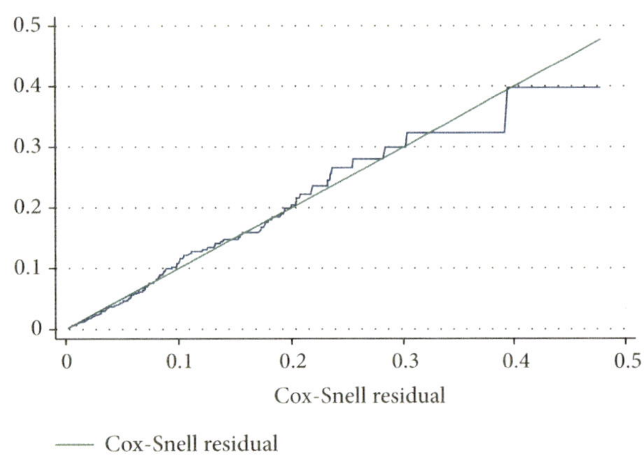

FIGURE 5: Cumulative hazard plot of the Cox-Snell residuals of the proportional hazards Cox regression model in Table 7. The 45-degree straight line through the origin is drawn for reference.

smear result, and type of TB were not significantly associated with factors that are affecting the survival of patients with tuberculosis.

A study by Oursler et al. [5] showed that a total of 29 (21%) of the 139 patients died during treatment; the median time to death among these patients was 39 days and follow up for survivors was 202 days. (Lo et al. [10]) showed that, 50% of deaths occurred within 2 months. In this study we found that out of 826 TB patients, 721 patients were censored (87.29%) and 105 patients died (12.71%) during treatment; the median follow-up time is 168 days for patients that are censored (range from 15 to 284 days), 25% of the patients had 176 days of follow up (upper quartile). The median time to death among those patients who died was 52 days (ranges from 1 to 190 days); this shows that most of the events/deaths occurred in the earlier months of TB treatment initiation.

The survival curves of TB patient among age groups are significantly different. There was no difference in the survival curves of male and female patients and according to type of disease [11]. A study by Getahun et al. [12] conducted in Addis Ababa showed that the survival status was significantly different between patient age, weight at initiation of anti-TB treatment, patient category, year of enrolment, and treatment centre. We also found a similar result, no differences among survivor curves of gender and type of disease. However, there was a difference among survivor curves of age category, body weight at initiation of treatment, TB patient category, and HIV status for TB patients.

Age has been identified as an important risk factor for death in tuberculosis patients. Different studies showed that age was a factor that is affecting the survival of TB patients. According to Horne et al. [13] in Washington State, mortality was independently associated with increasing age. A study in Maryland, community-based cohort of patients with drug-susceptible pulmonary TB, showed age was strongly associated with the risk of death [5]. A study in Brazil showed that age was statistically significant in the multivariable Cox regression model [14, 15]. Another study also showed that age has been identified as an important risk factor for death in tuberculosis patients [10–12, 16–18] (Lo et al.). Our study also found that age was statistically a significant risk factor for death.

A study was carried out in Brazil aimed at analyzing survival probability and identifying risk factors for death from tuberculosis in a cohort of patients living in Recife who started treatment for tuberculosis. During follow up HIV-positive was statistically significant in the multivariable Cox regression model [14]. Also HIV coinfection was statistically

TABLE 9: The six highest differences in the parameter estimates of the variables included in the model in Table 7 when the data value for each patient is in turn deleted from the model, approximate delta-betas for age ($\widehat{\beta}_1$), TBC ($\widehat{\beta}_2$), HIV ($\widehat{\beta}_3$), and age by HIV ($\widehat{\beta}_4$).

(a)

Deleted Obs. (i)	$\Delta_i\widehat{\beta}_1$	% change parameter of the std. error	Deleted Obs. (i)	$\Delta_i\widehat{\beta}_2$	% change parameter of the std. error
730	0.0023234	30.57	413	−0.0439987	18.94
162	−0.0021205	27.90	585	−0.0428435	18.44
262	−0.0020957	27.58	343	−0.0427599	18.41
421	−0.0017624	23.20	368	−0.0423473	18.23
542	0.0017002	22.37	544	−0.04214	18.14
580	0.001611	21.20	447	−0.041601	17.91
Sd. error ($\widehat{\beta}_1$) of full model = 0.00760			Sd. error ($\widehat{\beta}_2$) of full model = 0.23231		

(b)

Deleted Obs. (i)	$\Delta_i\widehat{\beta}_3$	% change parameter of the std. error	Deleted Obs. (i)	$\Delta_i\widehat{\beta}_4$	% change parameter of the std. error
133	0.1185484	23.61	548	0.0042068	31.07
548	−0.1155908	23.02	63	0.0032745	24.18
204	0.1146464	22.83	133	−0.0031662	23.38
244	−0.1056003	21.03	204	−0.0030298	22.38
162	−0.1008921	20.10	244	−0.0027001	19.94
262	−0.098443	19.60	282	−0.0024873	18.37
Sd. error ($\widehat{\beta}_3$) of full model = 0.50215			Sd. error ($\widehat{\beta}_4$) of full model = 0.01354		

associated with an increased risk of death in TB patients during treatment [5, 13, 15, 19]. We have also found a similar result; that is, HIV coinfection was a statistically significant risk factor for death in TB patient, and this means the risk of death in TB patients with HIV infection was higher than in those without HIV infection (hazard ratio = 9.888 P value ≤ 0.0001) in multivariable Cox proportional hazard regression model.

Similar to our finding, other studies have also shown that TB patient category (TBC) was statistically associated with death of patients with tuberculosis [14, 15, 20, 21] (Mathew et al.).

The present study identified that body weight at initiation of treatment was not the risk factor for death in tuberculosis patients in multivariable Cox proportional regression model during antituberculosis treatment period (hazards ratio = 0.991, P value = 0.2659). However, studies by [12, 14, 20] reported that body weight at initiation of treatment was a risk factor for death from TB and is associated with survival of patients who begin treatment for tuberculosis.

In this study, the covariates gender and type of TB (TTB) were not found to be factors that affect the survival of patients with TB. But, different studies reported that males were at higher risk factor for death in TB patients [13, 16, 19, 22, 23] (Low et al.) and types of tuberculosis (positive pulmonary, negative pulmonary, and extrapulmonary tuberculosis) were identified as the significant factors for mortality of tuberculosis patients [15, 18, 19].

In this study age with HIV interaction was found a risk factor associated with death of tuberculosis patients. This study is consistent to the study conducted by (Lo et al.) [10]; the study revealed that HIV infection is a significant factor among younger age groups of tuberculosis patients.

Limitations of the study are as follows. The study is conducted based on secondary data which might have incomplete and biased information. Also information might have been missed in case of many censored observations. In many tuberculosis patients, multiple causes of death may act simultaneously, so the cause of death may not be determined accurately.

References

[1] "Global Tuberculosis Control: Surveillance, Planning, Financing," WHO Report, World Health Organization, Geneva, Switzerland, 2010.

[2] "Treatment of Tuberculosis: Guidelines for National Programmes," WHO Report, World Health Organization, Geneva, Switzerland, 2009.

[3] C. Kolappan, R. Subramani, K. Karunakaran, and P. R. Narayanan, "Mortality of tuberculosis patients in Chennai, India," *Bulletin of the World Health Organization*, vol. 84, no. 7, pp. 555–560, 2006.

[4] A. Faustini, A. J. Hall, and C. A. Perucci, "Tuberculosis treatment outcomes in Europe: a systematic review," *European Respiratory Journal*, vol. 26, no. 3, pp. 503–510, 2005.

[5] K. K. Oursler, R. D. Moore, W. R. Bishai, S. M. Harrington, D. S. Pope, and R. E. Chaisson, "Survival of patients with pulmonary tuberculosis: clinical and molecular epidemiologic factors," *Clinical Infectious Diseases*, vol. 34, no. 6, pp. 752–759, 2002.

[6] R. S. Gore, "Kentucky Epidemiologic Notes and Reports: TB Control Program Condensed from CDC National Center for HIV, STD and TB Prevention, Division of TB Elimination," Presented on World Tuberculosis Day, vol. 40, no. 2, 2005.

[7] D. W. Hosmer and S. Lemeshow, *Applied Survival Analysis Regression Modeling of Time to Event Data*, John Wiley and Sons, New York, NY, USA, 1999.

[8] D. Collett, *Modelling Survival Data in Medical Research*, Chapman and Hall, London, UK, 2nd edition, 2003.

[9] E. Arjas, "A graphical method for assessing goodness of fit in Cox's proportional Hazards model," *Journal of the American Statistical Association*, vol. 83, pp. 204–212, 1988.

[10] H. Y. Lo, J. Suo, H. J. Chang, S. L. Yang, and P. Chou, "Risk factors associated with death in a 12-month cohort analysis of tuberculosis patients: 12-month follow-up after registration," *Asia-Pacific Journal of Public Health*. In press.

[11] G. Pardeshi, "Survival analysis and risk factors for death in tuberculosis patients on directly observed treatment-short course," *Indian Journal of Medical Sciences*, vol. 63, no. 5, pp. 180–186, 2009.

[12] B. Getahun, G. Ameni, S. Biadgilign, and G. Medhin, "Mortality and associated risk factors in a cohort of tuberculosis patients treated under DOTS programme in Addis Ababa, Ethiopia," *BMC Infectious Diseases*, vol. 11, article 127, 2011.

[13] D. J. Horne, R. Hubbard, M. Narita, A. Exarchos, D. R. Park, and C. H. Goss, "Factors associated with mortality in patients with tuberculosis," *BMC Infectious Diseases*, vol. 10, article 258, 2010.

[14] M. D. F. P. M. de Albuquerque, J. D. L. Batista, R. A. D. A. Ximenes, M. S. Carvalho, G. T. N. Diniz, and L. C. Rodrigues, "Risk factors associated with death in patients who initiate treatment for tuberculosis after two different follow-up periods," *Revista Brasileira de Epidemiologia*, vol. 12, no. 4, pp. 513–522, 2009.

[15] M. P. Domingos, W. T. Caiaffa, and E. A. Colosimo, "Mortality, TB/HIV co-infection, and treatment dropout: predictors of tuberculosis prognosis in Recife, Pernambuco State, Brazil," *Cadernos de Saude Publica*, vol. 24, no. 4, pp. 887–896, 2008.

[16] T. Vasankari, P. Holmström, J. Ollgren, K. Liippo, M. Kokki, and P. Ruutu, "Risk factors for poor tuberculosis treatment outcome in Finland: a cohort study," *BMC Public Health*, vol. 7, article 291, 2007.

[17] A. D. Harries, N. J. Hargreaves, F. Gausi, J. H. Kwanjana, and F. M. Salaniponi, "High early death rate in tuberculosis patients in Malawi," *International Journal of Tuberculosis and Lung Disease*, vol. 5, no. 11, pp. 1000–1005, 2001.

[18] M. Muñoz-Sellart, L. E. Cuevas, M. Tumato, Y. Merid, and M. A. Yassin, "Factors associated with poor tuberculosis treatment outcome in the Southern Region of Ethiopia," *International Journal of Tuberculosis and Lung Disease*, vol. 14, no. 8, pp. 973–979, 2010.

[19] M. W. Borgdorff, J. Veen, N. A. Kalisvaart, and N. Nagelkerke, "Mortality among tuberculosis patients in the netherlands in the period 1993–1995," *European Respiratory Journal*, vol. 11, no. 4, pp. 816–820, 1998.

[20] M. Vasantha, P. G. Gopi, and R. Subramani, "Survival of tuberculosis patients treated under DOTS in a rural Tuberculosis Unit (TU), south India," *The Indian journal of tuberculosis*, vol. 55, no. 2, pp. 64–69, 2008.

[21] T. A. Mathew, T. N. Ovsyanikova, S. S. Shin et al., "Causes of death during tuberculosis treatment in Tomsk Oblast, Russia," *International Journal of Tuberculosis and Lung Disease*, vol. 10, no. 8, pp. 857–863, 2006.

[22] M. Demissie and D. Kebede, "Defaulting from tuberculosis treatment at the Addis Abeba tuberculosis centre and factors associated with it," *Ethiopian Medical Journal*, vol. 32, no. 2, pp. 97–106, 1994.

[23] S. Low, L. W. Ang, J. Cutter et al., "Mortality among tuberculosis patients on treatment in Singapore," *International Journal of Tuberculosis and Lung Disease*, vol. 13, pp. 328–334, 2009.

16

Gender-Related Barriers and Delays in Accessing Tuberculosis Diagnostic and Treatment Services: A Systematic Review of Qualitative Studies

Lakshmi Krishnan,[1] Tokunbo Akande,[2] Anita V. Shankar,[2] Katherine N. McIntire,[1] Celine R. Gounder,[1] Amita Gupta,[1,2,3] and Wei-Teng Yang[2]

[1] *Department of Medicine, Johns Hopkins University School of Medicine, Baltimore, MD 21287, USA*
[2] *Johns Hopkins Bloomberg School of Public Health, Baltimore, MD 21205, USA*
[3] *Center for Clinical Global Health Education, Johns Hopkins University, 600 North Wolfe Street, Phipps 540B, Baltimore, MD 21287, USA*

Correspondence should be addressed to Amita Gupta; agupta25@jhmi.edu

Academic Editor: Edward A. Graviss

Background. Tuberculosis (TB) remains a significant global public health problem with known gender-related (male versus female) disparities. We reviewed the qualitative evidence (written/spoken narrative) for gender-related differences limiting TB service access from symptom onset to treatment initiation. *Methods.* Following a systematic process, we searched 12 electronic databases, included qualitative studies that assessed gender differences in accessing TB diagnostic and treatment services, abstracted data, and assessed study validity. Using a modified "inductive coding" system, we synthesized emergent themes within defined barriers and delays limiting access at the individual and provider/system levels and examined gender-related differences. *Results.* Among 13,448 studies, 28 studies were included. All were conducted in developing countries and assessed individual-level barriers; 11 (39%) assessed provider/system-level barriers, 18 (64%) surveyed persons with suspected or diagnosed TB, and 7 (25%) exclusively surveyed randomly sampled community members or health care workers. Each barrier affected both genders but had gender-variable nature and impact reflecting sociodemographic themes. Women experienced financial and physical dependence, lower general literacy, and household stigma, whereas men faced work-related financial and physical barriers and community-based stigma. *Conclusions.* In developing countries, barriers limiting access to TB care have context-specific gender-related differences that can inform integrated interventions to optimize TB services.

1. Introduction

Tuberculosis (TB) comprises a major portion of the global disease burden and is associated with significant gender-related disparities, defined using binary male/female gender categories. In 2011, an estimated 33% of incident TB (2.9 million cases) occurred among women worldwide [1]. While the global case notification rate of TB is lower for women than men, TB is among the top three most significant causes of death among women aged 15 to 44 years [1]. Despite the gender-based disparities in TB statistics and the considerable disease burden among both genders, relatively little attention has been focused on gender-related differences in the epidemiology, diagnosis, treatment, outcomes, or socioeconomic costs of TB [2].

Gender-related disparities in TB and TB care may stem from gender-based differences in the barriers and delays that limit access to TB services. Several reviews suggest that gender differences in barriers that limit access to TB services exist at the individual and provider/system levels. These barriers include the direct and indirect costs of seeking TB services; casual or consistent employment; distance to TB services and access to transportation; stigma surrounding TB diagnosis and its association with HIV; TB-related knowledge and education; distinct gender-specific roles and status in the family; provider degree of suspicion for TB; number and types of providers seen; adherence with national TB program guidelines; and patient satisfaction with TB services [3–11].

Analyses of both qualitative data (primarily based on written or spoken narrative) and quantitative data (primarily based on numbers, frequencies, or mathematical equations) are needed to develop a comprehensive understanding of gender-related differences in the barriers and delays that limit access to TB care. Although previous reviews have found quantitative evidence [3–12], none have systematically reviewed the qualitative evidence. Qualitative data can uniquely inform the nature of quantitative gender-based differences, clarify formative pathways, and may reveal gender-related differences where no quantitative differences were found. Thus, qualitative gender analyses may provide critical insights to inform effective gender-specific interventions.

Our systematic review aims to assess the qualitative evidence for gender-related differences in barriers and delays that limit access to TB diagnostic and treatment services as reported by untreated patients and community members with suspected TB, persons who have presented for TB care, the general population, and health care providers. Using an inductive coding system for qualitative research synthesis, we examined emergent, gender-related themes within defined barriers and delays at the individual and provider/system levels, and our findings have implications for the development and prioritization of integrated gender-specific interventions to optimize the global impact of TB services.

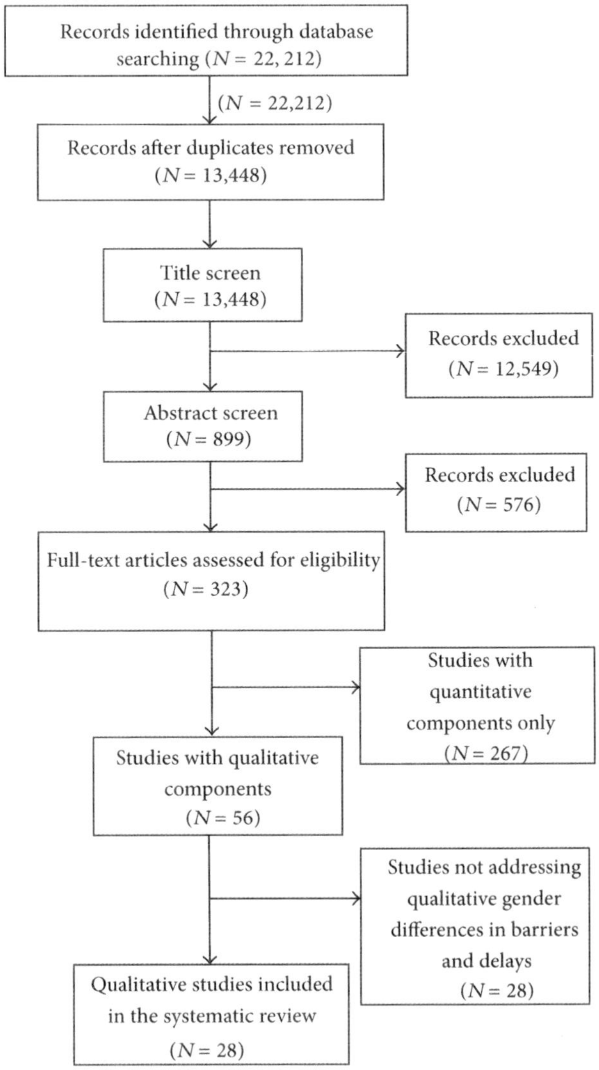

FIGURE 1: Study selection process.

2. Methods

2.1. Systematic Review Process

2.1.1. Search Strategy. We searched 12 electronic databases for human and English-language articles published between January 1953 and October 2010. Our search strategy was developed for MEDLINE using PubMed with a combination of controlled vocabulary and keyword terms and phrases (see Supplementary Material available online at http://dx.doi.org/10.1155/2014/215059). The strategy was then translated for the Excerpta Medica Database (EMBASE), the Cumulative Index to Nursing and Allied Health Literature (CINAHL), Global Health, Popline, Africa Wide, LILACS, Web of Science, and the inclusive databases of The Cochrane Library using their respective thesaurus terms, synonyms, and keywords. Citations from each database were imported into a reference management system, and duplicates were removed.

2.1.2. Study Selection Criteria. We included qualitative studies that reported on gender-related differences in barriers to and/or delays in accessing TB diagnostic and treatment services and studied human participants aged 15 years or older. We excluded studies that did not provide a gender comparison as well as case reports, editorials, review articles, commentaries, practice guidelines, and studies of treatment compliance and/or outcomes. Participants were defined as persons with diagnosed or suspected TB, persons from either the general population or high-risk populations (e.g., HIV-infected, homeless, and prisoner), or health care providers. Diagnosed TB included both pulmonary and extrapulmonary forms, and TB diagnosis could be made by sputum smear microscopy, culture, or chest X-ray using histopathological or clinical criteria.

2.1.3. Study Selection Process. Following deduplication, studies were screened sequentially by title and abstract and in full-text form (Figure 1). At each stage, two reviewers independently evaluated each study against our study selection criteria. Articles were included or excluded only when both reviewers were in agreement, and conflicts were resolved by a third, independent reviewer (AS). To ensure sufficient concordance between reviewers, a pilot review and reviewer discussion were conducted at each stage before proceeding with the remaining studies. Following the full-text screen, included articles underwent a full-text assessment, which included data abstraction and a study validity assessment.

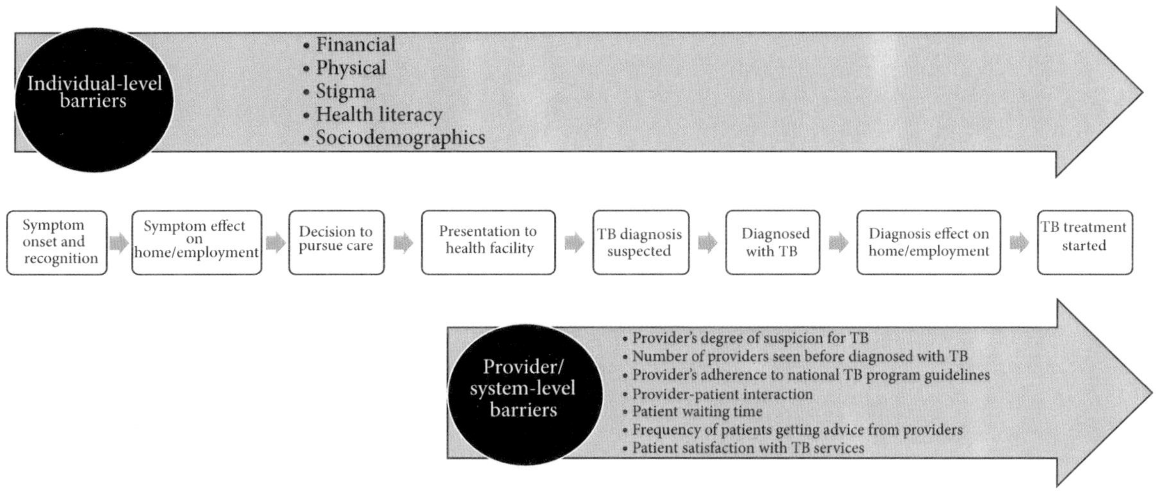

FIGURE 2: Conceptual framework illustrating barriers and delays that limit access to TB diagnostic and treatment services. Figure 2 illustrates the conceptual framework of the TB care continuum from symptom onset to treatment initiation that was used to define the barriers and delays that limit access to TB diagnostic and treatment services at the individual and provider/system levels. Individual-level barriers impact access to TB services along the full continuum of TB care, and the provider/system-level barriers impact TB service access from patient presentation to any health care provider through TB treatment initiation. Barriers may contribute to delays between each step along the TB care continuum. Accordingly, we define individual-level delay as the delay between symptom onset and presentation to any health care provider; provider/system delay as the delay between presentation to any health care provider and diagnosis, the delay between presentation to any health care provider and treatment initiation, or the delay between diagnosis and treatment initiation; and combined individual/provider/system delay as the delay between symptom onset and diagnosis or the delay between symptom onset and treatment initiation.

2.1.4. Data Abstraction and Synthesis. Three reviewers (Lakshmi Krishnan, Tokunbo Akande, and Wei-Teng Yang) independently abstracted data from each included full-text article in duplicate, and any conflicts were resolved through discussion with an additional independent reviewer (AS). Qualitative data were abstracted using a method similar to the "thematic synthesis" approach proposed by Thomas and Harden [13], which includes systematic data extraction involving the translation of concepts between studies, data analysis, and a quality assessment. Study design characteristics were abstracted and summarized, and we used a modified "inductive coding" system for qualitative research synthesis to develop "descriptive" and "analytical" themes within outcomes (our defined barriers and delays). Accordingly, we took findings to be text characterized as "results" or "study findings," and data were abstracted based on our review questions regarding gender-related differences and barriers to accessing TB diagnostic and treatment services. The general themes from these questions were categorized by outcome type (barrier or delay) and level of impact (individual or provider/system level).

2.1.5. Validity Assessment. We used the validity assessment to examine the quality of studies that inform our review; the assessment was not used to exclude studies. We examined several quality criteria for qualitative research [14–16], and, based on factors determined to critically inform our review process, we developed an adapted version of the Critical Appraisal Skills Programme (CASP) quality assessment tool to assess each study. Our validity assessment tool evaluated research design and purpose, study implementation, and the strength of the evidence used to support the conclusions of the study (Table 1).

2.2. Outcomes and Definitions. Outcomes were qualitative associations between gender and both barriers and delays that limit access to TB services along the full continuum of TB care from symptom onset through diagnosis and treatment initiation. Figure 2 presents the conceptual framework that was used to define barriers and delays at the individual and provider/system levels at various time points along the continuum of TB care. Individual-level barriers were defined as follows: financial (the direct or indirect costs of TB care, including costs of travel, diagnosis, and/or treatment as well as the opportunity costs of lost employment, compensation, or household work); physical (distance, travel logistics, and/or access to TB care facilities); stigma (TB-specific sociocultural barriers arising from community or individual prejudice related to TB diagnosis or treatment, including social isolation, marriage prospects, fertility concerns, and association with HIV); health literacy (TB-related knowledge and education); and sociodemographic (age, race, rural versus urban residence, social caste, norms of practice, and social hierarchies). Provider/system-level barriers were defined as any of the following: provider degree of suspicion for TB, number of providers seen before TB diagnosis, provider adherence to national TB program guidelines, provider-patient interaction, patient waiting time, frequency of getting advice, and patient satisfaction with TB services. Delay was defined as any time period between points along the TB care pathway under our conceptual framework, namely, the time period from symptom onset to presentation, diagnosis, or

Table 1: Quality of included studies.

Validity assessment tool[a]		Score		
Item number	Question	Yes (n)	No (n)	Unclear (n)
1	Is there a clear statement of research aims?	28	0	0
2	Is the research design appropriate to address the aims?	21	0	7
3	Are the data collection methods appropriate to obtain the aims?	23	2	3
4	Are the recruitment/sampling strategies appropriate for the aims?	21	0	7
5	Is the study context clearly described?	27	1	0
6	Have ethical considerations been addressed?	17	0	11
7	Is there a clear description of the data collection procedures?	26	2	0
8	Is the data analysis appropriate for research questions?	26	0	2
9	Are the findings clearly presented?	23	5	0
10	Are the claims made supported by sufficient evidence?	24	4	0

[a] After examining several quality criteria for qualitative research [14–16], we developed an adapted 10-question version of the Critical Appraisal Skills Programme (CASP) quality assessment tool based on factors determined to critically inform our review process. Our validity assessment was used to examine the quality of data from the included studies informing this review, not to exclude studies. For questions 1, 4, 5, 6, 7, and 8, studies were scored based on the presence (yes), absence (no), or insufficient information (unclear) regarding the stated criteria. For questions 2, 3, 9, and 10, a subjective review and assessment was performed to determine if the study had any minor or major issues related to compliance with the stated criteria. Accordingly, studies were scored "yes" if either no issues or minor issues were found, "no" if major issues were found, and "unclear" if there was insufficient information.

treatment initiation; presentation to diagnosis or treatment initiation; or diagnosis to treatment initiation.

3. Results

3.1. Study Characteristics. Our search strategy yielded 13,448 citations. Of these, 323 articles were screened in full-text form, and 28 studies [17–44] were included in our review (Figure 1). Overall, the included study characteristics were heterogeneous (Table 2). Studies ranged in size from 22 to 750 participants with women comprising 23–58% of the study population. Regarding study participants, 18 (64%) studies included TB cases or suspects presenting for care, 12 (43%) included community members, and 8 (29%) included health care providers or workers. All studies were published between 1995 and 2010 and were most commonly conducted in the World Health Organization (WHO) Southeast Asian (43%), Western Pacific (32%), and African Regions (25%).

3.2. Quality of Qualitative Research Reporting. Based on the validity assessment used to assess the included studies, we found a wide range of quality in methods, experimental design, and result reporting (Table 1). Several studies relied on only one form of data collection, and others based conclusions on a small number of participants (or groups) sampled for the study. In addition, some studies examined normative beliefs related to perceived stigma or barriers based on non-TB patient reports, which may not be representative of the actual barriers experienced by those with TB. There were several issues with qualitative studies including limited sample sizes and conclusions based on insufficient data. The studies that used multiple methods or a mix of qualitative and quantitative methods provided the strongest evidence to inform this review.

3.3. Outcomes. All of the included studies reported on individual-level barriers to accessing TB diagnostic and treatment services, and 11 (39%) studies also reported on provider/system-level barriers. Only two studies included data on individual-level delays. Community-based studies tended to report on individual-level barriers, whereas health facilities-based studies provided more provider/system-level evidence. No clear differences emerged between urban and rural environments or between types of health facilities. Emergent gender-related themes were synthesized and summarized by outcome type (barrier or delay) and level of impact (individual level or provider/system level) (Table 3). Key findings are discussed in depth below.

3.4. Individual-Level Barriers. Overall, prominent gender-related differences emerged within financial, physical, stigma, and health literacy barriers, and gender-specific sociodemographic themes (i.e., sociocultural norms associated with the status and roles of men and women) were found to directly affect each barrier type (Table 3). Emergent themes are discussed in depth by barrier type with illustrative quotations pertaining to each (Boxes 1, 2, 3, 4, 5, and 6).

3.4.1. Financial. The financial burden of obtaining TB care and pursuing treatment was a widespread theme that affected both genders. Among 10 (36%) studies [17–21, 23, 24, 30, 32, 36], only one [17] found that the direct costs for treatment incurred by women tended to be slightly higher than those incurred by men, suggesting a quantitative systems-based difference in treatment cost by gender. However, there was no gender difference in debt. While most studies described a universal financial cost, a gender differential limited access to TB care. Men tended to experience the financial burden of TB both indirectly and directly because illness limited their ability as breadwinners [18], and seeking TB treatment drained their financial resources [19]. In contrast, women lacked financial independence, which limited access to care. Resource allocation within families was another key concern. As the primary earners, men's health is prioritized. While

Table 2: Characteristics of included studies.

First author Year	Country WHO region[a]	Number of participants	Percentage of females	Participant characteristics	Research setting	Data collection methods	Type of barrier reported
Atre 2011 [24]	India SEARO	160	50	Community members	Rural	Interviews	Individual-level
Deribew 2010 [27]	Ethiopia AFRO	750	58	Community members	Rural and urban	Questionnaires; FGDs	Individual-level
Mavhu 2010 [42]	Zimbabwe AFRO	40	45	Community members	Urban	Interviews; FGDs	Individual-level
Onifade 2010 [20]	Peru AMRO	53	NR	TB patients; health workers	Urban	Interviews; FGDs	Individual-level Provider-/system-level
Rundi 2010 [34]	Malaysia WPRO	58	53	TB patients; family members; health workers	Rural	Interviews	Individual-level Provider-/system-level
Skordis-Worrall 2010 [44]	South Africa AFRO	8 FGD 6–8 each	NR	TB patients; community members	Urban	FGDs	Individual-level Provider-/system-level
Gosoniu 2008 [28]	Bangladesh, India, Malawi SEARO, AFRO	329	49	TB patients	Rural and urban	Interviews	Individual-level
Jaggarajamma 2008 [29]	India SEARO	276	31	TB patients	Rural and urban	Interviews; FGDs	Individual-level
Somma 2008 [35]	Bangladesh, India, Malawi, Colombia SEARO, AMRO	400	50	TB patients	Rural and urban	Interviews	Individual-level
Weiss 2008 [39]	Bangladesh, India, Malawi SEARO, AFRO	329	49	TB patients	Rural and urban	Interviews	Individual-level Provider-/system-level
Baral 2007 [26]	Nepal SEARO	34	NR	TB patients; family members; community members	Kathmandu Valley	Interviews	Individual-level
Ganapathy 2008 [41]	India SEARO	16 FGD	NR	Community members	Urban	FGDs	Individual-level Provider-/system-level
Karim 2007 [31]	Bangladesh SEARO	102	49	TB patients	Rural	Interviews	Individual-level
Yan 2007 [37]	China WPRO	16–22 FGD 82 interviews	NR	TB patients; community members	Rural	Questionnaires; interviews; FGDs	Individual-level Provider-/system-level
Zhang 2007 [23]	China WPRO	714	50	Rural farmers	Rural	FGDs	Individual-level Provider-/system-level
Fochsen 2006 [40]	India SEARO	22	23	Health care providers	Rural and urban	Interviews	Individual-level Provider-/system-level
Atre 2004 [25]	India SEARO	160	50	Community members	Rural	Interviews	Individual-level
Eastwood 2004 [19]	The Gambia AFRO	45	40	TB patients; health workers	Medical unit	Questionnaires; FGDs	Individual-level Provider-/system-level
Rodríguez-Reimann 2004 [43]	USA AMRO	166	53	Community members w/TB positive family member	Urban	Questionnaires	Individual-level

Table 2: Continued.

First author Year	Country WHO region[a]	Number of participants	Percentage of females	Participant characteristics	Research setting	Data collection methods	Type of barrier reported
Sanou 2004 [21]	Burkina Faso AFRO	28 FGD 8–12 each 68 interviews	NR	TB patients; non-TB patients; community members; traditional healers	Rural and urban	Interviews; FGDs	Individual-level
Thorson 2004 [22]	Vietnam WPRO	5 FGD 7-8 each 3 interviews	33	Physicians	General hospital; TB units	Interviews; FGDs	Individual-level
Xu 2004 [36]	China WPRO	16 FGD	31	TB patients; health workers; health providers	Rural	FGDs	Individual-level Provider-/system-level
Long 2001 [32]	Vietnam WPRO	16 FGD 8–10 each	NR	TB patients; non-TB patients	Rural and urban	FGDs	Individual-level
Johansson 2000 [30]	Vietnam WPRO	4 FGD 8–10 each	NR	TB patients; community members	Rural and urban	FGDs	Individual-level Provider-/system-level
Ngamvithayapong 2000 [33]	Thailand WPRO	85	33	Community members; healthcare staff	Rural and urban	FGDs	Individual-level
Long 1999 [38]	Vietnam WPRO	16 FGD 8–10 each	NR	TB patients; non-TB patients	Rural and urban	FGDs	Individual-level
Rajeswari 1999 [17]	India SEARO	304	39	TB patients; non-TB patients	Rural and urban	Interviews; FGDs	Individual-level
Liefooghe 1995 [18]	Pakistan SEARO	48	50	TB patients	Mission hospital	FGDs	Individual-level

FGD: focus group discussion; NR: not reported; TB: tuberculosis; WHO: World Health Organization.
[a]WHO regions: AFRO (African Region), AMRO (Americas Region), SEARO (Southeast Asian Region), and WPRO (Western Pacific Region).

TABLE 3: Summary of emergent gender-related themes by barrier type.

Barrier type	Gender-related themes[a]	
	Gender similarities	Gender differences
Individual level		
Financial	Both genders cite finances as a key barrier to seeking care; cost of TB treatment and diagnosis is a shared burden; economic burden affects both genders; cost of healthcare is a gender-wide deterrent to seeking services; and no gender difference in debt is incurred for treatment	Finances have a greater burden on men since they are breadwinners; TB treatment means time away from work and lost earning potential. Less financial independence for women reliant upon families or in-laws; family resource allocation preferring men and children's health above that of women; women's lack of financial autonomy a barrier to accessing care and care decision-making; men with greater access to money and treatment decision-making power; direct treatment costs for women sometimes greater than those for men
Physical	Distance from work and home to treatment facilities was reported as a barrier to accessing care; long traveling times to hospitals is a barrier	Distance from work to treatment affects men more heavily
Stigma	Adverse marital impact of TB-related stigma for both men and women (prospects and spousal support); both genders naming young unmarried people as the group at highest risk of stigma; both genders reporting hiding their diagnosis or describing their disease vaguely for fear of stigma; fear of social isolation reported by both genders; TB stigmatized, but not as much as AIDS; TB stigma not eliminated after treatment	Females expect more stigma in family and reported more isolation, psychosocial consequences, fear of divorce, losing spouses, or compromised marital prospects for unmarried children; TB in women is associated with loose and immoral behavior, leading to greater burden of stigma and more difficulty getting married; women are more likely to hide their diagnosis or delay seeking treatment because of stigma Men expect more stigma at work, sexual relationships, ability to marry
Health literacy	Low education level correlating with greater fear of TB and social isolation; widespread community beliefs that TB is incurable or that TB patients cannot have healthy children; community perceptions that even treated TB can harm offspring, leading to limited marriage prospects	Higher proportion of females displaying prejudice towards TB due to limited knowledge; women and the young with less knowledge than men and the elderly; men with greater formal education and TB knowledge than young and older women; women more likely to regard TB as fatal or incurable; women with limited knowledge in health seeking; men knowing more about HIV/TB transmission than women
Sociodemographic barriers	None	Women need to ask permission from husbands or elders to seek treatment; treatment of children and men is prioritized; diagnosed women receive less family support than men; women are expected to care for husbands with TB, whereas men are not expected to care for wives with TB; more males report that family members have a positive attitude towards their disease; men in societies where masculine resilience is valued are more likely to delay seeking treatment
Provider/system level	Both genders report long waiting times and poor conditions of TB facilities, unreliability of TB diagnostics as barriers; several studies reported government facilities as gender-neutral and fair	Women are more affected by lack of privacy in health facilities; women are more likely to perceive female health care workers as sympathetic and adhere to treatment; DOTS is more distressing for women; women are more likely to consult traditional healers, self-medicate, or use private physicians over government facilities

AIDS: autoimmune deficiency syndrome; DOTS: directly observed therapy; HIV: human immunodeficiency virus; TB: tuberculosis.
[a]Several independent reviewers identified qualitative gender-related themes using "inductive coding" and extracted specific barriers (i.e., individual-level financial, stigma, physical, health literacy, sociodemographic, and provider/system-level barriers). Emergent themes were compiled and then synthesized in Table 3.

"My husband told me to go to my parent's home. He refused to give me money for the cost of treatment. My neighbor did not help me that much either." (female) [28]

"He gave me medicines for every two weeks. Earlier on, he asked me to come every day but I told him, I am a poor man; I do not have my own transport. Everyday I have to spend RM 12 (about US$3) for transportation, how can I bear this financial burden, I told the doctor." (male) [34]

"Men have money to spend on their own, but women have to get it from the husband or from the family" (female) [18]

"He will feel ashamed of himself. He will think 'who will keep me in the job? What is my use if I cannot earn?'" (male) [24]

Box 1: Financial issues.

"Many people come from remote areas. They have neither resources nor available facilities for treatment. They die as 'victims of injustice.'" (male) [29]

"The county hospital has good equipment. The doctors can make correct diagnosis. . .[However,] we need to spend more than 1 day and a lot of money if we travel to the county hospital, because there is only one coach per day going back and forth from the county hospital" (female) [23]

Box 2: Physical factors.

"I was 18 years when I got married and my husband was only a child. After our marriage he went to school and he finished his matric. I had a daughter and a son. Now I am sick and my husband has taken a second wife" (female) [18]

"He will think if this disease is known to other people, they will have less respect for me. Hence he will try to hide it." (male) [24]

"If a girl gets TB, community people will be reluctant to arrange marriage with her, because TB is also perceived in community that it is a divine curse to the person and family, comes from wrong things they did in the past. This belief is so strong in the community. . ." (male) [26]

"If the other party would come to know that I had TB, then they would not be interested to give me the girl that had been agreed upon for me to marry. They would think that the girl might get this disease from me." (male) [31]

Box 3: Stigma.

"If a mother has it, then it will pass on to the next generation. Once it is in the family, it will continue" (female) [25]

"Yes, (TB is more of a problem for women) because of pregnancy. When a woman is pregnant, blood and water become one. Previous wounds come open again" (female) [18]

Box 4: Health literacy.

"Yes, his wife will support him, as she will not have any other alternatives besides him. It is her fate for life. She will serve him two meals. Physically also, she will help him (by trying to avoid sexual relations)." (male) [24]

"In the case of my dad, when my mother was ill, my dad didn't ask how she felt, he didn't take her to the health post. . .but when he was ill for any pain at all, he would go straight to the post and wouldn't be concerned about the expenses. . .but when my mom felt bad, he didn't ask her anything, didn't even buy her a pill. He just took care of himself. " (male) [20]

Box 5: Women's status and roles in society.

> "The first time I came here, I could not believe that this was where TB was treated. The conditions were very poor, but the doctors were very gentle and kind hearted." (male) [30]
>
> "Our lab is very poor. The ultra-violet lamp was borrowed from another hospital. The agents for tests were given by another hospital. And the patients used some antibiotics before coming to our hospital. So the sputum smear-positive rate is very low...The self protection funding is 'Zero.' No ventilation tunnel, poor equipment. I'm afraid of being infected. So I do it as quickly as possible. Of course, many mistakes are made." (female) [36]
>
> "We are visible to other patients when we go to take our medication. The place is very small." (female) [20]

Box 6: Provider/system-level factors.

men and children receive the lion's share of resources, women's lack of financial autonomy and lower status within households deprioritizes their health [20–22], leaving them dependent on spouses, families, or social services.

3.4.2. Physical. Only two (7%) studies explored physical barriers to accessing TB services [20, 23], which are generally linked to financial issues. In both studies, participants reported that the direct and indirect costs of traveling to healthcare facilities (including travel time and inflexible hours of health facilities) affected both men and women. One study [20] reported that men were more heavily affected than women since they are employed outside of their communities and, therefore, experience a greater burden due to travel time, seeking care within their communities, and inflexible clinic hours.

3.4.3. Stigma. Stigma pervasively affects both genders and was reported as a major barrier to accessing TB diagnostic and treatment services. Of 28 studies, 20 (71%) investigated gender-related differences in TB-related stigma [17–20, 22–37]. Among these, 9 (45%) studies found that women experienced greater stigma than men [17, 18, 20, 22, 28, 31–33, 35], 8 (40%) studies found no gender-related difference [19, 24–26, 29, 30, 34, 36], two (10%) studies reported that men faced a greater stigma burden than women [23, 37], and one study reported that women in the community had higher prejudice toward TB patients [27].

Several studies highlighted gender differences in the nature of TB-related stigma. Men reported greater workplace, community, and marital prospect-related stigma, whereas women reported greater stigma with family members as well as psychosocial consequences, feelings of isolation, and lack of proper care from the family [28, 30, 31, 35]. Women were also described as more likely to be stigmatized in communities where the level of family stigma was reported as low, but the community perception of TB as associated with immoral behavior was high [26]. The impact of TB-related stigma on marriage was noted in six studies. Many of these [23, 34, 36, 37] found that TB-related stigma affected the marriage prospects of both genders, with men having a slightly more difficult time finding a wife in areas with a low female/male ratio [23, 37]. Two studies [18, 32] discussed divorce as a direct consequence of TB to be more likely to affect females, and, of these, one study [18] reported that TB-infected females were more likely than TB-infected males to face difficult marital prospects. Another study [27] found that a higher percentage of females had high prejudice towards TB patients compared to males (AOR = 1.4; CI = 1.0–1.9). Notably, TB-related stigma overlapped with health literacy issues. Communal lack of knowledge regarding TB transmission and the concern that TB is incurable or can be passed down to offspring lead to stigma that stymies the marital prospects of all TB patients, regardless of gender.

3.4.4. Health Literacy. Men outstripped women in the domain of TB-related knowledge and education. Of 28 studies, 12 (43%) described gender-related differences in health literacy as barriers to accessing TB services [19, 20, 22, 23, 26, 27, 31–33, 37–39]. Among these, six (50%) found that men had higher levels of TB-related knowledge than women [22, 23, 27, 32, 37, 39]. This finding was largely due to higher male educational attainment and reflects gender-related differences in general literacy. Several studies examined gender-related differences in general education attainment and literacy [20, 31, 37], and two found that men were more educated and/or had higher literacy rates than women [31, 37]. No studies reported that women had higher levels of TB-related knowledge than men. However, one study [20] found that women had more knowledge about accessing health services than men. Two studies found that neither men nor women had much knowledge of TB or its transmission [19, 38].

3.4.5. Sociodemographic. Of 28 studies, 18 (64%) revealed sociocultural factors acting at the individual level. In all studies, the sociocultural context of women's roles and status in society permeated the observed gender differences, clearly demonstrating that norms of practice and social hierarchies lead men and women to face different barriers to accessing TB services [17–20, 22, 23, 28–30, 34–37, 39–43]. Specifically, men exhibited an unwillingness to access health care due to social perceptions described below or inability to leave work. Financial burdens as discussed above also play a role. One study [42] found that cultural beliefs (men believed that the body should be resilient and only sought care when it had succumbed to disease) and the perception that healthcare actions carry few benefits [43] affected male willingness to access treatment. Men were also less likely to access healthcare in situations where their work interfered [34]. For women, the primary barriers included the lack of autonomy, the need to seek permission from family [19, 20, 28], the requirement to be chaperoned to a consultation [40], lack of family support [18, 20, 22, 23, 29, 30, 37, 41], the prioritization of men and children's health [23, 41], and the expectation that an ill wife must take care of her husband, but not vice versa [20, 24]. Notably, when women were able to access healthcare, they often utilized healthcare services more than men because they perceived greater benefits from accessing treatment [43].

3.5. Provider/System-Level Barriers. Of 28 studies, 11 (39%) assessed gender-related barriers to accessing TB services at the provider/system level [19, 20, 23, 30, 34, 36, 37, 39–41, 44]. Although these combined barriers were felt by community members and patients to affect women more than men, one study found that all participants agreed that subsidized care played a major role in removing some of these barriers [36], and both genders complained that long waiting times, poor facilities [30], diagnostic unreliability or delay, and deferred or inappropriate treatment [36] hindered health-seeking behavior and treatment initiation. The lack of privacy in health clinics with the use of directly observed therapy (DOTS) posed a particular problem for women who experienced greater embarrassment and anxiety than men and reported this as a barrier to seeking treatment [19, 20]. However, in two studies, both men and women reported that, overall, the treatment at TB centers and government facilities was non-gender-discriminatory and fair [20, 34].

Among studies that surveyed health care providers versus the general community or TB patients, health workers who cared for TB patients believed that system-level barriers such as long waiting times, poor health care facilities, and lack of privacy were the most significant factors preventing their patients from accessing care. In contrast, community members or patients perceived greater individual barriers, especially those centered in the domains of finance and stigma. According to Eastwood et al., health workers felt that women experienced more difficulties than men as a result of such barriers (including cost, travel, and lack of privacy at treatment centers). Onifade et al. corroborated this finding, reporting that healthcare workers overwhelmingly stated that women experienced greater barriers (including stigma) to accessing care than men [20]. One study found that healthcare workers assumed a higher health literacy level among their patients than was actually the case, but this applied to both genders [34].

3.6. Individual-Level Delays. Only two studies reported on individual-level delays in TB diagnosis and treatment initiation [36, 44]. One study reported that delays affect both genders [36], and one study reported that men tended to delay communication about a suspected illness, which, in turn, appeared to delay treatment seeking [44].

4. Discussion

Understanding gender-related differences in barriers and delays that limit access to TB care is important to inform interventions designed to optimize the impact of TB services. Our systematic review aimed to assess the qualitative evidence for gender-related differences in the barriers and delays that limit access to TB diagnostic and treatment services at the individual and provider/system levels. Collectively, the 28 studies that informed our review represented developing countries within four WHO regions (AFRO, AMRO, WPRO, and SEARO) and reported on each of our defined individual-level barriers (financial, physical, stigma, health literacy, and sociodemographic), with a subset of 11 studies that also reported on provider/system-level barriers. Our review revealed the nature of gender-related differences found within individual-level barriers, which appear to arise from underlying gender-specific sociodemographic themes. Gender-specific themes were particularly pervasive within financial, stigma, and health literacy barriers, and provider/system-level barriers were also found to disproportionately affect women. Our findings may be used to inform interventions that may be integrated with provider/system-level strategies to improve access to TB services.

Our review revealed that gender-specific barriers to accessing TB diagnostic and treatment services are closely related to sociocultural structures. Approximately two-thirds of the included studies mentioned the imbalance in social norms and power between men and women, and gender-specific sociodemographic themes (i.e., gender-specific social norms, roles, and status) were found to impact all barrier types. In contrast, a systematic review of quantitative studies found that less than 5% of studies addressed sociodemographic barriers to accessing TB services [12]. This disparity between qualitative and quantitative evidence may reflect, in part, the difficulty of quantifying such an intangible concept. Specifically, our review revealed that women experienced barriers due to financial dependence, lack of physical independence, the deprioritization of their health in households, stigma within the household, and relatively low general and TB-related literacy, whereas men primarily experienced community-based stigma and work-related financial and physical barriers, which reflect their higher status/power and role as the primary earner. These findings support the prioritization of the gender empowerment framework as advocated by WHO, UNFPA, and other international organizations, which, in addition to balancing research, aims to create a more balanced power structure between men and women in health care and more broadly [45–47]. Overcoming gender-specific sociocultural barriers is an overarching problem that requires intervention but is a large and challenging task. Thus, understanding that the roles and status of women affect each of the individual-level barrier types, we propose that financial, physical, stigma, and health literacy barriers may be more amenable to direct intervention.

Among the individual-level barriers that limit access to TB services, TB-related stigma was particularly pervasive. The majority of included studies (70%) assessed TB-related stigma, and our review revealed that women faced greater stigma than men when gender-related differences were found. Specifically, men faced more prejudice in the workplace and community, whereas women faced prejudice in the household and experienced more psychosocial consequences of isolation. In addition, stigma was found to impact marriage in gender-specific ways. For men, diminished marriage prospects appeared to be linked to the potential inability to work and support the family, whereas women faced concerns with fertility before marriage and threats of divorce after marriage due to fear of contagion and the inability to perform household chores. Importantly, stigma and health literacy are related, and gender-specific interventions to improve TB-related health literacy may overcome some barriers due to individual-level stigma.

Regarding health literacy, our review revealed a clear gender disparity in TB-related knowledge. Several studies reported that men had a higher level of TB-related health literacy than women, and this disparity corresponded with a gender-related difference in general literacy. This finding has implications for health literacy interventions, which will also impact TB-related stigma. The lack of accurate TB-related knowledge impacts individual and community perceptions of disease and can perpetuate stigma [48]. In addition, both general literacy and health literacy are important predictors of health status [48]. Accordingly, community-level programs that provide education on TB symptomatology, risks, and treatment options will continue to be important. However, to prompt more women to seek TB diagnosis and treatment, existing strategies such as educating trusted traditional healers, using community gatherings as a mode of TB education delivery, and providing early childhood education within schools will need to be supplemented with novel gender-specific approaches. For example, interventions that increase the general literacy of women might expand the uptake and impact of existing TB education campaigns that use written materials to explain TB disease mechanisms and treatment. In addition, to optimize the access and uptake of general literacy and TB education programs among women, tailored health communication strategies need to be developed that take into account the financial dependence, lack of autonomy, deprioritization of care, and household roles that impact women's lives. Integrating health education programs with innovative interventions that foster intrinsic motivation and self-advocacy among women may also help overcome the substantial sociodemographic challenges that women face when seeking TB care.

Gender-specific interventions that address individual-level stigma and health literacy barriers are critical to improve access to TB services. However, overcoming interrelated individual-level financial/physical barriers and provider/system-level barriers must also be prioritized, and a decentralized approach to TB service delivery may be required. Currently, the traditional "top-down" structure delivers TB treatment through government centers, centralized National Government Organization clinics, and community clinics and leaves large gaps in treatment. Our review identified that both genders experience physical barriers due to travel time and inflexible hours of centralized health facilities, which also manifest as gender-specific financial barriers. As the primary household earner, men reported work-related financial barriers, whereas women faced barriers arising from their lower social status, including financial dependence, physical dependence, and

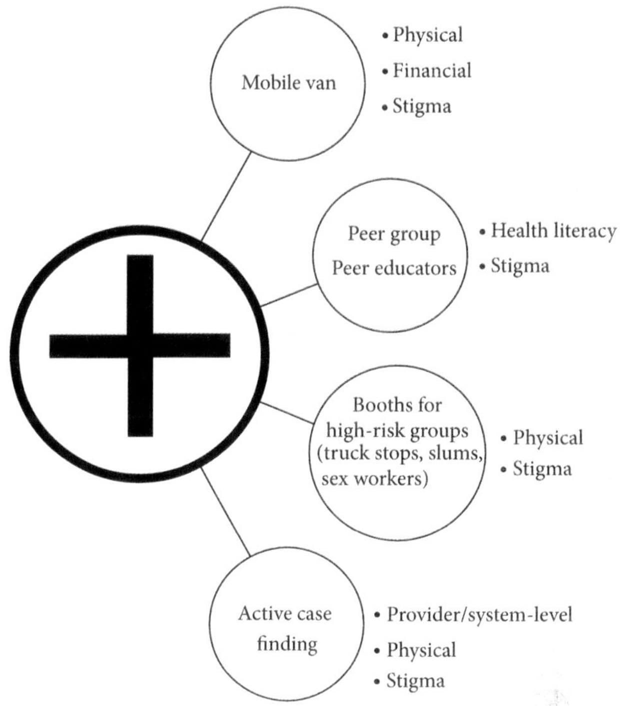

Figure 3: Decentralized model of TB care delivery highlighting suggested interventions to target identified barriers. Figure 3 illustrates the transition from the traditional, centralized model of TB care delivery (central circle with the cross), which uses primary, secondary, and tertiary facility-based TB care (including government hospitals as well as community and nongovernmental organization clinics), to a decentralized model of TB service delivery that incorporates several interventions to overcome the individual-level and provider/system-level barriers identified in this review. Suggested interventions are listed with the specific barriers that each may address.

the deprioritization of their health care in households. In addition, although fewer studies assessed provider/system-level barriers, our review found that, particularly for women, large central hospitals pose a threat to privacy and may substantiate stigma. Overall, both genders also reported that long wait times, poor facilities, diagnostic delays/unreliability, and deferred/inappropriate treatment hindered access to TB services. Accordingly, we might propose a decentralized TB service delivery structure that integrates provider/system-level treatment options with interventions targeting the gender-specific barriers that limit access to those services (Figure 3). Thus, many financial, physical, stigma, health literacy, and provider/system-level barriers may be overcome by reorienting the way in which TB service delivery interacts with the overarching sociocultural issues that dictate community perceptions of TB.

Strong models of integrated interventions exist and have been designed to address several of our identified individual-level thematic areas as well as the overarching sociocultural context of women's roles and status. Operation ASHA, a program begun in India that is expanding worldwide, addresses financial, physical, stigma, and health literacy barriers and "fills gaps" in treatment by departing from the traditional

DOTS model of TB treatment. The program establishes community centers in underserved areas (including slums), provides extensive counseling to destigmatize TB diagnosis and treatment, and leverages trusted community members to assist with education and treatment provision [49]. In Pakistan, programs have engaged the private sector with novel approaches that use laypeople, mobile phone software and incentives, and communication campaigns and have been found to substantially increase TB case notification in urban settings [50]. Overall, these integrated systems of case detection are able to overcome provider/system-level and sociodemographic barriers.

Another possible approach involves leveraging existing HIV programs. In areas where TB-HIV coinfection is prevalent, government and NGO TB treatment programs might adapt strategies used by HIV programs, which, in many communities, have successfully destigmatized the use of government antiretroviral (ARV) treatment centers. Successful strategies include offering HIV counseling at local, community, and public health centers; offering mobile HIV testing and treatment resources in vans or trucks; and providing HIV education in general and neutral community spaces such as schools, community centers, shopping areas, or other gathering places. In addition, one program, the Avahan India AIDS Initiative, has targeted high-risk groups such as male truck drivers and female sex workers by using peer educators and community mobilization to disperse preventive efforts (condoms, education, etc.) and establishing clinical services at gathering points such as truck stops or through a franchised network of private sexually transmitted infection (STI) providers [51]. Tailoring TB intervention efforts to high-risk groups may improve resources allocation and community mobilization, destigmatize TB, and, through the use of peer educators of both genders, may help to neutralize gender-related differences in accessing care.

Further research is urgently needed in the area of gender-related differences in barriers to accessing TB diagnostics and treatment services. The systematic nature of literature identification was the strength of this review but was limited by the number of English-language qualitative studies available in the area of gender-related differences in barriers to TB care. Overall, after a rigorous study selection, we were left with 28 studies from which to extrapolate themes that covered a range of gender-specific issues. Because developed countries were not represented among the included studies, our review may not be globally representative.

However, our review protocol did not exclude developed countries, and the included studies do reflect the regions with the greatest global TB burden. Finally, our study selection criteria excluded studies that lacked a gender comparison. Therefore, studies of pregnant women were largely excluded because only women were involved.

5. Conclusions

TB continues to be a significant global public health threat. Moving forward with the post 2015 Millennium Development Goals agenda, the WHO and Stop TB Partnership have proposed a set of interim goals, namely, a 75% reduction of TB mortality and a 40% reduction of TB incidence by 2025 [52]. Improving access to TB care by addressing gender-related barriers will be a key step in this direction. To this end, our systematic review revealed the gender-variable nature and impact of several barriers and their overlapping relationships, thus identifying high-impact targets for interventions that may be tailored to the specific sociocultural context and integrated into decentralized models of TB service delivery. However, to optimize the impact of global TB services, our review also highlights a clear need for further studies. Prospectively designed qualitative gender analyses and standardized methods to study and address gender issues are needed in TB research. In addition, the majority of reviewed studies did not survey HIV-TB coinfected populations. Because both diseases individually cause significant stigma, studies examining the compound effect are critical, including studies to investigate the impact of TB and HIV service programs on barriers and delays in the diagnosis and treatment of both diseases and how TB and HIV service efforts might be coordinated. Lastly, an ongoing focus on gender as a variable affecting access to care must be maintained in both research and intervention, and future work must adopt a broader perspective on gender and address complex gender differences rather than assuming that women alone face greater barriers to treatment than men.

Conflict of Interests

The authors declare that there is no conflict of interests regarding the publication of this paper.

Authors' Contribution

Lakshmi Krishnan, Wei-Teng Yang, and Katherine N. McIntire wrote the paper and analyzed the data. Lakshmi Krishnan, Tokunbo Akande, and Wei-Teng Yang abstracted the data and made tables. Anita V. Shankar edited the paper, assessed study quality, and reviewed study methods and data abstraction. Amita Gupta and Celine R. Gounder wrote the grant for funding from the World Health Organization. All authors commented on and approved the paper and this submission.

Acknowledgment

This study was funded in part by a grant from the World Health Organization. The funders had no role in study design, data collection and analysis, preparation of the paper, or decision to publish.

References

[1] WHO, "Global Tuberculosis Control," 2012.

[2] WHO, "Tuberculosis Women and TB," http://www.who.int/tb/womenandtb.pdf.

[3] I. Bates, C. Fenton, J. Gruber et al., "Vulnerability to malaria, tuberculosis, and HIV/AIDS infection and disease. Part 1:

determinants operating at individual and household level," *The Lancet Infectious Diseases*, vol. 4, no. 5, pp. 267–277, 2004.

[4] M. Connolly and P. Nunn, "Women and tuberculosis," *World Health Statistics Quarterly*, vol. 49, no. 2, pp. 115–119, 1996.

[5] C. B. Holmes, H. Hausler, and P. Nunn, "A review of sex differences in the epidemiology of tuberculosis," *International Journal of Tuberculosis and Lung Disease*, vol. 2, no. 2, pp. 96–104, 1998.

[6] P. Hudelson, "Gender differentials in tuberculosis: the role of socio-economic and cultural factors," *Tubercle and Lung Disease*, vol. 77, no. 5, pp. 391–400, 1996.

[7] J. Ogden, S. Rangan, M. Uplekar et al., "Shifting the paradigm in tuberculosis control: illustrations from India," *International Journal of Tuberculosis and Lung Disease*, vol. 3, no. 10, pp. 855–861, 1999.

[8] D. G. Storla, S. Yimer, and G. A. Bjune, "A systematic review of delay in the diagnosis and treatment of tuberculosis," *BMC Public Health*, vol. 8, article 15, 2008.

[9] A. Thorson and V. K. Diwan, "Gender inequalities in tuberculosis: aspects of infection, notification rates, and compliance," *Current Opinion in Pulmonary Medicine*, vol. 7, no. 3, pp. 165–169, 2001.

[10] M. W. Uplekar, S. Rangan, M. G. Weiss, J. Ogden, M. W. Borgdorff, and P. Hudelson, "Attention to gender issues in tuberculosis control," *International Journal of Tuberculosis and Lung Disease*, vol. 5, no. 3, pp. 220–224, 2001.

[11] B. Vissandjee and M. Pai, "The socio-cultural challenge in public health interventions: the case of tuberculosis in India," *International Journal of Public Health*, vol. 52, no. 4, pp. 199–201, 2007.

[12] C. Gounder, W. -T Yang, T. Akande et al., "Gender-related barriers to and delays in accessing tuberculosis diagnostic and treatment services: a systematic review of quantitative studies," in *Proceedings of the 43rd Union World Conference on Lung Health*, Kuala Lumpur, Malaysia, 2012.

[13] J. Thomas and A. Harden, "Methods for the thematic synthesis of qualitative research in systematic reviews," *BMC Medical Research Methodology*, vol. 8, article 45, 2008.

[14] S. Atkins, S. Lewin, H. Smith, M. Engel, A. Fretheim, and J. Volmink, "Conducting a meta-ethnography of qualitative literature: lessons learnt," *BMC Medical Research Methodology*, vol. 8, article 21, 2008.

[15] K. Malterud, "Qualitative research: standards, challenges, and guidelines," *The Lancet*, vol. 358, no. 9280, pp. 483–488, 2001.

[16] Programme CAS, "Making sense of evidence: the ten questions to help you make sense of qualitative research".

[17] R. Rajeswari, R. Balasubramanian, M. Muniyandi, S. Geetharamani, X. Thresa, and P. Venkatesan, "Socio-economic impact of tuberculosis on patients and family in India," *International Journal of Tuberculosis and Lung Disease*, vol. 3, no. 10, pp. 869–877, 1999.

[18] R. Liefooghe, N. Michiels, S. Habib, M. B. Moran, and A. De Muynck, "Perception and social consequences of tuberculosis: a focus group study of tuberculosis patients in Sialkot, Pakistan," *Social Science and Medicine*, vol. 41, no. 12, pp. 1685–1692, 1995.

[19] S. V. Eastwood and P. C. Hill, "A gender-focused qualitative study of barriers to accessing tuberculosis treatment in The Gambia, West Africa," *International Journal of Tuberculosis and Lung Disease*, vol. 8, no. 1, pp. 70–75, 2004.

[20] D. A. Onifade, A. M. Bayer, R. Montoya et al., "Gender-related factors influencing tuberculosis control in shantytowns: a qualitative study," *BMC Public Health*, vol. 10, article 381, 2010.

[21] A. Sanou, M. Dembele, S. Theobald, and J. Macq, "Access and adhering to tuberculosis treatment: barriers faced by patients and communities in Burkina Faso," *International Journal of Tuberculosis and Lung Disease*, vol. 8, no. 12, pp. 1479–1483, 2004.

[22] A. Thorson and E. Johansson, "Equality or equity in health care access: a qualitative study of doctors' explanations to a longer doctor's delay among female TB patients in Vietnam," *Health Policy*, vol. 68, no. 1, pp. 37–46, 2004.

[23] T. Zhang, X. Liu, H. Bromley, and S. Tang, "Perceptions of tuberculosis and health seeking behaviour in rural Inner Mongolia, China," *Health Policy*, vol. 81, no. 2-3, pp. 155–165, 2007.

[24] S. Atre, A. Kudale, S. Morankar, D. Gosoniu, and M. G. Weiss, "Gender and community views of stigma and tuberculosis in rural Maharashtra, India," *Global Public Health*, vol. 6, no. 1, pp. 56–71, 2011.

[25] S. R. Atre, A. M. Kudale, S. N. Morankar, S. G. Rangan, and M. G. Weiss, "Cultural concepts of tuberculosis and gender among the general population without tuberculosis in rural Maharashtra, India," *Tropical Medicine and International Health*, vol. 9, no. 11, pp. 1228–1238, 2004.

[26] S. C. Baral, D. K. Karki, and J. N. Newell, "Causes of stigma and discrimination associated with tuberculosis in Nepal: a qualitative study," *BMC Public Health*, vol. 7, article 211, 2007.

[27] A. Deribew, G. Abebe, L. Apers et al., "Prejudice and misconceptions about tuberculosis and HIV in rural and urban communities in Ethiopia: a challenge for the TB/HIV control program," *BMC Public Health*, vol. 10, article 400, 2010.

[28] G. D. Gosoniu, S. Ganapathy, J. Kemp et al., "Gender and socio-cultural determinants of delay to diagnosis of TB in Bangladesh, India and Malawi," *International Journal of Tuberculosis and Lung Disease*, vol. 12, no. 7, pp. 848–855, 2008.

[29] K. Jaggarajamma, R. Ramachandran, N. Charles, V. Chandrasekaran, M. Muniyandi, and S. Ganapathy, "Psycho-social dysfunction: perceived and enacted stigma among tuberculosis patients registered under revised national tuberculosis control programme," *The Indian Journal of Tuberculosis*, vol. 55, no. 4, pp. 179–187, 2008.

[30] E. Johansson, N. H. Long, V. K. Diwan, and A. Winkvist, "Gender and tuberculosis control: perspectives on health seeking behaviour among men and women in Vietnam," *Health Policy*, vol. 52, no. 1, pp. 33–51, 2000.

[31] F. Karim, A. M. R. Chowdhury, A. Islam, and M. G. Weiss, "Stigma, gender, and their impact on patients with tuberculosis in rural Bangladesh," *Anthropology and Medicine*, vol. 14, no. 2, pp. 139–151, 2007.

[32] N. H. Long, E. Johansson, V. K. Diwan, and A. Winkvist, "Fear and social isolation as consequences of tuberculosis in Vietnam: a gender analysis," *Health Policy*, vol. 58, no. 1, pp. 69–81, 2001.

[33] J. Ngamvithayapong, A. Winkvist, and V. Diwan, "High AIDS awareness may cause tuberculosis patient delay: results from an HIV epidemic area, Thailand," *AIDS*, vol. 14, no. 10, pp. 1413–1419, 2000.

[34] C. Rundi, "Understanding tuberculosis: perspectives and experiences of the people of Sabah, East Malaysia," *Journal of Health, Population and Nutrition*, vol. 28, no. 2, pp. 114–123, 2010.

[35] D. Somma, B. E. Thomas, F. Karim et al., "Gender and socio-cultural determinants of TB-related stigma in Bangladesh, India, Malawi and Colombia," *International Journal of Tuberculosis and Lung Disease*, vol. 12, no. 7, pp. 856–866, 2008.

[36] B. Xu, G. Fochsen, Y. Xiu, A. Thorson, J. R. Kemp, and Q. W. Jiang, "Perceptions and experiences of health care seeking and access to TB care—a qualitative study in Rural Jiangsu Province, China," *Health Policy*, vol. 69, no. 2, pp. 139–149, 2004.

[37] F. Yan, R. Thomson, S. Tang et al., "Multiple perspectives on diagnosis delay for tuberculosis from key stakeholders in poor rural China: case study in four provinces," *Health Policy*, vol. 82, no. 2, pp. 186–199, 2007.

[38] N. H. Long, E. Johansson, V. K. Diwan, and A. Winkvist, "Different tuberculosis in men and women: beliefs from focus groups in Vietnam," *Social Science and Medicine*, vol. 49, no. 6, pp. 815–822, 1999.

[39] M. G. Weiss, D. Somma, F. Karim et al., "Cultural epidemiology of TB with reference to gender in Bangladesh, India and Malawi," *International Journal of Tuberculosis and Lung Disease*, vol. 12, no. 7, pp. 837–847, 2008.

[40] G. Fochsen, K. Deshpande, and A. Thorson, "Power imbalance and consumerism in the doctor-patient relationship: health care providers' experiences of patient encounters in a rural district in India," *Qualitative Health Research*, vol. 16, no. 9, pp. 1236–1251, 2006.

[41] S. Ganapathy, B. E. Thomas, M. S. Jawahar, K. J. A. Selvi, S. Sivasubramaniam, and M. Weiss, "Perceptions of gender and tuberculosis in a south Indian urban community," *The Indian Journal of Tuberculosis*, vol. 55, no. 1, pp. 9–14, 2008.

[42] W. Mavhu, E. Dauya, T. Bandason et al., "Chronic cough and its association with TB-HIV co-infection: factors affecting help-seeking behaviour in Harare, Zimbabwe," *Tropical Medicine and International Health*, vol. 15, no. 5, pp. 574–579, 2010.

[43] D. I. Rodríguez-Reimann, P. Nicassio, J. O. Reimann, P. I. Gallegos, and E. L. Olmedo, "Acculturation and health beliefs of Mexican Americans regarding tuberculosis prevention," *Journal of Immigrant Health*, vol. 6, no. 2, pp. 51–62, 2004.

[44] J. Skordis-Worrall, K. Hanson, and A. Mills, "Confusion, caring and tuberculosis diagnostic delay in Cape Town, South Africa," *International Journal of Tuberculosis and Lung Disease*, vol. 14, no. 2, pp. 171–180, 2010.

[45] WHO, "Strategy for integrating gender analysis and actions into the work of WHO," 2009.

[46] "Gender Equality: A Cornerstone of Development," http://www.unfpa.org/gender/.

[47] UNAIDS, "UNAIDS Action Framework: Addressing Women, Girls, Gender Equality and HIV," 2009.

[48] I. S. Kickbusch, "Health literacy: addressing the health and education divide," *Health Promotion International*, vol. 16, no. 3, pp. 289–297, 2001.

[49] Operation ASHA, "Fighting Tuberculosis Worldwide," http://www.opasha.org/.

[50] A. J. Khan, S. Khowaja, F. S. Khan et al., "Engaging the private sector to increase tuberculosis case detection: an impact evaluation study," *The Lancet Infect Diseases*, vol. 12, no. 8, pp. 608–616, 2012.

[51] "Avahan-The India AIDS Initiative," http://docs.gatesfoundation.org/avahan_factsheet.pdf.

[52] M. C. Raviglione and L. Ditiu, "Setting new targets in the fight against tuberculosis," *Nature Medicine*, vol. 19, no. 3, p. 263, 2013.

17

Quality of Tuberculosis Care in Private Health Facilities of Addis Ababa, Ethiopia

Gezahegn Gebrekidan,[1] Gezahegn Tesfaye,[2] Mitiku Teshome Hambisa,[2] and Negussie Deyessa[3]

[1] *Policy and Planning Directorate, Federal Ministry of Health (FMOH), P.O. Box 50332, Addis Ababa, Ethiopia*
[2] *Department of Public Health, College of Health and Medical Sciences, Haramaya University, P.O. Box 235, Harar, Ethiopia*
[3] *School of Public Health, College of Medical Sciences, Addis Ababa University, P.O. Box 3253, Addis Ababa, Ethiopia*

Correspondence should be addressed to Gezahegn Gebrekidan; gezahegn_kidan@yahoo.com

Academic Editor: Luis E. Cuevas

Ensuring provision of good quality tuberculosis (TB) care, especially in private for profit health facilities, is an important component of TB control strategy to reduce poor medical practice which results in multidrug resistant TB (MDR-TB). The aim of this study was to investigate quality of TB care in private health facilities of Addis Ababa. A facility based cross-sectional study was conducted based on Donabedian's structure-process-outcome model of health care quality. Quality of care was determined by adherence to National TB Program guidelines, treatment success rate, and client satisfaction. Exit interview was conducted on 292 patients on the intensive phase of treatment and 384 patient records were reviewed in eight private health facilities. Initial diagnostic AFB test was done for 95.4% of pulmonary TB patients. Most important components of TB care recommended by national guidelines were delivered for a significant proportion of patients. Majority (75%) of the clients were found to be satisfied with each component of TB care. The treatment success rate was 90.9%. The quality of TB care was fairly good. However, only 77.7% of the patients were counseled for HIV testing. Strengthening HIV counseling and testing, tackling shortage of streptomycin and laboratory reagent at private TB clinic is crucial.

1. Introduction

Tuberculosis (TB) remains a major global health problem. It causes ill-health among millions of people each year and ranks as the second leading cause of death from an infectious disease worldwide, after the human immune deficiency virus (HIV) [1]. The latest estimates indicate that there were 8.6 million new TB cases and 1.3 million TB deaths in 2012. Short-course regimens of first-line drugs can cure around 90% of cases, if the right treatment with recommended quality of care is provided [1].

DOTS (directly observed treatment, short course) is the internationally recommended control strategy for TB [2, 3]. This strategy includes the delivery of a standard short course of drugs to individuals diagnosed with TB. The delivery includes the direct observation of therapy (DOT), either by a health worker or by someone nominated by the health worker and the patient for this purpose (sometimes called a DOT supporter) [3].

The global target for TB control through full DOTS expansion was the attainment of 70% case detection and attainment of 85% cure rate by 2005 [4]. Though critical, these targets are insufficient in achieving the TB-related millennium development goals (MDGs) target of halting the spread and beginning to reverse the incidence of TB by 2015. Unfortunately, even these targets were not achieved, especially in Africa by the year 2005 and still only 82% [1, 5]. One major constraint identified as limiting the attainment of these targets is the noninvolvement of the private sector in the TB control programs. Thus, WHO observed that the target of 70% case detection would not be reached unless DOTS programs continue to expand geographically as well as involve the private sector consequently, and the current stop TB strategy that includes calls for promotion of public-private partnership was started in 2006 [5].

In 2011, the global TB treatment success rate was 87% among all new TB cases, while it was 89% in Ethiopia [1]. Ethiopia is one of the 22 high burden countries. According to the WHO global TB report 2011, there were an estimated 261 per 100,000 incident cases of TB in Ethiopia in 2010. According to the same report the prevalence of TB was estimated to be 394 per 100,000. During the year 2010/11, a total of 159,017 TB cases were notified in Ethiopia. Among these 151,866 (95.5%) were new cases of TB. The proportion of new smear-positive, smear negative, and EPTB among all new cases is 32.7%, 34.8%, and 32.5%, respectively. Only about 45% of TB patients have undergone HIV test and 15% were tested HIV positive [6].

To intensify the access and case detection rate, the Federal Ministry of Health (FMOH) has expanded DOTs services in line with WHO's global recommendation to involve the private sector in the delivery of TB services since 2006 which is known as public-private mix directly observed therapy-short course (PPM-DOTS) [6, 7].

Expanding TB care to the private sector increases access to care, particularly for clients who are reluctant to patient load at crowded public facilities and expand access to care for migrant populations who do not have local identity cards necessary to access care at public facilities [8].

Improving access to high-quality services also means reducing the harmful effects of poor medical practice. Inappropriate medical practices for TB diagnosis, treatment, and case management contribute to unnecessary suffering for patients, diagnostic delays, continuous spread of TB, high health-care costs for patients and society, and development of MDR-TB. Despite the increment of case detection rate through the engagement of private health facilities in TB care provision being encouraging, the emergence of drug resistance tuberculosis (MDR-TB) becomes a major public health problem in a number of countries including Ethiopia and an obstacle to the global TB control efforts [9].

Involvement of private sector for DOTS strategy in Ethiopia has been started since 2006 and this initiative increases access to service and case detection rate for TB control [8]. But to date, in Ethiopia, there is no study assessing the quality of provision of TB service in private health facilities. So assessing the quality TB care service is important to determine whether standards are being practiced in private health facility, to identify potential areas for improvement and to strengthen and implement better TB care in private health facilities.

2. Methods and Materials

2.1. Study Area. The study was conducted in Addis Ababa, the capital city of Ethiopia, which serves as the social, political, and economic center of the country. It is located at the geographic center of the country and covers a landmass of 540 km^2 and has a total population of around 3 million. The city has 30 hospitals of which 25 are private, 29 health centers, 8 not-for-profit clinics, and 442 for-profit private clinics. In the city 25 private health facilities (10 hospitals and 15 higher clinics) provide DOTS service for more than two years during the study period [8].

2.2. Study Design and Period. A facility based cross-sectional study involving both quantitative and qualitative method was conducted. The study was based on the Donabedian's framework of health care quality assessment. Three dimensions of quality of TB care based on Donabedian's structure-process-outcome model were assessed [10]. The specific structural and process elements of TB care were identified from the National-TLCP manual and PPM-DOTS guidelines [6, 7] where availability of resources required to provide TB care and supervision are included for structural assessment, while technical performances, use of equipment and supplies for TB control activities, interpersonal relations, and convenience of TB care to patients are included for processes of care assessment. Patients' satisfaction level and treatment success rate were taken for outcome quality assessment (Figure 1). The study was conducted from March 11 to 22, 2011.

2.3. Sample Size and Sampling. A "rule of thumb" was used for the rough estimation of sample size. According to this rule, for quality assessment of health care, if the numbers of units are less than 50, 30–50% of the sample will be taken [11]. Hence, eight private health facilities (five higher clinics and three hospitals), that is, 30% sample from a sampling frame of 15 higher clinic and 10 hospitals, were included in this study. Selection of eight private health facilities from sampling frame is done by simple random sampling (Figure 2).

With the purpose of assessing recent practices, patients who had completed their treatment in the previous one year in TB clinic were included for record review. The sample size for record review was determined by single population proportion formula based on the assumption that 50% of the patient record was complete, marginal error of 5% and CI 95% which yields a sample of 384. Health facility TB registration book was used for the sampling frame. A number of sampled TB patient who completed their treatment in the previous one year for each health facility were allocated proportionally based on the determined sample size and systematic random sampling technique was employed to select TB patient from TB registration book (Figure 2).

For exit interview, TB patients on intensive phase of treatment were included since they are available on daily basis for medication in the health facilities. Patients who visited the health facilities for the first time were excluded as they may not have adequate prior experience with the health facility to provide valid information. The total numbers of TB clients on intensive phase in the selected health facilities during the study period were 292. Hence, to get maximum sample size, all patients on the intensive phase of treatment in these eight private health facilities were included. In addition, observations on 71 patients were done to assess patient-provider interaction. TB control activities in the eight private

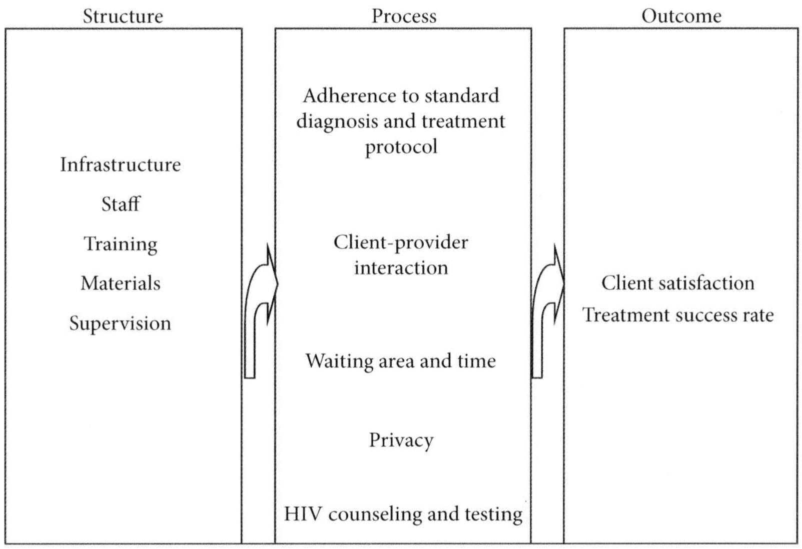

FIGURE 1: The conceptual framework for assessing quality of TB care in private health facilities of Addis Ababa, Ethiopia 2011.

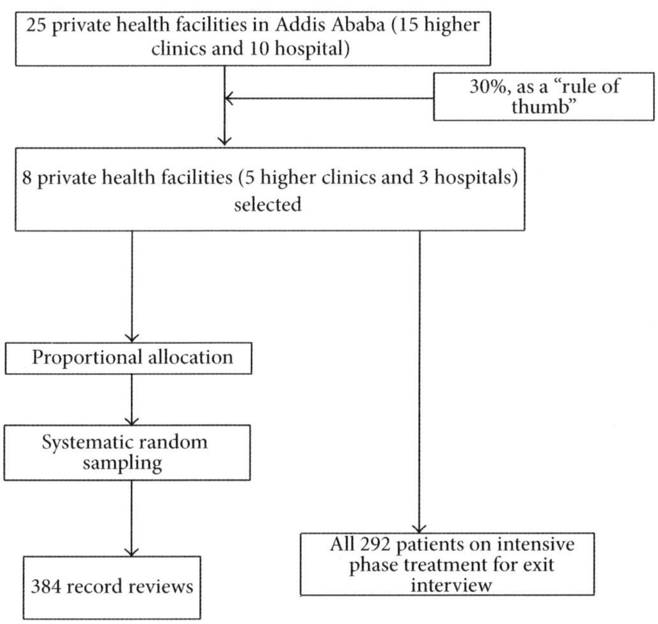

FIGURE 2: Schematic presentation of selection of health facilities and sampling strategies in private health facilities of A. A, 2011.

health facilities were observed; heads and health workers in TB clinics were interviewed (Figure 2).

2.4. Measurements. The main outcome variables were patient satisfaction and treatment success rate, while independent variables include sociodemographic and socioeconomic variables such as age, sex, educational level, marital status, occupation, monthly income, availability and accessibility of services, adequacy of information, providers' competence in providing different services, initial diagnostic AFB test and result, HIV test and result, and classification of TB patient.

2.5. Data Collection

2.5.1. Structural Assessment. National TB and leprosy control program (TLCP) performance monitoring checklist was used to assess availability of different materials, drugs, equipment, and supplies for TB control activities by the principal investigator. Data on staff assignment, training on tuberculosis control activities like AFB microscopy procedures, and patterns of service delivery and supervision were collected by interviewing heads of the health facilities.

2.5.2. Process Quality Assessment. The principal investigator observed the process of care and reviewed record. Observations and health care providers' interview using guiding questions were made on some TB control activities like whether health education on TB is given in the health facility, time at which TB clinics opened, adequacy of information given to TB patients, patient's participation in decision-making process, and utilization of equipment in TB clinics and the level of provider-patient interaction. In addition to this, health workers in charge of TB clinic and laboratory technicians were also interviewed by the principal investigator on any procedures/norms followed in the health facility in the case detection, AFB microscopy procedures, treatment, monitoring and follow-up of TB patients, and use of guidelines, manuals, and so forth.

2.5.3. Outcome Assessment. For the patient satisfaction level trained nurses conducted the exit interview using standard questionnaire among TB patients' on the intensive phase of treatment. Client's sociodemographic and socioeconomic characteristics, organization of treatment services, provider-client interaction, provider's competence, and adequacy of information were included in the interview. For the treatment success rate data from the record review was used.

2.6. Data Quality Assurance. Data collectors were trained for one day and the completeness, accuracy, and consistency of the collected data were checked on daily basis during data collection by the principal investigator. Incomplete, inaccurate and inconsistent questionnaires were returned back for data collectors to be filled again.

2.7. Data Processing and Analysis. Data were coded, cleaned, and entered into EPI info then transferred and analyzed using SPSS version 16 software for windows. Descriptive statistics were used to describe the structural, process, and outcome quality assessment results. Bivariate analysis was done by logistic regression to see any association between the outcome variables and independent variables. Since no variable was found to be significant on the bivariate analysis, further multivariate analysis was not done.

2.8. Ethical Considerations. Ethical clearance was obtained from University of Gondar institutional review board (IRB). Based on the ethical clearance, permission was obtained from A. A regional health bureau and the respective health institutions. Respondents were informed of the purposes, procedures, risks, and benefits of the study before making the interview. The privacy and confidentiality of the study participants were kept. Anonymity was maintained for all those records reviewed. For those patients less than 18 years old, oral consent was obtained from their parents and information has been collected from their parents.

3. Results

3.1. Sociodemographic Characteristics of Respondents. Exit interview of clients at TB service delivery outlet was carried out to assess their satisfaction level with the medical care for which the response rate of the study was 100%. All 292 clients on intensive phase of treatment were included in the study. More than half of respondents 52.4% were male, 63% were in the age group 1–35 years, 55.1% were grade 12 completed and above, majority 32.5% were private workers, 68.8% of them have income of less than 1500 Ethiopian birr, and more than half of them (51.7%) were in the first month of intensive phase (Table 1).

Regarding their means of transportation to get TB clinic, 56.8% got to the TB clinic by walking on foot and the remaining 43.2% clients used car/public bus to get TB clinic. The median time taken to reach the health facilities was 10 minutes, and the median waiting time to see their health care provider was 10 minutes, while the minimum and maximum waiting time was 1 and 40 minutes, respectively.

3.2. Resource Availability. TB care in all health facilities is provided in a separate room (Table 2). The TB rooms in each health facilities have light, ventilation, water supply, chair, table, and waiting space for TB clients. DOT service is opened throughout Monday to Friday from 8.30 am to 4.30 pm in all health facilities.

All the eight health facility has full time staffs assigned for TB clinic and TB care was run by trained TB nurses.

Table 1: Sociodemographic characteristics of TB patients in private health facilities of A. A, 2011.

Variables	Number (n = 292)	Percent
Age group		
≤35	184	63.0
35^+	108	37.0
Sex		
Male	153	52.4
Female	139	47.6
Marital status		
Single	131	44.9
Married	116	39.7
Divorced	32	11.0
Widowed	13	4.5
Educational status		
Illiterate	16	5.5
Elementary	48	16.4
Secondary	67	22.9
Grade 12 completed	98	33.6
Higher education	63	21.6
Occupation		
Government employee	95	32.5
Private worker	83	28.4
House wife	19	6.5
Merchant	49	19.5
Student	33	11.3
Others	13	4.5
Treatment duration		
On 1st month	151	51.7
On 2nd month	141	48.3
Income		
1–1500 Ethiopian birr	201	68.8
>1500 Ethiopian birr	91	31.2

Each health facility has at least one staff that had been trained on TB control activities and all of them had received refreshment trainings in the last 12 months (Table 2). All health facilities had at least one laboratory technician who had received AFB microscopy techniques where only four of health facilities had a laboratory technician who received refreshment trainings in the last 12 months.

Recent version of TLCP manual, TLCP laboratory manual, TB unit registration book, TB referral and transfer form, TB sputum examination request form, and TB control activity report form is available in all health facilities (Table 2). Only three health facilities have posted and used TB flip chart and flow chart for diagnosis of PTB+ and four health facilities had TB posters in different languages in a visible place. Except shortage of streptomycin, all of the health facilities had the recommended anti-TB drugs, namely, rifampicine, isoniazide pyrazinamide, and ethambutol, in the stock adequately during study period. As to the laboratory materials for TB diagnosis and control activities all of the health facilities provide routine laboratory tests, including

TABLE 2: Summary of selected structure indicators in private health facilities of A. A, 2011.

Variables	Number (facility)	Percent
Separate TB room		
Yes	8	100
No	0	0
Presence of trained TB care provider		
Yes	8	100
No	0	0
Availability of standard monitoring tools		
Yes	8	100
No	0	0
Posted TB poster in different languages		
Yes	4	50.0
No	4	50.0
Recommended anti-TB drugs		
Rifampicine	8	100
Isoniazide	8	100
Pyrazinamide	8	100
Ethambutol	8	100
Streptomycine	0	0
Presence of HIV and AFB test		
Yes	8	100
No	0	0
Supervisory support in the last 6 months		
Yes	8	100
No	0	0

HIV testing, microscopy for TB diagnosis (Table 2). All the required laboratory supplies based on the National TLCP implementation guideline are available in all health facilities except for a shortage of staining reagents due to inconsistent supply.

All health facilities, 8 (100%) had been supervised once in the last 6 months by Addis Ababa regional health bureau and other program supporters (Table 2). The supervision involved observation of TB registration book, discussion, and guidance in all health facilities; besides all supervised health facilities received written feedback timely.

3.3. Compliance with the National Guideline and Protocol. In depth interview with head of the health facility was done on service provision and all selected health facilities use the WHO recommended spot morning spot (SMS) sputum collection for AFB microscopic test. Besides, all the health facilities were using the recommended anti-TB drugs and their dosage based on NTLCP manual. Concerning drug provision to clients, on intensive phase, all eight health facilities provide the drugs to most of TB clients on daily basis under supervision, while some patient took the anti-TB drugs for 2–4 days for self-administration and came back after finishing. All health facilities monitored patients' treatment compliance by daily filling patient's TB registration form, pill count, and checking on monthly basis during continuation phase and all health facilities communicate contact person to trace absentee and defaulter. However, all health facilities had no health education program that addresses tuberculosis to their clients as part of their routine daily activities.

Record review was conducted on 384 patients who have completed their treatment in the previous one year. All of them were found to have a registered unique TB registration number. Out of 384 patients, 238 (61.8%) were pulmonary TB and 146 (38.2%) were extrapulmonary TB patients. Initial diagnostic AFB test was done for 59.1% of all TB patients (PTB and EPTB), where 37.4% were positive for AFB. From the pulmonary TB patients initial AFB test was done for 95.4%. During the continuation phase, weight was recorded for all patients, while drugs and their dosages given were recorded for 383 (99.7%) patients. Besides, follow-up AFB microscopy on the 5th/7th months of treatment were done for 78 (96.3%) of the 81 PTB+ patients, where one (1.23%) was found to be positive, 77 (95.1%) were negative, and it was unrecorded for one (3.7%) patient (Table 3).

Exit interview was done to assess anti-TB drug collection during intensive phase and HIV counseling and testing status. Of 292 TB clients, 227 (77.7%) were counseled and 65 (22.3%) were not counseled on HIV testing. Among TB clients counseled on HIV, 202 (89.0%) were tested, while the remaining 25 (11%) were not tested where the main reasons mentioned by clients were nonvoluntariness, laboratory cost, and tested before. Concerning anti TB drug collection, from the total of TB patient on intensive phase, 199 (68.2%) clients were collecting anti-TB drugs on daily basis under supervision from TB clinic, while the remaining 93 (31.8%) took the drugs home for self-administration and came back after finishing during the study period (Table 3).

Observation on 71 clients was done to assess provider-patient interactions while they receive the service in TB clinic. It was observed that all health workers in TB room of all health facilities demonstrate greeting, respectful, and encouraging attitude to their patients when they were receiving their drugs. Patients were seen in privacy in TB room and participated in part of decision making processes in the process of service delivery in each facility. Health information on the need to comply with treatment is provided in all health facilities.

3.4. Patient Satisfaction and Treatment Outcome. Clients' degree of satisfaction was assessed using different questions. It was found out that 10.3%, 7.5%, and 6.8% of study participants were dissatisfied in the adequacy and appropriateness of working hours, comfort of waiting area, and waiting time, respectively. Meanwhile, a higher proportion of study participants were satisfied with provider's competence/skill (99.3%), the measures taken to assure privacy (99.3%), and completeness of information given 98.3% (Table 4).

Scaling was done using the twelve satisfaction's related equations. The rating was determined using the count value with in cases' in the transform menu of SPSS software. Those TB clients who answered satisfied for each of the satisfaction related questions were taken as fully satisfied. Thus, the total clients who were satisfied fully in their stay at the day of their TB care visit were 219 (75%).

TABLE 3: Summary of selected process indicators in private health facilities of A. A, 2011.

Variables	Number	Percent
Record review (384)		
Initial AFB test done		
Yes	227	59.1
No	157	40.9
HIV test done		
Yes	230	59.9
No	154	40.1
Follow-up AFB microscopy done on 2nd month of Rx (85)		
Yes	84	95.3
No	1	4.7
Follow-up AFB microscopy done on 5/7th month of Rx (81)		
Yes	78	96.3
No	16	3.7
Completeness of information on TB registration		
Complete	373	97.1
Incomplete	11	2.9
Client exit interview (292)		
HIV counseling done		
Yes	227	77.7
No	65	22.3
HIV testing done (227)		
Yes	202	89.0
No	25	11
Health education program on TB		
Yes	0	0
No	8	100
DOT (collecting anti-TB drugs on daily basis under supervision)		
Yes	199	68.2
No	93	31.8

TABLE 4: TB patients' satisfaction level with different components of services in private health facilities of A. A, 2011.

Aspects of the variable	Satisfied	Neutral	Dissatisfied
Adequacy and appropriateness of working hours	262 (89.7%)	0 (0.0%)	30 (10.3%)
Waiting time	271 (92.8%)	1 (0.3%)	20 (6.8%)
Time spent with HW	281 (96.2%)	3 (1.0%)	8 (2.7%)
Cleanliness of waiting area	276 (94.5%)	4 (1.4%)	12 (4.1%)
Comfort of waiting area	265 (90.8%)	5 (1.7%)	22 (7.5%)
Cleanliness of examination/treatment room	269 (92.1%)	7 (2.4%)	16 (5.5%)
Cleanliness of treatment/diagnosis equipment	268 (91.8%)	16 (5.5%)	8 (2.7%)
Respect offered by health provider	287 (98.3%)	3 (1.0%)	2 (0.7%)
Measures taken to assure privacy	289 (99.0%)	2 (0.7%)	1 (0.3%)
Provider's competence/skill	290 (99.3%)	1 (0.3%)	1 (0.3%)
Cost incurred	286 (97.9%)	0 (0.0%)	6 (2.1%)
Completeness of information given	288 (98.3%)	2 (0.7%)	2 (0.7%)

With respect to treatment outcome, out of all 384 patients, 79 (20.6%) were cured cases and 270 (70.3%) completed treatment, defaulter constituted 1 (0.3%), and the treatment success rate (those cured + treatment completed) was 349 (90.9%).

On the bivariate analysis there was no significant association between patients' satisfaction level and different sociodemographic characteristics of the patients. Again, there was no significant association between treatment success rate and the independent variables.

4. Discussion

This study showed that a significant proportion of patients attending TB clinic in the private health facilities have got important components of TB care recommended by the national guidelines. All of the health facilities had the recommended anti-TB drugs except shortage of streptomycin. Quantity and the qualities of staffing were satisfactory. Initial diagnostic AFB test was done for 59.1% of patients. Follow-up AFB microscopy on the 5th/7th months of treatment was done for 96.3% of the PTB+ patients, where only one was found to be positive. Majorities (75%) of the clients were found to be satisfied with each component of TB care they received and the treatment success rate was 90.9%.

Even though both the quantity and the qualities of staffing were satisfactory, only half of the health facilities have a laboratory technician who received refreshment training on TB control activities which is consistent with a study in Afar region where both the quantity and the qualities of staffing were not satisfactory in that almost half of the health facilities lacked laboratory technicians who received on the job training on TB control activities [12]. Staff development in general is a critical component of any DOTS program. The challenges of maintaining a competent and sufficient workforce remain problematic in TB high-burden countries [13]. This problem is confounded by high staff turnover. Like the public sector, the private sector is observed to be in great need of in-service training activities to update providers on new activities such as the Stop TB Strategy, including the management of TB linked to HIV/AIDS, multidrug resistant TB, and PPM-DOTS.

The supervision pattern seems good in all health facilities where all got a chance of being supervised in the last six months. The supervision pattern was also scheduled, consistent, and involves observation of TB registration book, discussion, and guidance in all health facilities and written feedback is given. This is consistent with the national recommendations where they recommend strong supportive supervision as a way of ensuring staff competence, effectiveness, efficiency, and satisfaction through observation, discussion, record reviewing, support, and guidance [6] as opposed to the study in Afar where no TLCP focal person had regular supervisor and supervisory schedule for TB control activities which may be due to the fact that there is usual strict follow up of quality service provision in the private health sector than the government sector [12].

All health facilities seem to be well equipped with the materials required for TB control activity as per the national standard. However, shortages of streptomycin drug and laboratory reagents were reported by providers despite the national TLCP guideline recommend adequate and consistent supply of TB drugs and other consumables [6]. This is in line with an evaluation assessment in Addis Ababa and Oromia which showed that the supply of the combination drug RH, INH, and E was not sufficient to last for more than three months and vitamin B6 was not available in all the facilities assessed and the available RHZE, E, and Streptomycin had a shelf life of less than three months [14]. In the same manner, in a study conducted in government health facilities in Jimma Zone, South West Ethiopia, shortage of laboratory reagents and slides for sputum smear microscopy were problems identified [15]. It is obvious that drug supply management and supply chain management are deficient and have the potential to hamper the delivery of quality TB services in the private sector [14]. However, it must also be noted that drug supply management is an inherent problem in the health care system in general and, as such, is faced by public health facilities as well.

The accuracy and completeness of the patient record may result in either underestimating or overestimating some of the indicators. The correct completion of patients' registration book is crucial to the patients monitoring and evaluation. This study revealed that the majority, 373 (97.1%) patient records', were found complete; that is, treatment for most patients was initiated and continued with proper recording of full information which is critical for patient monitoring. This finding was almost similar to study in Tigray where 93.2% of patients' records were found to be complete but higher than study conducted in Afar (11.5%) [12, 16]. The difference might be explained in terms of geographical, health infrastructure, and staffing difference between these areas as Addis Ababa is the capital of the country where there is high health infrastructure and highly qualified health professionals.

Sputum microscopy is the main diagnostic tool for pulmonary tuberculosis (PTB). All suspected TB cases should have sputum microscopy as their first diagnostic tool. But in our case, initial diagnostic AFB test was done only for 59.1% of patients. This finding is slightly lower than study conducted in Jimma in which 1st smear sputum microscopy was done for all 399 (100.0%) pulmonary TB patients [15]. This could be attributed to the fact that in our study there is the lack of laboratory reagent and lack of refresher training for laboratory technicians. Followup on the 2nd months of treatment seems good (95.3%) in that almost all initially diagnosed PTB+ cases received follow-up AFB microscopy which is in line with the national guideline, where it recommends that all PTB+ patients should get follow-up AFB microscopy services. Similarly, follow-up AFB microscopy at the 5th/7th months of treatment was done for 78 (96.3%) of diagnosed PTB+ patients, which is again in line with the FMOH's recommendations [6].

Information Education Communication (IEC) activities for TB control activities were found to be poor as even no one health facility was giving health education that addresses TB. Only half of health facilities have TB posters in different languages being posted in visible public places, despite its cost effectiveness. Similarly, a study in Jimma revealed absence of health education for TB patients, flip charts, and TB posters in local language were major identified problems [15]. Moreover, the research conducted in Afar showed that IEC activities for TB control activities were absent as only small proportion of health facilities were giving health education that address TB and had TB posters in different languages being posted in visible public places [12]. This again opposes the national guideline where every treatment facility is expected to deliver health education to patients and the public [6] as this is found to be the most effective and efficient strategy in health care programs implementation and interventions. The findings in the above studies show that IEC activities are ignored and less utilized in both private and public health facilities.

The patterns of patient-provider interactions were good in that almost all TB patients were greeted politely, participated in parts of decision making, advised to comply with treatment, and speak the same language with the providers. This seems that the processes of care were patient centered services which are in favor to the principles of quality health care and continuous quality improvement approaches [17]. Adequate communications between providers and patients are expected phenomenon in private health facility setup unlike the public health facilities and can be taken as an advantage to potentiate TB control activities.

Getting patients regularly to collect their drugs daily under supervision during intensive phase is recommended by the national TLCP manual. However, it is reported by providers and TB clients that a relatively high number of TB patients took drugs for 2 to 3 days home for self-administration and come back after finishing which affects TB control activities. This may be due to poor physical access to health facility, transport cost by clients, work load by providers, trust between clients and providers, and time inconvenience by client. Supporting bodies of evidence have reported from a study conducted in Gambia in which high defaulter rate was found among those patients that incurred significant time traveling to receive treatment [18].

Monitoring treatment adherence of TB clients is strongly recommended by WHO and national TB guideline [6] for implementing effective treatment compliance; the findings of this study showed that monitoring for treatment compliance was practiced in all health facilities through pill count, ensuring followup and providing accurate information, which could be again due to having relatively high number of trained health care providers and having strong regular supportive supervision from the respective bodies. This was supported by the study in Ethiopia which shows that patients tended to interrupt and default from treatment when their care provider had been inadequately supervised by district TB control experts [19].

The synergy between TB and HIV/AIDS is strong. In high HIV prevalence populations, TB is a leading cause of morbidity and mortality, and HIV is fuelling the tuberculosis epidemic in Ethiopia [20]. World Health Organization recommended package of collaborative TB/HIV activities to reduce the burden of TB/HIV includes HIV testing for TB patients [21]. However, record review of this study revealed that only 59.9% TB clients who had completed treatment in the previous one year got HIV test. On the other hand, from exit interview, 202 (69%) were tested. This finding is relatively high as compared to the national (45%) [6]. This high achievement as compared to the national may be due to free availability of HIV test kits to private health facilities and the trainee's motivation heightens through training of health worker on TB/HIV service. But still the target to reach the recommended 80% HIV testing rate among TB patients in Ethiopia is not yet achieved [22].

Satisfied client is more likely to comply with prescribed medical treatment and completion of treatment which is of utmost priority for TB control programs. Client satisfaction with the services and perceived quality tend to influence utilization of service as well as compliance with practitioner recommendation [23]. In this study the majority (75%) of the respondents were satisfied with all components of TB care that they received. But study conducted in Sidama zone, South Ethiopia, revealed that 90% of the study participants were satisfied with TB treatment service. [24]. This might be due to the difference in study setting and measuring clients' satisfaction might overestimate the satisfaction level in Sidama study, since the patients may respond in a relatively positive way fearing being recognized and similarly mostly satisfied patients usually visit public health facility. However, relatively higher proportions of TB clients were dissatisfied in the adequacy and appropriateness of working hours 133 (63.6%). Similarly most studies showed that waiting time or time spent with the provider strongly influence the level of client satisfaction [25–27], which can lead to service rejections by the patients and defaulting which can lead to incomplete treatment, treatment failure, and drug resistances.

The treatment success rate in this study was 90.9% which is similar with the national figure (89%) and a bit higher than the treatment success rate in Africa in 2011. This finding is also above the international target which is 85% [1]. This higher treatment success rate might be due to the good quality and quantity of staffs in private health facility, rational diagnosis, standard treatment, and successful followup (adherence to the national guideline).

The strength of this study was that it involves different approaches of data collection such as exit interview, record review, and observation, based on the Donabedian framework of health care quality assessment and focused on private for profit health facilities. Nevertheless, the study has the following limitations: reviewed records lack important variables and the study includes only private health facilities in A. A, so it may not represent all private facilities in Ethiopia.

5. Conclusion

All health facilities have adequate resources to provide TB care. However, there is shortage of streptomycin TB drugs and inconsistent supply of laboratory reagent for AFB in all facilities. Adherence to national TLCP guidelines was high in all private health facilities as all health facilities were used SMS sputum collection for AFB test, monitor clients' treatment adherence, follow-up AFB test at 2nd and 5/7th for PTB+, and maintaining a standardized recording and reporting TB activities which are the most important aspect of DOTS to prevent and control TB and the development of MDR-TB. IEC activity on TB control, HIV counseling, and testing in TB clinic was poor. Majority of TB clients were found satisfied with each component of TB care. The treatment success rate was very good. Strengthening TB/HIV collaboration activity through offering HIV counseling and testing actively and routinely to all TB patients, tackling shortage of streptomycin and laboratory reagent in private TB clinics is crucial.

Authors' Contribution

Gezahegn Gebrekidan has conceived the study, carried out the overall design and execution of the study, and performed data collection and statistical analysis. Negussie Deyessa has participated in the critical revision of the design of the study, data collection techniques, and helped the statistical analysis. Gezahegn Tesfaye and Mitiku Teshome Hambisa have participated in the drafting of the paper and assisted in the design of the study and data analysis. All authors read and finally approved this paper for submission.

Acknowledgments

The authors' sincere thank, goes to Addis Ababa City Administration Council Health Bureau Ethical Committee for reviewing of the proposal, issuing ethical clearance, and writing a letter for the cooperation to the respective private health facilities. The authors are grateful to all studied private health facility owners and TB clinic focal person for their full cooperation during data collection. The authors would like to extend their special thanks to all data collectors and study participants for their willingness to participate in the study.

References

[1] World Health Organization (WHO), Global tuberculosis report, 2013.

[2] World Health Organization's (WHO's) Global TB Report, 2009.

[3] WHO, "Global tuberculosis control, surveillance, planning and financing," WHO Report, STOP TB Department WHO, Geneva, Switzerland, 2006.

[4] WHO, "Global tuberculosis control, surveillance, planning and financing (121–123)," WHO Report, STOP TB Department WHO, Geneva, Switzerland, 2007.

[5] African Union Update on Tuberculosis Control in Africa, Special Summit of the African Union on HIV/AIDS, Tuberculosis and Malaria (ATM) Sp/Ex.CL/ATM/4 (1) Abuja, 2006.

[6] Federal Ministry of Health (FMOH) of Ethiopia, *Tuberculosis/Leprosy and TB/HIV Prevention and Control Program Manual*, 5th edition, 2012.

[7] FMOH-Ethiopia PPM-DOTS implementation Guideline, Addis Ababa, Ethiopia, 2006.

[8] Private Sector Program-Ethiopia (PSP-E), "Assessing the foundation for a continuum focused on public private health sector collaboration in addressing HIV/AIDS and tuberculosis in Ethiopia," Private Sector Partner Report, 2009.

[9] Federal Ministry of Health of Ethiopia, *Guideline for Program and Clinical Management of Drug Resistant Tuberculosis*, Federal Ministry of Health of Ethiopia, Addis Ababa, Ethiopia, 1st edition, 2009.

[10] A. Donabedian, "The quality of care. How can it be assessed?" *The Journal of the American Medical Association*, vol. 260, no. 12, pp. 1743–1748, 1988.

[11] A. Donabedian, "Methods for deriving criteria for assessing the quality of medical care," *Medical Care Review*, vol. 37, no. 7, pp. 653–698, 1980.

[12] A. Girma, D. Hailemariyam, and K. Deribe, "Quality of tuberculosis care in six health facilities of Afar Region, Ethiopia," *Ethiopian Medical Journal*, vol. 48, no. 3, pp. 195–203, 2010.

[13] J. Figueroa-Munoz, K. Palmer, M. R. Dal Poz, L. Blanc, K. Bergström, and M. Raviglione, "The health workforce crisis in TB control: a report from high-burden countries," *Human Resources for Health*, vol. 3, article 2, 2005.

[14] A. Wasihun, G. Kombe, A. Leykun, W. Assefa, D. Assefa, and F. Hussein, *A Summartive Evaluation of Pilot Sites Providing TB-DOTS Services in the Private Sector in Ethiopia*, Private Sector Program for HIV and TB-Ethiopia, Abt Associates Inc., Bethesda, Md, USA, 2008, http://shopsproject.org/sites/default/files/resources/5183_file_ TbEthiopia.pdf.

[15] T. Geremew, C. Jira, and F. Girma, "Assessment of quality of care delivered for infectious pulmonary tuberculosis patients in Jimma Zone, South West Ethiopia," *Ethiopian Journal of Health Sciences*, vol. 21, supplement 1, pp. 39–48, 2011.

[16] M. M. Mengiste, W. T. Tesfaye, and J. R. Madley, "The quality of TB diagnosis in district of Tigray region of Northern Ethiopia," *Ethiopian Journal of Health Development*, vol. 19, no. 1-34, pp. 12–20, 2005.

[17] B. B. Longest, J. S. Rakich, and K. Darr, *Managing Health Service Organizations and Systems*, Health Professionals Press, Baltimore, Md, USA, 3rd edition, 2003.

[18] P. C. Hill, W. Stevens, S. Hill et al., "Risk factors for defaulting from tuberculosis treatment: a prospective cohort study of 301 cases in the Gambia," *International Journal of Tuberculosis and Lung Disease*, vol. 9, no. 12, pp. 1349–1354, 2005.

[19] M. M. Mesfin, J. N. Newell, J. D. Walley et al., "Quality of tuberculosis care and its association with patient adherence to treatment in eight Ethiopian districts," *Health Policy and Planning*, vol. 24, no. 6, pp. 457–466, 2009.

[20] Federal Ministry of Health Ethiopia, *Tuberculosis, Leprosy and TB/HIV Prevention and Control Programme Manual*, Federal Ministry of Health Ethiopia, Addis Ababa, Ethiopia, 4th edition, 2008.

[21] "WHO policy on collaborative TB/HIV activities: guidelines for nation-al programs and other stakeholders," WHO, Geneva, Switzerland, (WHO/HTM/TB/2012.1), 2012.

[22] World Health Organization, "Global tuberculosis control: epidemiology, strategy, financing," WHO Report WHO/HTM/TB/2009.411, 2009, http://www.who.int/tb/publications/global_report/2009/en/.

[23] M. H. Bernhart, I. G. P. Wiadnyana, H. Wihardjo, and I. Pohan, "Patient satisfaction in developing countries," *Social Science and Medicine*, vol. 48, no. 8, pp. 989–996, 1999.

[24] Z. S. Nezenega, Y. H. M. Gacho, and T. E. Tafere, "Patient satisfaction on tuberculosis treatment service and adherence to treatment in public health facilities of Sidama zone, South Ethiopia," *BMC Health Services Research*, vol. 13, article 110, 2013.

[25] C. Yildirim, H. Kocoglu, S. Goksu, N. Gunay, and H. Savas, "Patient satisfaction in a university hospital emergency department in Turkey," *Acta Medica*, vol. 48, no. 1, pp. 59–62, 2005.

[26] J. Bain, H. Kelly, D. Snadden, and H. Staines, "Day surgery in Scotland: patient satisfaction and outcomes," *Quality in Health Care*, vol. 8, no. 2, pp. 86–91, 1999.

[27] C. T. Lin, G. A. Albertson, L. M. Schilling et al., "Is patients' perception of time spent with the physician a determinant of ambulatory patient satisfaction?" *Archives of Internal Medicine*, vol. 161, no. 11, pp. 1437–1442, 2001.

18

An Evaluation of Treatment Outcomes in a Cohort of Clients on the DOTS Strategy, 2012–2016

Ato Kwamena Tetteh,[1] **Edward Agyarko**,[2] **Joseph Otchere**,[3] **Langbong Bimi**,[4] **and Irene Ayi**[3]

[1] *Laboratory Department, Metropolitan Hospital, P.O. Box 174, Cape Coast, Ghana*
[2] *Department of Community Medicine and Health, Anglican University College of Technology, P.O. Box 74, Nkoranza, Ghana*
[3] *Noguchi Memorial Institute for Medical Research, Department of Parasitology, College of Health Sciences, University of Ghana, Legon, Accra, Ghana*
[4] *Department of Animal Biology and Conservation Sciences, University of Ghana, Legon, Accra, Ghana*

Correspondence should be addressed to Ato Kwamena Tetteh; aktetteh@outlook.com

Academic Editor: William N. Rom

We present, for the first time, an evaluation of treatment outcomes in a cohort at a TB referral centre in the Central Region of Ghana. Of the 213 clients placed on DOTS, 59.2% (126/213) were sputum smear-positive. An overall cure rate of 90.2% (51.6% cured + 37.6% completed) and a death rate of 8.5% (18/213) were estimated. Of the number of clients who died, 5.7% (12/213) were males ($\chi^2 = 2.891$, $p = 0.699$; LR = 3.004, $p = 0.699$). Deaths were only recorded among clients who were > 19 years old ($\chi^2 = 40.319$, $p = 0.099$; LR = 41.244, $p = 0.083$). Also, 0.9% (2/213) was lost to follow-up, while 1.4% (3/213) had treatment failure. In total, 13.6% (7.0%, 15/213 males, and 6.6%, 14/213 females) of clients who were placed on DOTS were HIV seropositive. Ages of 40–49 years had the highest number, 13/213 (6.1%), infected with HIV, though the difference among the remaining age groups was not statistically significant ($\chi^2 = 9.621$, $p = 0.142$). Furthermore, 7.0% (15/213) had TB/HIV coinfection. Out of them, 9 were cured and 5 died at home, while 1 had treatment failure. Tuberculosis/HIV infection prevention advocacy and interventions that address sociodemographic determinants of unfavourable treatment outcomes are urgently required to augment national efforts towards control.

1. Introduction

Successful tuberculosis (TB) treatment has a positive significant effect on the control of TB. Therefore, completing prescribed medication in active cases is of prime importance to TB control programmes [1]. Globally, the Directly Observed Therapy Short-course (DOTS) has been accepted as a strategy to the cure of tuberculosis [2]. The DOTS strategy has been used in Ghana since 1994, and it remains the medication strategy of choice [3]. This strategy aims at improving patients' commitment to medication and therefore minimizes development of drug resistance to contemporary remedies [4]. With this strategy, it is expected that 80 to 90% of patients will undergo smear conversion within two to three months of treatment [5].

The change in bacterial infection status of sputum of patients from initial Acid-Fast Bacilli (AFB) positive to negative after treatment is referred to as sputum smear conversion (SSC). Smear conversion rate (SCR) at two months of intensive phase (IP) and at three months of IP (extended IP) is a significant operational indicator, as it shows the capacity of the programme to maintain the patients on treatment. It also provides an objective verification for the client's response to therapy and consequently the treatment outcome [5].

The Global TB Report (2011) estimated 86 smear-positive pulmonary TB cases per 100,000 people per year [6]. It has been established that one untreated infectious tuberculosis patient is likely to infect 10 to 15 persons annually [7]. Also, a number of factors have been acknowledged as delaying the time to smear and culture conversion. These include

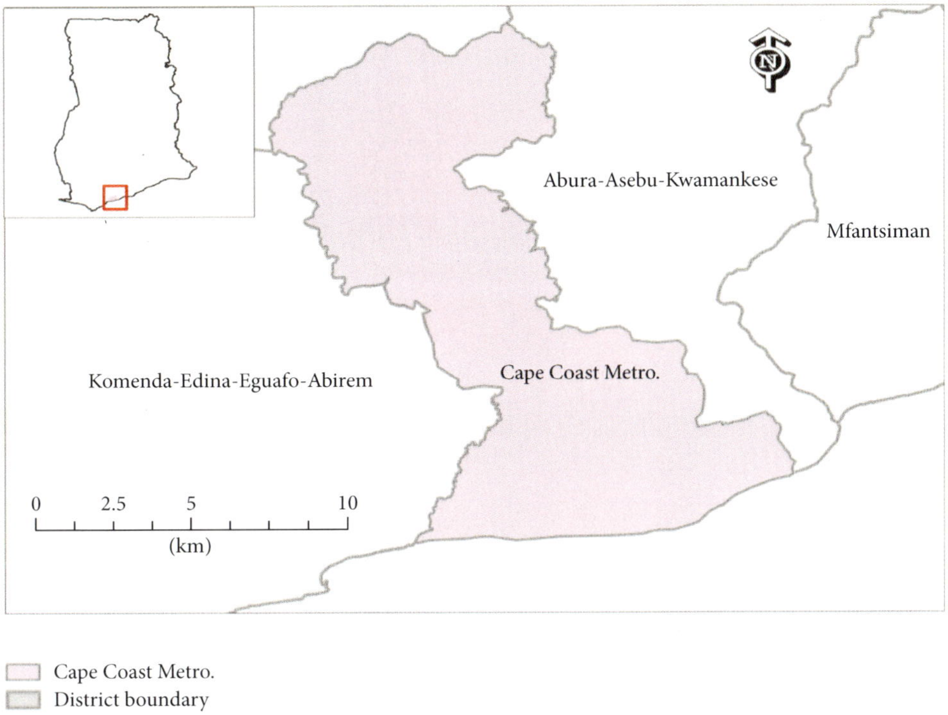

FIGURE 1: *Map of Cape Coast Metropolitan Area (credit: Dr. Charles Gyamfi, Department of Civil Engineering, Tshwane University of Technology, Pretoria, South Africa).*

high intensity initial sputum smear AFB grade, cavitary lesion, uncontrolled hyperglycaemia/diabetes mellitus, old age, certain ethnic population (e.g., Hispanic), multidrug-resistant tuberculosis, initial treatment with less than four antitubercular drugs, and non-rifampicin-based treatment regimens [8–14].

Generally, only sputum culture confirms noncontagious clients. However, lack of culture facilities in most TB centres, except for Regional/Teaching Hospitals in Ghana, necessitates the use of serial negative smears (SNS) before removal of infection control measures. Sputum examination has been described worldwide as the most definite, cost-effective, and dependable test for the diagnosis of pulmonary TB. It confirms the diagnosis and provides information on whether there is positive and progressive response to treatment. At the end of treatment, it shows if clients have been cured. The Metropolitan Hospital (MH), located within the Cape Coast Metropolitan Area (CCMA), has a TB testing centre and it is the only TB referral centre in the Central Region of Ghana. Yearly, about 250–400 new diagnostic cases are referred for testing from within CCMA and adjoining communities. A third of these return test results to treatment centres within their communities for management. The remaining, who reported to MH for consultation, may be recruited onto the DOTS strategy, which is comprehensively elaborated in the Tuberculosis Case Management Desk Aide. Over the past decades, no on-site assessment has been done regarding the conversion rates and performance of the current DOTS strategy. This study presents the outcome of a five-year retrospective evaluation of TB-confirmed and TB-suggestive clients placed on the DOTS strategy.

2. Materials and Methods

2.1. Setting. The entire Cape Coast Metropolis covers an area of 122 km^2 and it is located on longitude $1^\circ 15'$W and latitude $5^\circ 06'$N (Figure 1). The Metropolitan Hospital, Cape Coast, was established in 1939 and it is located on the Beulah Road (Beach Road) between the Nursing and Midwifery Training College and St. Augustine's College. The hospital serves the entire Metropolis and it is the first referral facility for all Government Health Centres and Clinics in the area, as well as the adjoining communities (https://www.google.com.gh/maps/@5.1038147,-1.2596938,587m/data=!3m1!1e3). The hospital has a separate special structure, christened "Chest Ward," where all clients diagnosed or suspected of having TB are admitted.

2.2. Study Design and Population. This was a five-year retrospective study comprising all diagnosed and suspected clients who were admitted and enrolled on the DOTS strategy from 1 January 2012 to 31 December 2016 (Table 1). In total, 213 male and female clients of all ages were included in the study. Compiled data included clients who were acid fast bacilli-(AFB-) positive or negative. All clients had persistent cough, with/without expectoration, increased axillary temperature, loss of appetite, and weight loss.

2.3. Data Collection. Secondary data were compiled from TB patients' registers at the Chest Ward. Client information collected included age, sex, form of tuberculosis (pulmonary or extrapulmonary), type of tuberculosis (smear-positive or smear-negative), category of tuberculosis (new cases

Table 1: Recommended DOTS treatment regimen for each category of tuberculosis in Ghana.

Patient category	Definition	Initial phase treatment[1*] Daily (28 doses/month)	Continuation phase treatment* Daily (28 doses/month)
I	*All new cases* (i) New smear-positive (ii) New smear-negative PTB (iii) Concomitant HIV disease (iv) Extrapulmonary TB	*2 (HRZE)*^{2} = 56 doses of HRZE	*4 (HR)* = 112 doses of HR
II	*Previously treated sputum smear-positive PTB* (i) Relapse (ii) Treatment after interruption (iii) Treatment failure	*2 (HRZE)S + 1 (HRZE)* = 84 doses of HRZE + 56 doses of S	*5 (HRE)* = 140 doses of HRE
III[3]	*Children below 12 years*	*2 (HRZ)* = 56 doses of HRZ	*4 (HR)* = 112 doses of HR

Table 1 is adopted from the National Tuberculosis Programme (NTP) Training Manual, 2012. [1]*Direct observation of treatment intake is required and always in regimens including rifampicin.* [2]*Streptomycin may be used instead of ethambutol. In meningitis, ethambutol should be replaced by streptomycin.* [3]*In children with meningitis, add streptomycin in the initial phase.* Category I: new clients; category II: previously treated clients; category III: children < 12 years. *TB drugs and codes*: H: *isoniazid;* R: *rifampicin;* Z: *pyrazinamide;* S: *streptomycin;* E: *ethambutol. Codes for Fixed Drug Combinations (FDC)*: (HR): isoniazid + rifampicin; (HRZ): isoniazid + rifampicin + pyrazinamide; (HRZE): isoniazid + rifampicin + pyrazinamide + ethambutol. * *The administration of these drugs has been expansively explained in the 2012 edition of the NTP Training Manual.*

or relapse or retreatment cases), and treatment outcome. Treatment outcome of clients was evaluated in harmony with World Health Organization reference and classified as cured, completed (treatment completed), default, treatment failure, death, and others. In this study, treatment was based on pretreatment sputum smear grading (PSSG) and/or TB-suggestive symptoms/sign, coupled with X-ray suggestive images. In addition, the HIV statuses of TB clients were confirmed from their medical records. Those whose status was not already known were tested using the preliminary First Response HIV® 1/2 and the confirmatory OraQuick® HIV 1/2.

2.4. Treatment Regimen. See Table 1.

2.5. Ethical Approval. Permission was sought from the Metropolitan Hospital and the Chest Centre to access TB clients' archived data. Path numbers of patients were not recorded at all in order to conceal their identity. It was emphasized that data presented in this study will strictly be for academic purposes only to help improve management of patients in the future and will cause no harm in accordance with the Declaration of Helsinki (1964).

2.6. WHO Operational Definitions. New smear-positive TB case is a patient who has never had treatment for TB or who has taken anti-TB drugs for less than one month. *Treatment outcome* was divided into six categories according to the National TB Control Programme guidelines: *cured*: a patient who was smear-positive at diagnosis and was smear-negative at the end of the last month of treatment and on at least one previous occasion; *treatment completed*: any patient who was smear-negative but with suggestive signs/symptoms of TB at the time of diagnosis and had completed treatment, with or without sputum smear results; *died*: any patient who died irrespective of the cause of death during the course of treatment; *treatment failure*: any patient who remained or became positive at the end of the fifth month or later during treatment; *treatment defaulter*: any patient who has interrupted treatment two consecutive months or more after the date of the last attendance during the course of treatment; *transfer-out*; a patient who was transferred to another treatment centre and whose treatment outcome is unknown.

2.7. Data Analysis. All records from TB patients' registers from 2012 to 2016 were recoded, concealing the identities of clients. Data were double-entered into Microsoft Excel® and then cleaned (checked and edited) of inconsistencies. Completeness of the TB patients' registers after cleaning was approximately 99.5%. Data were later transported into SPSS (version 20) for analysis. Results were expressed as absolute frequencies (n) and percentages (%). Proportions with 95% confidence intervals and Chi-square test were employed to compare different groups and p value less than 0.05 was considered statistically significant. Smear conversion was estimated as the time (in weeks) from initiation of treatment to first of the two serial negative smears for AFB. Cure rate was deduced according to the WHO cure rate/treatment success rate definition as follows: the proportion of new smear-positive TB cases registered under DOTS in a given year that successfully completed treatment, whether with ("cured") or without ("treatment completed") bacteriologic evidence of success. The study consolidated the respective yearly data to obtain overall rates for the period under review.

3. Results

3.1. Sociodemographic Characteristics. In total, 213 clients whose data were available in tuberculosis (TB) treatment registers from 2012 to 2016 (2012 = 44; 2013 = 55; 2014 = 48;

TABLE 2: Age and sex distribution of clients from 2012 to 2016.

Age group (years)	Sex of clients*		Total**
	Female (%)	Male (%)	
<10	2 (0.9)	—	2
10–19	5 (2.3)	6 (2.8)	11
20–29	12 (5.6)	23 (10.8)	35
30–39	14 (6.6)	30 (14.1)	44
40–49	9 (4.2)	42 (19.7)	51
50–59	9 (4.2)	31 (14.6)	40
≥60	3 (1.4)	27 (12.7)	30
Total	*54 (25.4)*	*159 (74.6)*	*213*

*Significantly *more males than females were recruited for treatment* (χ^2 = 16.9, p = 0.013). **Total number of clients on the *Directly Observed Treatment Short-course* (DOTS).

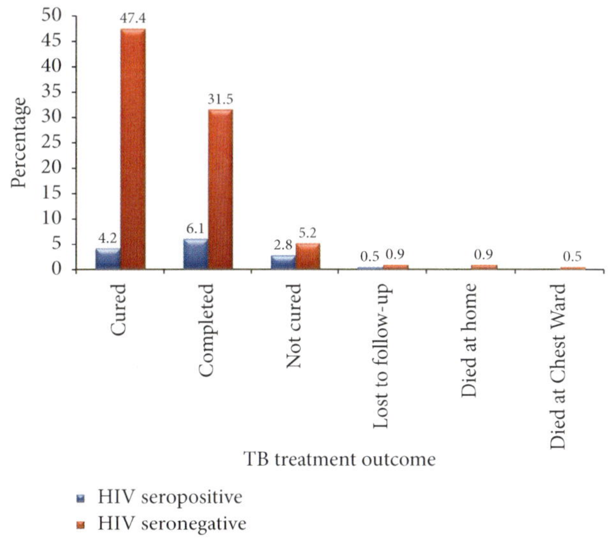

FIGURE 2: *Treatment outcomes for TB/HIV coinfected clients.*

2015 = 44; 2016 = 22) were included in the analysis. These consisted of 54 females and 159 males (χ^2 = 16.9, p = 0.013), aged between 4 and 79 years (mean age = 42.37 ± 15.33) (Table 2). Of the total, 38.0% were from Cape Coast, while 62.0% were from adjoining rural communities.

3.2. Pretreatment Sputum Smear Grade and Treatment Outcome among Clients. Of the total number of clients on DOTS, 40.8% (87/213) were sputum smear-negative (SSN), while the remaining 59.2% (126/213) were sputum smear-positive (SSP) (Table 3). In all, 173 were placed in category I, 38 in category II, and 2 in category III (table not shown). Percentage distribution of the pretreatment sputum smear grade (PSSG) among clients is as indicated in Table 4. Out of the total SSP clients, 77.0% (97/126) were males and 23% (29/126) were females. The overall cure rate, 90.2%, was determined by adding the percentage cured to the percentage that completed the treatment.

3.3. Death Rate for TB Clients from 2012 to 2016. According to the records, two clients were lost to follow-up (Table 3). Of these, one was SSN, while the other was SSP. In total, 8.5% (18/213) of clients on DOTS died (17 at home and 1 at the Chest Ward) during the period under review. The annual death distribution over the entire period is as follows: 2012, 0.5% (1/213); 2013, 1.9% (4/213); 2014, 2.8% (6/213); 2015, 2.4% (5/213); and 2016, 0.9% (2/213). Among the sexes, six females (2.8%) died compared to 12 males (5.7%) (χ^2 = 2.891, p = 0.699; likelihood ratio = 3.004, p = 0.699). With regard to the age groups, no death was recorded among clients ≤ 19 years; in the age group of 20–29 years, one death was recorded; in the age group of 30–39 years, three deaths were recorded; in the age group of 40–49 years, six deaths were recorded; in the age group of 50–59 years, six deaths were recorded; and in the age group of ≥60 years, one death was recorded (χ^2 = 40.319, p = 0.099; likelihood ratio = 41.244, p = 0.083).

3.4. HIV-Infected TB Clients on DOTS from 2012 to 2016. In total, 13.6% (29/213) who were HIV seropositive were placed on DOTS (Table 4). This was based on either a positive PSSG or a TB-suggestive sign/symptom, coupled with an X-ray image. Although more males were placed on DOTS as seen in the entire evaluation, an approximately equal number of males (7.0%, 15/213) and females (6.6%, 14/213) were found to be infected with HIV. Among the age groups, the age group of 40–49 years had the highest number (6.1%, 13/213) of HIV infections; however, the distribution among the remaining age groups was statistically insignificant (χ^2 = 9.621, p = 0.142, likelihood ratio = 9.584, p = 0.143). The annual trend of HIV infection among clients on DOTS for the period is as indicated in Table 4 (χ^2 = 2.742, p = 0.602, likelihood ratio = 2.995, p = 0.559).

3.5. Treatment Outcome of TB/HIV Coinfected Clients. Pretreatment sputum smear grading among these HIV-infected clients showed that 14 out of the 29 (48.3%) infected had no AFB. The remaining 15 were coinfected with TB. Of the 29 clients with TB and HIV coinfection, nine were cured, 13 completed the treatment, and 6 were not cured, while 1 was lost to follow-up (Figure 2). The fate of the one who was lost to follow-up could not be traced in the TB register. None of the clients with the HIV infection died during the period under review.

3.6. Analysis on TB/HIV Coinfection. Out of the 126 clients whose PSSG was positive (sc, 1+, 2+, or 3+), 15 were coinfected with HIV. This number represents 7.0% (15/213) of the total number of clients evaluated. The distribution of TB/HIV coinfection with regard to PSSG is as shown in Figure 3. With regard to their treatment outcome, 9 got cured and 5 died at home, while 1 had treatment failure (not cured). There was no default among the TB/HIV coinfected clients.

4. Discussion

A comprehensive evaluation of treatment outcomes is of supreme importance to the National TB Control Programme. Significant among strategic schemes to reduce the prevalence of TB infection worldwide is the annual evaluation

TABLE 3: Pretreatment sputum smear grade and treatment outcome among clients.

	Pretreatment sputum smear grade (%)					Total
	Negative	Scanty (sc)	(1+)	(2+)	(3+)	
Age range (years)						
<10	2 (0.9)	—	—	—	—	2
10–19	4 (1.9)	1 (0.5)	2 (0.9)	1 (0.5)	3 (1.4)	11
20–29	9 (4.2)	2 (0.9)	4 (1.9)	8 (3.8)	12 (5.6)	35
30–39	17 (8.0)	4 (1.9)	3 (1.4)	10 (4.7)	10 (4.7)	44
40–49	16 (7.5)	4 (1.9)	13 (6.1)	4 (1.9)	14 (6.6)	51
50–59	17 (8.0)	5 (2.3)	6 (2.8)	4 (1.9)	8 (3.8)	40
≥60	22 (10.3)	—	—	2 (0.9)	6 (2.8)	30
Total	*87 (40.8)*	*16 (7.5)*	*28 (13.1)*	*29 (13.6)*	*53 (24.9)*	*213*
Sex						
Female	25 (11.7)	6 (2.8)	4 (1.9)	7 (3.3)	12 (5.6)	54
Male	62 (29.1)	10 (4.7)	24 (11.3)	22 (10.3)	41 (19.2)	159
Total	*87 (40.8)*	*16 (7.5)*	*28 (13.1)*	*29 (13.6)*	*53 (24.9)*	*213*
Treatment outcome						
Cured	—	13 (6.1)	25 (11.7)	27 (12.7)	45 (21.1)	110 (51.6)
Completed	80 (37.6)	—	—	—	—	80 (37.6)
Treatment failure	—	1 (0.5)	2 (0.9)	—	—	3 (1.4)
Lost to follow-up	1 (0.5)	—	—	1 (0.5)	—	2 (0.9)
Died at home	6 (2.8)	2 (0.9)	1 (0.5)	1 (0.5)	7 (3.3)	17 (8.0)
Died at Chest Ward	—	—	—	—	1 (0.5)	1 (0.5)
Total	*87 (40.8)*	*16 (7.5)*	*28 (13.1)*	*29 (13.6)*	*53 (24.9)*	*213*

Negative: *no Acid-Fast Bacilli (AFB) seen in at least 100 fields*; scanty (sc): *1–9 AFB found in 100 fields*; (1+): *10–99 AFB found in 100 fields*; (2+): *1–10 AFB found per field in at least 50 fields*; (3+): *more than 10 AFB per field in at least 20 fields.*

TABLE 4: HIV infection status among TB clients.

	HIV infection		Total
	Positive (%)	Negative	
Sex			
Male	15 (7.0)	144	159
Female	14 (6.6)	40	54
Age			
<10	—	2	2
10–19	1 (0.5)	10	11
20–29	4 (1.9)	31	35
30–39	6 (2.8)	38	44
40–49	13 (6.1)	38	51
50–59	2 (0.9)	38	40
≥60	3 (1.4)	27	30
Year			
2012	3 (1.4)	41	44
2013	10 (4.7)	45	55
2014	7 (3.3)	41	48
2015	6 (2.8)	38	44
2016	3 (1.4)	19	22

of treatment outcomes in sputum smear-positive TB cases and among individuals with TB/HIV coinfection. This study sought to do that evaluation.

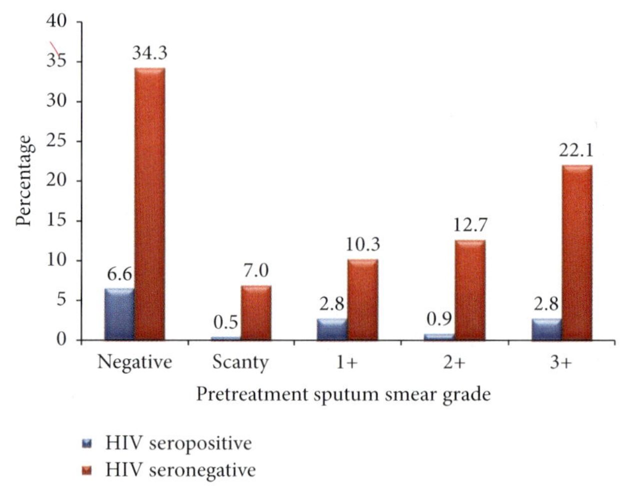

FIGURE 3: *TB/HIV coinfection.* Negative: *no Acid-Fast Bacilli (AFB) seen in at least 100 fields*; scanty (sc): *1–9 AFB found in 100 fields*; (1+): *10–99 AFB found in 100 fields*; (2+): *1–10 AFB found per field in at least 50 fields*; (3+): *more than 10 AFB per field in at least 20 fields.*

Out of the total, 51.6% clients were "cured," while 37.6% completed their medication. In total, 90.2%, which equals the WHO 2011–2015 updated cure rate target of 87.0%, was achieved from 2012 to 2016 at the treatment site of the Metropolitan Hospital. This study's results suggest an improvement in treatment outcome. However, further studies are required to explain the factors associated with unfavourable outcomes, such as death and treatment failures at this TB treatment site as these could threaten the success of the National TB Control Programme in future.

Default rate throughout the entire period was 0.9% compared to the WHO interventional target of 5.0%. This has been achieved through establishment of zonal treatment sites to maximize reach and supervision of adherence to medication. For example, all TB clients who accessed diagnostic services at our treatment site were referred back to treatment sites within their respective locations. Only clients within the Cape Coast Metropolitan Assembly were offered treatment, and this could have led to such an outcome. In addition, the treatment site adopts a facility based DOTS backed by a community strategy involving intensive defaulter tracing through house address and telephone number calling. These could have contributed to the increased adherence. The study, however, documented an 8.5% death rate in total. Death rate ranges from 7% to 35% worldwide [15–17]. Our results and interactions with nursing staff suggest that clients could have died at home due to lack of proper care and poor adherence to treatment regimen. Counselling, sustained supervision, home visits, and health education have been used successfully as interventions to reduce defaulter rate/loss to follow-up of TB patients [18].

This study showed that sex was not significantly associated with treatment outcome but two times more of the males died compared to females. Males are known to have poor health seeking behavior than females and usually seek medical attention late at advanced stages of the disease. Males are known to have poor adherence to treatment and often default treatment compared to females [19, 20].

Sputum smear-positive clients are infectious to close contacts and the general population throughout the treatment period. Following commencement of treatment, patients have a reduction in AFB load; however, they continue to expel viable bacilli for a variable period of time. In the present study, 8.4% [(sc: 9, 1+: 6, 2+: 1, and 3+: 2)/213] still had AFB after 2-3 months of treatment. At the end of the 5th month up till the 8th month, 1.9% [(sc: 1, 1+: 2, and 3+: 1)/213] remained not cured and would continue to expel viable bacilli. Treatment failure was seen in the age groups of 20–29 (0.9%, 2/213) and 50–59 (0.5%, 1/213) years. Two clients were lost to follow-up, one each in the age groups of 20–29 and $\geq$ 60 years, respectively. Our findings are contrary to a study in Thailand, which showed that an age $\geq$ 60 years significantly correlated with treatment interruption and/or treatment failure [21]. Furthermore, the assertion in other studies [21–23] that an older age is a risk factor for death in pulmonary TB is incongruent with findings of this study. Out of 30 who died at home in this study, only one person was $\geq$60 years old. Further studies are required in TB clients on DOTS to bring finality to inconsequential outcomes.

This study found 13.6% of clients on DOTS strategy within the period to be infected with HIV. Out of this, 6.1% was among the age group of 40–49 years. Although males constituted the majority on DOTS, HIV prevalence of females, 6.6%, almost equaled that of males, 7.0%.

It is known that increased risk, as well as multidrug-resistant (MDR) tuberculosis, is mostly found in clients who are HIV positive. In this study, two MDRs were identified: one was HIV positive, while the other was HIV negative. Although studies in Ethiopia have shown high default likelihood among TB/HIV coinfected clients [19, 20], our study did not show any default among this category. In total, the number of clients with TB/HIV coinfection was 15 (7.0%). TB/HIV coinfection was highest (7/15) among the age group of 40–49 years. The potential of this age group being economically and sexually active cannot be substantiated without further studies. Since the overall number of HIV positive patients in the study is small, we could not establish the impact of HIV on sputum smear conversion. Literature search is yet to establish any effect in clients with TB/HIV coinfection [9, 24, 25]. Overall, the DOTS strategy has performed well, requiring continuous modifications and reviews to enhance its outcome.

5. Conclusion

We found a high treatment success rate among clients treated at our site. The relevant strategies to ensure early detection and treatment are under implementation. As expected, administration of medication on the wards is supervised by trained staff. Provision has also been made for trained staff to administer the DOTS and SLDs in communities where clients live. The information currently lacking is the potential negative sociodemographic/economic factors that result in unfavourable outcomes not controlled by the DOTS strategy.

Authors' Contributions

Ato Kwamena Tetteh and Edward Agyarko conceived and designed the study. They both participated in data analysis and the drafting of the manuscript. Irene Ayi, Langbong Bimi, and Joseph Otchere provided technical advice and contributed immensely to the writing of the manuscript.

Acknowledgments

The authors would like to thank the Officer in Charge of the Chest Centre and supporting Staff Nurses for cooperating with them during data collation and entry. They acknowledge their unrelenting patience in explaining all technical definitions regarding tuberculosis management at the facility. The authors' profound gratitude also goes to Dr. Charles Gyamfi, Department of Civil Engineering, Tshwane University of Technology, Pretoria, South Africa, for providing them with the map of Cape Coast Metropolitan Area.

References

[1] W. Wobeser, L. Yuan, and M. Naus, "The Tuberculosis Treatment Completion Study Group. Outcome of pulmonary tuberculosis treatment in the tertiary care setting-Toronto 1992/93,"

Canadian Medical Association Journal, vol. 160, pp. 789–794, 1999.

[2] *Global tuberculosis Control, Surveillance, Planning, Financing-WHO Report 2005: WHO/HTM/TB/2005*, vol. 49, WHO, Geneva, Switzerland, 2005.

[3] E. Owusu-Dabo, O. Adjei, C. G. Meyer et al., "Mycobacterium tuberculosis Drug Resistance, Ghana. Letter to the Editor," *Emerging Infectious Diseases*, vol. 12, no. 7, pp. 1170–1172, 2006.

[4] A. Trebueq and H. L. Reider, "Two excellent management tools for national tuberculosis programmes; history of prior treatment and sputum status at two months," *International Journal of Tuberculosis and Lung Disease*, vol. 2, pp. 184–186, 1998.

[5] F. Torman, Ed., *Tomans tuberculosis case detection, treatment, and monitoring—questions and answers*, World Health Organisation, Geneva, Switzerland, 2nd edition, 2004.

[6] TB. Global Report, 2011.

[7] S. P. Agarwal and L. S. Chauhan, "Tuberculosis control in India," in *Directorate general of Health services , Ministry of Health and Family Welfare, government of India*, New Delhi, India, 2005.

[8] R. Long, K. Bochar, S. Chomyc et al., "Relative Versus Absolute Noncontagiousness of Respiratory Tuberculosis on Treatment," *Infection Control and Hospital Epidemiology*, vol. 24, no. 11, pp. 831–838, 2003.

[9] E. E. Telzak, B. A. Fazal, C. L. Pollard, G. S. Turett, J. E. Justman, and S. Blum, "Factors influencing time to sputum conversion among patients with smear- positive pulmonary tuberculosis," *Clinical Infectious Diseases*, vol. 25, no. 3, pp. 666–672, 1997.

[10] M. S. Al-Moamary, W. Black, E. Bessuille, R. K. Elwood, and S. Vedal, "The significance of the persistent presence of acid-fast bacilli in sputum smears in pulmonary tuberculosis," *CHEST*, vol. 116, no. 3, pp. 726–731, 1999.

[11] P. G. Gopi, V. Chandrasekaran, R. Subramani et al., "Association of conversion & cure with initial smear grading among new smear positive pulmonary tuberculosis patients treated with Category I regimen," *Indian Journal of Medical Research*, vol. 123, no. 6, pp. 807–814, 2006.

[12] R. Singla, M. M. Osman, N. Khan, N. Al-Sharif, M. O. Al-Sayegh, and M. A. Shaikh, "Factors predicting persistent sputum smear positivity among pulmonary tuberculosis patients 2 months after treatment," *International Journal of Tuberculosis and Lung Disease*, vol. 7, pp. 58–64, 2003.

[13] J.-Y. Wang, L.-N. Lee, C.-J. Yu, Y.-J. Chien, and P.-C. Yang, "Factors influencing time to smear conversion in patients with smear-positive pulmonary tuberculosis," *Respirology*, vol. 14, no. 7, pp. 1012–1019, 2009.

[14] T. H. Holtz, M. Sternberg, S. Kammerer et al., "Time to sputum culture conversion in multidrug-resistant tuberculosis: Predictors and relationship to treatment outcome," *Annals of Internal Medicine*, vol. 144, no. 9, pp. 650–659, 2006.

[15] C. Dye, S. Scheele, P. Dolin, V. Pathania, and M. C. Raviglione, "Global burden of tuberculosis: estimated incidence, prevalence, and mortality by country. WHO Global Surveillance and Monitoring Project," *Journal of the American Medical Association*, vol. 282, no. 7, pp. 677–686, 1999.

[16] P. J. Dolin, M. C. Ranglione, and A. Kochi, "Global tuberculosis incidence and mortality during," *Bulletin of the World Health Organization*, vol. 72, Article ID 19902000, pp. 213-20, 1994.

[17] M. C. Ranglione, D. E. Snider Jr., and A. Kochi, "Global epidemiology of tuberculosis: morbidity and mortality of a worldwide epidemic," *Journal of the American Medical Association*, vol. 273, no. 3, pp. 220–226, 1995.

[18] G. Berhe, F. Enquselassie, and A. Aseffa, "Treatment outcome of smear-positive pulmonary tuberculosis patients in Tigray Region, Northern Ethiopia," *BMC Public Health*, vol. 12, no. 1, article 537, 2012.

[19] G. Mitike, D. Kebede, and H. Yeneneh, "HIV infection and antituberculosis drug resistance among pulmonary tuberculosis patients in Harar tuberculosis centre, Ethiopia," *East African Medical Journal*, vol. 74, no. 3, pp. 154–157, 1997.

[20] S. Vijay, P. Kumar, L. S. Chauhan, S. V. Rao, and P. Vaidyanathan, "Treatment outcome and mortality at one and half year follow-up of HIV infected TB patients under TB control programme in a district of South India," *PLoS ONE*, vol. 6, no. 7, Article ID e21008, 2011.

[21] S. Anunnatsiri, P. Chetchotisakd, and C. Wanke, "Factors associated with treatment outcomes in pulmonary tuberculosis in northeastern Thailand," *Southeast Asian Journal of Tropical Medicine and Public Health*, vol. 36, no. 2, pp. 324–330, 2005.

[22] K. C. Takarinda, A. D. Harries, S. Srinath, T. Mutasa-Apollo, C. Sandy, and O. Mugurungi, "Treatment outcomes of adult patients with recurrent tuberculosis in relation to HIV status in Zimbabwe: A retrospective record review," *BMC Public Health*, vol. 12, no. 1, article no. 124, 2012.

[23] M. A. Yassin, L. Takele, S. Gebresenbet et al., "HIV and tuberculosis coinfection in the southern region of Ethiopia: a prospective epidemiological study," *Infectious Diseases*, vol. 36, no. 9, pp. 670–673, 2004.

[24] A. Dominguez-Castellano, M. A. Muniain, J. Rodriguez-Bano et al., "Factors associated with time to sputum smear conversion in active pulmonary tuberculosis," *Int J Tuberc Lung Dis*, vol. vol 7, pp. 432–438, 2003.

[25] R. Bwire, M. W. Borgdorff, V. Sticht-Groh et al., "Tuberculosis chemotherapy and sputum conversion among HIV sero-positive and HIV sero-negative patients in south-earthern uganda," *East African Medical Journal*, vol. 76, pp. 307–313, 1999.

19

Histopathological Findings in Immunohistological Staining of the Granulomatous Tissue Reaction Associated with Tuberculosis

Shirin Karimi,[1] Masoud Shamaei,[2] Mihan Pourabdollah,[3] Makan Sadr,[4] Mehrdad Karbasi,[3] Arda Kiani,[4] and Moslem Bahadori[5]

[1] *Mycobacteriology Research Center, National Research Institute of Tuberculosis and Lung Diseases (NRITLD), Shahid Beheshti University of Medical Sciences, Tehran, Iran*
[2] *Clinical Tuberculosis and Epidemiology Research Center, NRITLD, Shahid Beheshti University of Medical Sciences, Tehran, Iran*
[3] *Pediatric Respiratory Diseases Research Center, National Research Institute of Tuberculosis and Lung Diseases (NRITLD), Shahid Beheshti University of Medical Sciences, Tehran, Iran*
[4] *Tracheal Diseases Research Center, National Research Institute of Tuberculosis and Lung Diseases (NRITLD), Shahid Beheshti University of Medical Sciences, Tehran, Iran*
[5] *Chronic Respiratory Diseases Research Center, National Research Institute of Tuberculosis and Lung Diseases (NRITLD), Shahid Beheshti University of Medical Sciences, Tehran, Iran*

Correspondence should be addressed to Mihan Pourabdollah; mihan_p@yahoo.com

Academic Editor: Juraj Ivanyi

Purpose. The histological diagnosis of Mycobacterium tuberculosis (MTB) remains a diagnostic challenge despite different methods. Immunohistochemistry (IHC) not only could confirm granulomatous tissue involvement but also can demonstrate MTB antigen immunolocalization. This study tries to clarify the details of immunohistochemical staining for MTB with pAbBCG. *Materials/Methods.* Twenty-three confirmed TB granulomatous tissue samples were studied by Ziehl-Neelsen and immunohistochemistry (IHC) staining with pAbBCG. Samples were selected from the archive of the Department of Pathology, National Research Institute of Tuberculosis and Lung Disease, Tehran, Iran. *Results.* IHC staining was positive in all samples, whereas Ziehl-Neelsen was positive in 9 cases out of 23 (39.1%). Tissue types used were pleural tissue, lymph nodes, and lung tissue. IHC showed positive coarse granular cytoplasmic and round, fragmented bacillary staining. In this study, epithelioid cells clearly showed more positive staining at the periphery of the granuloma rather than the center of granuloma. There is also positive staining in endothelial cells, fibroblasts, plasma cells, lymphocytes, and macrophages outside the granuloma. *Conclusion.* Considering the criteria of positive immunohistochemical staining of TB granulomatous reactions, this stain not only highlights the presence of mycobacterial antigens for tissue diagnosis, but also could morphologically localize its distribution in different cells.

1. Introduction

Histological diagnosis of tuberculosis (TB) has long been an important issue in anatomical pathology. On the other hand, extrapulmonary TB comprises 10–15% of infections with Mtb. Following HIV prevalence increase, extrapulmonary TB is rising as well [1, 2].

Considering the limitations in sensitivity and specificity of Ziehl-Neelsen staining [3], mycobacterial evaluation, mycobacterial culture, and molecular and serological techniques [4–6], histomorphological analysis appears to be the only feasible technique for field diagnosis of TB in some patients [7, 8].

Granulomatous reactions, and in some cases, nongranulomatous reactions such as the presence of foamy macrophages [9] or mycobacterial spindle cell pseudotumour [10] in some types of mycobacterial infections are indicative of TB only if the presence of TB bacilli has been confirmed in the tissue. Recently, it has been stated that PCR results are acceptable only if the presence of TB bacilli can be confirmed in the tissue [11].

Detection of beaded bacilli (which are more commonly observed in the necrotic zone) by Ziehl-Neelsen staining of tissue specimens [12] indicates the association of tissue reaction with mycobacterial infection. However, Ziehl-Neelsen stain has a relatively low sensitivity for detecting Mtb with sensitivity range of zero to 44% for this infection [13]. Furthermore, presence of a minimum of 10^4 bacilli per each slide is required to reach diagnosis.

Considering the mechanism of Ziehl-Neelsen staining and its relatively low sensitivity and specificity, this staining technique has limited diagnostic value and inadequate ability for pathophysiological assessment of Mtb antigens in the tissue. Searching for mycobacterial antigens using IHC is a well-recognized technique with special application in research projects. This technique is based on the production of a variety of polyclonal and monoclonal antibodies in tissue reactions. Several studies have reported the sensitivity of this technique can be 64 to 100% for the detection of mycobacterial antigen. Limited numbers of studies have discussed in depth positive tissue staining method for Mtb [14]. However, these techniques have only been briefly mentioned in the pathology reference books and textbooks do not provide a standard for morphological assessment with regard to IHC staining of granulomatous reactions.

Recent studies on the variable morphology of TB bacilli emphasize the importance of IHC in searching for different morphological variations of TB antigens in the tissue.

The present study compares the sensitivity and specificity of the two techniques of Ziehl-Neelsen and IHC staining for field diagnosis of TB. It also evaluates the value of accurate description of IHC staining with pAbBCG in tissues with granulomatous reaction due to TB with regard to diagnosis, immunolocalization, and morphology of TB bacilli in this technique.

2. Materials and Methods

A total of 50 patients undergoing simultaneous biopsy and tissue culture with positive tissue culture for Mtb during 2005–2009 were selected from the MRC Department Masih Daneshvari Hospital. Using the archives of the Pathology Department of this hospital, which is a referral center for pathological lung lesions, H&E slides of the selected patients were evaluated. Cases with small number of granulomatous lesions or tissue volume were excluded from the study. Eventually, 23 tissue samples of 23 TB patients with adequate tissue and number of granuloma were chosen for different staining techniques. Characteristics and type of samples were retrieved from the pathology reports. Paraffin-embedded blocks were stained using Ziehl-Neelsen and IHC staining. Seven control tissue specimens were also selected from the archives of the Pathology Department. These specimens had granulomatous reactions due to foreign body, fungi, or hydatid cyst. These specimens were also stained similar to the abovementioned samples. Mycobacteriology Research Center of Masih Daneshvari Hospital is the national reference center and educational collaborating center of the WHO office in Eastern Mediterranean Region. The study conducted after Masih Daneshvari Hospital ethic committee.

For immunohistochemical staining, 3-4 micron sections were cut from the tissue block and incubated overnight at room temperature. After deparaffinization and fixation with 99–70% alcohol, specimens were rinsed with distilled water and PBS. In order to remove endogenous peroxidase, methanol and 3% H_2O_2 were used for 10 minutes.

After retrieval and cooling down the tissues, they were rinsed with distilled water and PBS and specimens were blocked with antiserum. Antibody was prepared with Tween 20 + Tris (Merck 1.088387) at a 1 : 1000 dilution. In the first phase, primary antibody (DAKO, code no. B 0124) (pAbBCG) was reacted in a wet environment at room temperature for 30 min and after rinsing the specimens with PBS, and secondary antibody (Envision K5007) was added. After staining with chromogen, hematoxylin was used as the contrast dye. For each staining, one negative and one positive control were also considered. Staining was done as fine granular cytoplasmic, coarse granular cytoplasmic and bacillus staining. Different areas and cells in tissue specimens were evaluated; type of granuloma (with or without necrosis), and presence of multi-nuclear giant cells, epithelioid cells, necrotic zones, lymphocytes, plasma cells, peri-granuloma macrophages and fibroblasts and perigranuloma endothelial cells were assessed by a junior and a senior pathologist. Positive staining was defined as staining of 10% of epithelioid cells in the granuloma. For other types of cells, any form of staining was considered as positive.

Ziehl-Neelsen staining was performed according to the standard protocol. In summary, tissue specimens were deparaffinized and rinsed with consecutive dilutions of alcohol (96% to 70% ethanol). After heat fixation, specimens were washed with carbol fuchsin for 4 minutes and incubated with HCL. Counterstaining was done using Brilliant Green for 20 s. After rinsing, samples were allowed to dry at room temperature.

3. Results

A total of 23 cases were evaluated, out of which 17 (73.9%) were males. Type of tissue in understudy cases was pleura (9 cases, 39.1%), lymph node (cervical, axillary, and thoracic) (9 cases, 39.1%), and lung tissue (5 cases, 21.7%). Granuloma, in the form of necrotizing poorly organized granuloma, was 9 cases (39.1%), necrotizing well-organized granuloma in 5 cases (21.7%), necrotizing nonpoorly organized granuloma in 4 cases (17.3%), and non-necrotizing well-organized granuloma observed in 3 cases (13%). In all biopsy samples, IHC staining yielded positive results for both fine and coarse granular cytoplasmic and round bacillary staining in epithelioid cells (Figures 1 and 2). Staining of other cells was also positive in varying percentages. These shapes were variable from fragmented bacilli to antigen dust. Ovoid and circular shapes were also observed. In granulomatous reactions in the control group (which were all non-TB), IHC staining was only in the form of fine granular cytoplasmic staining in epithelioid cells and focal staining was also seen in some other cells

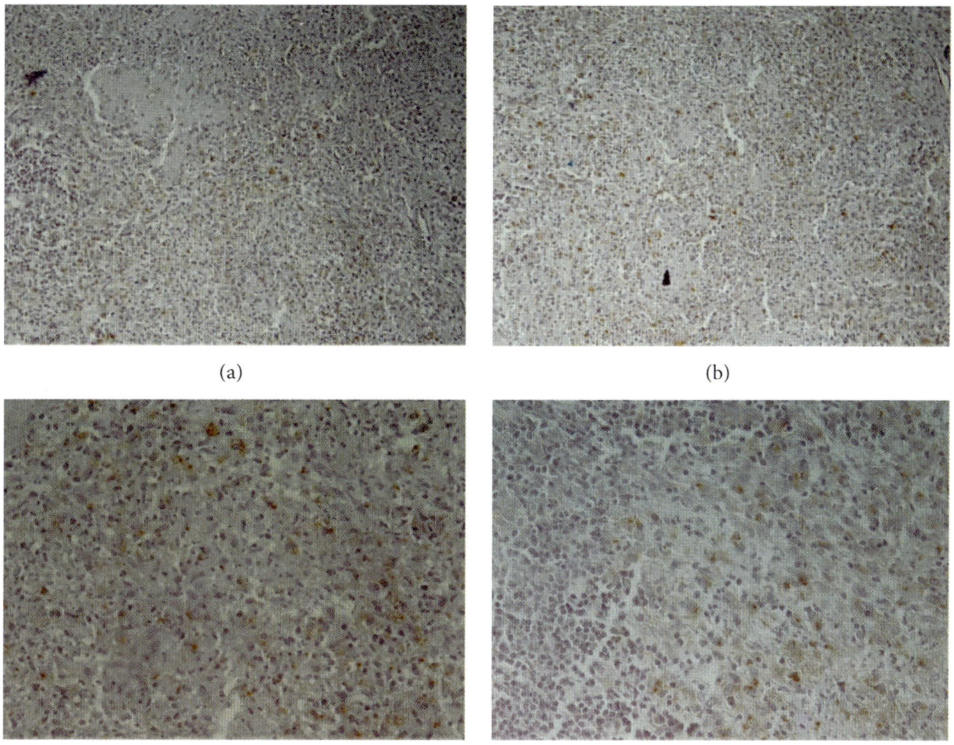

(a) (b) (c) (d)

FIGURE 1: Necrotizing granulomatous reaction with course granular cytoplasmic positioning in epithelioid histiocyte ((a) and (b) ×10, (c) ×20, and (d) ×40).

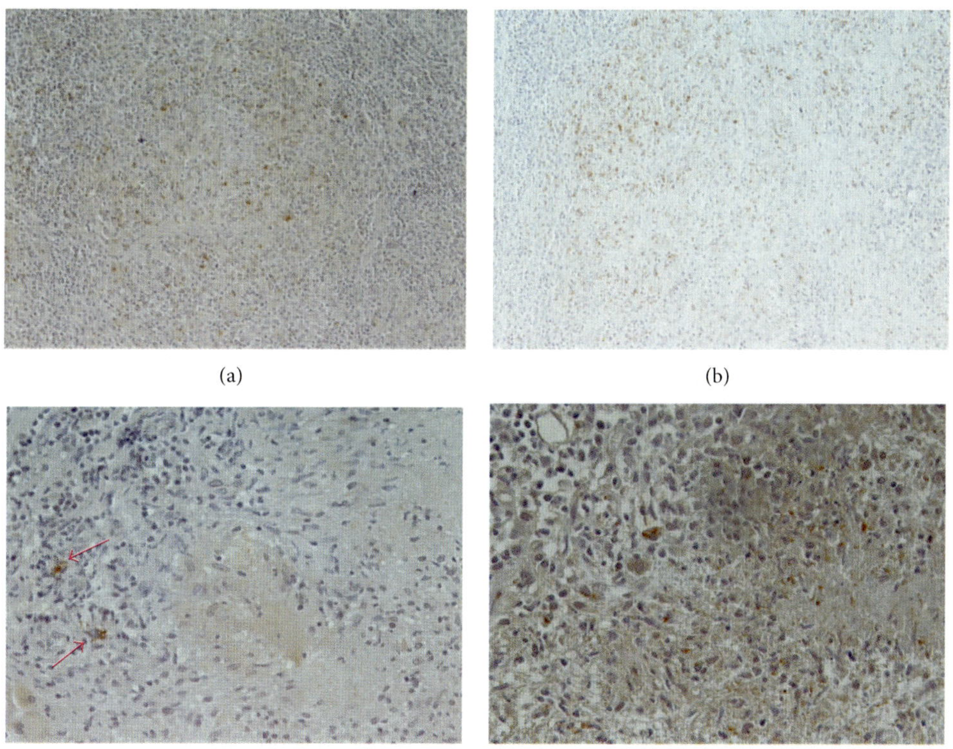

(a) (b) (c) (d)

FIGURE 2: IHC for pAbBCG (×20): course cytoplasmic positivity of epithelioid macrophage without background in epithelioid histiocyte in nongranulomatous reaction in lymph node ((a) and (b)). Course granular cytoplasmic positivity of macrophage outside the granulomatous process ((c) and (d)).

Table 1: Comparison of the sensitivity and specificity of pAbBCG and Ziel-Neelsen.

Variable	No. (%)	Positive finding	Culture positive	Sensitivity (%)	Specificity (%)	Positive predictive value (%)	Negative predictive value (%)
pAbBCG							
Case	23	23	23	100	100	100	33/3
Control	7	0	0				
Ziel-Neelsen							
Case	23	9	9	39/1	100	100	33/3
Control	7	0	0				

outside the granuloma. Coarse granular cytoplasmic staining, fragmented or round bacillary staining, was not observed in any of the cases. Ziehl-Neelsen staining of all control cases was negative. In test patients, 9 out of 23 (39.1%) had positive Ziehl-Neelsen staining. Table 1 shows the positive results and comparison of the sensitivity and specificity of pAbBCG and Ziehl-Neelsen.

In all 23 cases, coarse granular cytoplasmic staining and stained intact bacilli along with lower degrees of fine granular cytoplasmic staining were observed in epithelioid cells. According to cell types, positive IHC staining was observed in endothelial cells, epithelioid cells, fibroblasts, giant cells, lymphocytes, macrophages, and plasma cells, 2 (8.7%), 19 (82.6%), 3 (13%), 5 (21.7%), 1 (4.3%), 8 (34.8%), and 1 (4.3%), respectively, (Figure 3). Necrotic zone was also positive in IHC staining in 5 cases (21.7%). In this study, epithelioid cells at the periphery of the granuloma were more positively stained than the epithelioid cells at the center or adjacent to the necrotic zone.

4. Discussion

Ziehl-Neelsen stain method for the diagnosis of TB is positive in one-third of cases with confirmed TB infection. Detection of tuberculosis in tissue slides is still based on the histological pattern of the granuloma that has several differential diagnoses with different treatments [13].

Presence of mycobacterial antigens and tissue morphology can be evaluated with IHC technique. Eliminating background with proper technique could provide 100% specificity if coarse granular cytoplasmic and bacillus staining are considered. These obtained results are comparable with the findings of a study by Goel and Budhwar, reporting 64–100% sensitivity for IHC and zero to 44% sensitivity for Ziehl-Neelsen staining [14].

Moreover, the results of monoclonal antibody testing [15] also show 100% sensitivity, which is in accordance with our obtained results. This agreement seems to be due to the appropriate staining and accurate consideration of positive staining results.

In order to achieve appropriate staining by this technique, great attention must be paid to dilution and technique of IHC with polyclonal antibodies. If adequate attention is not paid, fine granular staining in the background can cause false positive reactions provided that the pathologist is not familiar with this technique. This is among the main limitations of working with this type of antibody. However, in case of positivity of this staining as coarse granular cytoplasmic staining, stained fragmented bacillia or stained bacilli form, percentage of specificity for this staining technique is highly increased. It should be emphasized that coarse granular cytoplasmic staining or positively stained fragmented bacilli of any degree were not observed in control samples. These findings are in accordance with those of Madhu Goel and Budhwar, describing small bacillary fragments and antigenic dusts [14].

On the other hand, new findings have demonstrated that morphological modifications of tubercle bacilli in circular or intermediate shapes even in the tissue can be live TB bacilli. This issue has been well described by Velayati et al. [16]. In the present study, stained fragments and other shapes indicate morphological alterations of TB bacilli in the tissue.

Another finding is the presence of fragments of TB bacilli in macrophages, fibroblasts, plasma cells, lymphocytes and even endothelial cells outside the granuloma indicating that the mentioned cells play an active role in histopathogenesis of TB.

A similar study [15] mentioned the presence of mycobacterium and intracellular mycobacterium material outside the granuloma and in macrophages and even lymphocytic fragments around the granuloma. Recent studies are also indicative of the active role of endothelial cells in immunologic tissue reactions [17]. Furthermore, the role of plasma cells [18] and fibroblasts [19] alongside the main cells in cell-mediated immune response to TB is a matter of discussion.

Thus, aside from the positivity of lymphocytes for the presence of TB bacilli antigens in IHC staining with pAbBCG, our study is uniquely important in revealing the presence of these antigens in plasma cells, endothelial cells, and fibroblasts. This issue needs to be further investigated in terms of TB pathogenesis.

Ziehl-Neelsen staining has low sensitivity and requires the presence of intact bacilli. Logani et al. [10] demonstrated that IHC staining with pAbBCG yields positive results even in tissues with 10 bacilli per slide. Thus, this technique can be applied even in cases with small number of bacilli for any reason (such as in paucibacillary extrapulmonary TB). This technique can be used in primary stages of TB infection and HIV as a routine pathology test.

Our study showed that the IHC technique has high sensitivity and specificity. It also indicates localization of cells infected with mycobacterium or cells containing TB bacilli

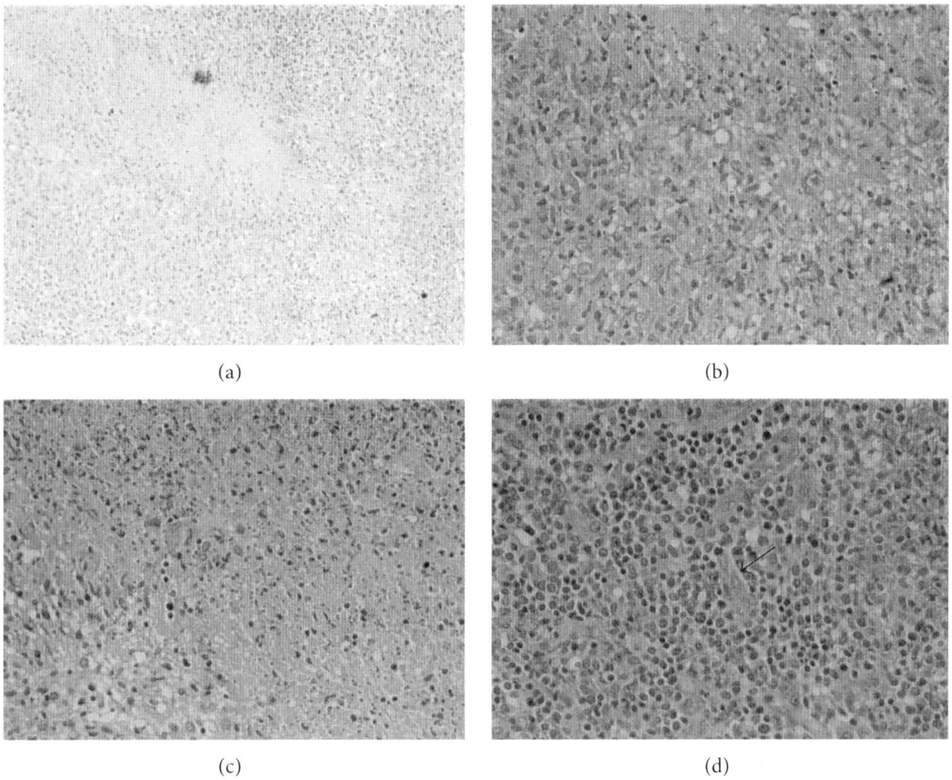

FIGURE 3: Fine antigen dust cytoplasmic positivity in plasma cell and lymphocyte, area of necrosis in the top without prominent positivity in contrast of coarse granular positivity of histiocyte. ((a) ×10, (b) and (c) ×20). Coarse granular and fine antigen dust in endothelial cells ((d) ×20).

antigens. It somehow reveals the dissemination of TB bacilli and its antigens in tissues as well. In this study, epithelioid cells in the periphery of granuloma were stained more positively than the epithelioid cells at the center of granuloma or adjacent to the necrotic zone. Using anti-MPT64 in tissues affected with TB granuloma, Purohit et al. [15] found that epithelioid cells outside the necrotic zone showed greater positivity than cells within the necrotic area. This finding is in contrast to Ziehl-Neelsen staining that mostly reveals intact bacilli at the center of necrotic zone.

There are some limitations to this study. First, we have selected 23 cases from 50 specimens that were culture positive for MTB; thus, the study has bias to show sensitivity and specificity exactly. Secondly, pAbBCG is polyclonal antibody for Mtb complex. Although we have compared the sensitivity and specificity of this method with Ziehl-Neelsen staining, the aim of study is illustration of immunolocalization of Mtb Ag for use in diagnostic or research field, not comparing sensitivity with specificity. Further studies should be carried out on suspected tissues involvement with Mtb bacilli through IHC and use of monoclonal antibodies.

Furthermore, pathologists must be acquainted with adequate staining pattern, elimination of background staining, and type of selected antibody. This method is especially important for use in countries with high prevalence of TB as a technique with early diagnostic value in tissue specimen. In early diagnosis, this technique can reduce related morbidity and mortality and decrease the rate of complications due to misdiagnosis and mistreatment of TB.

Conflict of Interests

There is no conflict of interests in this study.

References

[1] G. T. Programme, *Global Tuberculosis Control: WHO Report: Global Tuberculosis Programme*, World Health Organization, 2010.

[2] E. L. Corbett, C. J. Watt, N. Walker et al., "The growing burden of tuberculosis: global trends and interactions with the HIV epidemic," *Archives of Internal Medicine*, vol. 163, no. 9, pp. 1009–1021, 2003.

[3] A. Trusov, R. Bumgarner, R. Valijev et al., "Comparison of LuminŮ LED fluorescent attachment, fluorescent microscopy and Ziehl-Neelsen for AFB diagnosis," *International Journal of Tuberculosis and Lung Disease*, vol. 13, no. 7, pp. 836–841, 2009.

[4] A. M. Attallah, C. A. A. Malak, H. Ismail, A. H. El-Saggan, M. M. Omran, and A. A. Tabll, "Rapid and simple detection of a Mycobacterium tuberculosis circulating antigen in serum using dot-ELISA for field diagnosis of pulmonary tuberculosis," *Journal of Immunoassay and Immunochemistry*, vol. 24, no. 1, pp. 73–87, 2003.

[5] J. M. Dora, G. Geib, R. Chakr et al., "Polymerase chain reaction as a useful and simple tool for rapid diagnosis of tuberculous meningitis in a Brazilian tertiary care hospital," *Brazilian Journal of Infectious Diseases*, vol. 12, no. 3, pp. 245–247, 2008.

[6] A. Mishra, A. Singhal, D. S. Chauhan et al., "Direct detection and identification of Mycobacterium tuberculosis and Mycobacterium bovis in bovine samples by a novel nested PCR assay: correlation with conventional techniques," *Journal of Clinical Microbiology*, vol. 43, no. 11, pp. 5670–5678, 2005.

[7] J. S. Pedersen, I. Clarke, and J. Mills, "Improved detection of mycobacteria species in formalin-fixed tissue sections," *Histopathology*, vol. 59, no. 5, pp. 993–1005, 2011.

[8] T. Mustafa, H. G. Wiker, S. G. M. Mfinanga, O. Mørkve, and L. Sviland, "Immunohistochemistry using a *Mycobacterium tuberculosis* complex specific antibody for improved diagnosis of tuberculous lymphadenitis," *Modern Pathology*, vol. 19, no. 12, pp. 1606–1614, 2006.

[9] H. D'Avila, C. M. Maya-Monteiro, and P. T. Bozza, "Lipid bodies in innate immune response to bacterial and parasite infections," *International Immunopharmacology*, vol. 8, no. 10, pp. 1308–1315, 2008.

[10] S. Logani, D. R. Lucas, J. D. Cheng, H. L. Ioachim, and N. V. Adsay, "Spindle cell tumors associated with mycobacteria in lymph nodes of HIV-positive patients: 'Kaposi sarcoma with mycobacteria' and 'mycobacterial pseudotumor'," *American Journal of Surgical Pathology*, vol. 23, no. 6, pp. 656–661, 1999.

[11] T. Ulrichs, M. Lefmann, M. Reich et al., "Modified immunohistological staining allows detection of Ziehl-Neelsen-negative Mycobacterium tuberculosis organisms and their precise localization in human tissue," *Journal of Pathology*, vol. 205, no. 5, pp. 633–640, 2005.

[12] Á. Somoskövi, J. E. Hotaling, M. Fitzgerald, D. O'Donnell, L. M. Parsons, and M. Salfinger, "Lessons from a proficiency testing event for acid-fast microscopy," *Chest*, vol. 120, no. 1, pp. 250–257, 2001.

[13] R. W. Smithwick, *Laboratory Manual For Acid-Fast Microscopy: Public Health Service, Center For Disease Control*, Bureau of Laboratories, 1976.

[14] M. M. Goel and P. Budhwar, "Immunohistochemical localization of mycobacterium tuberculosis complex antigen with antibody to 38 kDa antigen versus Ziehl Neelsen staining in tissue granulomas of extrapulmonary tuberculosis," *The Indian journal of tuberculosis*, vol. 54, no. 1, pp. 24–29, 2007.

[15] M. R. Purohit, T. Mustafa, H. G. Wiker, O. Mørkve, and L. Sviland, "Immunohistochemical diagnosis of abdominal and lymph node tuberculosis by detecting Mycobacterium tuberculosis complex specific antigen MPT64," *Diagnostic Pathology*, vol. 2, no. 1, article 36, 2007.

[16] A. A. Velayati, P. Farnia, M. R. Masjedi, and G. Konstantinovich, "Morphological modification by tubercle bacilli: no time for denial," *Journal of Infection in Developing Countries*, vol. 6, no. 1, pp. 97–99, 2012.

[17] K. M. Dobos, E. A. Spotts, F. D. Quinn, and C. H. King, "Necrosis of lung epithelial cells during infection with *Mycobacterium tuberculosis* is preceded by cell permeation," *Infection and Immunity*, vol. 68, no. 11, pp. 6300–6310, 2000.

[18] S. A. Oracki, J. A. Walker, M. L. Hibbs, L. M. Corcoran, and D. M. Tarlinton, "Plasma cell development and survival," *Immunological Reviews*, vol. 237, no. 1, pp. 140–159, 2010.

[19] G. González-Avila, C. Sandoval, M. T. Herrera et al., "Mycobacterium tuberculosis effects on fibroblast collagen metabolism," *Respiration*, vol. 77, no. 2, pp. 195–202, 2009.

20

Characteristics and Treatment Outcomes of "Transfer-Out" Pulmonary Tuberculosis Patients in Gondar, Ethiopia

Tadesse Belayneh,[1] Afework Kassu,[2] Desalgne Tigabu,[3] Gashaw Asmare,[4] Sofanit Tilaye,[4] and Eveline Klinkenberg[5,6]

[1] *Department of Medical Anesthesiology, CMHS, University of Gondar, P.O. Box 196, Gondar, Ethiopia*
[2] *Department of Microbiology Immunology and Parasitology, CMHS, University of Gondar, P.O. Box 196, Gondar, Ethiopia*
[3] *Institute of Public Health, CMHS, University of Gondar, P.O. Box 196, Gondar, Ethiopia*
[4] *University of Gondar Hospital, P.O. Box 196, Gondar, Ethiopia*
[5] *KNCV Tuberculosis Foundation, The Hague, Netherlands*
[6] *Department of Global Health, Academic Medical Center, Amsterdam Institute for Global Health and Development, University of Amsterdam, Amsterdam, Netherlands*

Correspondence should be addressed to Tadesse Belayneh; tadbel20@gmail.com

Academic Editor: David C. Perlman

Background. During tuberculosis treatment, patients may transfer to continue treatment at another health facility. To ensure adherence until treatment completion, keeping track of patients is paramount. This study aimed to investigate treatment outcomes of patients who transferred out from the University of Gondar Hospital. *Methods.* This was a retrospective cohort evaluation of patients registered from 2009 to 2013. Treatment outcomes were collected from the TB registers of receiving units using a standardized data capture format. *Results.* During the study period 3,707 patients initiated treatment and 47.5% (1,760) transferred out. The study evaluated the outcome of 26% (457/1,760) patients, of whom 403 (88%) arrived in the receiving units. Overall, 79% were successfully treated and 13.8% transferred out for a second time. For all transferred-out cases, treatment outcomes were not reported to the referring unit. *Conclusion and Recommendation.* About half of the patients were transferred out to complete treatment elsewhere. Although successful treatment outcome was obtained in 79% of patients, these results were not fed back to the referring unit. Implementing a clear mechanism to communicate the arrival of and treatment outcome for transfer-out patients and appropriate patient education on treatment unit selection before treatment and during transfer-out are recommended.

1. Introduction

In Ethiopia, tuberculosis (TB) remains a major public health problem [1]. According to the Global TB Report 2015, Ethiopia is one of the 30 high TB burden countries and one of the 14 that have a high burden of TB, TH-HIV, and MDR-TB [2]. The directly observed treatment short course (DOTS) strategy has been implemented in the country since 1994 to control the TB epidemic [3]. Despite 100% geographical and 92% health facility coverage of the DOTS programme [3], noncompliance, low case detection, a high transfer-out rate, and deficient recording and reporting systems are still a challenge [4].

Globally, all national TB control programmes experience the challenges of intracountry movement of patients from one treatment center to another [2]. A transfer-out patient is a patient who has been transferred out at any time during treatment to continue treatment at another facility [5]. The proportion of transferred-out patients varies from one country to another. Reports indicate that in Sub-Saharan Africa it can range from 1% to 26% [6, 7]. In Ethiopia figures from 31% to 66% have previously been reported [8–10].

Treatment outcome is a key indicator in TB control and serves as a proxy of quality of TB treatment in a health care system [11]. A study in the UoGH showed that between 2003 and 2008, 42% of TB patients were transferred out to continue their treatment at nearby health units [9]. The Ethiopian Clinical and Programmatic Management of TB, TB/HIV and Leprosy guidelines [2] indicate that the outcome for transferred-out patients should be reported to the national surveillance system by the transferring unit, as this unit notified and initiated treatment for this patient. Monitoring treatment outcomes is essential in order to evaluate the effectiveness of the DOTS program [12]. This would make it possible to recognize and amend system failures before the incidence and proportion of resistant isolates rise [11]. However, there are limited studies conducted to assess the treatment outcome of PTB patients who are transferred out. Moreover, in view of the large number of transferred out patients in UoGH, it is important to know what their final treatment outcomes are and whether they are available at the transferring facility for them to be captured in the TB surveillance system. Therefore, this study was conducted to assess the TB treatment outcomes of transferred-out PTB patients who were registered and started treatment at UoGH.

2. Methods

2.1. Study Area. UoGH is a tertiary hospital serving the population of Gondar town and the remote hilly areas of northwest Ethiopia. The hospital has a DOTS clinic that has been operational since 2000 [13]. Around 740 TB patients are diagnosed and treated according to the national guidelines annually. The primary aim of the study was to evaluate treatment outcomes of PTB patients who had been transferred out from UoGH and who had arrived at their receiving centers. For logistic and resource reasons, only centers which were within a 180 km radius of Gondar town were included; these were fifteen centers.

2.2. Study Design and Data Collection. A retrospective analysis of the profile of transferred-out PTB patients registered at DOTS clinic of UoGH in the years 2009 to 2013 was conducted. Data were collected from March to June 2014. The registration documents reviewed contained basic information, such as age, sex, and sputum status, type of TB by history, HIV status, and phase of treatment at the time of transfer. Patients whose names, father's names, age, and sex matched between the registers at the UoGH and the receiving units and were classified as "transfers-in" in the receiving units were defined as "arrivals." Patients whose names did not appear in the receiving units were defined as "nonarrivals." For "arrivals," treatment outcome was collected from the TB treatment registers of the receiving centers.

2.3. Definitions. The treatment outcome was categorized according to National TB and Leprosy Control Program (NTLCP) guidelines [13]. These categories were being cured (finished treatment with negative bacteriology result at the end of treatment), completed treatment (finished treatment, but without bacteriology result at the end of treatment for those who are smear-positive), failure (remaining smear-positive at five months despite correct intake of medication), default (patients who interrupted their treatment for two consecutive months or more after registration), death (patients who died from any cause during the course of treatment), transfer-out (patients whose treatment results are unknown due to transfer to another health facility), and successful treatment (a patient who was cured or completed treatment).

2.4. Statistical Analyses and Ethical Considerations. Data were entered, cleaned, and analyzed using the statistical package SPSS for Windows, version 20. Inconsistencies in data entry were randomly checked by reentering 10% of the raw data. Frequencies and percentages were used to describe patient characteristics and treatment outcomes. The study was approved by the Institutional Review Board of the University of Gondar. In addition, official permission was secured from the Regional Health Bureau of Amhara region as well as the involved treatment units.

3. Results

3.1. Characteristics of Transferred-Out Patients. During the study period 3,707 PTB patients were registered and initiated the treatment at UoGH DOTS clinic. Among these, 47.5% (1,760/3,707) were transferred out to complete their treatment in different treatment units after his/her transfer request.

Of these patients, 25.9% (457/1,760) were transferred to the fifteen selected units and their outcome was evaluated. Most of these transferred-out patients (see Table 1) were smear-negative (76.4%), male (59.3%), and new (91.9%) and in the age group of 19–34 years (40.0%). All the transferred-out patients were offered Provider Initiated HIV Testing and Counseling (PITC) at UoGH and accepted to be tested. The TB-HIV coinfection rate was 37.9% (173/457) and 44 of those patients (27.1%) were on cotrimoxazole prophylaxis and 54 (33.3%) on antiretroviral therapy at the time of transfer. About two-thirds of the patients (309/457, 68%) were transferred out during the intensive phase. The median time between treatment initiation and transfer-out was 46 days (range 9 to 140 days).

In the TB registers of the receiving units, only 88.2% (403/457) patients were traced and classified as "arrivals." The remaining 54 (11.8%) were classified as "nonarrivals." Of the "nonarrivals," 9 (16.6%) were pulmonary smear-positive and 17 (31.5%) were HIV positive (Table 1).

3.2. Treatment Outcomes of Transferred-Out PTB Patients. TB treatment outcomes were analyzed for the 403 "arriving" patients only (Table 2). More than three-quarters, 78.8% (318/403), of patients had a successful treatment outcome (18.8% cured and 60.0% completed treatment) while 85 (21.1%) had an unsuccessful outcome (1.7% defaulted, 4.9% died, 0.5% failed, and 13.8% transferred out). For all 457 transferred-out patients, feedback on treatment outcomes was not reported to UoGH by the receiving units.

4. Discussion

Monitoring treatment outcomes is essential in order to evaluate the effectiveness of the DOTS program [12]. Many patients are diagnosed and initiate treatment at large hospitals. To

Table 1: Characteristics of transferred-out PTB patients at the University of Gondar Hospital and those who arrived and did not arrive at selected receiving units, respectively, Ethiopia, 2009–2013.

Characteristics	Transfer-out (N = 457) number (%)	Arriving (N = 403) number (%)	Nonarriving (N = 54) number (%)
Sex			
Male	271 (59.3)	244 (90.0)	27 (10.0)
Female	186 (40.7)	159 (85.5)	27 (14.5)
Age (years)			
≤18	137 (30.0)	111 (81.1)	26 (18.9)
19–34	183 (40.0)	168 (91.8)	15 (8.2)
35–54	106 (23.2)	98 (92.5)	8 (7.5)
≥55	31 (6.8)	26 (83.9)	5 (16.1)
Sputum status (pulmonary TB type)			
Smear-positive	108 (23.6)	99 (91.7)	9 (8.3)
Smear-negative	349 (76.4)	304 (87.1)	45 (12.9)
Type of TB by history			
New	420 (91.9)	368 (87.6)	52 (12.4)
Relapse	27 (5.9)	26 (96.3)	1 (3.7)
Return after default	4 (0.9)	4 (100.0)	0 (0.0)
Failure	6 (1.3)	5 (83.3)	1 (16.7)
HIV status			
Negative	284 (62.1)	247 (86.9)	37 (13.1)
Positive	173 (37.9)	156 (90.2)	17 (9.8)
Duration in which the patient transferred out after initiation of treatment			
<4 weeks	85 (18.6)	79 (92.9)	6 (7.1)
4–12 weeks	365 (79.9)	317 (86.8)	48 (13.2)
>12 weeks	7 (1.5)	7 (100.0)	0 (0.0)

enhance treatment adherence, these hospitals often transfer out patients to a clinic closer to the patients' homes, which has obvious benefits for patients and their families [14, 15]. Different studies have shown that receiving care at only one health facility improves patient compliance thereby reducing the risk of default [9, 10]. Moreover, receiving care close to home is also a key factor for compliance, as when people travel far for daily/weekly DOT they are more likely to default [10, 16]. The current study showed that nearly half of the patients were transferred out after being started on treatment. Other similar studies in the same region reported proportions in the 31.4%–42.0% range [8, 9]. The proportion of transferred-out patients in the current study was slightly higher than observed at a previous study in UoGH reporting 42% of patients were transferred out [9] and another study in the region that reported 31.4% [8]. The current observed higher proportion could be due to the establishment and expansion of treatment units, securing supplies of TB medicines in several health facilities and improving management in the TB program. These all lead patients to seek continued TB treatment in the nearby institutions. The result of current study is lower compared to a study conducted at one hospital in the same region (Felege Hiwot Hospital in Bahir Dar) in which 65.6% of patients were transferred out [10].

No patient should be lost when transferred out between treatment units. However, in the current study, 12% of patients were classified as "nonarrivals" as their names could not be identified in the register of the receiving unit. This proportion of 12% was higher compared to studies conducted in Laos and Afghanistan in which 4% and 10% of patients did not arrive and continue treatment at receiving units correspondingly [14, 17]. For these "nonarrivals" it could not be ensured whether they had continued their treatment. If not they continue to spread TB, especially when they are pulmonary smear-positive. In addition, such treatment interruption could favor the development of drug resistant TB. The possible reasons for these "nonarrivals" might be self-referral to another preferred facility before reaching the destined receiving unit or they may have died or discontinued treatment. This could be linked to patients not following instructions from the health care providers or providers not communicating clearly enough with patients or a combination of both. This needs further investigation.

A high transfer-out rate often results in a lower treatment success rate as for those for whom the result is not reported back the result is listed as not-evaluated.

This could jeopardize achieving the set TB control targets. The Ethiopian National Strategic Plan (2010–2015) has set a

TABLE 2: Treatment outcomes of transferred PTB patients who arrived at their receiving facility in northwest Ethiopia, 2009–2013 ($N = 403$).

Characteristics	Treatment outcomes *n* (%)					
	Cured	Treatment completed	Default	Failure	Death	Transfer-out
Age (years)						
≤18	17 (22.4)	72 (29.8)	0 (0)	0 (0)	6 (30.0)	16 (28.6)
19–34	29 (38.2)	96 (39.7)	6 (85.7)	2 (100.0)	8 (40.0)	27 (48.2)
35–54	24 (31.6)	57 (23.6)	1 (14.3)	0 (0)	4 (20.0)	12 (21.4)
≥55	6 (7.9)	17 (7.0)	0 (0)	0 (0)	2 (10.0)	1 (1.8)
Sex						
Male (=244)	43 (17.6)	145 (59.4)	4 (1.6)	1 (0.4)	14 (5.7)	37 (15.2)
Female (=159)	33 (20.7)	97 (61.0)	3 (1.9)	1 (0.6)	6 (3.8)	19 (11.9)
Sputum status (pulmonary type of TB)						
Smear-positive	42 (42.4)	35 (35.3)	2 (2.0)	0 (0)	4 (4.0)	16 (16.2)
Smear-negative	34 (11.2)	207 (60.1)	5 (1.6)	2 (0.6)	16 (5.3)	40 (13.1)
Categories of TB at start						
New	66 (17.9)	223 (60.6)	6 (1.6)	2 (0.5)	19 (5.2)	52 (14.1)
Relapse	8 (30.8)	14 (53.8)	0 (0)	0 (0)	1 (3.8)	3 (11.5)
Default	1 (25.0)	2 (50.0)	0 (0)	0 (0)	0 (0)	1 (25.0)
Failure	1 (20.0)	3 (60.0)	1 (20.0)	0 (0)	0 (0)	0 (0)
HIV status						
Positive (=155)	23 (14.8)	96 (61.9)	1 (0.6)	1 (0.6)	11 (7.1)	23 (14.8)
Negative (=248)	53 (21.4)	146 (58.8)	6 (2.4)	1 (0.4)	9 (3.6)	33 (13.3)
Time period between transfer-out and transfer-in (363)						
Same to 2nd day	31 (19.3)	91 (56.8)	3 (1.8)	1 (0.6)	13 (8.1)	21 (13.1)
3rd day	35 (19.2)	110 (60.4)	4 (2.2)	1 (0.5)	5 (2.7)	27 (14.8)
≥4th day	5 (23.8)	14 (66.6)	0 (0)	0 (0)	1 (4.8)	1 (4.8)
Phase of TB treatment at time of transfer-out						
Intensive	59 (21.1)	163 (58.2)	5 (1.9)	1 (0.3)	14 (5.0)	38 (13.5)
Continuation	17 (13.8)	79 (64.2)	2 (1.6)	1 (0.8)	6 (4.8)	18 (14.6)
Overall	**76** (18.9%)	**242** (60.0%)	**7** (1.7%)	**2** (0.5%)	**20** (4.9%)	**56** (13.8%)

treatment success target of 90% [1], equal to the global set target by the WHO [18]. In this study, the overall treatment success rate for PTB patients who were transferred out was 79% which is lower than both the national and the global target. Currently, Ethiopia reports a treatment success rate of 91% for new cases registered in 2012, while for previously treated cases this is 43% [1]. The study result of 79% treatment success is below this and also lower than previously reported treatment success rates in northwest Ethiopia ranging from 86% to 95% [19–21] and than Amhara region which reported a treatment success rate of 87.5% in 2014 [22].

If TB control activities function, all patients who transfer out to other units should be recorded as transfers-in and the treatment outcome results communicated back to the referring units via feedback reports and by telephone [15, 23]. In the current study, none of the transferred-in TB patients had an outcome communicated to their referral institution. This suggests that TB reporting systems might not function optimally with regard to communication on treatment outcome of transferred patients. Reasons for this were unclear but it could be due to unawareness of the need for the procedure, negligence, expecting the other to report, and/or lack of communication modalities [24]. Lack of clear guidance and communication between referring and accepting DOTS clinics requires evaluation and immediate attention. The primary DOTS clinic should have collected treatment outcome data from the accepting clinics. Efficient counseling and follow-up of transferred-out patients are mandatory to avoid poor treatment outcomes. Developing clear guidance on how to trace and report transferred-out cases is essential to avoid spillover of TB and MDR-TB [24]. Telecommunication facilities are an area in need of improvement as many of the DOT clinics lack this. Also, the reporting of transferred patients may cause double counting of patients during routine quarterly reporting to central units if both the referring and receiving facility are notifying the patient. This should be looked into.

5. Limitations of the Study

The current study had several limitations: Firstly, it is specific to one setting which may make it difficult to extrapolate the findings to other settings. Secondly, due to the inherent features of a retrospective study design missing data/incomplete records may have influenced the results. Thirdly, the study unfortunately did not include a control group of patients that were not transferred out for comparison purposes. Fourthly, the linking between facility records was done using name matching and not with a unique identifier. Also, TB treatment outcomes were not available for the "nonarrivals" and their exclusion might have biased the treatment success rate. Despite the above limitations, the study result provided important insights into TB control for policy makers and TB program managers and identified the need to strengthen communication for transferred-out cases to ensure the surveillance data accurately reflect the number of patients on treatment as well as treatment outcomes of all TB cases.

6. Conclusion and Recommendation

In conclusion, at UoGH about half of TB patients were transferred out to complete treatment elsewhere while 14% of them were transferred out for a second time. Successful treatment outcome was obtained in 79% of transferred-out patients. However these results are not fed back to the referring facilities that should formally report the outcomes for these cases. This results in underreporting of successful treatment outcomes. A clear mechanism should be implemented to communicate the arrival of and treatment outcomes for transfer-out patients to ensure all patient information is up to date for adequate monitoring of TB control activities. Appropriate patient education on treatment unit selection before treatment and during transfer-out is also recommended.

Abbreviations

DOTS: Directly observed treatment short course
HIV: Human Immunodeficiency Virus
TB: Tuberculosis
UoGH: University of Gondar Hospital
WHO: World Health Organization.

Ethical Approval

Retrospective data were collected from TB registers after approval and permission from UoG Ethics Review Board.

Disclosure

The contents are the responsibility of the authors and do not necessarily reflect the views of USAID or the United States Government.

Competing Interests

No competing interests exist regarding the publication of this paper.

Authors' Contributions

Tadesse Belayneh conceived the idea, designed the research, analyzed and interpreted the data, and drafted and critically revised the paper. Afework Kassu, Desalgne Tigabu, and Eveline Klinkenberg advised on the protocol and participated in statistical analysis and drafting and critical reviewing of the paper for important intellectual content. Gashaw Asmare and Sofanit Tilaye handled supervision of overall work and revised the paper critically for important intellectual content. All authors read and approved the final paper.

Acknowledgments

This study was conducted under the Ethiopia Operational Research Capacity Building Initiative of TRAC/FMOH supported by USAID/TB CARE I project. The authors thank the Global Health Bureau, Office of Health, Infectious Disease and Nutrition (HIDN) of the US Agency for International Development, which financially supported this study through the TB CARE I mechanism under the terms of Agreement no. AID-OAA-A-10-00020. This study was made possible by the generous support of the American people through the United States Agency for International Development (USAID). The authors also sincerely thank Dr. Riitta Dlodlo from the International Union against Tuberculosis and Lung Disease, for her constructive comments on the paper. The authors also sincerely thank the data collectors, health facility managers, and TB focal persons for their cooperation.

References

[1] World Health Organization, *Global Tuberculosis Report 2014*, WHO/HTM/TB/2014.08, World Health Organization, Geneva, Switzerland, 2014.

[2] World Health Organization, *Global Tuberculosis Report 2015*, World Health Organization, Geneva, Switzerland, 20th edition, 2015, http://www.who.int/tb/publications/global_report/en/.

[3] Ministry of Health of Ethiopia, *Tuberculosis, Leprosy and TB/HIV Prevention and Control Programme Manual*, MOH, Addis Ababa, Ethiopia, 2011.

[4] Federal Democratic Republic of Ethiopia, *Health Sector Development Programme IV 2010/11–2014/15*, 2010.

[5] World Health Organization, *Definitions and Reporting Framework for Tuberculosis—2013 Revision*, WHO/HTM/TB/2013.2, World Health Organization, Geneva, Switzerland, 2013.

[6] World Health Organization, *Treatment of Tuberculosis: Guidelines for National Programmes*, WHO/HTM/TB/2009.420, World Health Organization, Geneva, Switzerland, 4th edition, 2009.

[7] World Health Organization (WHO), *Global Tuberculosis Control: Epidemiology, Strategy, Financing: WHO Report 2009 WHO/HTM/TB/2009.411*, World Health Organization, Geneva, Switzerland, 2009.

[8] A. Esmael, G. Tsegaye, M. Wubie, H. Abera, and M. Endris, "Treatment outcomes of TB patients in Debre Markos Referral Hospital, North West Ethiopia: a five year retrospective study," *International Journal of Pharmaceutical Sciences and Research*, vol. 5, no. 4, pp. 1500–1505, 2014.

[9] B. Tessema, A. Muche, A. Bekele, D. Reissig, F. Emmrich, and U. Sack, "Treatment outcome of tuberculosis patients at Gondar University Teaching Hospital, Northwest Ethiopia. A five—year retrospective study," *BMC Public Health*, vol. 9, article 371, 2009.

[10] F. Biadglegne, B. Anagaw, T. Debebe et al., "A retrospective study on the outcomes of tuberculosis treatment in Felege Hiwot Referral Hospital, Northwest Ethiopia," *International Journal of Medicine and Medical Sciences*, vol. 5, no. 2, pp. 85–91, 2013.

[11] T. Vasankari, P. Holmström, J. Ollgren, K. Liippo, M. Kokki, and P. Ruutu, "Risk factors for poor tuberculosis treatment outcome in Finland: a cohort study," *BMC Public Health*, vol. 7, article 291, 2007.

[12] J. Veen, M. Raviglione, H. L. Rieder et al., "Standardized tuberculosis treatment outcome monitoring in Europe. Recommendations of a Working Group of the World Health Organization (WHO) and the European Region of the International Union Against Tuberculosis and Lung Disease (IUATLD) for uniform reporting by cohort analysis of treatment outcome in tuberculosis patients," *European Respiratory Journal*, vol. 12, no. 2, pp. 505–510, 1998.

[13] Ministry of Health of Ethiopia, *Tuberculosis, Leprosy and TB/HIV Prevention and Control Program Manual*, MOH, Addis Ababa, Ethiopia, 4th edition, 2012.

[14] T. Arnadottir, B. Phongosa, P. Chittamany, and H. Soukaseum, "Decentralizing tuberculosis treatment: follow-up of patients during the transitional period," *International Journal of Tuberculosis and Lung Disease*, vol. 6, no. 7, pp. 609–614, 2002.

[15] S. Meijnen, M. M. Weismuller, N. J. M. Claessens, J. H. Kwanjana, F. M. Salaniponi, and A. D. Harries, "Outcome of patients with tuberculosis who transfer between reporting units in Malawi," *International Journal of Tuberculosis and Lung Disease*, vol. 6, no. 8, pp. 666–671, 2002.

[16] B. Getahun, G. Ameni, S. Biadgilign, and G. Medhin, "Mortality and associated risk factors in a cohort of tuberculosis patients treated under DOTS programme in Addis Ababa, Ethiopia," *BMC Infectious Diseases*, vol. 11, pp. 127–134, 2011.

[17] M. Zhuben, F. M. Delawer, A. H. Andar, F. Salimi, and J. Ngamvithayapong-Yanai, "High tuberculosis treatment success in Kabul, Afghanistan despite high patient transfers out," *Eastern Mediterranean Health Journal*, vol. 19, no. 8, pp. 694–697, 2013.

[18] World Health Organization, *Global Tuberculosis Report 2012*, World Health Organization, Geneva, Switzerland, 2012.

[19] M. G. Beza, T. W. Moges, D. T. Mulat, S. G. Yenework, M. B. Sisay, and S. B. Tefera, "A five years Tuberculosis treatment outcome at kolla diba health center, dembia district, northwest ethiopia: a retrospective cross-sectional analysis," *Journal of Infectious Diseases and Therapy*, vol. 1, article 101, 2013.

[20] S. Tadesse and T. Tadesse, "Treatment success rate of tuberculosis patients in Dabat, northwest Ethiopia," *Health*, vol. 6, no. 5, pp. 306–310, 2014.

[21] M. Endris, F. Moges, Y. Belyhun, E. Woldehana, A. Esmael, and C. Unakal, "Treatment outcome of tuberculosis patients at Enfraz Health Center, Northwest Ethiopia: a five-year retrospective study," *Tuberculosis Research and Treatment*, vol. 2014, Article ID 726193, 7 pages, 2014.

[22] Amhara Regional State Health Bureau, Tenth National TB Research Conference, Adama Town, October 2014, http://www.etharc.org/resources/download/finish.

[23] Federal Ministry of Health, "Overview of national TB control implementation status," in *Proceedings of the Sixth National TB Research Workshop*, Gondar University, June 2011.

[24] I. Shabbir, R. Iqbal, M. Anwar, E. Qadeer, and N. Ahmed, "An improved record system for tracing outcome of 'transferred-out' DOTS patients," *Eastern Mediterranean Health Journal*, vol. 17, no. 2, pp. 88–92, 2011.

21

Qualitative Assessment of Challenges in Tuberculosis Control in West Gojjam Zone, Northwest Ethiopia: Health Workers' and Tuberculosis Control Program Coordinators' Perspectives

Senedu B. Gebreegziabher,[1,2] Solomon A. Yimer,[1,2,3,4] and Gunnar A. Bjune[2]

[1]*Amhara Regional State Health Bureau, P.O. Box 495, Bahir Dar, Ethiopia*
[2]*Institute of Health and Society, University of Oslo, P.O. Box 1130, Blindern, 0318 Oslo, Norway*
[3]*Oslo University Hospital, 0424 Oslo, Norway*
[4]*Norwegian Institute of Public Health, P.O. Box 4404, Nydalen, 0403 Oslo, Norway*

Correspondence should be addressed to Senedu B. Gebreegziabher; sinidu_bekele@yahoo.com

Academic Editor: Jacques Grosset

Background. Weak health systems pose many barriers to effective tuberculosis (TB) control. This study aimed at exploring health worker's and TB control program coordinator's perspectives on health systems challenges facing TB control in West Gojjam Zone, Amhara Region, Ethiopia. *Methods.* This was a qualitative descriptive study. Eight in-depth interviews with TB control program coordinators and two focus group discussions among 16 health workers were conducted. Purposive sampling was used to recruit study participants. Thematic analysis was used to identify and analyse main themes. *Results.* We found that intermittent interruptions of laboratory reagents and anti-TB drugs supplies, absence of trained and motivated health workers, poor TB data documentation, lack of adherence to TB treatment guideline, and lack of access to TB diagnostic tools at peripheral health institutions were challenges facing the TB control program performance in the study zone. *Conclusions.* Ensuring uninterrupted supply of anti-TB drugs and laboratory reagents to all health institutions is essential. Continuous refresher training of health workers on standard TB care and data handling and developing and implementing a sound retention strategy to attract and motivate health professionals to work in rural areas are necessary interventions to improve the TB control program performance in the study zone.

1. Introduction

Tuberculosis (TB) remains a major threat to human beings, with the majority of cases occurring in the developing world. The burden of TB has shown significant decline over the past two decades. The implementation of the Stop TB strategy has played a key role in the global reduction of the TB burden. As reported by the World Health Organization (WHO), an estimated 43 million lives have been saved between 2000 and 2014. The Millennium Development Goal target of halting and reversing TB incidence has been achieved on a global scale. Mortality from TB has fallen by 47% since 1990 [1]. Despite these gains, however, TB still remains a major global health threat. According to a recent WHO report, there were 9.6 million new TB cases and 1.5 million deaths from TB worldwide [1]. The 22 high-TB burden countries collectively accounted for 80% of all estimated incident cases.

Ethiopia is among the 22 high-TB burden countries in the world. The directly observed treatment short course strategy (DOTS) has been implemented in the country since 1994 to control the TB epidemic. The prevalence, incidence, and mortality from TB in the country are currently estimated at 200/100,000 people, 207/100,000 people, and 33/100,000 people, respectively [1]. These indicators show that the TB burden in Ethiopia is still enormous and suggest that the National TB Control Program should be functioning very well to achieve significant reduction in morbidity and mortality resulting from TB.

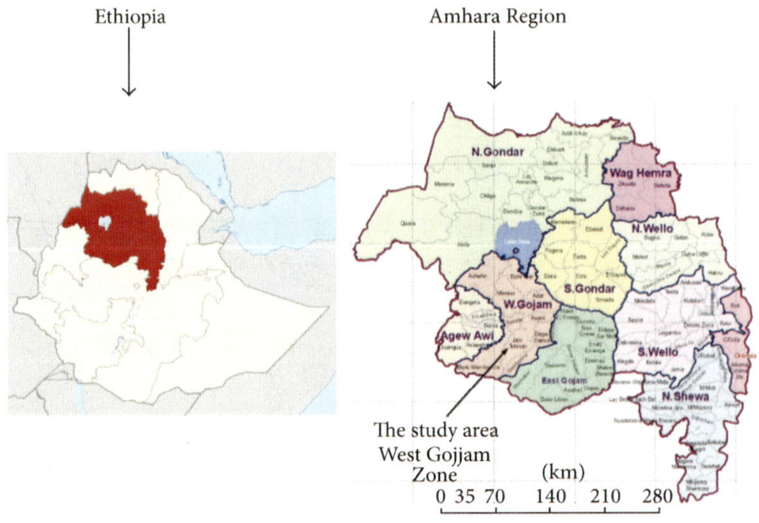

FIGURE 1: Map of Ethiopia, Amhara Region, and the study zone.

Recently, a study was conducted in West Gojjam Zone of Amhara Region, Ethiopia, to assess trends in case notifications and treatment outcomes [2]. The study revealed a number of interesting results that require further assessment. Among others, poor TB data documentation, poor sputum smear examination follow-ups at the 2nd, 5th, and 7th months of treatment, and considerable proportion of deaths were observed during the study period. These findings may indicate that there were challenges affecting the success of the TB control program performance in the study zone. Weak health systems pose many barriers to effective TB control [3]. Understanding the challenges affecting the TB control program is crucial to improve performance and ultimately reduce the TB burden.

Various studies in Ethiopia and other countries investigated TB control program challenges from patients' perspectives [4–10]. However, the number of studies that explored the challenges from health worker's and TB control program manager's perspectives is limited [11–13]. Challenges facing TB control program may vary within different context. Lack of actual understanding of the challenges in context would limit subsequent improvement. Therefore, in-depth understanding of the challenges affecting the TB control activities is crucial to identify potential areas for improvement. This study was thus conducted to explore health worker's and TB control program coordinator's perspectives on health systems challenges facing the TB control program performance in West Gojjam Zone, Amhara Region, Ethiopia.

2. Materials and Methods

2.1. Setting. The study area, West Gojjam Zone, is one of the ten zones in the Amhara Region of Ethiopia (Figure 1). The total population is estimated at 2,382,497 million and more than 90% of the people reside in rural areas [14]. Agriculture is the main source of livelihood for the community. The zone covers an area of 13,669 Km^2 and is administratively divided into 13 rural districts and five town administrations.

Health service in West Gojjam Zone is provided by one government hospital, 90 health centers, 76 private health facilities (hospitals and higher clinics), and 363 health posts. TB control program is decentralized in all districts and town administrations of the zone. One government hospital, 73 government health centers, and six private health institutions have TB diagnostic and treatment facilities. In addition, 276 health posts in the study zone are serving as treatment centers for implementing DOTS. A health post is the lowest level health facility and is staffed by two female health extension workers (HEWs). HEWs play an important role in identifying and referring TB suspects to the next level of health care, that is, health centers for diagnosis and initiation of treatment. Health posts are not equipped with TB diagnostic tools.

Sputum smear microscopy is the only TB diagnostic tool used in peripheral health centers. Thus, all sputum smear-negative pulmonary TB (PTB-) and extrapulmonary TB (EPTB) cases must be referred to hospitals and private clinics for chest radiography and other necessary investigations for TB.

2.2. Study Design, Participants, and Data Collection. This was a descriptive qualitative study conducted from January 2015 to March 2015. Qualitative data were collected using individual interviews and focus group discussions (FGDs). The in-depth interviews were conducted with eight TB control program coordinators who were recruited based on their experience in TB control program management at district, zonal, and regional levels. Two participants were recruited from Town Administration Health Offices, four were selected from District Health Offices, one was represented from West Gojjam Zone Health Department, and another one was selected from Amhara Regional State Health Bureau.

In-depth interview guide with open ended questions was employed to generate the relevant data. Key issues discussed were the regularity of anti-TB drug and laboratory supplies, availability of trained health workers at health facilities, and data quality in TB control program. In addition, respondents were requested to describe their perceptions regarding other challenges facing the TB control program performance in their context. The interviews were continued until saturation was reached. Saturation was reached during the 7th interview and there was no new information that was coming out other than repetition. The 8th interview was conducted to only verify whether there could be any new insights that might emerge, but this was not the case. All interviews were undertaken face-to-face. To ensure privacy and comfort, the interviews were conducted in a place convenient to the participants. The in-depth interviews were conducted by the principal investigator.

After the in-depth interviews were completed, preliminary analysis was conducted and major themes emerging from the data were identified. Subsequently, two FGDs were conducted with a total of 16 health workers. Eight participants took part in each discussion. Participants for the FGDs were selected with the assistance of health programs manager at the Zonal Health Department and TB control program coordinators at zonal, district, and health facility levels. Participants were purposively selected based on the responsibilities they have in relation to TB control activities at the respective health facilities where they were selected. The selected participants included were health workers involved in TB diagnosis and treatment. They were focal persons assigned for TB related activities at TB clinics and outpatient, laboratory, and pharmacy departments. In order to get a broad insight into the subject under study, professional diversity was considered in the composition of selected participants. Accordingly, four laboratory technologists, three pharmacy professionals, four health officers, and five nurses were recruited for the study. Participants were selected from health institutions (hospital and health centers) located in town administrations and rural districts of the study zone. A FGD guide was used and similar topics were explored in all the sessions. Issues that arose in the in-depth interviews were brought up during the FGDs for further discussion. We used this triangulation of data sources in order to increase the validity of findings in our study. Additional information was not coming out in the second FGD other than repetition of ideas.

Throughout the interviews and FGDs, follow-up questions using probes were asked in order to acquire a deeper understanding when an explanation was unclear. The interviews and FGDs were conducted in Amharic (the local language) for all participants. Each in-depth interview and FGD on average lasted 60 and 120 minutes, respectively, and was audio-taped with the consent of participants. All participants of the FGD hold a B.S. degree in their professions. The principal investigator and a trained assistant facilitated the FGDs. All participants actively participated and freely discussed the challenges facing the TB control program in their context.

2.3. Analysis. The audio-taped in-depth interviews and FGDs were transcribed verbatim and translated into English. The principal investigator thoroughly read the transcripts several times until she became familiar with the data. Thematic analysis was used to identify and analyse important themes [15]. The analysis focused on developing coding categories where narrative information was organized according to emerging themes. NVivo version 10 computer software program was used to code the transcripts. Coding of the data was done without fitting it into a preexisting coding frame. Equal attention was given to all data sets during coding. All coded data relevant to each theme was collated into potential themes. The themes that were identified through coding were further refined and developed. Quotes from respondents were included in the text in order to illustrate the findings.

2.4. Ethics. The Regional Committee for Medical Research Ethics (REK Øst) in Eastern Norway and the Ethiopian Ministry of Science and Technology in Ethiopia approved this study. Permission was obtained from respective local administrations. Informed-verbal consent was obtained from all participants before data collection. Confidentiality was ensured by not disclosing the identity of participants.

3. Results

Intermittent supply of anti-TB drugs, intermittent supply of laboratory reagents, trained health workers shortage, poor TB data documentation, and inadequate diagnostic tools were the most important themes identified from the analysis. Other themes identified were poor commitment of health workers and lack of adherence to TB treatment guideline. The themes are described below in detail with illustrative quotes from the data.

3.1. Intermittent Supplies of Anti-TB Drugs. As participants described, the Pharmaceuticals Fund and Supply Agency (PFSA) has been supplying anti-TB drugs to health facilities in the study zone. Health workers working in the TB clinics, the pharmacy professionals, and some of the TB control program coordinators mentioned that anti-TB drugs were intermittently supplied to health facilities. Participants also considered this issue as a common problem in their area.

Illustrations of this idea were mentioned as follows.

> *There is TB drugs shortage, specifically pediatric fixed drug dose combinations are not regularly supplied. The supply is also not balanced. If ethambutol is provided, rifampicin, isoniazid, pyrizinamide (RHZ) may not be there. If RHZ is provided, ethambutol may not be supplied. There was a time that we treated children using adult form tablets of these drugs. (Participant #10)*

Health workers working in TB clinics expressed their concern about shortage of drugs for IPT. They described that isoniazid is recommended to children under five years of age who have contact history with smear-positive pulmonary TB patients. However, they reported that they had been experiencing shortage of IPT.

> *Isoniazid should be given for all families of* smear-positive pulmonary TB *patients especially for children who are under the age of five years. However, there is no adequate supply of IPT. Previously, we had borrowed from Wegedad health center since we did not have the drug in our health center. (Participant #12)*

Participants were asked to clarify why supplies of anti-TB drugs were interrupted. They mentioned that PFSA did not timely deliver supplies to health facilities. In addition, TB control program coordinators stated that health facilities did not timely send drug consumption reports to PFSA based on the integrated pharmaceutical logistics system (IPLS) guideline. They also did not timely request the required amount of supplies for health facilities.

3.2. Intermittent Supplies of Laboratory Reagents. In addition to anti-TB drugs, intermittent supplies of reagents for performing Ziehl-Neelsen staining for acid-fast bacilli (AFB) were reported by majority of the TB control program coordinators and laboratory technicians. This was mentioned as a challenge for failing to regularly perform follow-up AFB microscopy test for sputum smear-positive cases. Participants were asked to clarify why laboratory reagent supplies for AFB test were interrupted. They mentioned the same reasons given for intermittent anti-TB drug supply as described above.

Illustrations of this idea were mentioned as follows.

> *I was transferred to this health center before six months. There is great reagent shortage. We reported this to the district TB focal person. We also told the store man at the health center. In addition, health workers working at the outpatient department are complaining about this. There is a great reagent shortage for TB test. (Participant #14)*

> *To get supplies at the right season, health centers must provide consumption reports for the previous supplies. We have provided training to health workers about IPLS and we are regularly discussing this issue when we go there for mentoring support. But sometimes, because of delay in sending consumption reports, laboratory reagent supplies are interrupted. (Participant #5)*

Some of the TB program coordinators reported that the follow-up sputum smear examination was not done regularly. Laboratory professionals also acknowledged the gaps in doing follow-up sputum smear examination for smear-positive pulmonary TB cases. Workload and lack of reagents were the suggested reasons for not regularly performing patient follow-up sputum smear examination.

> *After completing the intensive phase therapy and before the continuation phase treatment begins, follow-up sputum smear examination should be done, but sometimes, either unknowingly or when they were busy or due to other reasons, health workers were not performing follow-up sputum smear examination for patients. (Participant #2)*

3.3. Trained Health Workers Shortage. As mentioned by majority of the participants, there were no adequate numbers of trained health workers for TB control program in most health facilities of the study zone. Some of the TB program coordinators reported that, due to lack of trained health workers, untrained health workers were assigned in TB clinics.

> *In the past, untrained health workers were assigned in TB clinics. Untrained health workers do not properly know how to give the treatment, how to follow patients and when follow-up AFB examination should be done for TB patients. (Participant #11)*

Majority of the participants mentioned that a partner organization called Management Sciences for Health (MSH) that is implementing a project entitled "Help Ethiopia Address the Low Tuberculosis Performance (HEAL-TB)" in the study zone has been providing TB training to health workers. However, due to workload and high turnover of staffs in the health facilities, some of the health workers said that the number of available trained health workers was not adequate and suggested that standard TB training must be given for all health care providers to address this challenge.

> *I don't think the available trained health workers are adequate for our health center. We are providing a number of health services, even dispensing TB drugs takes half a day. (Participant #9)*

> *In places where two or more trained health workers are available, better services are provided, while in health centers where only one trained health worker is present, the TB service may be interrupted whenever the health worker is absent for various reasons. (Participant #2)*

Most participants expressed their concerns about the high turnover of trained staff in all health programs including TB control. Looking for work in health facilities located in urban areas and opting for further education and better payment were suggested reasons by most participants when they were asked to explain why high turnover of staff occurred.

> *The turnover of staff is high and frequent. Whenever health workers get better opportunities, they may not stay in their current job. This is their right! We cannot force them. Unless TB training is given regularly, the problem will continue. (Participant #1)*

Lack of laboratory technicians at some rural health facilities of the study zone was a concern mentioned by some of the TB control program coordinators. They said that they had posted vacancy to hire laboratory personnel for these health facilities; however, nobody showed up to compete for the post. Due to lack of laboratory personnel, laboratory services have not been started in some rural health facilities of the study zone.

> *For the time being, due to lack of laboratory personnel, we are not providing TB diagnostic service at four health centers. (Participant #2)*

Lack of interest in working in rural areas was the suggested reason for not finding applicants for the vacant post.

> *In our zone, there are remote areas such as Sekela, Damot, Quarit, Wonberma, North Achefer and Gonji. Health workers may not want to go and work there, but we are trying our very best to encourage them to go there and work. (Participant #1)*

3.4. Poor TB Data Documentation. The TB control program coordinators reported poor recording and reporting of TB related activities at health facility level. They said that health workers do not give enough attention for data management and do not consider recording activities as part of their responsibilities. Lack of capacity on data management and lack of attention were the suggested reasons for poor TB data recording and reporting. TB control program coordinators further stated that they regularly discussed the problem with health care providers during supportive supervision and review meetings; however, they noted that the problem of poor data quality is still persisting.

The following was the illustration.

> *Generally, there is a gap in monitoring and evaluation activities at all levels. Specifically to TB, there is a problem on data quality in recording and reporting of treatment outcomes. We have tried to solve this through supportive supervision, but even now, we are not sure to say that the data quality has been improved. (Participant #5)*

3.5. Lack of Diagnostic Tools. Few TB control program coordinators reported unavailability of diagnostic tools for diagnosing PTB- and EPTB cases at peripheral health institutions. They mentioned that smear microscopy has been used to diagnose smear-positive pulmonary TB cases in health centers. They further explained that suspected PTB- and EPTB cases are referred to the nearby hospitals and private clinics where better diagnostic tools are available. The TB program coordinators perceived lack of access to diagnostic tools at peripheral health facilities as one of the contributing factors to low TB case detection.

> *We are examining TB patients mostly using a microscope, however, microscope's sensitivity is very low i.e. 40–60%. Due to this, we can only diagnose 40–60% of the TB cases out of 100 patients screened for active TB. The rest of the patients can be examined using culture, chest X-ray and other methods. But in our region, only government hospitals and limited number of private health institutions have chest X-ray facilities. (Participant #5)*

3.6. Health Workers Commitment. Health workers' commitment was a concern mentioned by participants. There were divergent views among them about health workers' dedication in performing TB control program activities. Some of the TB program coordinators perceived that some health workers lack commitment and are not devoted to their job. They complain of the workload they have. In contrast, majority of the participants described that, despite the workload, health workers are doing their jobs with good commitment. The study participants felt that health workers are at risk of TB infection unless they prevent and control the disease. Moreover, they noted that their families may be at risk of infection if they are infected. Some participants also mentioned that many health professionals have become very concerned about their job after the emergence of MDR-TB.

> *If health workers don't work properly on TB prevention and control activities, they will be affected by the disease. The main transmission of TB infection is through air. Patients are coming to health facilities to seek care, unless we treat them, we can't stop disease transmission. (Participant #5)*

3.7. Lack of Adherence to TB Treatment Guideline. Majority of the participants generally acknowledged the necessity of strict DOT in TB management. However, they mentioned that TB treatment provision was not done according to the national TB treatment guideline. For example, when patients complained of showing up on daily bases at health facilities to take their anti-TB medication, some health workers were just providing them with anti-TB medications to take them at their home without being supervised by either a health worker or treatment supporter. Majority of the TB control program coordinators mentioned health worker's negligence as a reason for not adhering to the treatment guideline.

> *There are principles to follow when providing ant-TB drugs during the two phases i.e. intensive and continuation phase treatment. However, health workers do not practice the treatment guideline according to DOTS. There is a problem of adhering to DOTS during the intensive phase, in particular. (Participant #17)*

> *There is patient follow-up problem. In DOTS, anti-TB drugs must be taken daily throughout the intensive phase treatment under health worker's direct supervision, but when patients sometimes complain of different reasons, health workers dispense TB drugs to patients so that they can take it at home on their own. In addition, patients complete their treatment without having the AFB follow-up test. (Participant #11)*

4. Discussion

This descriptive qualitative study explored health workers' and TB control program coordinators' views on challenges facing the TB control program performance in the study zone. Most of the challenges the participants described were health system based. We suggested possible measures that may help to overcome these challenges in the study zone.

4.1. Intermittent Supplies of Reagents and Anti-TB Drugs. As reported by TB control program coordinators and laboratory technicians, there were interruptions in the supply of AFB reagents. Shortage and interruptions of AFB reagents supplies were reported from previous studies [12, 13, 16]. Sputum smear microscopy is widely used for TB diagnosis and monitoring of treatment progress in the study area [17]. Treatment monitoring is an essential component of TB treatment. Patient response to the treatment regimens is evaluated in the 2nd, 5th, and 7th month of treatment and corrective measures are taken based on the results. Continuous supply of reagents to all health facilities is mandatory to perform this task. Health facilities that lack reagents cannot monitor patient treatment response according to the treatment monitoring guideline, and this may increase the risk of unfavorable treatment outcome, that is, death, treatment failure, and also dissemination of drug resistant TB. In addition, intermittent reagents supplies may affect the routinely performed AFB smear microscopy test to diagnose patients in health facilities. This may discourage patients who seek health care and subsequently contributes to delay in diagnosis and treatment and increased transmission of TB.

Intermittent supplies of anti-TB drugs were also reported as a challenge. Patients' adherence to treatment is seriously affected in such conditions [18, 19]. It could also delay treatment initiation after diagnosis has been made and subsequently results in severe illness and increased transmission of TB. The National TB Control Program recommends isoniazid preventive therapy (IPT) for children [20]. Due to shortage of isoniazid, however, health care providers could not implement IPT. IPT has high efficacy in reducing mortality [21] and risk of developing TB among exposed children [22].

As part of a major intervention to improve the supply chain management in Ethiopia, PFSA, in partnership with its collaborators, has been implementing integrated pharmaceuticals logistics system (IPLS) since 2009 [23]. Failure to timely report consumption status and requesting new supplies based on IPLS guideline were reasons for irregular supplies of anti-TB drugs and AFB laboratory reagents in the study zone. Routine monitoring reports show that IPLS is improving information recording and reporting and storage and distribution systems as well as the availability of essential commodities at service delivery points [24]. Inappropriate implementation of IPLS may contribute to irregular supply of anti-TB drugs and reagents. Our findings suggest that strengthening IPLS implementation is needed to ensure uninterrupted anti-TB drugs and laboratory reagents supplies to health facilities. Enhancing a dialogue between health workers who are responsible for reporting and requesting anti-TB drugs and reagents and the PFSA staffs who are accountable for ensuring continuous supply of the requested supplies may help to solve the problem.

4.2. Trained Health Workers Shortage. As mentioned by the TB control program coordinators, there were conditions where TB patients had been treated by health workers who had not received standard TB training. Previous studies from Ethiopia and other countries highlighted this experience [13, 25–27]. Due in part to the high turnover and lack of adequate number of trained health workers, health facilities were providing TB care by untrained staffs. Without adequate TB training, health care workers are not able to provide proper counseling to TB patients and this will have a negative effect on patient adherence to treatment [26]. Managing TB patients by inadequately trained health workers could generally compromise the quality of TB care and may contribute to poor treatment outcome. This finding indicates that measures should be taken for ensuring the availability of adequate amount of trained health care workforce for TB at all times.

In addition to this, this study highlighted lack of laboratory personnel in some rural health facilities of the study zone. As mentioned by the TB control program coordinators, the District Health Offices had allocated the required budget to hire laboratory technicians. However, the remoteness of the health facilities seemed to have been the reason for laboratory technicians not applying for the vacant job. This may impede accessing TB diagnostic services to the rural community. Adequate number of skilled and motivated health workers at the right place and time is critical to deliver effective health services [28]. We suggest that the study Zone Health Department and the Amhara Regional State Health Bureau have to develop and implement a sound retention strategy that may attract and motivate health workers to work in rural and remote health facilities.

4.3. Poor Recording of TB Activities. TB control program coordinators acknowledged poor recording of TB activities as a challenge. Evidence from a recently conducted records review in the study zone supports this opinion [2]. Treatment outcomes in the unit TB registers were not documented for 13.9% of TB patients and follow-up sputum smear examination results were not available for more than 30% of smear-positive pulmonary TB patients. This evidence indicates that health workers were not properly recording the required patient data in the unit TB registers. Lack of health workers' capacity and poor perceptions about the importance of assuring data quality were possible reasons suggested by respondents. Inappropriate documentation of data seriously affects TB data quality, that is, accuracy, reliability, completeness, timeliness, and integrity of the data [29]. We suggest that strengthening or establishing internal mentoring is necessary. For example, internal mentoring using District Health Offices monitoring and evaluation officers and TB control program coordinators may be a practical and less resource intensive approach to improve data quality. In addition, adequate time allocation and attention for monitoring and evaluation part of the standard TB training may also be helpful.

4.4. Health Workers Lack of Adherence to TB Treatment Guideline. Supervised treatment, which includes direct observation of therapy, helps patients to regularly take their drugs and complete treatment, thus achieving cure and prevention of drug resistant TB [30]. As majority of the respondents said, DOTS was not properly implemented in health facilities. Health workers were not managing TB patients by adhering to the treatment guideline according to DOTS. Similarly, a former study showed health worker's poor adherence to the TB treatment guideline [11, 31]. This may be related to lack of understanding among health workers about the consequences of not adhering to DOTS during TB treatment.

As the TB control program coordinators indicated, this may have resulted due to health workers' negligence to adhere to the treatment guideline. Provision of regular-refresher training on TB, strengthening of regular program monitoring and evaluation, and supportive supervision may be useful to appropriately implement DOTS in the study area.

4.5. Diagnostic Tool Shortage. In high-incidence countries, TB control relies on passive case finding among individuals self-presenting to health care facilities, followed by either diagnosis based on clinical symptoms or laboratory diagnosis using sputum smear microscopy which has very low sensitivity [32]. Inability to rapidly diagnose and treat TB patients leads to increased morbidity, mortality, and ongoing transmission of TB [33]. Like other developing countries, most peripheral health facilities in Ethiopia widely use sputum smear microscopy to diagnose TB [17]. This study highlighted lack of diagnostic tool at the peripheral health facilities of the study zone for laboratory diagnosis of PTB- and EPTB cases. The TB program coordinators acknowledged this as a reason for diagnostic delay and low TB case detection in their context. Globally, emphasis has been given for timely diagnosis and treatment of all TB cases [34]. However, accurate TB diagnosis is difficult, particularly in peripheral health facilities where there are limited diagnostic tools and poor clinical experiences among health workers. In such situations, PTB- and EPTB suspects are often referred to hospitals and higher level private health institutions where better diagnostic tools are available. We suggest that improving the diagnostic capacity by availing better diagnostic tools for TB at peripheral health institutions expedites timely diagnosis and treatment of TB.

Our study has limitations. We only assessed the challenges of TB control program performance in the study area from TB control program coordinators' and health workers' perspectives. Because of limited time and resource, we did not assess the challenges from the patients' perspectives. Otherwise, this descriptive qualitative study provides valuable insights regarding the health system challenges of the TB control program in the study zone from a range of different health care providers' and TB control program coordinators' perspectives. We believe that the suggested recommendations may contribute to the improvement of TB control program performance in the study area.

5. Conclusions

From health workers' and TB control program coordinators' perspectives, the study identified a number of challenges affecting the success of TB control program performance in the study area. Most of the challenges were health system based and require adequate attention and intervention by health authorities in the study area. Among others, ensuring uninterrupted anti-TB drugs and laboratory reagents supplies to all health facilities in the study area is essential for the success of the TB control program performance. In addition, the health authorities should develop and implement a sound retention strategy to attract and motivate health professionals to work in rural and remote health facilities. Regular training of health workers on standard TB care and health management information system is mandatory. Moreover, improving the diagnostic capacity by availing better diagnostic tools at peripheral health facilities expedites timely diagnosis and treatment of TB. Last but not least, regular monitoring and evaluation of program performance is imperative to identify the real challenges and improve TB control program performance in the study area.

Acknowledgments

The authors would like to thank the University of Oslo for funding this study. They also would like to thank the Amhara Regional State Health Bureau, the West Gojjam Zone Health Department, and the Districts and Town Administration Health Offices for facilitating this study. The authors are grateful to all participants and to the assistant moderator for their participation and help.

References

[1] World Health Organization, *Global Tuberculosis Report 2015*, World Health Organization, Geneva, Switzerland, 2015, http://www.who.int/tb/publications/global_report/en/.

[2] S. B. Gebreegziabher, S. A. Yimer, and G. A. Bjune, "Tuberculosis case notification and treatment outcomes in West Gojjam Zone, Northwest Ethiopia: a five-year retrospective study," *Journal of Tuberculosis Research*, In press.

[3] World Health Organization (WHO), "Stop TB policy paper: contributing to health system strengthening; guiding principles for national tuberculosis programmes," Tech. Rep. WHO/HTM/TB/2008.400, WHO, 2008.

[4] T. Tadesse, M. Demissie, Y. Berhane, Y. Kebede, and M. Abebe, "Long distance travelling and financial burdens discourage tuberculosis DOTs treatment initiation and compliance in Ethiopia: a qualitative study," *BMC Public Health*, vol. 13, article 424, 2013.

[5] A. A. Gele, M. Sagbakken, F. Abebe, and G. A. Bjune, "Barriers to tuberculosis care: a qualitative study among Somali pastoralists in Ethiopia," *BMC Research Notes*, vol. 3, article 86, 2010.

[6] M. Sagbakken, J. C. Frich, and G. Bjune, "barriers and enablers in the management of tuberculosis treatment in addis ababa, ethiopia: a qualitative study," *BMC Public Health*, vol. 8, article 11, 2008.

[7] W. Xu, W. Lu, Y. Zhou, L. Zhu, H. Shen, and J. Wang, "Adherence to anti-tuberculosis treatment among pulmonary tuberculosis patients: a qualitative and quantitative study," *BMC Health Services Research*, vol. 9, article 169, 2009.

[8] M. H. Soomro, E. Qadeer, and O. Mørkve, "Barriers in the management of tuberculosis in Rawalpindi, Pakistan: a qualitative study," *Tanaffos*, vol. 12, no. 4, pp. 28–34, 2013.

[9] J. G. Ayisi, A. H. Van't Hoog, J. A. Agaya et al., "Care seeking and attitudes towards treatment compliance by newly enrolled tuberculosis patients in the district treatment programme in rural western Kenya: a qualitative study," *BMC Public Health*, vol. 11, article 515, 2011.

[10] E. Hasker, M. Khodjikhanov, S. Sayfiddinova et al., "Why do tuberculosis patients default in Tashkent City, Uzbekistan? A qualitative study," *International Journal of Tuberculosis and Lung Disease*, vol. 14, no. 9, pp. 1132–1139, 2010.

[11] J. Amo-Adjei, "Views of health service providers on obstacles to tuberculosis control in Ghana," *Infectious Diseases of Poverty*, vol. 2, article 9, 2013.

[12] J. F. Cowan, J. G. Cowan, S. Barnhart et al., "A qualitative assessment of challenges to tuberculosis management and prevention in Northern Ethiopia," *International Journal of Tuberculosis and Lung Disease*, vol. 17, no. 8, pp. 1071–1075, 2013.

[13] A. Cattamanchi, C. R. Miller, A. Tapley et al., "Health worker perspectives on barriers to delivery of routine tuberculosis diagnostic evaluation services in Uganda: a qualitative study to guide clinic-based interventions," *BMC Health Services Research*, vol. 15, article 10, 2015.

[14] Central Statistics Autority of Ethiopia, *Summary and Statestical Report of the 2007 Population and Housing Census*, Central Statestic Autority of Ethiopia, Addis Ababa, Ethiopia, 2008.

[15] V. Braun and V. Clarke, "Using thematic analysis in psychology," *Qualitative Research in Psychology*, vol. 3, no. 2, pp. 77–101, 2006.

[16] M. B. Shiferaw, H. A. Hailu, A. A. Fola et al., "Tuberculosis laboratory diagnosis quality assurance among public health facilities in west Amhara region, Ethiopia," *PLoS ONE*, vol. 10, no. 9, Article ID e0138488, 2015.

[17] T. Getachew, A. Bekele, A. Defar et al., "Tuberculosis service provision in Ethiopia: health facility assessment ," *American Scientific Research Journal for Engineering, Technology, and Sciences*, vol. 13, no. 1, pp. 145–159, 2015.

[18] A. Inotu and F. Abebe, "Assessment of defaulting from directly observed treatment short course (DOTS) and its determinants in Benin City, Nigeria," *Journal of Tuberculosis Research*, vol. 2, no. 1, pp. 30–39, 2014.

[19] Z. S. Nezenega, Y. H. M. Gacho, and T. E. Tafere, "Patient satisfaction on tuberculosis treatment service and adherence to treatment in public health facilities of Sidama zone, South Ethiopia," *BMC Health Services Research*, vol. 13, article 110, 2013.

[20] Federal Democratic Republic of Ethiopia Ministry of Health, *Guidelines for Clinical and Programmatic Management of TB, Leprosy and TB/HIV in Ethiopia*, Federal Democratic Republic of Ethiopia Ministry of Health, Addis Ababa, Ethiopia, 5th edition, 2012.

[21] V. F. Gomes, A. Andersen, G. Lemvik et al., "Impact of isoniazid preventive therapy on mortality among children less than 5 years old following exposure to tuberculosis at home in Guinea-Bissau: a prospective cohort study," *BMJ Open*, vol. 3, Article ID 001545, 2013.

[22] J. Ayieko, L. Abuogi, B. Simchowitz, E. A. Bukusi, A. H. Smith, and A. Reingold, "efficacy of isoniazid prophylactic therapy in prevention of tuberculosis in children: a meta-analysis," *BMC Infectious Diseases*, vol. 14, article 91, 2014.

[23] A. Shewarega, D. Paul, N. Welelaw, T. Sami, and Y. Yared, *Ethiopia: National Survey of the Integrated Pharmaceutical Logistics System*, USAID, Arlington, Va, USA, 2015, DELIVER PROJECT, Task Order 4, and Pharmaceuticals Fund and Supply Agency (PFSA), 2015.

[24] The Federal Democratic Republic of Ethiopia Pharmaceuticals Fund and Supply Agency (PFSA), *Integrated Pharmaceutical Logistics System: Changing the Supply Chain System of Ethiopia to Impact the Health Outcomes*, PFSA, 2014.

[25] M. M. Mesfin, J. N. Newell, J. D. Walley et al., "Quality of tuberculosis care and its association with patient adherence to treatment in eight Ethiopian districts," *Health Policy and Planning*, vol. 24, no. 6, pp. 457–466, 2009.

[26] L. M. Ibrahim, I. S. Hadjia, P. Nguku et al., "Health care workers' knowledge and attitude towards TB patients under Direct Observation of Treatment in Plateau state Nigeria, 2011," *Pan African Medical Journal*, vol. 18, supplement 1, 2014.

[27] A. Wynne, S. Richter, L. Banura, and W. Kipp, "Challenges in tuberculosis care in Western Uganda: health care worker and patient perspectives," *International Journal of Africa Nursing Sciences*, vol. 1, pp. 6–10, 2014.

[28] World Health Organization (WHO), *Increasing Access to Health Workers in Remote and Rural Areas Through Improved Retention. Global Policy Recommendations*, World Health Organization, 2010.

[29] J. H. Ledikwe, J. Grignon, R. Lebelonyane et al., "Improving the quality of health information: a qualitative assessment of data management and reporting systems in Botswana," *Health Research Policy and Systems*, vol. 12, article 7, 2014.

[30] World Health Organization, *The Global Plan to Stop TB 2011–2015: Transforming the Fight towards Elimination of Tuberculosis*, WHO, Geneva, Switzerland, 2010.

[31] G. Mala, A. Moser, G.-J. Dinant, and M. Spigt, "Why tuberculosis service providers do not follow treatment guideline in Ethiopia: a qualitative study," *Journal of Evaluation in Clinical Practice*, vol. 20, no. 1, pp. 88–93, 2014.

[32] L. M. Parsons, Á. Somoskövi, C. Gutierrez et al., "Laboratory diagnosis of tuberculosis in resource-poor countries: challenges and opportunities," *Clinical Microbiology Reviews*, vol. 24, no. 2, pp. 314–350, 2011.

[33] N. W. Yusuf, S. Iram, A. Zeenat, S. Hussain, and M. Aslam, "Rapid diagnosis of tuberculosis using Xpert MTB/RIF assay—report from a developing country," *Pakistan Journal of Medical Sciences*, vol. 31, no. 1, pp. 105–110, 2015.

[34] World Health Organization (WHO), "Improving the diagnosis and treatment of smear-negative pulmonary and extra pulmonary tuberculosis among adults and adolescents. Recommendations for HIV-prevalent and resource-constrained settings," Tech. Rep. WHO/HTM/TB/2007.379, WHO/HIV/2007.01, WHO, 2007.

22

Prevalence and Drug Resistance Patterns of *Mycobacterium tuberculosis* among New Smear Positive Pulmonary Tuberculosis Patients in Eastern Ethiopia

Berhanu Seyoum,[1] Meaza Demissie,[2] Alemayehu Worku,[2] Shiferaw Bekele,[3] and Abraham Aseffa[3]

[1] *Haramaya University, College of Health and Medical Sciences, P.O. Box 982, Harar, Ethiopia*
[2] *Addis Continental Institute of Public Health, Addis Ababa, Ethiopia*
[3] *Armauer Hansen Research Institute, P.O. Box 1005, Addis Ababa, Ethiopia*

Correspondence should be addressed to Berhanu Seyoum; seyoumbe07@gmail.com

Academic Editor: José R. Lapa e Silva

The study aimed at determining the prevalence and drug resistance patterns of *Mycobacterium tuberculosis* among new smear positive pulmonary tuberculosis patients visiting TB diagnosis and treatment facilities at selected health facilities in eastern Ethiopia. A cross-sectional study was conducted between October 2011 and May 2013. A total of 408 new adult pulmonary TB patients (≥ 18 years) were enrolled in this study. Three consecutive sputum samples (spot, morning, and spot) were collected from each patient and transported to the Armauer Hansen Research Institute TB laboratory located in Addis Ababa for culture on Lowenstein Jensen slant media. DST was performed on 357 (87.5%) of the patient samples for isoniazid (H), rifampicin (R), ethambutol (E), and streptomycin (S) using the standard proportion method. The rate of resistance to any one drug was 23%. Any resistance to H, S, R, and E was 14%, 11.5%, 2.8%, and 0.3%, respectively. The highest proportion of monoresistance was observed against H (9.5%). MDRTB was detected in 1.1% of the patients. Any drug resistance was associated with HIV infection (COR = 3.7, 95% CI 1.905–7.222) ($P = 0.000$). Although the prevalence of MDRTB is relatively low in the study area, high prevalence of H resistance is a serious concern demanding close monitoring. Expanding diagnostic capacity for mycobacterial culture and DST is a vital step in this regard.

1. Introduction

Tuberculosis (TB) is an infectious disease caused by strains belonging to the *Mycobacterium tuberculosis* complex. Multidrug resistant TB (MDR TB), defined as resistance to at least isoniazid and rifampicin, has been spreading rapidly in recent years. In 2012, 3.6% of newly diagnosed and 20% of retreatment cases were estimated to have MDR TB globally with noticeable geographical variations in prevalence [1]. Various reports demonstrated that, in Africa, resistance to one or more anti-TB and MDR-TB ranges from 3% to 37.3% [2, 3] and 1.4% to 11.6% [4–7], respectively. Besides, extensively drug resistant TB (XDR-TB) has been reported by 92 countries (including Ethiopia) and about 9.6% of MDRTB patients have XDRTB globally. Therefore, the rapid spread of MDRTB and XDRTB especially in new TB patients is challenging the effectiveness of TB control programmes in many low income countries [1, 5].

Development of TB drug resistance is mainly associated with ineffective TB control programmes due to inadequate therapy, poor patient compliance, interrupted drug supply, and inappropriate treatment regimens. This circumstance has adversely affected the control efforts being made by several countries with limited access to second line anti-TB drugs [8]. Therefore, early diagnosis and treatment, improving treatment outcomes, and expanding diagnostic capacity for mycobacterial culture (the international gold standard for the diagnosis of TB disease) and drug susceptibility test (DST) are crucial to limit the spread of drug resistant TB strains, especially MDRTB [1].

Ethiopia ranks the 7th among the world's 22 high TB burden countries. According to WHO 2013 report, the prevalence, incidence, and mortality rates in the country were 224/100,000, 247/100,000, and 18/100,000 populations, respectively. The same report showed that 1.6% of new TB patients and 12% of previously treated patients had MDRTB. Determining the proportion of drug resistance among new cases is vital in the assessment of the effectiveness of national TB control programme [9].

Ethiopia is working towards interrupting transmission dynamics of TB, reducing morbidity and mortality, and preventing emergence and spread of drug resistance in the general population. A total of 122 hospitals, 1,450 health centers, 642 clinics, and 1,253 health posts were providing directly observed treatment short course (DOTS) [10]. To strengthen the TB control programme, the Ministry of Health established one National Reference Laboratory at the Ethiopian Health and Nutrition Research Institute, five laboratories with TB culture facilities, five with line probe assay, and seven laboratories equipped with Gene Xpert MTB/RIF (to identify rifampicin resistance, which is a proxy marker for MDRTB) [1].

Despite all these efforts, in Ethiopia, the capacity of laboratories to perform TB culture and DST is very limited. For instance, WHO estimated that the number of patients tested for MDR TB in Ethiopia in the year 2012 was below 1% of new and 4% of retreatment cases [1]. As a consequence, many of MDR TB patients remain undiagnosed [10]. Moreover, most of the studies on TB drug resistance were conducted in only few regions of the country. Because of the absence of a regular monitoring program, the available data are often outdated and do not reflect the existing status of the problem [11–13].

The eastern part of Ethiopia is known for its high TB case load and anti-TB drugs have been in use for long time in the area before the implementation of directly observed treatment short course [3]. However, there is a paucity of data on prevalence and pattern of anti-TB drug resistance in this part of the country. Therefore, this study was conducted to determine the prevalence and drug resistance patterns of *Mycobacterium tuberculosis* among new smear positive pulmonary tuberculosis patients in eastern Ethiopia.

2. Materials and Methods

2.1. Study Design and Setting. This is a health facility based cross-sectional study conducted in three major towns (Dire Dawa, Haraar, and Jigjiga) found in the eastern part of Ethiopia. The study was conducted between October 2011 and May 2013. According to the 2007 national census conducted by the Central Statistical Agency, the total population of the three towns was about 529,383 [14]. New smear positive pulmonary TB patients from five health facilities, namely, Dil Chora Referral Hospital, Legehare Health Centre, and Sabian Health Centre found in Dire Dawa town; Hiwot Fana Specialized University Hospital and Karamara Regional Hospital found in Harar and Jigjiga towns, respectively, were included in this study. These facilities were selected because of the fact that they represented the largest centres for TB diagnosis and treatment in their respective regions.

Diagnosis and treatment of TB patients in Dire Dawa, Harar, and Jigjga towns are mainly provided by government hospitals and health centres following the national guidelines of the Federal Ministry of Health of Ethiopia [10]. Basic TB diagnostic facilities including smear microscopy and X-ray are available in all the three hospitals but only smear microscopy service is offered in the health centres.

Detection of TB without investigating for drug resistance can lead to poor treatment outcomes and further spread of drug-drug resistant *M. tuberculosis* strains. Therefore, WHO recommends one TB culture facility with drug susceptibility testing for 5 million people. In Ethiopia, however, due to inadequate laboratory capacity, there is only one public reference centre per 50 million people located in Addis Ababa performing TB culture and DST [1]. Therefore, the service is not currently available in other regions in which eastern part of Ethiopia is not an exception.

2.2. Population. The study population was all consecutive, consenting new smear positive outpatient pulmonary tuberculosis (PTB) patients aged ≥18 years visiting the selected public health facilities during the study period. Patients with previous history of anti-TB treatment for more than 4 weeks and relapses and smear-negative and extrapulmonary TB cases were excluded.

2.3. Sample Size. The sample size was determined by taking the prevalence of rifampicin resistance of 1.6% from a previous study [3], desired precision of 1%, a 95% confidence level and a nonresponse rate of 20%. The sample size was calculated based on the sampling method recommended by WHO for drug resistance survey in tuberculosis [15]. The final sample size calculated was 408.

2.4. Selection of Patient Population. A total of three public hospitals and two health centres were purposively selected based on high patient flow to the health facilities.

In Ethiopia, majority of TB patients visit public health facilities compared to private wings. This is due to the limited number of private health institutions in various regions of the country. Besides, they also demand high health care cost compared to public facilities. Hence, in this study, we focused on public health facilities in order to obtain the required number of patients, to minimize duration of the study and for effective utilization of resources.

The total number of new smear positive PTB patients registered in each study site in the year 2010 was 218, 297, and 265 in Dire Dawa, Harar, and Jigjiga, respectively. Thus, in total 780 new smear positive PTB patients were registered in the same year. Based on this patient load, the sample size proportionally allocated for each site was 155, 139, and 114 for Harar, Jigjiga, and Dire Dawa, respectively.

2.5. Sample Collection and Transportation. Three consecutive sputum specimens (spot, morning, and spot) were collected by a laboratory technologist from each study participant as recommended by WHO [15]. Those samples positive for acid fast bacilli (AFB) by Ziehl-Neelsen (ZN) staining technique were collected and transported to the Armauer Hansen Research Institute (AHRI) TB laboratory at Addis Ababa, Ethiopia, in a cold box (at +4°C) within three days of collection. At AHRI, the samples were pooled into one 20 mL sterile screw capped bottle for each patient and processed for Mycobacterial culture within 24 hours [8].

A pretested structured questionnaire was used to collect sociodemographic data, history of contact with known TB patients, HIV serostatus, history of hospitalization, history of imprisonment, and other relevant data from each study participant.

2.6. Sample Processing, Mycobacterial Culture, and Isolation. A volume of 2.5–10 mL sputum sample was decontaminated, digested, and homogenized using standard Petroff's method [16]. Briefly, the organisms were concentrated by centrifugation at 800 g for 15 minutes. The pellet (sediment) was reconstituted using few drops of sterile phosphate buffer saline (PBS). The pellet was inoculated into Lowenstein-Jensen (LJ) slant tubes (containing 0.75% glycerol and 0.6% pyruvate) for primary isolation of the organisms. Afterwards, the tubes were incubated at 35–37°C and inspected for growth of Mycobacteria for a period of 8 weeks. The isolates were confirmed by combination of microscopic observation of AFB using Ziehl-Neelsen (ZN) staining method and Region of difference nine (RD9) deletion typing as previously described [17].

2.7. Preparation of Drug Containing and Drug-Free Middlebrook 7H10 Media. Middlebrook 7H10 (Becton Dickinson, France) media containing the four first line anti-TB drugs, namely, rifampicin (R), isoniazid (H), streptomycin (S), and ethambutol (E) with the final concentration of 1 μg/mL, 0.2 μg/mL, 2 μg/mL, and 5 μg/mL (Sigma, St. Louis, USA) were prepared as recommended by the manufacturer, respectively.

2.8. Drug Susceptibility Testing. Drug susceptibility testing for streptomycin (S, 2 μg/mL), isoniazid (H, 0.2 μg/mL), ethambutol (E, 5 μg/mL), and rifampin (R, 1 μg/mL) was performed using the indirect proportion method on LJ media as previously described [18]. In brief, bacterial suspensions were prepared and inoculated on DST plates. Subsequently, the plates were sealed with par film and incubated at 35–37°C. A strain was considered resistant when bacterial growth on a drug containing well was equal to or greater than 1%.

2.9. HIV Testing. All study participants were tested for HIV-1 and HIV-2 antibodies after counseling using rapid test kit (Stat pack, KHP, and Unigold) as recommended by the National Guide Line [10].

2.10. Quality Control. Mycobacterium Tuberculosis H37Rv reference strain (ATCC 27294) which is susceptible to all anti-TB drugs tested was included in each test batch as positive and one distilled water inoculated well as negative control. For data obtained through interview, the questionnaire was pretested before use and data were collected by trained data collectors under close supervision by the investigators.

2.11. Statistical Analysis. Data obtained through questionnaire and laboratory test results were double entered into Epi data 3.1 software. Data analysis was performed using STATA version 12. Descriptive analysis, frequencies, and odds ratios (OR) with 95% confidence interval were calculated. Logistic regression analysis was used to assess the association between drug resistance and independent factors. A significance level of $P < 0.05$ was considered statistically significant.

2.12. Ethical Considerations. This study was reviewed and approved by the Institutional Ethics Review Committee of Haramaya University, College of Health Sciences and Armauer Hansen Research Institute (AHRI)/All Africa Leprosy, and Tuberculosis and Rehabilitation Training Centre (ALERT) ethics review committee.

Written consent was obtained from all study participants. Drug susceptibility test results were reported to the respective health facilities for further management of the patients.

3. Results

3.1. Sociodemographic Characteristics. A total of 408 smear positive sputum samples were collected from new PTB patients. Of these, 51 (12.5%) were either culture negative or contaminated and thus excluded from further analysis. Among the 357 patients included in this study, 215 (60.2%) were male, 183 (51.3%) were married, 253 (70.9%) were literate, 285 (79.8%) were urban residents, and 89 (24.9%) were students. The mean age of the patients was 28.8 (SD ± 11.9) (range: 18 to 75 years) and 270 (75.6%) were in the age group of 18–34 years. Forty-two patients (11.8%) were HIV positive (Table 1).

3.2. Drug Susceptibility Pattern. Drug sensitivity test was performed for a total of 357 *Mycobacterium tuberculosis* isolates for the first line anti-TB drugs (H, R, S, and E). Prevalence of any resistance to one drug was 82 (23%, 95% CI: 18.58–27.35). MDR was observed in 4 (1.1%) of the isolates. Any resistance to H, S, R, and E was 50 (14%), 41 (11.5%), 10 (2.8%), and 1 (0.3%), respectively. The highest proportion of monoresistance was observed against H, 34 (9.5%), followed by S, 25 (7.0%), R, 6 (1.7%), and E, 1 (0.3%). There was no strain resistant to all the drugs tested (Table 2). There was a statistically significant association between HIV infection and any drug resistance (COR = 3.7, 95% CI: 1.905–7.222) ($P = 0.000$). HIV-positive patients were 3.7 times more likely to develop resistance to any one of anti-TB drugs compared with those HIV negative patients (Table 3).

4. Discussion

To our knowledge, this is the first report in its kind on the prevalence and drug resistance patterns of *Mycobacterium*

TABLE 1: Sociodemographic characteristics and HIV status of study participants in Eastern Ethiopia, 2013 ($n = 357$).

Characteristics	N (%)
Sex	
Male	215 (60.2)
Female	142 (39.8)
Age group (in years)	
18–24	170 (47.6)
25–34	100 (28.0)
35–44	45 (12.6)
≥45	42 (11.8)
Marital status	
Married	183 (51.3)
Single	156 (43.7)
Divorced	8 (2.2)
Widowed	10 (2.8)
Educational status	
Illiterate	104 (29.1)
Literate	253 (70.9)
Occupational status	
Civil servant	32 (9.0)
Housewife	79 (22.1)
Daily labourer	74 (20.7)
Unemployed	20 (5.6)
Student	89 (24.9)
Merchant	25 (7.0)
Farmer	22 (6.2)
Pensioner	10 (2.8)
Others	6 (1.7)
Place of residence	
Urban	285 (79.8)
Rural	72 (20.2)
HIV serostatus	
Yes	42 (11.8)
No	315 (88.2)

HIV: human immunodeficiency virus.

TABLE 2: Resistance pattern to primary anti-TB drugs among new smear positive pulmonary TB patients in eastern Ethiopia, 2013 ($n = 357$).

Drug resistance pattern	N (%)	95% CI
Any resistance to one drug	82 (23)	18.58–27.35
Any H	50 (14)	10.39–17.62
Any R	10 (2.8)	1.08–4.52
Any S	41 (11.5)	8.16–14.81
Any E	1 (0.3)	
Resistance to only one drug		
H only	34 (9.5)	6.64–12.58
R only	6 (1.7)	0.34–3.02
S only	25 (7.0)	4.34–9.66
E only	1 (0.3)	
Resistance to only two drugs		
H + R only	0	
H + S only	12 (3.4)	1.48–5.24
H + E only	0	
Resistance to only three drugs		
H + R + E only	0	
H + R + S only	4 (1.1)	0.02–2.22
H + S + E only	0	
Resistance to four drugs		
H + R + S + E		0

MDR: multidrug resistant, H: isoniazid, R: rifampicin, S: streptomycin, E: ethambutol.

tuberculosis particularly in Dire Dawa and Jigjiga towns in eastern Ethiopia. The study showed that nearly a quarter of the patent isolates were resistant to any one or more anti-TB drugs tested. Besides, two thirds of the isolates were resistant to only one drug, commonly to isoniazid or streptomycin. There was also a link between HIV seropositivity and any drug resistance.

In this study, resistance to one or more first line anti-TB drugs was 23%. This is relatively higher than previous reports from other parts of Ethiopia, such as Jimma (18.4%) [19], Arsi, (18.2%) [20], and Gondar (10.7%) [21]. A comparable rate of resistance (21%) [22] was reported from Addis Ababa, whereas higher rates of resistance (32.5%) [3], (30.1%) [23], and (25%) [24] have also been reported from similar surveys in the country in the previous years. Studies from Uganda [25] and Nairobi, [26] reported a higher resistance level of (28.6%) and (30%), respectively. The variations in overall prevalence of drug resistance among the different study settings could be due to difference in sample size (small sample size could overestimate the proportion), irregular supply of antituberculosis drugs, poor TB case management (inadequate diagnosis, treatment, and follow-up), and poor treatment compliance.

In the present study, the highest rate of monoresistance was associated with isoniazid (9.5%). Previous studies in Ethiopia reported that the proportion of resistance to isoniazid was within a range of 1.9%–21.4% [3, 11]. Our finding is similar to a rate of resistance 10.0% and 9.9% reported in other African countries such as Nigeria, Abuja [27], and Tanzania [28], respectively while studies in Central African Republic [29], Somalia [30], and Zambia [31] reported a lower resistance rate of 5.8%, 5.7%, and 4.5%, respectively. The relatively high proportion of isoniazid resistance in this study might be due to the common use of the drug in the national TB control programme for longer time because of its accessibility. This reflects that the precursors of isoniazid resistance are accumulating in the study setting which can increase the likelihood of MDRTB if rifampicin resistance rises. Therefore, monoresistance to isoniazid should be properly monitored in order to minimize the spread of MDRTB strains in the study area.

The detected streptomycin monoresistance in this study was 7.0%. This is lower than similar studies conducted in other parts of Ethiopia [22–24] while a lower proportion of resistance was reported elsewhere [19, 21]. But, investigators from sub-Saharan African countries reported a higher rate

TABLE 3: Bivariate analysis for selected risk factors for any resistance to one drug among new smear positive pulmonary TB patients in eastern Ethiopia, 2013 (n = 357).

Characteristic	Any resistance to one drug		COR (95% CI)	*P*-value
	Yes, *n* (%)	No, *n* (%)		
Sex				
Male	49 (59.8)	166 (60.4)	1	
Female	33 (40.2)	109 (39.6)	1.026 (0.620–1.696)	0.921
Age group (in years)				
≥45	10 (12.2)	32 (11.6)	1	
18–24	34 (41.5)	136 (49.5)	1.381 (0.839–2.275)	0.204
25–34	26 (31.7)	74 (26.9)	1.261 (0.738–2.156)	0.396
35–44	12 (14.6)	33 (12)	1.257 (0.617–2.563)	0.529
HIV status				
Negative	62 (75.6)	253 (92.0)	1	
Positive	20 (24.4)	22 (8.0)	3.710 (1.905–7.222)	0.000
Place of residence				
Rural	15 (18.3)	57 (20.7)	1	
Urban	67 (81.7)	218 (79.3)	0.856 (0.455–1.610)	0.630
Contact with known TB cases				
No	60 (73.2)	192 (69.8)	1	
Yes	22 (26.8)	83 (30.2)	0.848 (0.488–1.473)	0.559
History of imprisonment				
No	75 (91.5)	248 (90.2)	1	
Yes	7 (8.5)	27 (9.8)	0.857 (0.359–2.047)	0.729
History of hospitalization				
No	79 (96.3)	264 (96.0)	1	
Yes	3 (3.7)	11 (4.0)	1.097 (0.299–4.031)	0.889

COR: crude odds ratio; CI: confidence interval; HIV: human immunodeficiency virus.

of 14.8% in Benin [32] and 12.9% in Uganda [33]. Though streptomycin is almost no longer considered as a first line drug in the treatment of TB (except when one or more of the primary anti-TB drugs is contraindicated because of toxicity or intolerance), the relatively high proportion of resistance to this drug in this study is probably due to the extensive use of the drug in the TB control programme in the previous years. Besides, erratic use of streptomycin in the treatment of other bacterial infections may also exacerbate the problem.

In this study, monoresistance to rifampicin was detected in 1.7% of the isolates. Studies conducted in Ethiopia between 1984 and 2012 indicated that primary resistance to rifampicin ranges from 0% to 1.9% [12, 13, 21, 34].

The present finding is comparable to a report in India (1.1%) [35], Myanmar (2%) [36], and Cameroon (2.1%) [7]. Lower proportion of rifampicin resistance in this study might be due to relatively recent introduction of the drug as compared to isoniazid and streptomycin. However, in most low income countries including Ethiopia, the drug is broadly used for the treatment of other bacterial infections other than TB. Since rifampicin plays a pivotal role in the management of TB, proper use of the drug should be monitored in order to limit the spread of resistant strains of *M. tuberculosis* to sustain the effectiveness of TB control programme.

In the present study, low rate of ethambutol monoresistance (0.3%) was detected. This is consistent with previous reports in Ethiopia (0%–1.5%) [11, 13, 23, 24]. But, a higher rate of resistance (3.5%) was described by other investigator [22]. A comparable proportion of resistance was also reported in other African countries such as Bukina Faso (0.3%) [9] and Uganda (0.2%) [33]. Low resistance to ethambutol in this study may be due to recent introduction of the drug as compared to isoniazid, streptomycin, and rifampicin. Besides, the drug is only used during the intensive phase unlike isoniazid and rifampicin which are in use both during intensive and continuation phases of TB management.

The prevalence of MDRTB in this study was 1.1%. This is in agreement with the previous survey conducted in other parts of Ethiopia [13, 19, 20, 34]. However, a higher rate of resistance was showed in other study [24]. Our finding is lower than the 7.7% prevalence reported in Swaziland [37], 5.8% in Mozambique [38], and 5.2% in Somalia [30]. This may reflect the variations in sample size, studied population, access to health care facilities, and effectiveness of TB control programmes. In this study, there is a lower proportion of MDR-TB than that in previous reports in Ethiopia. This may possibly due to effective functioning of TB Control Programmes which include regular supply of antituberculosis drugs, well-organized patient diagnosis, treatment, and follow-up and good patient adherence that may contribute to the low prevalence of MDR strains in the study settings.

The association between HIV infection and anti-TB drug resistance remains controversial. Studies showed that more associations were reported in North America than in Africa [37]. In the present study, HIV infection is associated with any drug resistance. Similar results were reported in other studies [22, 23, 39]. Whereas other studies from different parts of Ethiopia showed lack of association between HIV infection and drug resistance [19, 21, 40].

Similar results were reported in other African countries [37, 38]. However, reports in Tanzania [8], in Central African Republic [29], and in Uganda [33] were not in agreement with our study. The possible association between HIV infection and anti-TB drug resistance could be explained from different perspectives. These may include malabsorption of anti-TB drugs among HIV-positive patients, poor treatment adherence, lack of access to proper treatment, exposure of HIV/ADS persons to MDR TB patients during hospitalizations, or frequent visits to health facilities and rapid progression of TB in HIV-infected patients compared with HIV-negative patients [41].

Primary drug resistance indicates the performance of TB control programme in the past. Therefore, information on drug resistance survey is an instrumental strategy in strengthening the existing National TB Control Programme. To maintain the validity of our data, we employed trained data collectors and pretested structured questionnaire and followed standard operating procedures. However, our study was not without limitations. One of the limitations was selection bias, not including all public health facilitates (hospitals and health centres) due to resource constraints. Besides, as the study was conducted among service seekers in health facilities, reported data may not be representative of TB patients in the geographical setting under study.

5. Conclusion

The current study reveals that the overall resistance to first line anti-TB drugs is high. The highest monodrug resistance is detected against H. While the proportion of MDRTB is relatively low, signifying conditions favouring the spread of MDR TB is on rising. HIV coinfected patients were more likely to develop resistance to any one of the drugs tested compared with HIV-negative patients. For early case detection and treatment, expanding diagnostic capacity for mycobacterial culture and DST is a vital step to limit further spread of drug resistant TB strains in the study area.

Authors' Contribution

Berhanu Seyoum, Meaza Demissie, Alemayehu Worku, Shiferaw Bekele, and Abraham Aseffa participated in designing the study, data collection, laboratory work, statistical analysis, and preparation and reviewing of the manuscript. All the authors read and approved the final paper.

Acknowledgments

The authors would like to acknowledge the Haramaya University and Armauer Hansen Research Institute for funding the study. The authors would like to thank Addis Continental Institute of Public Health for offering various forms of support for the primary author. They would also like to extend their heartfelt gratitude to all the study participants who participated in this study. Last but not least, they are very grateful to their data collectors for their dedication during data collection.

References

[1] World Health Organization, *WHO Report 2013. Global Tuberculosis Report 2013*, World Health Organization, Geneva, Switzerland, 2013.

[2] F. Dias, S. Ghebre Michael, S. E. Hoffner, L. Martins, R. Norberg, and G. Kallenius, "Drug susceptibility in Mycobacterium tuberculosis of a sample of patients in Guinea Bissau," *Tubercle and Lung Disease*, vol. 74, no. 2, pp. 129–130, 1993.

[3] G. Mitike, D. Kebede, and H. Yeneneh, "Prevalence of antituberculosis drug resistance in Harar Tuberculosis Centre, Ethiopia," *East African Medical Journal*, vol. 74, no. 3, pp. 158–161, 1997.

[4] J. R. Glynn, A. C. Crampin, H. Traore et al., "Mycobacterium tuberculosis Beijing genotype, Northern Malawi," *Emerging Infectious Diseases*, vol. 11, no. 1, pp. 150–153, 2005.

[5] J. Lin, A. N. Sattar, and T. Puckree, "An alarming rate of drug-resistant tuberculosis at Ngwelezane Hospital in Northern KwaZulu Natal, South Africa," *International Journal of Tuberculosis and Lung Disease*, vol. 8, no. 5, pp. 568–573, 2004.

[6] E. Kassa-Kelembho, G. Bobossi-Serengbe, E. C. Takeng, T. B. Nambea-Koisse, F. Yapou, and A. Talarmin, "Surveillance of drug-resistant childhood tuberculosis in Bangui, Central African Republic," *International Journal of Tuberculosis and Lung Disease*, vol. 8, no. 5, pp. 574–578, 2004.

[7] C. Kuaban, R. Bercion, J. Noeske, P. Cunin, P. Nkamsse, and S. Ngo Niobe, "Anti-tuberculosis drug resistance in the West Province of Cameroon," *International Journal of Tuberculosis and Lung Disease*, vol. 4, no. 4, pp. 356–360, 2000.

[8] W. Urassa, F. Mugusi, E. Villamor et al., "Primary antimicrobial resistance among Mycobacterium tuberculosis isolates from HIV seropositive and HIV seronegative patients in Dar es Salaam Tanzania," *BMC Research Notes*, vol. 1, article 58, 2008.

[9] S. Diandé, L. Sangaré, S. Kouanda, B. I. Dingoumda, and A. S. Traoré, "Drug resistance of Mycobacterium tuberculosis complex among newly diagnosed tuberculosis cases in Burkina Faso," *West African Journal of Medicine*, vol. 28, no. 6, pp. 353–357, 2009.

[10] Federal Ministry of Health of Ethiopia, *Manual for National Tuberculosis and Leprosy Control Programme*, Ministry of Health, Addis Ababa, Ethiopia, 2008.

[11] E. Lemma, J. A. Valdivia Alvarez, G. Gebre-Tsadik, and M. E. Font, "Drug sensitivity patterns of Mycobacterium tuberculosis isolated in Addis Ababa," *Ethiopian Medical Journal*, vol. 22, no. 2, pp. 93–96, 1984.

[12] E. Lemma, M. Niemi, B. Lindtjorn, and G. Dubrie, "Bacteriological studies of tuberculosis in Sidamo Regional Hospital," *Ethiopian Medical Journal*, vol. 27, no. 3, pp. 147–149, 1989.

[13] M. Demissie, M. Gebeyehu, and Y. Berhane, "Primary resistance to anti tuberculosis drug in Addis Ababa, Ethiopia," *International Journal of Tuberculosis and Lung Disease*, vol. 1, no. 1, pp. 64–67, 1997.

[14] Central Statistic Authority, *Population Census of Ethiopia*, 2007.

[15] World Health Organization, *Guidelines for Surveillance of Drug Resistance in Tuberculosis*, WHO/HTM/TB/2009.422, WHO, Geneva, Switzerland, 4th edition, 2009.

[16] P. Kent and G. Kubica, *Public Health Mycobacteriology: A Guide for the Level III Laboratory*, U. S. Department of Health and Human Services. Centers for Disease Control, Atlanta, Ga, USA, 1985.

[17] R. C. Huard, L. C. De Oliveira Lazzarini, W. R. Butler, D. Van Soolingen, and J. L. Ho, "PCR-based method to differentiate the subspecies of the Mycobacterium tuberculosis complex on the basis of genomic deletions," *Journal of Clinical Microbiology*, vol. 41, no. 4, pp. 1637–1650, 2003.

[18] G. Canetti, W. Fox, A. Khomenko et al., "Advances in techniques of testing mycobacterial drug sensitivity, and the use of sensitivity tests in tuberculosis control programmes," *Bulletin of the World Health Organization*, vol. 41, no. 1, pp. 21–43, 1969.

[19] G. Abebe, K. Abdissa, A. Abdissa et al., "Relatively low primary drug resistant tuberculosis in southwestern Ethiopia," *BMC Research Notes*, vol. 5, article 225, 2012.

[20] M. Gebeyehu, E. Lemma, and G. Eyob, "Prevalence of drug resistant tuberculosis in Arsi Zone, Ethiopia," *Ethiopian Journal of Health Development*, vol. 15, no. 1, pp. 11–16, 2001.

[21] B. Tessema, J. Beer, F. Emmrich et al., "First- and second-line anti-tuberculosis drug resistance in Northwest Ethiopia," *International Journal of Tuberculosis and Lung Disease*, vol. 16, no. 6, pp. 805–811, 2012.

[22] D. Asmamaw, B. Seyoum, E. Makonnen et al., "Primary drug resistance in newly diagnosed smear positive tuberculosis patients in Addis Ababa, Ethiopia," *Ethiopian Medical Journal*, vol. 46, no. 4, pp. 367–374, 2008.

[23] S. A. Yimer, M. Agonafir, Y. Derese, Y. Sani, G. A. Bjune, and C. Holm-Hansen, "Primary drug resistance to anti-tuberculosis drugs in major towns of Amhara region, Ethiopia," *APMIS*, vol. 120, no. 6, pp. 503–509, 2012.

[24] M. Agonafir, E. Lemma, D. Wolde-Meskel et al., "Phenotypic and genotypic analysis of multidrug-resistant tuberculosis in Ethiopia," *International Journal of Tuberculosis and Lung Disease*, vol. 14, no. 10, pp. 1259–1265, 2010.

[25] E. Sanchez-Padilla, E. Ardizzoni, D. Sauvageot et al., "Multidrug- and isoniazid-resistant tuberculosis in three high HIV burden African regions," *International Journal of Tuberculosis and Lung Disease*, vol. 17, no. 8, pp. 1036–1042, 2013.

[26] P. W. Ndung'u, S. Kariuki, Z. Ng'ang'a, and G. Revathi, "Resistance patterns of Mycobacterium tuberculosis isolates from pulmonary tuberculosis patients in Nairobi," *Journal of Infection in Developing Countries*, vol. 6, no. 1, pp. 33–39, 2012.

[27] L. Lawson, M. A. Yassin, S. T. Abdurrahman et al., "Resistance to first-line tuberculosis drugs in three cities of Nigeria," *Tropical Medicine and International Health*, vol. 16, no. 8, pp. 974–980, 2011.

[28] G. S. Kibiki, B. Mulder, W. M. V. Dolmans et al., "M. tuberculosis genotypic diversity and drug susceptibility pattern in HIV-infected and non-HIV-infected patients in northern Tanzania," *BMC Microbiology*, vol. 7, article 51, 2007.

[29] F. Minime-Lingoupou, A. Manirakiza, F. Yango, G. Zandanga, A. Le Faou, and L. Rigouts, "Relatively low primary resistance to anti-tuberculosis drugs in Bangui and Bimbo, Central African Republic," *International Journal of Tuberculosis and Lung Disease*, vol. 15, no. 5, pp. 657–661, 2011.

[30] I. Sindani, C. Fitzpatrick, D. Falzon et al., "Multidrug-resistant tuberculosis, somalia, 2010-2011," *Emerging Infectious Diseases*, vol. 19, no. 3, pp. 478–480, 2013.

[31] C. Mulenga, A. Chonde, I. C. Bwalya et al., "Low occurrence of tuberculosis drug resistance among pulmonary tuberculosis patients from an urban setting, with a long-running DOTS program in Zambia," *Tuberculosis Research and Treatment*, vol. 2010, Article ID 938178, 6 pages, 2010.

[32] D. Affolabi, O. A. B. G. Adjagba, B. Tanimomo-Kledjo, M. Gninafon, S. Y. Anagonou, and F. Portaels, "Anti-tuberculosis drug resistance among new and previously treated pulmonary tuberculosis patients in Cotonou, Benin," *International Journal of Tuberculosis and Lung Disease*, vol. 11, no. 11, pp. 1221–1224, 2007.

[33] D. Lukoye, F. G. J. Cobelens, N. Ezati et al., "Rates of anti-tuberculosis drug resistance in kampala- Uganda are low and not associated with HIV infection," *PLoS ONE*, vol. 6, no. 1, Article ID e16130, 2011.

[34] J. Bruchfeld, G. Aderaye, I. B. Palme et al., "Molecular epidemiology and drug resistance of Mycobacterium tuberculosis isolates from ethiopian pulmonary tuberculosis patients with and without human immunodeficiency virus infection," *Journal of Clinical Microbiology*, vol. 40, no. 5, pp. 1636–1643, 2002.

[35] S. K. Sharma, G. Kaushik, B. Jha et al., "Prevalence of multidrug-resistant tuberculosis among newly diagnosed cases of sputum-positive pulmonary tuberculosis," *Indian Journal of Medical Research*, vol. 133, no. 3, pp. 308–311, 2011.

[36] S. Phyu, T. Ti, R. Jureen et al., "Drug-resistant Mycobacterium tuberculosis among new tuberculosis patients, Yangon, Myanmar," *Emerging Infectious Diseases*, vol. 9, no. 2, pp. 274–276, 2003.

[37] E. Sanchez-Padilla, T. Dlamini, A. Ascorra et al., "High prevalence of multidrug-resistant tuberculosis, Swaziland, 2009-2010," *Emerging Infectious Diseases*, vol. 18, no. 1, pp. 29–37, 2012.

[38] E. A. Nunes, E. M. De Capitani, E. Coelho et al., "Patterns of anti-tuberculosis drug resistance among HIV-infected patients in Maputo, Mozambique, 2002-2003," *International Journal of Tuberculosis and Lung Disease*, vol. 9, no. 5, pp. 494–500, 2005.

[39] M. Demissie, E. Lemma, M. Gebeyehu, and B. Lindtjorn, "Sensitivity to anti-tuberculosis drugs in HIV-positive and -negative patients in Addis Ababa," *Scandinavian Journal of Infectious Diseases*, vol. 33, no. 12, pp. 914–919, 2001.

[40] G. Mitike, D. Kebede, and H. Yeneneh, "HIV infection and antituberculosis drug resistance among pulmonary tuberculosis patients in Harar Tuberculosis Centre, Ethiopia," *East African Medical Journal*, vol. 74, no. 3, pp. 154–157, 1997.

[41] S. Suchindran, E. S. Brouwer, and A. Van Rie, "Is HIV infection a risk factor for multi-drug resistant tuberculosis? A systematic review," *PLoS ONE*, vol. 4, no. 5, Article ID e5561, 2009.

23

Socioeconomic Factors Associated with Knowledge on Tuberculosis among Adults in Ethiopia

Sifrash Meseret Gelaw[1,2]

[1]*Unit 12 A, Tuscany Condo, Ayala Avenue 6751, Makati City, 1226 Metro Manila, Philippines*
[2]*24th Floor Citibank Tower, Paseo De Roxas 8741, Makati City, 1226 Metro Manila, Philippines*

Correspondence should be addressed to Sifrash Meseret Gelaw; sifrashm@yahoo.com

Academic Editor: Isamu Sugawara

Background. Ethiopia is among highly tuberculosis affected countries. This might be related to low level of awareness on the disease in the population. The objective of the study was to determine the level of tuberculosis knowledge and socioeconomic factors associated with it. *Methods.* The 2011 Ethiopia health and demographic survey data were used. Overall tuberculosis knowledge score was computed to evaluate the outcome variable. Multivariable logistic regression was employed to identify independent socioeconomic factors associated with low tuberculosis knowledge. *Results.* The overall tuberculosis knowledge was low, 44.05% (95% CI: 42.05–46.24%) among women and 32.3% (95% CI: 30.34–34.32%) among men. Rural women (AOR = 1.22) and youth, no formal education (women: AOR = 3.28, men: AOR = 7.42), attending only primary education (women: AOR = 1.95, men: AOR = 3.49), lowest wealth quintiles (women: AOR = 1.4, Men: AOR = 1.28), unskilled female manual workers (AOR = 4.15), female agricultural employee (AOR = 2.28), and lack of access to media (women: AOR = 1.52, men: AOR = 1.71) are significantly associated with low tuberculosis knowledge. *Conclusion.* The level of tuberculosis knowledge among adults in Ethiopia is low and varied by socioeconomic groups. Tuberculosis control programs should consider appropriate strategies for tuberculosis education, promotion, communication, and social mobilization to address the rural women, youths, the poor, less educated people, and unskilled workers.

1. Introduction

Tuberculosis (TB) is a widely recognized high-burden infectious disease in the world. It is a bacterial infection caused by a member *Mycobacterium* TB complex, commonly *Mycobacterium tuberculosis*. TB is transmitted by respiratory route when a patient is coughing or sneezing, and one strain of TB, *Mycobacterium bovis*, can be caused by drinking unboiled milk [1]. Risk of TB is high among population living in poverty, low socioeconomic groups, low income, immune-suppressed (including AIDS), and extreme age (old age and children) groups, certain ethnicity, migrants, and those exposed to animals (*Mycobacterium bovis*) [1, 2]. The risk of TB transmission also increases with the intimacy and duration of contact to TB patients and infectiousness of the TB patients [1].

Ethiopia is the second populous country in Africa with a population size of 88 million (July 2014 projection). Only 16% of the population lives in urban areas and the literacy rate is 42.7% [3, 4]. The country is one of the tuberculosis high-burden countries, standing on rank 8 under the 22 high TB burden countries in the world with an estimated prevalence and incidence rate of 394 and 261 cases per 100,000 inhabitants, respectively [5, 6]. The country begun to implement DOTS strategy in 1992. However, only approximately 60 to 70% of the population has access to DOTS services by 2005 [7, 8]. One of the major problems in controlling the TB burden is the poor awareness and knowledge of the population on TB [9, 10].

Low level of knowledge on TB can lead to complications and worse health outcomes increasing the transmission and delaying health seeking behavior, lack of adherence, resulting in multidrug resistance, treatment failure, and disease complication and death [11–13].

TB control could be significantly improved if more consideration was given to the population's knowledge and attitudes about TB and related health care-seeking behavior by directing efforts towards making individuals more informed and aware of all aspects of TB [14–16]. Advocating for the health of patients and developing policy to increase health literacy among the general public as well as health care professionals will create a supportive environment where optimal TB-related outcomes can be achieved [12, 17–20].

Different studies from different countries show the significance of the problem of low TB knowledge and the different socioeconomic factors associated with low TB knowledge in the different study populations. But on the other hand most studies done on TB knowledge in Ethiopia [9, 10, 17–22] as well as studies in different other high TB burden countries [23–29] are done among restricted population subgroups and are mainly health facility based studies which may overestimate the magnitude of the level of knowledge on TB and may not reflect the actual situation in the general population. Moreover, the TB knowledge components considered in these studies were not comprehensive items. These demonstrated the need for exploring large scale comprehensive community level study to recognize the different factors associated with knowledge on TB with the context of Ethiopian culture and socioeconomic status. Further detail analysis of large scale data will help to understand the level of knowledge on TB and associated factors at the country level, which will further guide to design evidence based country appropriate policy, strategy, intervention, service provision, and advocacy to enhance the TB control program. The aim of this study is to identify level of knowledge and socioeconomic factors associated with TB awareness and knowledge about TB transmission, TB symptoms, and TB treatment among adult population of Ethiopia.

2. Methods

To address the objectives of the study, secondary analysis of the 2011 Ethiopia Demographic and Health Survey (EDHS) was employed. The survey has used a cross-sectional study design. The survey interviewed a nationally representative sample population in 18,500 households involving 16,515 women aged 15–49 and 14,110 men aged 15–59 from all selected households. A stratified, two-stage cluster sampling method was used. Stratification was achieved by separating each region into urban and rural areas. In the first stage, 624 Enumeration Areas (EAs) were selected with probability proportional to the EA size and with independent selection in each sampling stratum. In the second stage, a fixed number of 30 households were selected for each EA. The survey used three questionnaires: the Household Questionnaire, the Woman's Questionnaire, and the Man's Questionnaire. The questionnaires were pretested, and consent was taken. Interviewers and supervisors were properly trained. A quality control team regularly visited the fieldwork to closely supervise and monitor field activities [3].

Due to the nonproportional allocation of the sample to the different regions and to their urban and rural areas, sampling weights are required for any analysis using 2011 EDHS data to ensure representativeness of the survey results at the national and regional level. Since the 2011 EDHS sample is a two-stage stratified cluster sample, sampling weights were calculated based on sampling probabilities separately for each sampling stage and for each cluster [3].

2.1. Data Management. Information on TB knowledge and socioeconomic factors was extracted from the large dataset. The different datasets for women and men were explored, variables relevant for the current study were identified, and the variables between the women and men dataset were harmonized. To have comparable age distribution between women and men, those with only 15–49 years were included in the analysis. Then the two datasets were matched to produce a subset of the original variables. The extracted data became the working dataset to address the objectives of the project.

2.2. Data Preparation. STATA version 12 was used to analyse the data. Exploration of the variables was made. Data were checked for errors by summarizing and producing frequencies and cross tabulations. Missing values were checked, identified, decoded, and excluded from the analysis.

2.3. Data Analysis Method

2.3.1. Descriptive Analysis. Background characteristics of respondents were summarized and presented in tables. Absolute numbers and percentages are displayed. The proportion of respondents who are aware of TB and who have correct knowledge on TB transmission, TB symptoms, and TB treatment was calculated.

2.3.2. Outcome Measure. The outcome variable, low comprehensive TB knowledge was measured as a composite indicator by considering responses related to TB awareness, modes of transmission, sign and symptoms, and treatment. Questions correctly answered were coded as "1" and incorrect answers as "0" during analysis. The lower terciles of the overall summary score were taken as low TB knowledge. The methodological approach in this study is based on different previous similar studies [9, 15]. In this study, the level of comprehensive TB knowledge was measured as the main outcome of interest. All the components of TB knowledge such as knowledge on TB transmissions, symptoms, and treatment are included as all the components are relevant with regard to their contribution to TB prevention and control as described above. Moreover, using an overall composite score allows straight forward comparison of TB knowledge among its different determinant factors. Since there was no study found on psychometric properties of DHS TB knowledge items, factor analysis was employed to examine the psychometric properties of the overall knowledge score.

2.3.3. Factor Analysis and Measuring the Reliability of the Summary Scores. The factor structure of the different knowledge question items was investigated using Principal Components Analysis (PCA), to get clearance on the different dimension of the overall score index. A total of 15 items regarding assessing

TB knowledge were included in the PCA. Factors with eigenvalue >1 were retained. Accordingly, five factors were identified and then rotation was done. Three variables with rotated loading factor less than 0.4 were omitted (these are transmission through sharing utensils, transmission through touching a person with TB, and the fact that tuberculosis can be cured). One variable which was loading on a factor but that was not interpretable was omitted (transmission through exposure to cold). In addition, an initial Cronbach Alpha was calculated (for the whole summary score) and for each variable an alternative alpha if a variable was sorted out was computed. One variable was omitted because the alternative alpha is higher than the initial alpha (transmission through sexual contact). A total of five variables were excluded. Cronbach's Alpha was calculated for checking consistency of the variables and found to be 0.62. This value is because an index of ten variables is quite small and alpha is dependent on the number of variables in the index. The value of alpha increased to 0.7 as the number of variables increased to fifteen. An overall summary score was calculated using raw values of the remaining variables with rotated factor loading greater than 0.4 on at least one interpretable factor. The lower terciles of the summary score were taken as the outcome measure (low TB knowledge).

From the above factor analysis result, four interpretable factors remained for the overall index construction. These factors are interpreted and qualitatively described as follows. The first component with three items is interpreted as "cough related symptoms and transmissions." The second component with two items is interpreted as "food related symptoms and transmissions." The third component with three items is interpreted as "key symptoms and transmissions." The last component with two items is interpreted as "misconceptions."

2.3.4. Independent Variables. The following different socioeconomic factors are taken as independent variables in the analysis in this study: gender categorized as female and male; age in ten-year intervals; regions categorized into accessible regions (Tigray, Amhara, Oromiya, and SNNPR), hard to reach regions (Afar, Somali, Gambela, and Benishangul Gumuz), and city administrations and regions (Addis Ababa, Dire Dawa, and Harari); residence classified as urban and rural; wealth index (which was already calculated in the primary study based on a standard set of household assets, dwelling characteristics, and ownership of consumer items) categorized in to five where the first quintile was the poorest 20% of the households and fifth quintile the wealthiest 20% of the households; marital status classified as never in union, married, living with partner, widowed, divorced, and no longer living together/separated; education categorized into no education, primary, secondary, and more than secondary; occupational status classified as not working, professional/technical/managerial, clerical, sales and services, agricultural employee, skilled manual, and unskilled manual; frequency of exposure to mass media classified as reading newspaper, watching television, and listening radio; and exposure to community conversation program as yes and no response [3].

2.3.5. Assessing Magnitude of Low TB Knowledge. Proportion of adults with low comprehensive TB knowledge was determined along with the corresponding 95% confidence interval (95% CI) at national and regional level as well as for urban and rural areas. The outcome measure, low comprehensive TB knowledge, was tabulated against socioeconomic factors. All analysis was stratified by sex, since there may be multiple interactions between sex and other independent variables.

2.3.6. Bivariate and Multivariate Analysis of Association. Crude odds ratios (OR) along with the corresponding 95% confidence intervals were estimated using Mantel-Haenszel method to assess the association between the outcome of interest and each exposure factor. STATA SVY prefix command and weights were used to account for the complex sampling nature of the survey.

Binary logistic regression was employed to further analyse the data. The variables for subsequent analysis in the logistic regression model were selected based on prior information from the literature and/or statistical plausibility ($p < 0.05$ in the bivariate analysis). Forward logistic regression strategy was used for building the multivariate logistic regression model step by step.

In addition, interaction terms for effect modifiers were checked. Multicollinearity between independent variables was resolved by computing the collinearity matrix index. The likelihood ratios and the pseudo-R^2 in the STATA output of the final fit of the multivariable logistic regression model were checked and recorded to see the improvement of the model due to the independent variables included and the estimation of proportion of variability explained by the model. Crude and adjusted odds ratios along with their 95% confidence interval were presented. Associations were declared significant, if $p < 0.05$.

2.3.7. Ethical Considerations. The project was approved by the Ethics Committee of LSHTM. The data source is a secondary human dataset from EDHS 2011. The primary EDHS 2011 has received clearance from the responsible bodies in Ethiopia. MEASRE DHS has given permission to further analyse the data and use it for the current study. There is no personal identifier attached to the dataset.

3. Results

3.1. Socioeconomic Characteristics. There were a total of 30,625 study participants in the dataset, of which 16,515 (53.9%) were women and 14,110 (46.1%) were men.

Majority, 68.8%, were from rural area and about half, 49.3%, were from the accessible regions (Tigray, Amhara, Oromia, and SNNPR). The age ranged from 15 to 49 years and 40.9% were 15 to 24 years of age. More than half (55.6%) were married and 32.9% have never been in union. About 41.6% of the participants had no formal education and 40.9% had only primary education. Almost one-third of the participants had no work and 38.3% were agricultural employees. About one in four (26.4%) had no access to newspaper, television, or radio. More than half (58.7%) of the participants have never heard of community conversions on various topics (Table 1).

TABLE 1: Background characteristics of respondents, Ethiopia 2011.

Characteristics	Category	Number	Percentage
Gender	Female	**16,515**	**53.9**
	Male	**14,110**	**46.1**
Residence	Urban	9,545	31.2
	Rural	21,080	68.8
Age	15–24	12,019	40.9
	25–34	9,241	31.5
	35–44	6,061	20.6
	45–49	2,062	7.0
Current marital status	Never in union	10,066	32.9
	Married	17,017	55.6
	Living with partner	1,117	3.7
	Widowed	679	2.2
	Divorced	1,220	4.0
	No longer living together/separated	526	1.7
Region	Accessible regions	15,092	49.3
	Hard to reach regions	8,388	27.4
	City administrations and Harari region	7,145	23.3
Education	No education	12,727	41.6
	Primary	12,529	40.9
	Secondary	3,021	9.9
	More than secondary	2,348	7.7
Wealth quintile	Lowest	6,558	21.4
	Second	4,511	14.7
	Middle	4,422	14.4
	Fourth	4,909	16.0
	Highest	10,225	33.4
Occupation	Not working	9,183	30.3
	Professional/technical/managerial	1,199	4.0
	Clerical/sales/services	5,517	18.2
	Agricultural employee	11,608	38.3
	Skilled manual	2,431	8.0
	Unskilled manual	404	1.3
Exposures to mass media	Accesses either newspaper, TV, or radio less than or at least once a week	22,455	73.6
	Access none of the three media	8,065	26.4
Heard of community conversation program	No	17,959	58.7
	Yes	12,652	41.3
Last time attended community conversation meeting	Never attended	2,977	23.6
	Within last 3 months	3,598	28.5
	4–11 months ago	1,478	11.7
	One year or more ago	1,657	13.1

3.2. Awareness and Correct Knowledge about TB. Awareness on TB is high, with 15,045 (89.9%) of women and 13,518 (95.1%) of men and overall 28,563 (92.3%) mentioning they had "heard of an illness called tuberculosis (TB)." But only 49.97% of women and 61.84% of men knew that TB is transmitted "by air when coughing or sneezing." There were misconceptions of TB transmission; the common misconception was TB transmission by "sharing utensils" and by "exposure to cold," with overall correct responses rate of 68.71% and 79.6%, respectively. Surprisingly, only 1.82% of females and 2.55% of males knew that drinking unboiled milk can cause tuberculosis. Very small proportion of participants

TABLE 2: TB awareness and respondents correct knowledge on TB transmission, symptoms, and treatment, Ethiopia 2011.

Characteristics	Characteristics (correct response)	Women n (%)	Men n (%)	Total n (%)
Awareness	Heard of tuberculosis or TB (yes)	15,045 (89.92)	13,518 (95.09)	28,563 (92.3)
Transmission: tuberculosis spread by	Air when coughing or sneezing (yes)	8,644 (49.97)	9,036 (61.84)	17,680 (55.44)
	Sharing utensils (no)	11,568 (71.6)	8,673 (65.33)	20,241 (68.71)
	Touching a person with TB (no)	14,864 (92.32)	12,587 (90.74)	27,451 (91.59)
	Food (no)	15,284 (93.5)	13,093 (93.03)	28,377 (93.29)
	Sexual contact (no)	15,656 (95.94)	13,513 (96.97)	29,169 (96.42)
	Mosquito bites (no)	16,379 (99.47)	13,958 (99.19)	30,337 (99.34)
	Drinking unboiled milk (yes)	312 (1.82)	423 (2.55)	735 (2.16)
	Exposure to cold (no)	12,894 (79.22)	11,124 (80.12)	24,018 (79.64)
Symptom/signs: symptoms of a person with TB	Persistent cough (>2 weeks) (yes)	11,354 (66.56)	11,141 (77.02)	22,495 (71.38)
	Weight loss (yes)	5,250 (28.44)	6,131 (42.54)	11,381 (34.94)
	Poor appetite (yes)	1,870 (9.304)	1,940 (15.15)	3,810 (12)
	Night sweating (yes)	905 (3.7)	853 (4.16)	1,758 (3.91)
	Chest pain (yes)	1,033 (6.16)	1,020 (5.57)	2,053 (5.89)
	Fever (yes)	2,121 (9.16)	1,974 (9.99)	4,095 (9.54)
Treatment	Tuberculosis can be cured (yes)	12,564 (79.8)	12,302 (89.45)	24,866 (84.38)
Attitude	Will keep TB patient in family a secret (no)	10,724 (72.12)	11,025 (81.25)	21,749 (76.47)

knew major symptoms of a person with tuberculosis: "night sweating" (3.7% of females and 4.16% of males), "chest pain" (6.16% of females and 5.57% of males), and "fever" (9.16% of females and 9.99% of males) (Table 2). The most commonly identified TB symptom is "persistent cough" (66.6% of females and 77.02 of males, overall: 71.38%). The majority of respondents (84.38%) knew that "TB can be cured." And 76.47% said they will not "keep TB patients in family a secret."

3.3. Magnitude of Low TB Knowledge. The overall prevalence of low TB knowledge is high, with higher proportion among women, 44.05% (95% CI: 42.05–46.24%), compared to men, 32.3% (95% CI: 30.34–34.32%). Rural residents (49.17% of females and 35.44% of males) have higher prevalence of low TB knowledge compared with urban residents (28.1% among females and 21.11% among males). For both female and male respondents, the magnitude of low TB knowledge is higher among the youths (15–24 years) (46.17%) compared with older age groups. Respondents from both hard to reach and accessible regions have similar level of low TB knowledge (Table 3).

3.4. Socioeconomic Factors Associated with Low TB Knowledge

3.4.1. Bivariate Analysis Results. At the bivariate analysis stage, the crude ORs showed that all the socioeconomic variables were significantly associated with low TB knowledge among both female and male study participants. After adjusting, all factors remained significant for females but residence, region, and occupation were not any more significantly associated with low TB knowledge in males (Tables 4 and 5).

3.4.2. Multivariate Analysis Results for Female Study Participants. Rural women are victims of having low TB knowledge. The odds of low TB knowledge was 1.22 (95% CI: 1.06–1.41, $p = 0.006$) times higher among rural female residents as compared to urban residents. Being in the age groups 25–34, 35–44, and 45–49 was negatively associated with low TB knowledge compare with 15–24 years females, AORs being 0.68 (95% CI: 0.62–0.75), 0.60 (95% CI: 0.54–0.67), and 0.62 (95% CI: 0.53–0.71), respectively, and $p < 0.0001$ in all. Not having any formal education (AOR = 3.28, 95% CI: 2.52–4.27, $p < 0.0001$) and having attended only primary education (AOR = 1.95, 95% CI: 1.51–2.51, $p < 0.0001$) had increased odds of low TB knowledge as compared to women participants who have attended more than secondary school. The odds of low TB knowledge were higher among participants with lowest wealth quintiles, second, middle, and fourth wealth quintiles, as compared to those participants from highest wealth quartiles, AORs = 1.4 (95% CI: 1.20–1.63, $p < 0.0001$), 1.25 (95% CI: 1.07, 1.46, $p = 0.005$), 1.23 (95% CI: 1.06–1.44, $p = 0.008$), and 1.17 (95% CI: 1.01–1.35, $p = 0.035$), respectively. "Unskilled female manual workers," being "agricultural employee," those "not working," "skilled manual" worker, and "clerical/sales and service workers" were associated with increased odds of low TB knowledge compared with professional/technical/managerial female workers, AORs being 4.15 (95% CI: 2.37–7.28, $p < 0.0001$), 2.28

TABLE 3: Prevalence of low comprehensive TB Knowledge, Ethiopia 2011.

Characteristics	Category	Women		Men	
		Prevalence	95% CI	Prevalence	95% CI
National total		44.14	(42.05, 46.24)	32.3	(30.34, 34.32)
Residence	Urban	28.1	(24.55, 31.95)	21.11	(18.29, 24.24)
	Rural	49.17	(46.69, 51.66)	35.44	(33.06, 37.9)
Age	15–24	46.31	(43.74, 48.9)	39.92	(37.18, 42.74)
	25–34	42.57	(39.72, 45.47)	27.6	(25.24, 30.08)
	35–44	41.5	(38.37, 44.71)	27.19	(24.61, 29.93)
	45–49	45.36	(41.02, 49.77)	27.42	(23.27, 32.0)
Region	Accessible regions	45.4	(43.07, 47.75)	33.14	(30.97, 35.37)
	Hard to reach regions	41.59	(8.09, 45.18)	34.31	(31.03, 37.75)
	City administrations	27.51	(24.79, 30.42)	17.95	(14.34, 22.23)
Current marital status	Never in union	42.11	(39.4, 44.87)	36.87	(34.24, 39.57)
	Married	44.66	(42.03, 47.32)	28.79	(26.66, 31.02)
	Living with partner	42.96	(37.22, 48.9)	31.87	(24.1, 40.8)
	Widowed	39.84	(34.23, 45.73)	37.95	(22.82, 55.84)
	Divorced	52.83	(47.14, 58.45)	41.79	(33.78, 50.27)
	No longer living together/separated	42.72	(35.54, 50.21)	22.6	(12.84, 36.65)
Education	No education	52.67	(50.01, 55.32)	44.01	(40.85, 47.21)
	Primary	40.09	(37.68, 42.56)	31.16	(28.84, 33.58)
	Secondary	22.41	(18.72, 26.59)	15.8	(13.16, 18.85)
	More than secondary	13.99	(10.36, 18.61)	8.251	(6.038, 11.18)
Wealth quintile	Lowest	55.31	(51.78, 58.8)	42.7	(38.29, 47.22)
	Second	50.77	(47, 54.53)	37.05	(33.63, 40.61)
	Middle	49.63	(45.9, 53.36)	35.66	(32.09, 39.39)
	Fourth	43.69	(40.33, 47.11)	30.15	(26.9, 33.62)
	Highest	27.93	(24.86, 31.23)	20.67	(17.8, 23.87)
Occupation	Professional/technical/managerial	9.023	(5.007, 15.73)	7.766	(5.317, 11.21)
	Not working	45.25	(42.51, 48.01)	34.94	(30.09, 40.12)
	Clerical/sales and services	36.02	(33.35, 38.78)	24.66	(20.87, 28.89)
	Agricultural employee	51.38	(48.06, 54.7)	35.84	(33.4, 38.35)
	Skilled manual	41.52	(35.84, 47.44)	21.01	(17.13, 25.5)
	Unskilled manual	55.6	(47.14, 63.74)	29.98	(20.37, 41.73)
Exposure to mass media	Accesses none of the three media at least once a week	57.17	(54.52, 59.77)	50.75	(46.78, 54.72)
	Accesses either newspaper, TV, or radio at least once a week	37.87	(35.66, 40.14)	28.31	(26.41, 30.3)
Heard of community conversation program	No	50.1	(47.62, 52.58)	42.1	(39.45, 44.79)
	Yes	30.71	(28.51, 32.99)	23.35	(21.24, 25.59)

(95% CI: 1.44–3.60, $p < 0.001$), 1.96 (95% CI: 1.25–3.08, $p = 0.004$), 1.81 (95% CI: 1.13–2.89, $p = 0.013$), and 1.70 (95% CI: 1.08–2.67, 0.023), respectively. Female participants who had no access to newspaper, television, or radio had 1.52 (95% CI: 1.41–1.64, $p \leq 0.0001$) times increasing odds of low TB knowledge as compared to those who had access to either of the three media at least once a week (Tables 4 and 5).

3.4.3. Multivariate Analysis Results for Male Study Participants. Not having any formal education and having attended primary education and secondary education had increased odds of having low TB knowledge as compared to male participants who have attended more than secondary school, AORs being 7.42 (95% CI: 5.70–9.66, $p < 0.0001$), 3.49 (95% CI: 2.71–4.48, $p < 0.0001$), and 1.55 (95% CI: 1.17–2.05,

TABLE 4: Factors associated with low TB knowledge among women, Ethiopia 2011.

Characteristics	Category	Low knowledge n (%)	Crude OR (95% CI)	p value (crude)	Adjusted OR (95% CI)	p value (adjusted)
Residence	Urban	1,344 (28.1)	1		1	
	Rural	5,253 (49.17)	2.48 (2.01, 3.05)	<0.0001	1.22 (1.06, 1.41)	0.006
Age	15–24	2,907 (46.31)	1		1	
	25–34	2,057 (42.57)	0.86 (0.76, 0.97)	0.016	0.68 (0.62, 0.75)	<0.0001
	35–44	1,212 (41.5)	0.82 (0.71, 0.95)	0.010	0.60 (0.54, 0.67)	<0.0001
	45–49	421 (45.36)	0.96 (0.80, 1.16)	0.688	0.62 (0.53, 0.71)	<0.0001
Current marital status	Never in union	1,673 (42.11)	1		1	
	Married	3,897 (44.66)	1.11 (0.96, 1.28)	0.152	0.82 (0.74, 0.91)	<0.0001
	Living with partner	275 (42.96)	1.04 (0.80, 1.34)	0.787	0.92 (0.77, 1.10)	0.362
	Widowed	216 (39.84)	0.91 (0.71, 1.17)	0.465	0.75 (0.61, 0.93)	0.009
	Divorced	400 (52.83)	1.54 (1.21, 1.96)	<0.0001	1.22 (1.04, 1.44)	0.017
	No longer living together/separated	136 (44.14)	1.03 (0.75, 1.40)	0.876	1.03 (0.81, 1.32)	0.807
Region	Accessible regions	3,578 (45.4)	2.19 (1.85, 2.60)	<0.0001	0.91 (0.77, 1.08)	0.293
	Hard to reach regions	2,013 (41.59)	1.88 (1.53, 2.30)	<0.0001	0.68 (0.54, 0.85)	0.001
	City administrations	1,006 (27.51)	1		1	
Education	No education	4,013 (52.67)	6.84 (4.80, 9.76)	<0.0001	3.28 (2.52, 4.27)	<0.0001
	Primary	2,227 (40.09)	4.12 (2.94, 5.76)	<0.0001	1.95 (1.51, 2.51)	<0.0001
	Secondary	260 (22.41)	1.78 (1.23, 2.56)	0.002	1.17 (0.89, 1.55)	0.261
	More than secondary	97 (13.99)	1		1	
Wealth quintile	Lowest	1,873 (55.31)	3.19 (2.59, 3.94)	<0.0001	1.40 (1.20, 1.63)	<0.0001
	Second	1,162 (50.77)	2.66 (2.14, 3.31)	<0.0001	1.25 (1.07, 1.46)	0.005
	Middle	1,094 (49.63)	2.541 (2.05, 3.15)	<0.0001	1.23 (1.06, 1.44)	0.008
	Fourth	1,058 (43.69)	2.00 (1.66, 2.42)	<0.0001	1.17 (1.01, 1.35)	0.035
	Highest	1,410 (27.93)	1		1	

TABLE 5: Factors associated with low TB knowledge among women, Ethiopia 2011, continued.

Characteristics	Category	Low knowledge n (%)	Crude OR (95% CI)	p value (crude)	Adjusted OR (95% CI)	p value (adjusted)
Occupation	Professional/technical/managerial	27 (9.02)	1		1	
	Not working	3,292 (45.25)	8.33 (4.45, 15.58)	<0.0001	1.96 (1.25, 3.09)	0.004
	Clerical/sales and services	1,138 (36.02)	5.68 (3.01, 10.69)	<0.0001	1.70 (1.08, 2.67)	0.023
	Agricultural employee	1,531 (51.38)	10.66 (5.58, 20.35)	<0.0001	2.28 (1.44, 3.60)	<0.0001
	Skilled manual	490 (41.52)	7.16 (3.63, 14.14)	<0.0001	1.81 (1.13, 2.89)	0.013
	Unskilled manual	57 (55.6)	12.62 (6.14, 25.96)	<0.0001	4.15 (2.37, 7.28)	<0.0001
Exposure to mass media	Accesses none of the three media at least once a week	2,987 (57.17)	2.19 (1.96, 2.44)	<0.0001	1.52 (1.41, 1.64)	<0.0001
	Accesses either newspaper, TV, or radio at least once a week	3,585 (37.87)	1		1	
Heard of community conversation program	No	5,203 (50.1)	2.27 (1.99, 2.57)	<0.0001	1.63 (1.52, 1.76)	<0.0001
	Yes	1,385 (30.71)	1		1	
Final model fit	Pseudo-R^2 = 0.08, Log Likelihood = −10360.78, LR χ^2 (25) = 1680.62, $p < 0.0001$					

$p = 0.002$), respectively. The odds of low TB knowledge were higher among participants with lowest and middle wealth quintiles as compared to those participants from highest wealth quintile, AORs being 1.28 (95% CI: 1.11–1.48, p = 0.001) and 1.19 (95% CI: 1.03–1.36, $p = 0.015$), respectively. Male participants who had no access to newspaper, television, or radio had 1.71 (95% CI: 1.54–1.90, $p < 0.0001$) times higher odds of low TB knowledge as compared to those who had

TABLE 6: Factors associated with low TB knowledge among men, Ethiopia 2011.

Characteristics	Category	Low knowledge n (%)	Crude OR (95% CI)	p value (crude)	Adjusted OR (95% CI)	p value (adjusted)
Residence	Urban	664 (21.11)	1			
	Rural	3,477 (35.44)	2.05 (1.67, 2.53)	<0.0001		
Age	15–24	1,871 (39.92)	1		1	
	25–34	1,010 (27.6)	0.57 (0.51, 0.65)	<0.0001	0.59 (0.52, 0.68)	<0.0001
	35–44	679 (27.19)	0.56 (0.49, 0.65)	<0.0001	0.54 (0.46, 0.63)	<0.0001
	45–49	244 (27.42)	0.57 (0.46, 0.71)	<0.0001	0.49 (0.40, 0.60)	<0.0001
Current marital status	Never in union	1,833 (36.87)	1		1	
	Married	2,061 (28.79)	0.69 (0.62, 0.78)	<0.0001	0.73 (0.64, 0.84)	<0.0001
	Living with partner	100 (31.87)	0.80 (0.54, 1.20)	0.280	1.17 (0.87, 1.57)	0.307
	Widowed	22 (37.95)	1.05 (0.51, 2.17)	0.901	0.74 (0.35, 1.60)	0.447
	Divorced	99 (41.79)	1.23 (0.87, 1.74)	0.245	1.14 (0.84, 1.54)	0.400
	No longer living together/separated	26 (22.6)	0.50 (0.25, 1.00)	0.050	0.57 (0.34, 0.96)	0.033
Region	Accessible regions	2,410 (33.14)	2.27 (1.70, 3.01)	<0.0001		
	Hard to reach regions	1,319 (34.31)	2.39 (1.76, 3.24)	<0.0001		
	City administrations	412 (17.95)	1	1		
Education	No education	1,834 (44.01)	8.74 (6.14, 12.44)	<0.0001	7.42 (5.70, 9.66)	<0.0001
	Primary	1,989 (31.16)	5.03 (3.54, 7.16)	<0.0001	3.49 (2.71, 4.48)	<0.0001
	Secondary	224 (15.8)	2.09 (1.39, 3.13)	<0.0001	1.55 (1.17, 2.05)	0.002
	More than secondary	94 (8.251)	1		1	
Wealth quintile	Lowest	1,144 (42.7)	2.86 (2.21, 3.70)	<0.0001	1.28 (1.11, 1.48)	0.001
	Second	785 (37.05)	2.26 (1.78, 2.87)	<0.0001	1.06 (0.92, 1.22)	0.390
	Middle	768 (35.66)	2.13 (1.67, 2.71)	<0.0001	1.19 (1.03, 1.36)	0.015
	Fourth	723 (30.15)	1.66 (1.31, 2.09)	<0.0001	1.01 (0.89, 1.16)	0.828
	Highest	721 (20.67)	1		1	

access to either of the three media at least once a week. The adjusted ORs for residence, occupation, and region did not show association in men and were excluded by the forward regression (Tables 6 and 7).

4. Discussion

In this study, though awareness of tuberculosis is high, specific knowledge on TB transmissions and symptoms is very low. Some major misconceptions on TB transmission are identified. The prevalence of low TB knowledge is high in the general adult population of Ethiopia, with higher magnitude among females than among males.

Rural women, younger people, less educated people, people from low socioeconomic status, those who have no access to mass media, and those who never heard of community conversation program on health and related topics have higher odds of low TB knowledge.

The level of low TB knowledge in the population in this study is in line with other small scale similar studies in different parts of Ethiopia [9, 14, 21, 22] and with studies done in other African countries and Asia [15, 16, 23, 30]. The high prevalence of low TB knowledge in the general population of Ethiopia might indicate that the current information and health education on TB is not sufficient and it is not properly addressing the target population. The situation is also exacerbated by the fact that majority of the population in Ethiopia live in low socioeconomic status and majority are from rural area (86.8%), with high rate of no formal education or only primary education (41.6% and 40.9%), no formal work (30.3%) or being only agricultural employees (38.3%), with lowest wealth index (21.4%), and no regular access to media (26.4%), or having not heard of community conversation (58.7%), which in turn are associated with low level of TB knowledge. As shown in the study by Gele et al. [18] and another study by Demissie et al. [17], low knowledge on TB is significantly associated with patient delay to seek health care, which is one of the major obstacles for controlling TB.

The finding regarding high misconception on TB transmission is comparable with other similar studies done in Africa and Asia [16, 31]. Understanding the misconceptions is very important as it might be the indication of the presence for delay of proper health seeking and refusal to take the right treatment decision and adherence to treatment. Misconception also may lead to stigma, which creates difficulty in engaging the community in TB control programs [11, 13]. Health education programs on TB need to address the common misconceptions in the community.

Table 7: Factors associated with low TB knowledge among Men, Ethiopia 2011, continued.

Characteristics	Category	Low knowledge n (%)	Crude OR (95% CI)	p value (crude)	Adjusted OR (95% CI)	p value (adjusted)
Occupation	Professional/technical/managerial	63 (7.77)	1			
	Not working	340 (34.94)	6.38 (4.03, 10.08)	<0.0001		
	Clerical/sales and services	403 (24.66)	3.89 (2.44, 6.19)	<0.0001		
	Agricultural employee	3,030 (35.84)	6.63 (4.42, 9.96)	<0.0001		
	Skilled manual	201 (21.01)	3.16 (1.99, 5.02)	<0.0001		
	Unskilled manual	64 (29.98)	5.08 (2.69, 9.60)	<0.0001		
Exposure to mass media	Accesses none of the three media at least once a week	1,096 (50.75)	2.61 (2.23, 3.05)	<0.0001	1.71 (1.54, 1.90)	<0.0001
	Accesses either newspaper, TV, or radio at least once a week	3,027 (28.31)	1		1	
Heard of community conversation program	No	5,203 (42.1)	2.39 (2.10, 2.71)	<0.0001	1.71 (1.57, 1.85)	<0.0001
	Yes	1,385 (23.35)	1		1	
Final model fit	Pseudo-R^2 = 0.104, Log Likelihood = −7164.00, LR χ^2 (17) = 1655.86, $p < 0.0001$					

The fact that the rural women are highly affected with low TB knowledge compared to urban women could be due to the fact that the majority of rural women in Ethiopia are housewives confined to household activities with fewer outside social interaction compared to male in the society. They are also exposed to different economic, cultural, geographical barriers to get access to proper information. Similar findings from North Ethiopia were reported by Mesfin [21] and other study from Vietnam [32]. Addressing the rural women will contribute to the success of the TB control program.

The poor (low wealth quintile) have high prevalence of low comprehensive TB knowledge and it is in line with the study from India [16]. As proved by the study from Manila [15], people with low income have association with low health seeking behavior. The low level of knowledge among the poor in our study worsens the low level of health seeking behavior among the poor [17]. The burden of TB is high among the poor with deprived living conditions, malnutrition, and exposure to other communicable diseases. The lack of knowledge on TB in this community will aggravate the situation as they will not know how to protect themselves from the disease, when to seek health care, the need for treatment, and the importance of adherence to treatment for TB. As a result, these would in turn create difficulty to have effective TB control program. The poor need to be addressed in the health education and information on TB and addressing the problems of the poor will contribute to the effectiveness of TB control programs.

Education is highly associated with the level of comprehensive TB knowledge, and the uneducated people and those who had only primary education had high odds of low comprehensive knowledge. This finding was supported by similar other studies [9, 15, 21, 23, 33]. The explanation might be that the educated people have more access to different sources of information and easily understand more complex messages. Increasing the level of education in the community will increase the general knowledge about infection control including TB and the general health of the people.

Access to mass media is an important factor associated with TB knowledge. Those study participants who have access to either newspaper, TV, or radios at least once a week had better TB knowledge. Increasing the access to mass media and community health education in TB control through mass media can play a key role in creating awareness and building knowledge on TB. This may encourage individuals to seek health care on timely fashion, to adhere to treatment to protect them from TB which will contribute in all over reduction of prevalence of TB.

The secondary data analysis employed in this study could have been influenced by any unknown limitations related to the primary data method of data collection and sampling procedures.

Some variables which may have effect on TB knowledge and at the same time which were not collected in the primary data are not analysed in the current study. There might also be unmeasured confounding factors affecting TB knowledge as primary data was collected for a different purpose. The TB knowledge questions collected in the primary data were not complete. Information such as knowledge on TB prevention methods and importance of adherence to treatment could have been included.

Moreover, the composite index of low TB knowledge was taken from ten variables after doing factor analysis for consistency. Due to the small number of variables included in the index construction, the Chronbach Alpha was relatively in the lower border. Including more TB prevention knowledge items such as ventilation of the households, avoiding overcrowding, avoiding of spiting in all places, protecting people from directly coughing and sneezing, and importance of using mask for contacts with infectious TB patients may increase the reliability of the overall index.

5. Conclusion and Recommendation

The result from this study produced useful information for policy makers to evaluate and shape the TB control programs and plan socioeconomic and public health measures to increase TB knowledge and further enhance the TB control programs.

Public health measures should thus focus on enhancing the health education to address the most affected population group and increase the level of TB knowledge among the general population. The education materials need to be target oriented and incorporate the basic knowledge gaps such as concepts on TB transmission, TB major symptoms, curability, prevention methods, and the importance of treatment, at the same time of addressing the misconceptions. Increasing the use of multiple mass media sources would help to improve the health education coverage and address the target populations. Increasing the regular education coverage to the population and incorporating TB to school curriculum would especially address the uneducated and the in-school youths. Most importantly, tuberculosis control programs and intervention prioritizations should consider appropriate strategies for tuberculosis education, promotion, communication, and social mobilization to address the rural women, the youth, the poor, less educated people, and unskilled workers. Additionally, the depth of the magnitude of the problem needs to be addressed by socioeconomic measures such as empowering rural women to make their own decision and to get access to information and reformulating poverty reduction strategies to improve the socioeconomic status of the people.

Further large scale study is recommended to address the unmeasured confounders and additional TB knowledge questions.

Acknowledgments

The author would like to highly acknowledge Mr. Alexander Rommel for his kind support during the study. The author would also like to thank her husband Professor Alemayehu Worku Yalew for his support and encouragement.

References

[1] N. Noah, "'Tuberculosis'. Controlling communicable disease. EnglandSL6 2QL, and Two Penn Plaza, New York, NY 10121–2289, USA," in *Understanding Public Health*, pp. 157–170, Open University Press, London School of Hygiene & Tropical Medicine, 2006.

[2] M. S. Jassal and W. R. Bishai, "Epidemiology and challenges to the elimination of global tuberculosis," *Clinical Infectious Diseases*, vol. 50, supplement 3, pp. S156–S164, 2010.

[3] Central Statistical Agency of Ethiopia and ICF International, *Ethiopia Demographic and Health Survey 2011*, MEASURE DHS Demographic and Health Surveys, Calverton, NY, USA, 2012, http://measuredhs.com/pubs/pdf/FR255/FR255.pdf, http://dhsprogram.com/Where-%20We-Work/Country%20Main.cfm?ctry_id=65&c=Ethiopia&Country=Ethiopia&cn=&r=1.

[4] CSA Ethiopia, *National Statistical Abstract,Population 2014*, Central Statistical Agency of Ethiopia, Addis Ababa, Ethiopia, 2012, http://www.csa.gov.et/index.php/2013-02-20-13-43-35/national-statistics-abstract/141-population.

[5] WHO, *Global Tuberculosis Control WHO Report 2011*, WHO, Geneva, Switzerland, 2011, http://whqlibdoc.who.int/publications/2011/9789241564380_eng.pdf.

[6] WHO, *Tuberculosis. Global Tuberculosis Report 2012*, WHO, Geneva, Switzerland, 2012, http://www.who.int/tb/publications/global_report/en/.

[7] Health Sector Development Programme IV Version 1, Annual Performance Report EFY 2003(2010/11), Ministry of Health of Federal Democratic Republic of Ethiopia, http://www.moh.gov.et/mwginternal/de5fs23hu73ds/progress?id=01qXHAb3CFDfsKf8GSMVCX7DhByQ8AysmcUH2iz6doM,&dl.

[8] WHO, *WHO and Stop TB Strategy, Building on and Enhancing DOTS to Meet the TB-Related Millennium Development Goals*, World Health Organization, Geneva, Switzerland, 2006, http://apps.who.int/iris/bitstream/10665/69241/1/WHO_HTM_STB_2006.368_eng.pdf.

[9] R. Abebe and M. Demissie, "Assessment of knowledge and practices related to tuberculosis and associated factors among HIV positive people in Addis Ababa, Ethiopia," *Global Journal of Medicine and Public Health*, vol. 1, no. 2, 2012, http://www.gjmedph.org/.

[10] E. B. Shargie and B. Lindtjørn, "Determinants of treatment adherence among smear-positive pulmonary tuberculosis patients in Southern Ethiopia," *PLoS Medicine*, vol. 4, no. 2, aticle e37, 2007.

[11] HATiP HIV & AIDS treatment in practice: TB/HIV treatment literacy, Issue 153/February 2010, http://www.aidsmap.com/.

[12] *BC Strategic Plan for Tuberculosis Prevention, Treatment and Control*, BC Communicable Disease Policy Advisory Committee, British Columbia, Canada, 2012.

[13] Fighting TB on the front lines: highlights and recommendations from the Stop-TB eForum 2005. A joint publication of Health and Development Networks and the AIDS-Care-Watch Campaign, Health and Development Networks, 2005.

[14] D. S. Abebe, D. Biffa, G. Bjune, G. Ameni, and F. Abebe, "Assessment of knowledge and practice about tuberculosis among eastern Ethiopian prisoners," *International Journal of Tuberculosis and Lung Disease*, vol. 15, no. 2, pp. 228–233, 2011.

[15] J. L. Portero Navio, M. Rubio Yuste, and M. A. Pasicatan, "Socio-economic determinants of knowledge and attitudes about tuberculosis among the general population of Metro Manila, Philippines," *The International Journal of Tuberculosis and Lung Disease*, vol. 6, no. 4, pp. 301–306, 2012.

[16] C. T. Sreeramareddy, H. N. Harsha Kumar, and J. T. Arokiasamy, "Prevalence of self-reported tuberculosis, knowledge about tuberculosis transmission and its determinants among adults in India: results from a nation-wide cross-sectional household survey," *BMC Infectious Diseases*, vol. 13, article 16, 2013.

[17] M. Demissie, B. Lindtjorn, and Y. Berhane, "Patient and health service delay in the diagnosis of pulmonary tuberculosis in Ethiopia," *BMC Public Health*, vol. 2, article 23, 2002.

[18] A. A. Gele, G. Bjune, and F. Abebe, "Pastoralism and delay in diagnosis of TB in Ethiopia," *BMC Public Health*, vol. 9, article 5, 2009.

[19] M. Belay, G. Bjune, G. Ameni, and F. Abebe, "Diagnostic and treatment delay among Tuberculosis patients in Afar Region, Ethiopia: a cross-sectional study," *BMC Public Health*, vol. 12, no. 1, article 369, 2012.

[20] D. G. Storla, S. Yimer, and G. A. Bjune, "A systematic review of delay in the diagnosis and treatment of tuberculosis," *BMC Public Health*, vol. 8, article 15, 2008.

[21] M. M. Mesfin, T. W. Tasew, I. G. Tareke, G. W. Mulugeta, and M. J. Richard, "Community knowledge, attitudes and practices on pulmonary tuberculosis and their choice of treatment supervisor in Tigray, Northern Ethiopia," *Ethiopian Journal of Health Development*, vol. 19, 2005.

[22] M. Legesse, G. Ameni, G. Mamo et al., "Knowledge and perception of pulmonary tuberculosis in pastoral communities in the middle and lower awash valley of afar region, Ethiopia," *BMC Public Health*, vol. 10, article 187, 2010.

[23] A. I. Mohamed, M. A. Yousif, P. Ottoa, and A. Bayoumi, "Knowledge of tuberculosis. A survey among tuberculosis patients in Omdurman, Sudan," *Sudanese Journal of Public Health*, vol. 2, no. 1, 2007.

[24] E. Kiefer, T. Shao, O. Carasquillo, P. Nabeta, and C. Seas, "Knowledge and attitudes of tuberculosis management in San Juan de Lurigancho district of Lima, Peru," *Journal of Infection in Developing Countries*, vol. 3, no. 10, pp. 783–788, 2009.

[25] M. A. Solliman, M. A. Hassali, M. Al-Haddad et al., "Assessment of knowledge towards tuberculosis among general population in North East Libya," *Journal of Applied Pharmaceutical Science*, vol. 2, no. 4, pp. 24–30, 2012.

[26] C. Gilpin, P. de Colombani, S. Hasanova, and U. Sirodjiddinova, "Exploring TB-related knowledge, attitude, behaviour, and practice among migrant workers in Tajikistan," *Tuberculosis Research and Treatment*, vol. 2011, Article ID 548617, 10 pages, 2011.

[27] M. Renuka and M. Dhar, "Knowledge and awareness of tuberculosis among high school students of Mysore City," *Al Ameen Journal of Medical Sciences*, vol. 5, no. 3, pp. 333–336, 2012.

[28] S. X. Jittimanee, S. Nateniyom, W. Kittikraisak et al., "Social stigma and knowledge of tuberculosis and HIV among patients with both diseases in Thailand," *PLoS ONE*, vol. 4, no. 7, Article ID e6360, 2009.

[29] A. A. Fatiregun and C. C. Ejeckam, "Determinants of patient delay in seeking treatment among pulmonary tuberculosis cases in a government specialist hospital in Ibadan, Nigeria," *Tanzania Journal of Health Research*, vol. 12, no. 2, 2010.

[30] P. Mweemba, C. Haruzirishe, S. Siziya et al., "Knowledge, attitude, compliance with TB treatment, Lusaka, Zambia," *Medical Journal of Zambia*, vol. 35, no. 4, 2008.

[31] J. A. Khan, M. Irfan, A. Zaki, M. Beg, S. F. Hussain, and N. Rizvi, "Knowledge, attitude and misconceptions regarding tuberculosis in Pakistani patients," *Journal of the Pakistan Medical Association*, vol. 56, no. 2, pp. 211–214, 2006.

[32] N. P. Hoa, A. E. K. Thorson, N. H. Long, and V. K. Diwan, "Knowledge of tuberculosis and associated health-seeking behaviour among rural Vietnamese adults with a cough for at least three weeks," *Scandinavian Journal of Public Health*, vol. 31, no. 6, supplement, pp. 59–65, 2003.

[33] E. A. Obuku, C. Meynell, J. Kiboss-Kyeyune et al., "Socio-demographic determinants and prevalence of Tuberculosis knowledge in three slum populations of Uganda," *BMC Public Health*, vol. 12, article 536, 2012.

Characteristics and Treatment Outcomes of Retreatment Tuberculosis Patients in Benin

Serge Ade,[1,2,3] Omer Adjibodé,[1] Prudence Wachinou,[1] Narcisse Toundoh,[1] Bérénice Awanou,[1] Gildas Agodokpessi,[1] Dissou Affolabi,[1] Gabriel Adè,[1] Anthony D. Harries,[3,4] and Séverin Anagonou[1]

[1] *National Tuberculosis Programme, 01 BP 321 Cotonou, Benin*
[2] *Faculté de Médecine, Université de Parakou, Parakou, Benin*
[3] *International Union against Tuberculosis and Lung Disease, Paris, France*
[4] *London School of Hygiene & Tropical Medicine, London, UK*

Correspondence should be addressed to Serge Ade; adeserg@yahoo.fr

Academic Editor: Isamu Sugawara

Objective. To determine among retreatment tuberculosis patients in Benin baseline characteristics, culture, and drug sensitivity testing (DST) results and treatment outcomes. *Materials and Methods.* A retrospective national cohort study of all retreatment tuberculosis patients in Benin in 2013 using registers and treatment cards. *Results.* Of 3957 patients with tuberculosis, 241 (6%) were retreatment cases. Compared to new pulmonary bacteriologically confirmed tuberculosis (NPBCT) patients, there were significantly higher numbers of males ($P = 0.04$), patients from "Atlantique-Littoral" ($P = 0.006$), patients aged 45–64 years ($P = 0.007$), and HIV-positive patients ($P = 0.04$) among those retreated. Overall, 171 (71%) patients submitted sputum for DST, of whom (163) 95% were positive for *Mycobacterium tuberculosis* on Xpert MTB/RIF and/or culture and 17 (10%) were rifampicin resistant (9 with MDR-TB and 8 monoresistant to rifampicin). For those without MDR-TB ($n = 224$), treatment success was 93%. Worse outcomes occurred in those with unknown HIV status (RR: 0.27; 0.05–1.45; $P < 0.01$) while better outcomes occurred in those who relapsed (RR: 1.06, 95 CI: 1.02–1.10, $P = 0.04$). *Conclusion.* In 2013, a high proportion of retreatment patients received DST. Treatment success was good although more needs to be done to systematically increase the final follow-up smear examination. Reasons of high losses to follow-up from "Oueme-Plateau" should be investigated.

1. Introduction

Patients with retreatment tuberculosis (TB) represent those who have been treated previously for one month or more with anti-TB drugs and who have been diagnosed once again with the disease. These patients mainly include relapses, treatment after failure, or loss to follow-up on a first-line treatment regimen [1]. The number of these patients is not negligible. In 2014, of the 6.3 million TB cases that were notified by National TB Programmes (NTPs) to the World Health Organization (WHO), approximately 700,000 patients were already previously treated [2].

Interest in this category of TB comes from the fact that patients are known to have a higher risk of drug resistance compared with new cases. Therefore, in addition to recommendations that all TB patients be screened for Human Immunodeficiency Virus (HIV) coinfection, NTPs have been advised since 2010 by WHO to systematically test at diagnosis all retreatment TB patients for culture and drug susceptibility (DST with genotypic and/or phenotypical methods), in order to detect resistance to rifampicin which is usually synonymous with multidrug resistance (MDR, strictly defined as resistance of *Mycobacterium tuberculosis* to both rifampicin and isoniazid) [3, 4]. Unfortunately, there is concern about implementation of this recommendation as only 58% of all retreatment TB patients in the world were tested for drug resistance in 2014 [2]. Improving this proportion in the future requires an analysis of the situation at country levels.

In Benin, a sub-Saharan country that reports approximately 40 incident TB cases per 100,000 people per year, retreatment patients account for less than 10% of all notified TB cases. Unfortunately, there is dearth of information on the epidemiological characteristics and HIV status of these patients in annual reports in the country [5]. Two previous studies, which were only conducted in Cotonou, the economic capital, and which had included retreatment patients diagnosed in the periods of 1992–2001 and 2005–2009, respectively, reported a high loss to follow-up of 12%, with a treatment success of retreatment cases significantly lower than new cases. Moreover, the majority of these patients recorded as "loss to follow-up" during the retreatment initially had also defaulted from their first-line treatment [6, 7]. DST in retreatment cases was also only performed in early 2003 in those patients registered in Cotonou that also houses the "Laboratoire de Référence des Mycobactéries (LRM)".

The current study was therefore undertaken in the whole country to determine the principal characteristics of retreatment patients, to assess how well DST was performed in this category of patients and whether there was any change in their treatment outcomes. Specific objectives were to determine among retreatment TB patients diagnosed and treated in 2013 in Benin: (i) the epidemiological, clinical and geographical characteristics and HIV status of these patients and compared to those registered with New Pulmonary Bacteriologically Confirmed TB (NPBCT); (ii) the proportion with DST results available along with the proportion showing resistance to rifampicin; (iii) treatment outcomes of these patients compared with NPBCT cases; and (iv) factors associated with a successful treatment outcome.

2. Materials and Methods

2.1. Study Design. This was a retrospective cohort study using routinely collected data.

2.2. General Setting and Study Sites

Country. Benin is a small low-income country in West Africa with a population of 10,315,244 inhabitants in 2015 [8]. The country shares borders with Burkina Faso and Niger in the north, Togo in the west, and Nigeria in the east. Benin is a low-income country with a gross national income per capita of US$1780 in 2013 and an under-five mortality rate of 85 per 1000 live births [9].

National TB Programme & Management of Patients with a Previous History of TB. The country follows the WHO DOTS strategy for diagnosis and treatment of TB patients [4]. All patients with a previous history of TB and who return to the health facility for presumptive symptoms of the disease are requested to provide two sputum samples on two consecutive days for acid-fast bacilli microscopy. Sputum samples are routinely examined using auramine-phenol staining and fluorescence microscopy. The diagnosis is confirmed by a positive result for acid-fast bacilli on sputum smears. Sputa of all confirmed retreatment TB cases in the 57 Basic Management Units (BMUs) are then sent by laboratory technicians using cetylpyridinium chloride solution to the LRM for both Xpert MTB/RIF and culture on Lowenstein-Jensen media. All retreatment TB patients, except those diagnosed in Cotonou, start on a standardised regimen of retreatment [3]. When the result of Xpert MTB/RIF is available (this usually takes some days or weeks), those who are found sensitive to rifampicin continue the standardised regimen. On the other hand, patients with resistance to rifampicin are switched to a MDR-TB treatment regimen.

Because of the closeness of the LRM, patients treated in Cotonou do not start TB treatment unless their Xpert MTB/RIF is available. This takes approximately 24 hours. The standardised retreatment regimen consists of an initial phase of rifampicin, isoniazid, ethambutol, and pyrazinamide for 3 months (with streptomycin added during the first 2 months) followed by a continuation phase using the first three anti-TB drugs for 5 months [3]. The treatment is strictly directly observed during the initial phase. Patients with resistance to rifampicin are treated with a shortened 9-month regimen recommended by the International Union against Tuberculosis and Lung Disease [10]. During retreatment of rifampicin sensitive patients, sputum samples are collected at 3 months, at 5 months, and at the end of the treatment for microscopy. Treatment is monitored through the use of treatment cards and registers. A quarterly supervision of all the 57 BMUs is systematically organized by the TB control programme coordination. All retreatment TB patients are systematically offered HIV testing at diagnosis. Those who are found coinfected receive co-trimoxazole, and Antiretroviral Therapy (ART) is provided within 2 weeks to 2 months after TB treatment initiation [11].

All molecular tests, culture, DST, TB treatment, co-trimoxazole, and ART are provided free of charge. Anti-TB and ARV drugs are not available in private pharmacies.

2.3. Study Population. All retreatment TB patients diagnosed and treated between January and December 2013 were included in the study.

2.4. Data Variables, Sources of Data, Data Collection Tools, and Definition of Variables. For each retreatment TB case, data were collected on epidemiological characteristics, region, HIV status, type of retreatment, ART status for HIV-positive patients, Xpert MTB/RIF results, culture and DST results, and treatment outcomes. Sources of data were TB registers and TB treatment cards. Xpert MTB/RIF, culture, and phenotypical DST results were extracted from a laboratory Excel file. For comparison, aggregate data of NPBCT patients were collected from the annual report. Data on patients were collected into a paper based questionnaire. Because of the retrospective nature of this study, data validation was not possible. The definitions of the NPBCT, the different types of previously treated patients, and the treatment and outcomes are explained in Table 1.

2.5. Analysis and Statistics. Data from the questionnaire were double entered into an electronic file using EpiData software and analysed using this software (EpiData version 3.1 for entry and version 2.2.2.182 for analysis, EpiData Association,

TABLE 1: New category of patients and treatment outcomes recommended by the WHO [1].

	Definitions
Category of TB patients	
New pulmonary bacteriologically confirmed patients	Patients never treated for TB (or treated for less than 1 month) and whose sputum is positive by smear microscopy, culture, or WHO-approved Rapid Diagnostic (such as Xpert MTB/RIF)
Previously treated patients	Patients have received 1 month or more of anti-TB drugs in the past
Relapse patients	Patients have previously been treated for TB, were declared *cured* or *treatment completed* at the end of their most recent course of treatment, and are now diagnosed with a recurrent episode of TB
Treatment after failure patients	Patients have previously been treated for TB and *failed treatment* during or at the end of their most recent treatment course
Treatment after loss to follow-up patients	Patients have previously been treated for TB and were declared *lost to follow-up* during or at the end of their most recent course of treatment
Other previously treated patients	Patients have previously been treated for TB but their outcome after their most recent course of treatment is unknown or undocumented
Patients with unknown previous TB treatment history	Patients do not fit into any of the categories listed above
Treatment outcomes	
Cured	A pulmonary TB patient with bacteriologically confirmed TB at the beginning of treatment who was smear- or culture-negative in the last month of treatment and on at least one previous occasion
Treatment completed	A TB patient who completed treatment without evidence of failure, but with no record to show that sputum smear or culture results in the last month of treatment and on at least one previous occasion were negative, either because tests were not done or because results were unavailable
Treatment failed	A TB patient whose sputum smear or culture is positive at month 5 or later during treatment
Died	A TB patient who dies for any reason before starting or during the course of treatment
Loss to follow-up	A TB patient who did not start treatment or whose treatment was interrupted for 2 consecutive months or more
Not evaluated	A TB patient for whom no treatment outcome is assigned; this includes cases "transferred out" to another treatment unit as well as cases for whom the treatment outcome is unknown to the reporting unit
Treatment success	The sum of *cured* and *treatment completed*

Odense, Denmark). Data were analysed by using frequencies and percentages. Comparisons between categorical variables were done using the chi-square test and risk ratios as appropriate with 95% confidence intervals. Levels of significance were set at 5%.

3. Results

In 2013, 241 retreatment TB patients were diagnosed and treated in Benin on the basis of a positive result for acid-fast bacilli using sputum smear microscopy. They represented 6% of the 3957 total TB cases notified in the country in the same time-period. Demographic characteristics and HIV status of these patients were compared to those reported from NPBCT and are shown in Table 2. There were significantly more males ($P = 0.04$), patients from the "Atlantique-Littoral" ($P = 0.006$), patients aged between 45 and 64 years ($P = 0.007$), and HIV-positive patients ($P = 0.04$) among retreatment TB cases compared to NPBCT patients. On the other hand, patients younger than 24 years were significantly less common among previously treated patients ($P < 0.001$). Demographic characteristics and HIV status of the different types of retreatment TB cases are compared in Table 3. "Oueme-Plateau" reported significantly more "treatment after loss to follow-up cases" ($P < 0.001$) while "Atlantique-Littoral" reported more "relapse cases" ($P = 0.04$). In addition, significantly more males were found in "treatment after loss to follow-up" ($P = 0.03$). Otherwise, no significant differences were found.

The results of Xpert MTB/RIF and/or *Mycobacterium tuberculosis* culture among retreatment TB patients and rifampicin sensitivity are presented in Table 4. Overall, 71% of the 241 retreatment TB patients submitted their sputum for DST, and 95% of these patients showed a positive result on Xpert MTB/RIF and/or culture for *M. tuberculosis.* Of these patients, 17 (10%) were found to have resistance to rifampicin (9 with MDR-TB and 8 with monoresistance to rifampicin) and they were redirected to a MDR-TB treatment regimen.

Treatment outcomes of the remaining 224 retreatment TB patients were compared with those for NPCBT cases and

TABLE 2: Demographic characteristics and HIV status of new pulmonary bacteriologically confirmed and retreatment tuberculosis patients, Benin, 2013.

	NPBCT*	Retreatment TB	*P* value
Total	3129	241	
Sex			
Male	2063 (65.9)	175 (72)	0.04
Female	1066 (34.1)	67 (28)	0.04
Age (years)			
00–24	600 (19.2)	21 (8.7)	0.00005
25–44	1705 (54.5)	136 (56.6)	0.55
45–64	676 (21.6)	70 (28.9)	0.007
65 and above	148 (4.7)	14 (5.8)	0.43
Region			
Atacora-Donga	199 (6.4)	14 (5.8)	0.72
Borgou-Alibori	231 (7.4)	13 (5.4)	0.24
Zou-Collines	416 (13.3)	33 (13.7)	0.86
Mono-Couffo	486 (15.5)	29 (12)	0.14
Oueme-Plateau	708 (22.6)	47 (19.5)	0.26
Atlantique-Littoral	1089 (34.8)	105 (43.6)	0.006
HIV status			
HIV positive	396 (13.5*)	43 (18.2**)	0.04
HIV negative	—	193 (82)	—
Unknown	—	5 (2.4)	—

Note: NPBCT: new pulmonary bacteriologically confirmed tuberculosis. TB: tuberculosis.
*Of the 2934 new pulmonary bacteriologically confirmed tuberculosis patients who underwent the HIV test, 396 were found positive.
**Of the 236 retreatment tuberculosis patients who underwent the HIV test, 43 were found positive.

the results are shown in Table 5. In 2013, the success rate of these patients was 93%. There were significantly more patients who completed their treatment without achieving the last follow-up examination, but otherwise there were no other differences between the groups. Factors associated with a successful outcome are presented in Table 6. Patients with relapse TB had a significantly higher chance of successful treatment outcome (RR: 1.06, 95 CI: 1.02–1.10, $P = 0.04$) while those with an unknown HIV status had a worse treatment outcome (RR: 0.27; 0.05–1.45; $P < 0.01$). In this cohort, in which all but one of the HIV-positive patients were on ART, no significant difference in treatment success was found between HIV-positive and HIV-negative patients.

4. Discussion

The main findings of this study were the predominance of males, adults aged between 45 and 64 years, and HIV-positive status among retreatment TB cases compared with NPBCT patients. Most of these previously treated TB patients were reported from "Atlantique-Littoral" where there were also predominately "relapse cases." The large majority of patients who were reported from "Oueme-Plateau" were recorded as "lost to follow-up" prior to treatment, which is a department close to "Atlantique-Littoral" in the southern part of the country. Rifampicin sensitivity-status was known in nearly three-fourths of patients with one-tenth of those tested having resistance to rifampicin and therefore requiring a MDR-TB treatment regimen. Treatment outcomes of patients who were found without resistance to rifampicin were excellent, although some did not achieve the last follow-up sputum smear examination after treatment completion. Patients who relapsed had a greater chance of a successful treatment outcome, while those with unknown HIV status had worse treatment outcomes.

The strengths of this study were the inclusion of all retreatment TB patients diagnosed in the country, and therefore there was no need for any sampling framework. The study report also followed Strengthening the Reporting of Observational Studies in Epidemiology (STROBE) guidelines [12]. Data used for this study had been checked and validated during regular quarterly supervision of the 57 BMUs from the central unit. Limitations include the operational nature of the study and the use of routine data from registers and quarterly reports. Some information such as time to relapse after a previous treatment is often missed and therefore could not be included in the study.

This is the first assessment one year after the NTP coordination decided as a policy to perform DST at diagnosis for all retreatment cases countrywide. Benefits from the implementation of such a recommendation can be seen from this study. MDR-TB patients can promptly start appropriate treatment without having to start and fail a retreatment regimen, which has individual benefits as well as preventing further transmission of drug-resistant TB in the community. Studies from India have also shown that this approach improves treatment outcomes among previously treated patients [13]. According to our study findings, one-quarter of the patients did not achieve this goal of DST. The proportion of previously treated patients in whom DST has been performed largely varies according to the study settings, from less than 10% in the midwest Nepal to 91% in Sri Lanka [14, 15].

One of the major challenges in achieving DST for all patients that arose from discussions with health workers and that has also been reported elsewhere is related to transportation issues of samples from laboratories in BMUs to the LRM. This is a key step for successful implementation of culture and DST, particularly in resources-limited countries. In Benin, several options of sample transportation have been tried. In the first option, sputum specimens once collected were appropriately packaged in specific boxes in BMUs; and, during quarterly supervisions, national teams had the opportunity to bring them back to the LRM for analysis with results communicated later to the TB health workers in the BMUs. The consequences of this approach, however, were the high likelihood of having a negative culture due to lengthy times between sputum collection and the plating of specimens on Lowenstein-Jensen culture media and the subsequent delays in diagnosing and treating patients requiring MDR-TB treatment. In the second option, laboratory technicians in BMUs were requested to bring to the LRM specimens from patients and they were reimbursed for transportation. Unfortunately the high cost of this option did not allow it to continue. The third option and the current strategy is to send

TABLE 3: Demographic characteristics and HIV status of the different types of retreatment tuberculosis patients, Benin, 2013.

	Relapse	Failure	Treatment after loss to follow-up	*P* value
Total	147	78	16	
Sex				
Male	102 (69.4)	56 (71.8)	16 (100)	0.03
Female	45 (30.6)	22 (28.2)	—	0.03
Age (years)				
00–24	10 (6.8)	10 (12.8)	1 (6.3)	0.29
25–44	86 (58.5)	42 (53.8)	8 (50)	0.69
45–64	42 (28.6)	22 (28.2)	6 (37.5)	0.74
65 and +	9 (6.1)	4 (5.1)	1 (6.3)	—
Regions				
Atacora-Donga	8 (5.4)	6 (7.7)	0	—
Borgou-Alibori	7 (4.8)	6 (7.7)	0	—
Zou-Collines	16 (10.9)	16 (20.5)	1 (6.3)	0.09
Mono-Couffo	16 (10.9)	12 (15.4)	1 (6.3)	0.46
Oueme-Plateau	27 (18.4)	10 (12.8)	10 (62.5)	0.00002
Atlantique-Littoral	73 (49.7)	28 (35.9)	4 (25)	0.04
HIV status				
HIV positive	27 (18.4)	14 (17.9)	2 (12.5)	0.84
HIV negative	116 (78.9)	63 (80.8)	14 (87.5)	0.70
Unknown	4 (2.7)	1 (1.3)	0	—

TABLE 4: Retreatment tuberculosis patients, drug susceptibility testing achieved, and bacilli sensitivity to rifampicin, Benin, 2013.

Total retreatment TB patients	241
Patients whose specimens were sent to the LRM for DST tests (∗)	171 (71)
MTB identification after culture and or Xpert MTB/RIF$	163 (95)
Xpert (+) Culture (+) ($)	86 (50)
Xpert (+) Culture (−) ($)	72 (42)
Xpert (−) Culture (+) ($)	5 (3)
Resistance to rifampicin ($)	17¥ (10)

Note: TB: tuberculosis; LRM: "Laboratoire de Références des Mycobactéries"; DST: drug susceptibility testing.
*The percentage was derived from the total tuberculosis patients retreated.
$The percentage was derived from the total tuberculosis patients whose sputa were sent and analysed in LRM.
¥Of the 17 patients with resistance to rifampicin, there were 9 multidrug resistant and 8 monoresistant.

TABLE 5: Treatment outcomes of new pulmonary bacteriologically confirmed and retreatment tuberculosis patients, Benin, 2013.

	NPBCT*	Retreatment TB	*P* value
Total	3124$	224£	
Successful outcome	2803 (89.7)	208 (92.9)	0.12
Cure	2587 (82.8)	184 (82.1)	0.79
Completion	216 (6.9)	24 (10.7)	0.03
Unsuccessful outcome	321 (10.3)	16 (7.1)	0.13
Failure	91 (2.9)	3 (1.3)	0.16
Death	170 (5.4)	9 (4)	0.37
Loss to follow-up	45 (1.4)	3 (1.3)	0.83
Not evaluated	15 (0.5)	1 (0.4)	0.72

Note: TB: tuberculosis.
*NPBCT: new pulmonary bacteriologically confirmed tuberculosis.
$Of the 3129 new smear positive TB patients treated, treatment outcomes were assessed for 3124 patients in 2013.
£Of the 241 retreatment tuberculosis patients treated, 18 were found multidrug resistant and did not continue the retreatment regimen.

Table 6: Factors associated with a successful treatment among retreatment tuberculosis patients, 2013, Benin.

	Successful outcome	Risk ratio	[95% CI]	*P* value
Sex				
Female	60/62 (97.8)	1		
Male	148/162 (91.4)	0.94	0.88–1.01	0.24
Age group				
00–24	19/19 (100)	1		
25–44	117/124 (94.4)	0.94	0.90–0.99	0.59
45–64	60/67 (89.6)	0.90	0.83–0.97	0.34
65 and +	12/14 (85.7)	0.86	0.69–1.06	0.17
Type of TB				
NPBCT	2803/3124 (89.7)	1		
Relapse	133/140 (95)	1.06	1.02–1.10	0.04
Failure	63/69 (91.3)	1.02	0.95–1.10	0.67
Treatment after loss to follow-up	12/15 (80)	0.89	0.69–1.15	0.19
HIV status				
HIV negative	169/181 (93.4)	1		
HIV positive	38/39 (97)	1.04	0.98–1.11	0.47
HIV status unknown	1/4 (25)	0.27	0.05–1.46	0.001
Region				
Atacora-Donga	13/14 (92.9)	1.01	0.86–1.18	1
Borgou-Alibori	9/11 (81.8)	0.89	0.67–1.10	0.26
Zou-Collines	28/30 (93.3)	1.02	0.91–1.14	1
Mono-Couffo	27/28 (96.4)	1.05	0.96–1.15	0.68
Oueme-Plateau	40/42 (95.2)	1.04	0.95–1.13	0.72
Atlantique-Littoral	91/99 (91.9)	1		

Note: NPBCT: new pulmonary bacteriologically confirmed tuberculosis; TB: tuberculosis.

sputum specimens as soon as these are collected to the LRM through public transportation with transportation charges immediately refunded at receipt in the LRM. This strategy seems to be working well and contributes to an increase in the proportion of retreatment TB patients being tested. For example, an assessment of the 2014 programme activities of diagnosis and treatment of TB by the International Union against Tuberculosis and Lung Diseases estimated that 85% to 92% of retreatment TB patients in that year submitted sputum specimens to the LRM (Unpublished data, V. Schwoebel, Benin; TB control Programme, Annual report number 30; International Union against Tuberculosis and Lung Diseases). Finally, the forthcoming decentralization of Xpert MTB/RIF machines in regional laboratories will undoubtedly increase the proportion of patients having sputum specimens tested and this should accelerate the achievement of 100% DST.

There are a few other points to note. The proportion of patients requiring a MDR-TB treatment regimen in the country in 2013 was not higher in comparison with previous years [16, 17]. A predominance of males among retreatment TB cases was found in this study and this has also been reported elsewhere, although the reasons for this are not known [18]. "Atlantique-Littoral," which houses Cotonou, the economic capital and the city with the highest density of population, always reports the highest number of TB cases in the country; and we are not surprised that this is also the case for retreatment TB cases. In terms of treatment outcomes and in comparison with previous reports, there have been improvements. We noticed that patients who were recorded as "lost to follow-up" are no longer at higher risk of defaulting during their retreatment [6, 7]. The treatment success is also higher than that observed elsewhere [13]. Furthermore, of the different types of retreatment TB patients, the highest success rate was reported in those who relapsed. Possible reasons for better outcomes include the following: (a) this is a new exogenous infection with drug-susceptible *Mycobacterium tuberculosis* rather than reactivation of a drug-resistant strain and (b) there is more awareness about TB symptoms and treatment management from the first experience with the disease resulting in earlier diagnosis. A worse treatment outcome was also reported in patients with unknown HIV status. In this group, it is possible that an HIV-positive status was known but the patient attempted to hide it with a consequent lack of appropriate HIV-care delivery.

The study has some implications for the programme. First, since the large majority of "loss to follow-up" patients retreated were from a specific region, there is a need to address the reasons why these patients stopped their first line treatment. Second, although the treatment success was good, we need to be stricter on ensuring that the last follow-up sputum examination is performed as these patients are being treated for the second time and are potentially at high risk of drug resistance. Third, although the proportion of TB patients with known HIV status is high (96%) in the country [5], it is important to try to screen all TB cases because of the poor treatment outcomes in those with unknown HIV status.

5. Conclusion

In 2013, the proportion of retreatment TB patients tested for culture and DST in Benin was 71%. Although the treatment success of these patients was encouraging, there is room for improvement. There is a need to increase the proportion of patients having the last follow-up sputum examination and to understand why one of the regions of the country has a sizeable number of patients recorded as "lost to follow-up."

Ethical Approval

The study was approved by the Benin NTP Coordination and the "Ethics Advisory Group" of the International Union against Tuberculosis and Lung Disease, Paris. Because of its retrospective nature, approval from the national ethics committee "Comité National d'Ethique pour la Recherche en Santé" was not required according to the country's recommendations.

Competing Interests

All authors declared no competing interests.

Acknowledgments

The authors thank all workers in the 57 health facilities involved in tuberculosis management in the country for their daily hard work. The authors also thank The Union for technical and financial support in this study. S. Ade is partly supported as a Union Operational Research Fellow.

References

[1] World Health Organization, "Definitions and reporting framework for tuberculosis—2013 revision," Tech. Rep. WHO/HTM/TB/2013.2, World Health Organization, Geneva, Switzerland, 2013, http://apps.who.int/iris/bitstream/10665/79199/1/9789241505345_eng.pdf.

[2] World Health Organization, *Global Tuberculosis Report 2015*, WHO/HTM/TB/2015.22, World Health Organization, Geneva, Switzerland, 2015, http://apps.who.int/iris/bitstream/10665/191102/1/9789241565059_eng.pdf?ua=1.

[3] World Health Organization, *Treatment of Tuberculosis: Guidelines for National Programmes*, WHO/HTM/TB/2009.420, World Health Organization, Geneva, Switzerland, 2009, http://apps.who.int/iris/bitstream/10665/44165/1/9789241547833_eng.pdf.

[4] TB CARE I, *International Standards for Tuberculosis Care*, TB CARE I, The Hague, Netherlands, 3rd edition, 2014, http://www.who.int/tb/publications/ISTC_3rdEd.pdf?ua=1.

[5] World Health Organization, *Tuberculosis Country Profiles: Benin*, World Health Organization, Geneva, Switzerland, 2015, https://extranet.who.int/sree/Reports?op=Replet&name=%2FTBCountryProfile&ISO2=BJ&LAN=EN&outtype=html.

[6] M. Gninafon, L. Tawo, F. Kassa et al., "Outcome of tuberculosis retreatment in routine conditions in Cotonou, Benin," *International Journal of Tuberculosis and Lung Disease*, vol. 8, no. 10, pp. 1242–1247, 2004.

[7] G. Agodokpessi, G. Ade, B. H. Mbatchou Ngahane et al., "Evaluation of tuberculous patient's management when retreated in Cotonou, Benin," *Revue des Maladies Respiratoires*, vol. 30, no. 9, pp. 774–779, 2013.

[8] Institut National de la Statistique et de l'Analyse Économique, *La Population Béninoise*, http://www.insae-bj.org/population.html.

[9] World Health Organization, *Benin: World Health Organization Statistical Profile*, World Health Organization, Geneva, Switzerland, 2014, http://www.who.int/gho/countries/ben.pdf?ua=1.

[10] J. A. Caminero, *Guidelines for Clinical and Operational Management of Drug-Resistant Tuberculosis*, International Union of Tuberculosis and Lung Disease, Paris, France, 2013.

[11] World Health Organization, *Antiretroviral Therapy for HIV Infection in Adults and Adolescents. Recommendations for a Public Health Approach*, World Health Organization, Geneva, Switzerland, 2010, http://apps.who.int/iris/bitstream/10665/44379/1/9789241599764_eng.pdf.

[12] E. Von Elm, D. G. Altman, M. Egger, S. J. Pocock, P. C. Gøtzsche, and J. P. Vandenbrouckef, "The strengthening the reporting of observational studies in epidemiology (STROBE) statement: guidelines for reporting observational studies," *Bulletin of the World Health Organization*, vol. 85, no. 11, pp. 867–872, 2007.

[13] P. Dave, B. Vadera, A. M. V. Kumar et al., "Has introduction of rapid drug susceptibility testing at diagnosis impacted treatment outcomes among previously treated tuberculosis patients in Gujarat, India?" *PLoS ONE*, vol. 10, no. 4, Article ID e0121996, 2015.

[14] M. B. Tharu, A. D. Harries, S. Goel et al., "Screening retreatment tuberculosis patients for drug resistance in mid-west Nepal: how well are we doing?" *Public Health Action*, vol. 4, no. 1, pp. 60–65, 2014.

[15] S. C. Abeygunawardena, B. N. Sharath, R. Van den Bergh, B. Naik, N. Pallewatte, and M. N. Masaima, "Management of previously treated tuberculosis patients in Kalutara district, Sri Lanka: how are we faring?" *Public Health Action*, vol. 4, no. 2, pp. 105–109, 2014.

[16] D. Affolabi, O. A. B. G. Adjagba, B. Tanimomo-Kledjo, M. Gninafon, S. Y. Anagonou, and F. Portaels, "Anti-tuberculosis drug resistance among new and previously treated pulmonary tuberculosis patients in Cotonou, Benin," *International Journal of Tuberculosis and Lung Disease*, vol. 11, no. 11, pp. 1221–1224, 2007.

[17] S. Ade, A. Trébucq, A. D. Harries et al., "MDR-TB treatment needs in patients previously treated for TB in Cotonou, Benin," *Public Health Action*, vol. 3, no. 2, pp. 160–165, 2013.

[18] S. S. Sarpal, N. K. Goel, D. Kumar, and A. K. Janmeja, "Gender disparities in retreatment patients of tuberculosis: a north Indian study," *Journal of Natural Science, Biology and Medicine*, vol. 6, no. 1, pp. 63–66, 2015.

25

TB Notification from Private Health Sector in Delhi, India: Challenges Encountered by Programme Personnel and Private Health Care Providers

Mahasweta Satpati,[1] Sharath Burugina Nagaraja,[2] Hemant Deepak Shewade,[3] Prabhakaran Ottapura Aslesh,[4] Blesson Samuel,[5] Ashwani Khanna,[6] and Sarabjit Chadha[3]

[1] *Population Services International (PSI), New Delhi, India*
[2] *ESIC Medical College and PGIMSR, Bangalore, India*
[3] *International Union Against Tuberculosis and Lung Disease (The Union), South-East Asia Regional Office, New Delhi, India*
[4] *Department of Community Medicine, Academy of Medical Sciences, Pariyaram, Kerala, India*
[5] *World Vision India, New Delhi, India*
[6] *State TB Office, New Delhi, India*

Correspondence should be addressed to Mahasweta Satpati; mahaswetasatpati@gmail.com

Academic Editor: Vincent Jarlier

Objective. To identify the challenges encountered by private health care providers (PHCP) to notify tuberculosis cases through a programme developed web-based portal mechanism called "NIKSHAY." *Study Design.* It is a descriptive qualitative study conducted at two revised national tuberculosis control programme (RNTCP) districts of New Delhi. The study included in-depth interviews of PHCP registered with "NIKSHAY" and RNTCP programme personnel. Grounded theory was used to conceptualise the latent social patterns in implementation of tuberculosis case notification process and promptly identifying their challenges. *Results.* The analysis resulted in identification of three broad themes: (a) system implementation by RNTCP: it emphasizes the TB notification process by the RNTCP programme personnel; (b) challenges faced by PHCP for TB notification with five different subthemes; and (c) perceived gaps and suggestions: to improvise the TB notification process for the private health sector. The challenges encountered by PHCP were mainly related to unsystematic planning and suboptimal implementation by programme personnel at the state and district level. The PHCP lacked clarity on the need for TB notification. *Conclusion.* Implementation of TB notification among private health care providers requires systematic planning by the programme personnel. The process should be user-friendly with additional benefits to the patients.

1. Introduction

In India, tuberculosis continues to be the major public health problem. It accounts for 27% (2.8 million) of the estimated global annual incidence of 10.4 million tuberculosis (TB) cases [1]. Inappropriate diagnosis and irrational, incomplete treatment have led to emergence of drug resistant TB cases which are estimated to be 99,000 cases annually in the country [1, 2]. Globally, one-third of the nearly nine million people are estimated to fall ill with TB each year and many out of them could not be reached by TB programme. This "missing" patient, of population over three million, has stubbornly remained unchanged since 2007 [3].

During the year 2012, the Government of India had made notification of TB mandatory for the public and private health sector [4]. In 2014, global reporting system created by WHO measured a marked increase in global TB notifications. The annual total of new TB cases increased globally to 6%, mostly due to a 29% increase in TB notifications in India [5]. The increase can be attributed to the increased TB notification which otherwise was not notified earlier to the programme.

TABLE 1: Notification profile of "NIKSHAY" registered PHCP in NDMC and GTB RNTCP districts of Delhi state, 2014.

Stratification of private health care providers	NDMC RNTCP district			GTB RNTCP district		
	Number registered in NIKSHAY	Number notifying patients with TB	Number of patients with TB notified	Number registered in NIKSHAY	Number notifying patients with TB	Number of patients with TB notified
Laboratories	2	2	**178**	16	0	**0**
Private practitioners clinic/single private practitioners	27	0	**0**	21	1	**90**
Hospitals/clinics/nursing home	3	0	**0**	5	3	**0**
Total	32	2	**178**	42	4	**90**

RNTCP: revised national tuberculosis control programme; NIKSHAY: web-based portal for notification and follow-up of patients with TB; NDMC: New Delhi Municipal Corporation; GTB: Guru Teg Bahadur Chest clinic.

The RNTCP is promoting and advocating a web-based online reporting mechanism called "NIKSHAY" for TB notification. To start notifying the disease the practitioner had to get registered in the "NIKSHAY" web-based system. Initially, this process of registration into the system was facilitated by the RNTCP programme personnel.

The public health sector had begun notifying the disease through "NIKSHAY": however, the notification from the private health sector remained suboptimal [1]. It is important considering more than 40% of TB cases are catered by private sector and nearly half of them are missed by the TB notification system [6]. In 2013, of all the total notified TB cases from New Delhi state no cases were notified by the private sector [7].

Due to expanding horizons and strategies under RNTCP, the programme managers and personnel were incapacitated by limited overburdened programme personnel [6, 8]. Conceptually, it was presumed that TB notification as a strategy in private health sector would be difficult to implement as there was no organized system in order to make notification a routine practice. There were only few studies on knowledge and gaps of private health care providers (PHCP) on TB notification, therefore, limiting information on the prevailing implementation issues related to notification system [8, 9]. Hence, we conducted this qualitative study to explore the challenges encountered by the RNTCP programme personnel and PHCP registered in "NIKSHAY" to routinely operationalize TB notification in New Delhi, India. The study finding has the potential to improve the manner in which the programme is implemented through PHCP at New Delhi, India.

2. Methods

2.1. Study Design. It is a qualitative study involving grounded theory approach. The data collection has been done through in-depth interviews for respondents selected through purposive sampling techniques. Content analysis was performed for data analysis.

2.2. Setting. The study was conducted at New Delhi during 1st December 2014 to 31st October 2015. A total of nine administrative districts are established and for the purpose of RNTCP programme implementation these are subdivided into 26 programme management units or RNTCP districts [10]. All the programme management units have similar human resources and logistics pattern for programme implementation. Based on the feasibility and convenience we purposively selected the following two RNTCP districts: New Delhi Municipal Corporation (NDMC) and the Guru Teg Bahadur (GTB) Chest clinic. These RNTCP districts have a population of 6.1 and 7.6 lakhs and had registered 1,417 and 1,914 TB patients, respectively, between October 2012 and September 2013 out of 1,52,181 TB cases registered at Delhi state [7]. The number of patients with TB notified by the PHCP in these two RNTCP districts during 2014 is shown in Table 1.

2.3. Study Participants and Sampling. A purposive sampling method with maximum variation was adopted depending on the respondents consent and availability. The aim of using a maximum variation in purposive sampling method was to purposively select heterogeneous population which maximize the diversity relevant for the research study. The RNTCP programme personnel and the PHCP registered in "NIKSHAY" between January 2014 and April 2015 at these two RNTCP districts constituted the study population. A total of 11 programme personnel and 19 PHCP were the respondents for in-depth interviews. The mean duration of time for the entire interviews was up to thirty minutes. The RNTCP programme personnel includes the District TB officer (DTO), who is overall in-charge for RNTCP implementation in the entire district, senior treatment supervisor (STS) who is responsible for TB treatment registration and supervision of patients with TB in 5,00,000 population, and the TB health visitor (TBHV) who is responsible for facilitating initiation of domiciliary treatment for patients with TB in 100,000 population.

The list of PHCP registered with "NIKSHAY" were obtained from the programme and for the purpose of sampling, the list of registered PHCP was further stratified into (a) laboratories, (b) private practitioners clinics/single private practitioners, and (c) hospitals/clinics/nursing homes. It was mainly done to obtain uniform representativeness from different type of health care providers. As it was a qualitative study the minimum numbers of sample size and sampling units were not required [11, 12]. Each of the RNTCP programme personnel cadre and the stratified PHCP were considered as sampling units [10].

2.4. Data Collection. Interview guides were prepared to elicit relevant information from RNTCP programme personnel and PHCP. Broadly, the programme personnel interview guide focused on the registration process of health facilities under RNTCP, their experiences in learning the phases of registration, and the web-based notification process. Emphasis was placed on challenges encountered for implementation and their plausible solutions [13]. Before interviewing the guides were pilot tested between January and June 2015. Informed consent was obtained from the respondents after explaining the purpose of the study and permission was sought to use audio recording during the interviews. Places for interviews were chosen by the respondents and interviews were conducted at a time which was convenient and comfortable for them. There were no repeat interviews and only the principal investigator (PI) engaged the respondents for interviews. The summary of the interviews were discussed with the respondents to ensure participant validation.

The PI stopped interviewing respondents once redundancy or consistency in responses was identified. The redundancy was defined as repetition of description of incidents for implementation of TB case notification process and its challenges.

2.5. Data Analysis and Management. To maintain consistency in data collection and in order to obtain respondent's concerns on TB notification, the grounded theory of data collection was adopted [13, 14]. The theory helped us to conceptualise the latent social patterns involved in implementation of TB case notification process and challenges. Interviews were transcribed and a constant comparative analysis was employed and an inductive analysis was carried out with focus on content to elicit codes and themes. Open type of coding method was employed, for the data analysis [15]. The analysis followed emergent codes from the responses of the individual respondents. To elicit codes the PI read and identified underlying meaning of the sentences and wrote them on the margins by clustering similar topics, unique topics, and other left over topics. The process was repeated till new codes emerged from the text [11]. After completing the process the PI identified themes for analysis [15]. Data relevant to each category was identified and examined using a process called constant comparison to establish analytical categories. The analysis of transcribed data was first performed by the PI and then independently analysed by the coinvestigators. For a common understanding of codes and establishing the intercoder reliability codes were discussed among two coinvestigators. Consultation within team was also held to decide about the next steps of data collection and to ensure the analysis followed the constant comparative steps of grounded theory to reach a saturation of details. To ensure descriptive validity and consistency both the researchers interpreted the data and made inferences about the findings [16]. The software Atlas Ti (version 6.0) was used for management of the data [17].

Complete, deidentified representative statements were included in the results to illustrate the main themes. The available themes from the programme personnel and PHCP interviews were conceptualised into broad categories, such as (a) system implementation by RNTCP; (b) challenges encountered by PHCP; (c) gaps and suggestions. A COREQ guideline was followed for reporting the qualitative aspects of the study [18].

2.6. Ethical Approval. Ethics Advisory Group, International Union Against Tuberculosis and Lung Disease (The Union), Paris, and Research Ethics Board of Population Services International approved this study. Administrative approval to conduct the study was obtained from RNTCP, Delhi, India. At times, when the programme personnel and private health providers were hesitant to provide written informed consent before speaking on sensitive issue such as "TB notification," we sought oral consent for the interviews. The Ethics Committees approved the consent procedure and recording of interviews.

3. Results

The complete process of how the activities were performed by RNTCP staff, flow of information, implementation of TB notification system and challenges faced by RNTCP and PHCP, gaps, and suggestions are discussed in this section. A theoretical model is represented showing interrelationships between themes (Figure 1). The themes have been organized into the building blocks of the emerging theoretical model. The relationships between the themes are visualized with arrows to show the direction in which the process proceeded. The themes and information areas are labeled under RNTCP and PHCP. The details of the thematic structure observed and analysed during the interviews are enumerated below with detailed select quotes exemplifying the content.

3.1. System Implementation by RNTCP. The implementation process for TB notification system was driven by the state RNTCP. The strategy involved introduction of "NIKSHAY" web site at state and district levels. As a process the line lists of PHCP were prepared at district level and they were to be motivated for registering into the newer reporting mechanism "NIKSHAY."

> *At first we received a mail from STO to DTO, and then we were informed. Then we informed tuberculosis health visitors that the private practitioner who does treatment of TB patients should be met, they met them took their registered number, contact number and prepared a list and submitted to office. (41 years, male, RNTCP programme personnel, Delhi)*

> *Initially there was a difference as the processes were not planned. It took a one whole year to process the discussion. (50 years, male, RNTCP programme personnel, Delhi)*

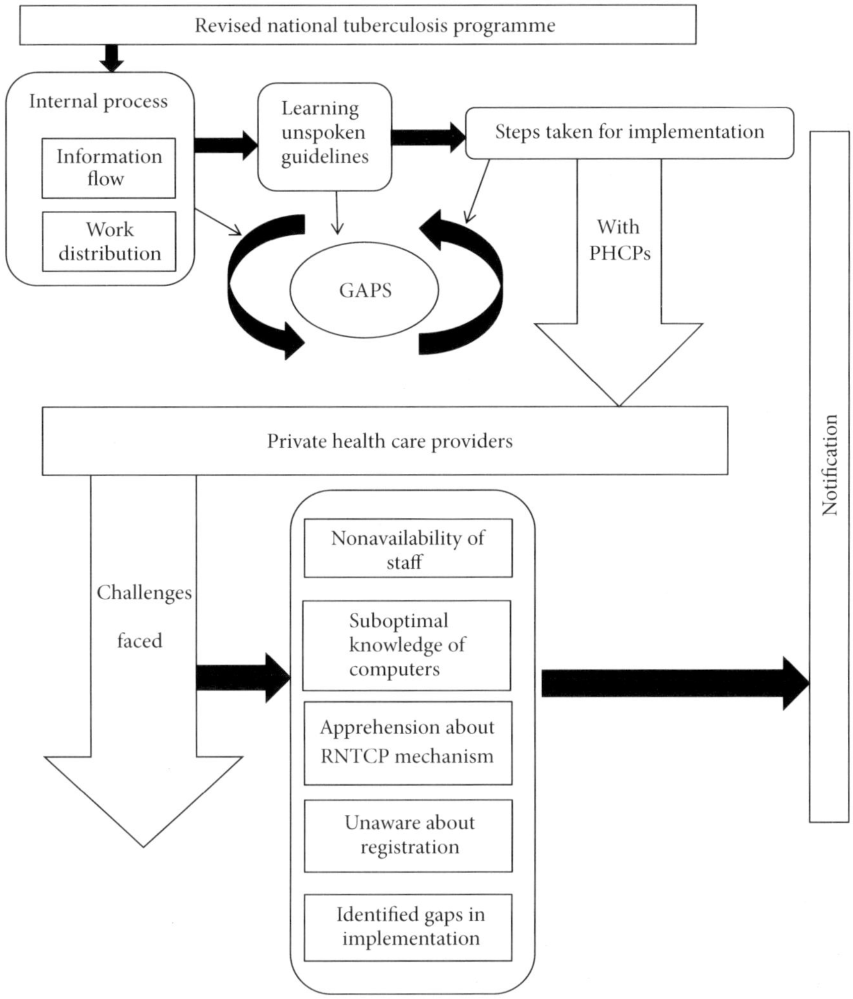

FIGURE 1: Theoretical model showing interrelationships of themes.

> *We were not informed that we have to enter about TB notification in the 'NIKSHAY' web site. (39 years, male, RNTCP programme personnel, Delhi)*

It was noticed that, at both of these RNTCP districts, there was a difference in the process of line list preparation, information that has to be disseminated to PHCP for TB notification, and registration in "NIKSHAY."

At GTB RNTCP district the PHCP were provided with two options for notification: (i) to directly notify TB in the website or (ii) to submit the filled form and later submitting to programme personnel for further data entry and onward submission. while, at the NDMC RNTCP district, the field staff had informed PHCP to notify patients with TB treated by them and no specific process that has to be followed for notification was briefed to them.

> *We [field staff] did line list and in next visit we took DTO for field visit and submitted the line list for registration. (24 years, male, RNTCP programme personnel, Delhi)*

> *We [field staff] had got line list provided by chest clinic which had Dr. Name alone in the list. We went there with one- one copy of format [notification format hard copy] and had told to private clinic that whatever TB patients come, about them you need to notify. (27 years, male, RNTCP programme personnel, Delhi)*

> *We had given them two options that you can directly do in the computer in the ID we had created. The second option was we had asked them to keep register where they can record and give us a list. (41 years, male, RNTCP programme personnel, Delhi)*

> *We informed them [PHCP] that if you are treating TB patients you have to inform us. If you face any problem you have to inform us. (41 years, male, RNTCP programme personnel, Delhi)*

Programme personnel had informed that support was required for better implementation of TB notification system.

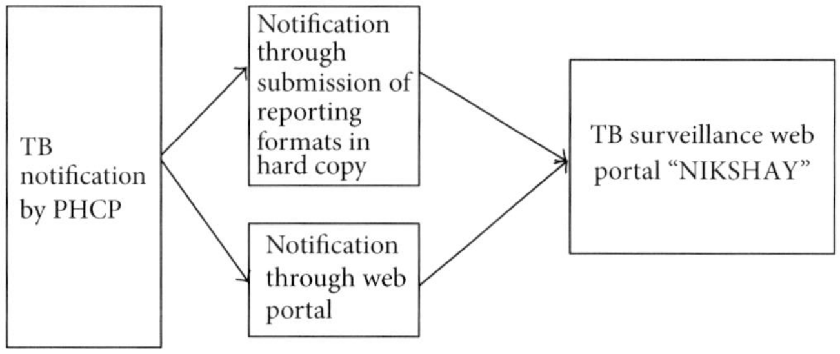

FIGURE 2: Schematic representation of TB notification process by PHCP in RNTCP system through "NIKSHAY" web portal. RNTCP: revised national tuberculosis control programme; NIKSHAY: web-based portal for notification and follow-up of patients with TB.

The field staff required support for microplanning of field activities, training to carry the activities, and support of higher officials in interaction with PHCP.

> *We should know beforehand what we have to do. Some training should be there in which we will learn what we have to speak? We also need some ID card. Nobody accepts if you don't have any identity card. People ask from where you come. (39 years, male, RNTCP programme personnel, Delhi)*

> *Someone needs to take the responsibility to speak to private Doctors, rest we can handle. People with higher position with higher responsibility can take initiative, as they have recognition in health as they have telephone number and cards. (25 years, male, RNTCP programme personnel, Delhi)*

3.2. Challenges Faced by PHCP. The notification process for PHCP involved notification of TB patient by submitting the hard copy formats to the government TB clinics or through direct notifying at web portal. The information through hard copies is filled by RNTCP staff and punched into the web portal. This information as either direct reporting or indirect reporting by PHCP goes to the TB notification web portal "NIKSHAY." These two submission processes enable the private health sector to enter the patients with TB details into the website (Figure 2). Themes identified as challenges for PHCP were as follows.

3.2.1. Incomplete Patients Address. PHCP stated that there were gaps in recording TB patient details as many patients with TB did not remember their exact postal house address, few were migrants with temporary house address, and few had come from unauthorized colonies with no house address. Hence, incomplete house details were not considered valid for getting notified and thus remained unnotified.

> *Whoever patients come to us we try to get address from patients and they write from their hand. Still many illiterate people comes to us who do not know to write their address, few don't know about their address, some know their address of their lane but does not know home number. Many of the patients come from unauthorized colonies where addresses are not proper. Even in birth and death certificate government has tried to enforce the address still you may find the addresses are not correct. (52 years, male, private health care provider, Delhi)*

3.2.2. Nonavailability of Staff. Quite often, the private health facility encountered shortage of human resources that led to poor maintenance of records and registers at the facility. PHCP emphasized that they had no manpower to fill the individual forms and to maintain records.

> *I don't have any paramedical staff to do the work [notification]. On behalf of management I have said I will give phone numbers, other particulars like fathers name and address of patient will be given. It is being one year the notification process has started. And these cards will go back to our trust and will get destroyed in few months. (65 years, female, private health care provider, Delhi)*

3.2.3. Suboptimal Knowledge of Computers. Motivation to notify was also determined by challenges faced by PHCP at their individual levels. Lack of time during their routine practice and relatively less knowledge to deal with computers demotivated them to continue notification.

> *I being a general practitioner I am not very well versed with computer. To do notification in computer I have to ask my son to do for me. (46 years, male, private health care provider, Delhi)*

> *I don't know much in computers as we are from earlier generation. People have not even given training on how to feed the data, once and twice they have informed us. There is a password and user identity, which we forget. (52 years, male, private health care provider, Delhi)*

3.2.4. Apprehension about RNTCP Mechanism. The prime source of earnings to the private health sector is patient's footfall to their health centers. Sharing details of the same patients to RNTCP gave them insecurity and a sense of loss of patients and monetary loss. They were also unhappy because they perceived that government might scrutinize

TABLE 2: Gaps identified by RNTCP Personnel during the process of PHCP "NIKSHAY" registration and continued notification at two RNTCP districts of Delhi state, 2105.

District TB officer	Delayed start and the process does not take place properly Lack of strategy planning No monthly or quarterly targets
STS/STLS	Burdened higher officials Lack of rapport building with private practitioners TBHV, STS/STLS have poor recognition amongprivate practitioners
TBHV	Vast areas to cover and short time for reporting information No transportation facilities No formal training on process

RNTCP: revised national tuberculosis control programme; NIKSHAY: web-based portal for notification and follow-up of patients with TB.

TABLE 3: Gaps perceived by RNTCP personnel and PHCP for smooth implementation of TB notification, at two RNTCP districts of Delhi state, 2015.

District TB officer	Double entries of the same TB cases at different places More chances of getting wrong information from field and wrong entries Difficulty in identification of entered address
Management information system personnel	Confusion with the process and reasons for data entry No clear information on indicators and which details to go where No guidance from superiors and miss communication on indicators
Private health care provider	No follow-up from RNTCP staff No proper information on the reasons of TB notification No perceived benefits are stated by RNTCP No trainings or meetings or communication materials given Confusion on intervention earlier done on public private mix strategy and TB notification

RNTCP: revised national tuberculosis control programme; NIKSHAY: web-based portal for notification and follow-up of patients with TB.

their efficiency on diagnosis and treatment. They felt discomfort with a situation to disclose their charges to the patient for the services offered and were ignorant about the benefits rendered to the notified patients.

> *If I am treating, after curing then why should I send the information to those people [RNTCP]? I have notified but I don't know what benefit happened to me or patients. I don't know why we are doing it? If there is no monetary benefit why people should do notification? (47 years, male, private health care provider, Delhi)*

> *There may be some apprehension in their mind (other PHCPs) that if they report about their patient directly then RNTCP will continue the treatment [DOTS] and the patient will go out of their hand. (65 years, female, private health care provider, Delhi)*

3.2.5. Unaware about Registration. Though the private health care providers were registered in "NIKSHAY" it was found that many of them were not aware about their name getting registered in the web site for treating TB patients.

> *I don't even know when they have registered me. I have no connections with them. They had come to meet us long back and have never come back. (32 years, female, private health care provider, Delhi)*

> *I have no idea how come my name has come in your registration sheet we don't refer any TB patient. We do diagnostic for diabetics. (27 years, female, private health care provider, Delhi)*

> *None of them had come to me. I would be very much interested to know more about it. (45 years, female, private health care provider, Delhi)*

3.3. Perceived Gaps and Suggestions. Gaps were identified by different level of personnel involved in implementation of TB notification. The identified gaps by different personnel were related to their role and responsibility for TB notification. Gaps related to TB notification information punching in "NIKSHAY" were also discussed (Table 2). There were some perceived gaps stated by PHCP which were related to the implementation process conducted by RNTCP staff (Table 3). The private health sector also opined for better implementation of TB notification; most of these suggestions were related

Table 4: Suggestions for smooth implementation of TB notification among "NIKSHAY" registered PHCP at two RNTCP districts of Delhi state, 2015.

Respondents	Suggestions
RNTCP personnel	
TBHV	Conduct prior meeting or workshop to give information on "NIKSHAY" and TB notification to TBHVs
	DTO should take steps and inform his staffs to collect data for 15 days or once in a month from private health care providers
	Conducting meeting with private health care providers on TB notification
STS/STLS	Government should provide a notice about TB notification to private practitioners and should be made a rule
	Indian Medical Association (IMA) at national and district level should inform all the doctors about this and should be sensitized on this
	Before making guideline at policy level ground reality should be understood
DTO	If notified once they should be known to others also in other district or state
	DTO should visit to meet private practitioners and vehicle can be hired for full time; many things can happen from DTOs part
	Duplication of TB numbers for same person at different places should be stopped
PHCP	DOT centers should be provided to private health care providers
	Follow-up process from RNTCP will be an effective solution to improve notification
	Notification process should be made convenient and easy
	Group for qualified and nonqualified PHCP should be build and educate them from RNTCP

RNTCP: revised national tuberculosis control programme; NIKSHAY: web-based portal for notification and follow-up of patients with TB; STS: senior treatment supervisor; STLS: senior TB laboratory supervisor; DTO: district tuberculosis officer; TBHV: TB health visitor; PHCP: private health care providers.

to training and conducting meetings and workshop for dissemination of information on notification among private health sector (Table 4).

4. Discussion

The TB notification in high-incidence countries is limited. A study based on literature search on notification system across high-incidence countries provided insights in private provider perceptions, including barriers to notification. Low notification rate was found in Republic of Korea, Pakistan, and Nigeria which was due to low knowledge associated with poor engagement of private providers on TB; lack of time was the major reason for not notifying while other concerns were confidentiality and poor knowledge of the reporting procedure. India is one among the few high-incidence countries, implementing electronic notification system recording details of TB patients [19].

In India, we conducted a qualitative study on TB notification which describes the challenges encountered by RNTCP programme personnel and PHCP. Our study findings revealed the operational issues in implementation of notification at various levels among PHCP starting from registration of PHCP in the notification system, the actual process of notification, and the perceptions associated with it among PHCP. The studies conducted elsewhere had evolved similar themes such as lack of complete knowledge about TB notification, lack of simplified operational mechanism of notification, and lack of trust and coordination with the government health system [9, 10, 20].

For implementation of TB notification by programme personnel at private health sector, the challenges faced by them were mainly the notification processes related issues and the differential strategies adopted by the programme at state and district levels. There appeared to be lack of microplanning at state and district level in terms of quantification of practitioners, planning, and implementation of systematic approach for involvement of practitioners and further mechanisms for regular follow-up of the involved practitioner. The component of TB notification for the programme at district level was perceived as another adjunct activity to the already existing RNTCP initiatives like TB-HIV (human immunodeficiency virus), drug resistance-TB, and TB-diabetes mellitus.

The programme had not prioritized the advocacy on the importance of TB notification upfront to providers and various myths prevailed among the private health care providers about TB notification [21]. There was also an apprehension among PHCP of delinking their patients from their services and sending them to RNTCP; the same was observed in a study conducted at Pune, Maharashtra [10]. The interaction with PHCP suggested that the bridge of faith and trust between RNTCP and PHCP was fragile and weak and it required attention to maintain transparency and developing dependency at both the sides. The PHCP had not experienced any gains either individually or to their patients upon notification [22].

Due emphasis of the programme should be concentrated on convincing the practitioners of the importance of TB notification [9, 23]. Awareness needs to be generated among the community for making the TB patients notified. This activity has to be widely publicized and supported through the involvement of community, NGOs, and social media. Innovative ideas need to be explored to make the tool user-friendly as the PHCP lacks clarity on functioning and usage of mobile phones and computers [23].

The gaps in the process of TB notification and suggestions to improvise the process as perceived by the programme personnel and the PHCP are enumerated in the tables. Though gaps are perceived at all levels by the programme personnel and PHCP, there are opinions for improvisation for notification. Accordingly, there is a need for the programme to popularise "NIKSHAY" as a notification tool. An advocacy forum of PHCP may be considered to motivate and streamline the notification among PHCP. The programme managers especially the district TB officers should judiciously take the initiative in meeting the PHCP by conducting meetings or workshops; thereafter, TBHV/STS should then follow up the PHCP at regular intervals. The programme personnel should also be adequately trained in the process with adequate transport facilities. It may be appropriate for the programme to collaborate with Indian Medical Association (IMA) which is the largest medical organization in the country to promote notification [23]. There is no universal successful formula to engage private health care providers; globally, there remains gaps in policy and practice for TB notification among the high burden TB countries [19].

4.1. Strength and Limitation of the Study. The strength of the study is that it was conducted under programmatic settings and reflected the ground reality. It represented the gaps and reasons behind poor notification, the detailed implementation process of TB notification, and strategies and challenges faced by PHCP. The limitations of the study included the following: (a) involvement of only two RNTCP districts of Delhi state may not reflect the challenges across the country and, hence, should be interpreted with caution; (b) although data saturation was achieved the additional themes might have emerged if additional nonregistered PHCP in "NIKSHAY" would have been interviewed to understand why other providers are not getting registered in "NIKSHAY" and interested to notify.

To conclude, the challenges in TB notification vary across the RNTCP personnel and PHCP. Notification of TB disease is an important monitoring and surveillance activity and the programme has to nurture its needs efficiently and establish a supportive environment for notification, while it is prudent that the importance and value of this tool are lost if not properly implemented. Implementation of TB notification among private health care providers requires systematic planning by the programme personnel and the process should be user-friendly with additional benefits to the patients and health care providers.

Disclosure

The authors alone are responsible for the views expressed in this publication and they do not necessarily represent the decisions or policies of the WHO, The Union, or the CDC.

Authors' Contributions

The study was conceived and designed by Mahasweta Satpati, Sharath Burugina Nagaraja, and Hemant Deepak Shewade; Mahasweta Satpati conducted the study; Mahasweta Satpati analysed the data; Mahasweta Satpati and Sharath Burugina Nagaraja contributed materials/analysis tools; Mahasweta Satpati, Sharath Burugina Nagaraja, and Hemant Deepak Shewade wrote the paper; Mahasweta Satpati, Sharath Burugina Nagaraja, Hemant Deepak Shewade, Prabhakaran Ottapura Aslesh, Blesson Samuel, Ashwani Khanna, and Sarabjit Chadha contributed to discussion.

Acknowledgments

The authors express their thanks to the District Tuberculosis Team and the private practitioners in NDMC and GTB RNTCP districts for their cooperation and support. They thank the National Operational Research Course (2014-15) conducted at National TB Institute, Bangalore. The study was undertaken as part of the TB Operations Research Training project conducted by the International Union Against Tuberculosis and Lung Disease (The Union), with funding support from The Global Fund through the Axshya project. This training project was conceived and implemented by The Union South-East Asia Regional Office (New Delhi, India) in collaboration with the Central TB Division of the Ministry of Health and Family Welfare (New Delhi, India), the National TB Institute (Directorate General of Health Services, Ministry of Health and Family Welfare, Government of India, Bangalore, India), the World Health Organization (WHO) India Country Office, and the US Centres for Disease Control and Prevention, Division of TB Elimination (CDC, Atlanta, GA, USA). They thank the Department for International Development (DFD), UK, for funding the Global Operational Research Fellowship Programme at the International Union Against Tuberculosis and Lung Disease (The Union), Paris, France.

References

[1] WHO, *Global Tuberculosis Report*, 2016, http://apps.who.int/iris/bitstream/10665/250441/1/9789241565394-eng.pdf?ua=1.

[2] World Health Organization, *Global Tuberculosis Control*, WHO, Geneva, Switzerland, 2010, http://apps.who.int/iris/bitstream/10665/44425/1/9789241564069_eng.pdf.

[3] Improving Tuberculosis Case Detection, A compendium of TB Reach Case Studies, Lessons learned and a monitoring and evaluation framework. Stop TB Partnership, Geneva, Switzerland, UNOPS, 2014, http://www.stoptb.org/assets/documents/news/TB_Case_Studies.pdf.

[4] Central TB Division, *TB Notification Order - Ministry of Health and Family Welfare*, 2016, http://www.tbcindia.nic.in/showfile.php?lid=3136.

[5] WHO, *Global Tuberculosis Report*, WHO, 2015, http://apps.who.int/iris/bitstream/10665/191102/1/9789241565059_eng.pdf.

[6] S. Satyanarayana, S. A. Nair, S. S. Chadha, R. Shivashankar, G. Sharma, S. Yadav et al., "From Where Are Tuberculosis Patients Accessing Treatment in India? Results from a Cross-Sectional Community Based Survey of 30 Districts," *PLoS ONE*, vol. 6, no. 9, p. e24160, 2011, http://dx.plos.org/10.1371/journal.pone.0024160.

[7] FW. TB India and FW. Central TB Division M of H, Central TB Division M of H and FW. TB India 2014, RNTCP, Annual Status Report [Internet]. New Delhi; 2014, http://tbcindia.nic.in/showfile.php?lid=3142.

[8] S. Philip, P. Isaakidis, K. D. Sagili, A. Meharunnisa, S. Mrithyunjayan, and A. M. V. Kumar, ""They know, they agree, but they don't do" - The paradox of tuberculosis case notification by private practitioners in Alappuzha district, Kerala, India," *PLoS ONE*, vol. 10, no. 4, Article ID e0123286, 2015.

[9] R. D. Yeole, K. Khillare, V. K. Chadha, T. Lo, and A. M. V. Kumar, "Tuberculosis case notification by private practitioners in Pune, India: how well are we doing?" *Public Health Action*, vol. 5, no. 3, pp. 173–179, 2015, The International Union Against Tuberculosis and Lung Disease.

[10] Central TB Division M of H and FW. TB India 2016, RNTCP, Annual Status Report [Internet]. New Delhi; http://tbcindia.nic.in/showfile.php?lid=3180.

[11] SAGE Publications, *The Coding Manual for Qualitative Researchers*, Johnny Saldana, London, UK, 2010 edition, 2009.

[12] S. Baker and R. Edward, *How Many Qualitative Interviews Is Enough? Expert Voices and Early Career Reflections on Sampling And Cases in Qualitative Research*, NCRM publisher, Southampton, UK, 2012, http://eprints.ncrm.ac.uk/2273/4/how_many_interviews.pdf.

[13] A. Strauss and J. Corbin, *Grounded Theory in Practice*, Sage publication, 1997.

[14] B. C. O'Brien, I. B. Harris, T. J. Beckman, D. A. Reed, and D. A. Cook, "Standards for Reporting Qualitative Research," *Academic Medicine*, vol. 89, no. 9, pp. 1245–1251, 2014, http://www.ncbi.nlm.nih.gov/pubmed/24979285.

[15] L. Burla, B. Knierim, J. Barth, K. Liewald, M. Duetz, and T. Abel, "From text to codings: Intercoder reliability assessment in qualitative content analysis," *Nursing Research*, vol. 57, no. 2, pp. 113–117, 2008.

[16] M. Sandelowski, "Focus on Research Methods-Whatever Happened to Qualitative Description?" *Journal Research in Nursing and Health*, vol. 23, pp. 334–340, 2000.

[17] ATLAS, ATLAS.ti 7 Quick tour [Internet]. Berlin; 2015, http://downloads.atlasti.com/quicktour/QuickTour_a7_en.pdf?_ga=1.161922108.187043838.1480643099.

[18] A. Tong, P. Sainsbury, and J. Craig, "Consolidated criteria for reporting qualitative research (COREQ): a 32-item checklist for interviews and focus groups," *International Journal for Quality in Health Care*, vol. 19, no. 6, pp. 349–357, 2007.

[19] M. Uplekar, S. Atre, W. A. Wells, D. Weil, R. Lopez, G. B. Migliori et al., "Mandatory tuberculosis case notification in high tuberculosis-incidence countries: policy and practice," *European Respiratory Journal*, vol. 48, no. 6, pp. 1571–1581, 2016.

[20] D. Kundu, K. Chopra, A. Khanna, N. Babbar, and T. J. Padmini, "Accelerating TB notification from the private health sector in Delhi, India," *Indian Journal of Tuberculosis*, vol. 63, no. 1, pp. 8–12, 2016.

[21] S. B. Nagaraja, S. Achanta, A. M. V. Kumar, and S. Satyanarayana, "Extending tuberculosis notification to the private sector in India: programmatic challenges?" *The International Journal of Tuberculosis and Lung Disease*, vol. 18, no. 11, pp. 1353–1356, 2014.

[22] N. Gawde, "Do we need notification of tuberculosis? A public health perspective," *Indian Journal of Medical Ethics*, vol. 10, no. 1, pp. 56-57, 2013.

[23] B. E. Thomas, B. Velayutham, K. Thiruvengadam et al., "Perceptions of private medical practitioners on tuberculosis notification: A study from Chennai, South India," *PLoS ONE*, vol. 11, no. 1, Article ID e0147579, 2016.

26

Acceptance of Provider Initiated HIV Testing and Counseling among Tuberculosis Patients in East Wollega Administrative Zone, Oromia Regional State, Western Ethiopia

Wakjira Kebede,[1] Fikru Keno,[2] Temesgen Ewunetu,[1] and Gutu Mamo[3]

[1] *Department of Medical Laboratory Sciences and Pathology, College of Public Health and Medical Sciences, Jimma University, Jimma, Ethiopia*
[2] *Oromia Regional Social and Labor Affairs Agency, Addis Ababa, Ethiopia*
[3] *Department of Pharmacy, College of Public Health and Medical Sciences, Nekemte Hospital, Jimma, Ethiopia*

Correspondence should be addressed to Wakjira Kebede; dandiwk2004@gmail.com

Academic Editor: Brian Eley

Human immunodeficiency virus (HIV) is a powerful risk factor for the development of tuberculosis. This study assessed the acceptance and associated factors that can affect provider initiated HIV testing and counseling (PITC) among tuberculosis patients at the East Wollega administrative zone, Oromia regional state, western Ethiopia, from January to August, 2010. A single population proportion formula is used to calculate the total sample size of 406 and the cluster sampling technique was used to select 13 health centers that provide PITC services. The sample size was proportionally allocated to each health center. The study participants were selected using a simple random sampling technique using the lottery method. Structured questionnaire was used for collection of sociodemographic data. From the total of study subjects, 399 (98.2%) TB patients were initiated for HIV test and 369 (92.5%) patients accepted the initiation. Of those, 353 (95.5%) patients had taken HIV test and received their results. According to the reviewed documents, the prevalence of HIV among tuberculosis (TB) patients in the study area was 137 (33.7%). The logistic regression result showed the PITC was significantly associated with their knowledge about HIV (AOR = 3.22, 95% CI: 1.3–7.97), self-perceived risk (AOR = 2.93, 95% CI: 1.12–7.66), educational status (AOR = 3.51, 95% CI: 1.13–10.91), and knowledge on transmission of HIV/AIDS (AOR = 7.56, 95% CI: 1.14–40.35) which were significantly associated with the acceptance of PITC among TB patients. Therefore, this study's results showed, the prevalence of HIV among TB patient was high; to enhance the acceptance of PITC among TB patients, health extension workers must provide health education during home-to-home visiting. TB treatment supervisors also provide counseling intensively for all forms of TB patients during their first clinical encounter.

1. Introduction

World Health Organization (WHO) estimates that one-third of the world's population is infected with *Mycobacterium tuberculosis*, resulting in an estimated nearly 8.7 million incident cases of tuberculosis (TB) and 1.4 million deaths in 2012. TB has been closely linked to human immunodeficiency virus (HIV) and is believed to account for 50–80% in parts of sub-Saharan Africa for 500,000 deaths; 25% of the total deaths occur in people living with HIV [1–3]. Worldwide, TB is the most common opportunistic infection affecting HIV-seropositive and it remains the most common cause of death and major threat in terms of its personal, family, and socioeconomic consequences [4].

WHO Global report of 2012 ranked Ethiopia as the seventh among the highest TB burden countries in the world, with an estimated incidence and prevalence of all forms of TB cases being 258, 237/100,000 population, respectively [5]. Ethiopia Ministry of Health Hospital statistics data show that TB is the third leading cause of outpatient morbidity and mortality and the fourth leading cause of hospital admission [6].

HIV is the main reason for failure to meet TB control targets in high HIV settings, because HIV infection has contributed to progressive decline in immune response and pathogenesis of TB, increasing the risk of coinfection leading to more frequent extrapulmonary disease [4, 7]. The risk of reactivating TB infection in HIV infected persons is 7–10% per year compared with 10% lifetime risk in those serum negative persons. In order to control TB in high HIV settings, the Stop TB strategy needs collaborative TB/HIV activities in the country [4, 5, 8].

Worldwide only 20% of people living with HIV know their status, and only one in four people estimated to be living with HIV and TB is detected and treated for both diseases [3]. In sub-Saharan Africa only 10–12% of people living with HIV know their serostatus [9]. In Ethiopia most of the adult segment of the population (95%) does not know their HIV status [10]. And ART has been accessed by only 13% of those who need ART [11].

Currently, acceptability of provider initiated HIV testing and counseling (PITC) among TB patients varies from place to place. In Ethiopia the acceptability of PITC may be influenced by different associated factors like fear of stigma and discrimination associated with having TB and HIV, sociodemographic factors, knowledge related to TB/HIV, the general perception of HIV infection, and attitude towards PITC may affect the acceptance and knowledge of TB patients. PITC is one of the main intervention areas to fight against failure to meet TB control targets in areas where HIV prevalence was high, particularly, for those coinfected patients with TB and HIV.

Therefore, the aim of this study was to assess the acceptance of PITC and factors affecting PITC acceptance among TB patients. Furthermore, the results of this study help to design and practice appropriate interventions that decrease the burden of HIV on TB patient by enhancing the utilization of PITC service and are also important to improve treatment outcome by preventing other infectious diseases and decrease life loss of AIDS cases secondary to tuberculosis.

2. Materials and Methods

An institution based, cross-sectional study was conducted from July to August 2010 among adult tuberculosis patients in the East Wollega administrative zone, Oromia regional state, western Ethiopia. It is located at 262 KMs from Jimma University and 331 KMs from Addis Ababa (the capital city). The expected population of the zone for 2005 was estimated to be 1,647,576. The zone was divided into 21 administrative districts. There were 2 hospitals, one zonal hospital and one district hospital, 15 health centers, 82 health stations, and 107 health posts; all were public [12]. All tuberculosis patients in selected health centers registered for directly observed treatment short course (DOTS) from October 8, 2009, to August 18, 2010, and TB cases encountered during the data collection period were included in the study and those TB patients below the age of 18 years and those critically ill patients are excluded from the study.

A single population proportion formula is used to calculate the total sample size of 406 and cluster sampling technique was used to select woredas based on their geographical location. The health center was selected from the total health centers using a simple random sampling technique. The number of participants was proportionally allocated to each health center. The identification number (ID number) of TB patients at each health center was written on a piece of paper and coiled and then the actual number of 406 study units was selected by using the lottery method. A structured questionnaire was used to obtain sociodemographic information (residence, ethnicity, sex, age, religion, marital status, educational status, occupation, and family size).

The study protocol was reviewed and approved by the Institutional Ethical Review Board of the Jimma University. The objective of the study was explained to the participants and verbal consent was obtained from each participant. Confidentiality of the result was kept by coding patient information. The data were checked for their completeness before entering for analysis; then all the data from study participants were imported into excel and analyzed by SPSS version 20 program software. Odds ratio, 95% confidence interval, and both bivariate and multivariate logistic regression were used to test the association between the outcome and independent variables.

3. Results

3.1. Sociodemographic. A total of 406 TB patients were included in the study and are with a 100% response rate. Of the total, 234 (57.6%) of the study participants were male with nearly 1.36 to 1 sex ratio. The mean age of the study populations was 35 years with 1.2 standard deviation (SD); more than half (68.2%) of the interviewed religions were Orthodox, followed by Protestant 120 (29.6%); 391 (96.3%) and 278 (68.5%) were identifying themselves as an Oromo ethnic group and live in urban areas, respectively. Marriage characteristics, educational status, family size, and monthly income per month were identified (Table 1).

3.2. Knowledge about TB/HIV/AIDS. Almost all study participants 404 (99.5%) believed that TB is a curable disease. 306 (75.4%) of the respondents believed that a person who lives with HIV/AIDS is at risk of acquiring tuberculosis 327 (80.1%). Likewise 359 (84.4%) participants agreed that controlling of HIV/AIDS is important in controlling process of TB infection. Study participants were able to identify the common means of HIV transmission and agreed that HIV/AIDS is not a curable disease. 87.9% of participants believed that they were at risk of getting a virus in the past, while the rest did not (Table 2). However, still there is a misconception on transmission of HIV/AIDS by mosquito bite accounting for 14.8% and wearing shared clothes (7.1%) with their friends.

3.3. Knowledge of Study Participants on Provider Initiated HIV Testing and Counseling (PITC) Services. The majority of the study participants had heard about PITC before the time of data collection and the primary health workers were cited as a source of this information accounting for 98.3% followed by friends (43.7%) (Figure 1).

Table 1: Sociodemographic characteristics of tuberculosis patients in East Wollega administrative zone at selected health centers, August 2010 ($N = 406$).

Variables	Frequency	Percentage (%)
Residence		
Urban	278	(68.5)
Rural	128	(31.5)
Ethnic group		
Oromo	391	(96.3)
Amharic	13	(3.2)
Others*	2	(0.5)
Sex		
Male	234	(57.6)
Female	172	(42.4)
Age		
19–34	236	(58.1)
35–50	125	(30.8)
>50	45	(11.1)
Religion		
Orthodox	277	(68.2)
Protestants	120	(29.6)
Others**	9	(2.2)
Marital status		
Single	80	(19.7)
Married	257	(63.3)
Divorced/widowed/separated	69	(17.0)
Educational status		
Not formal education	230	(56.7)
Formal education	176	(43.3)
Occupational status		
Government employee	37	(9.1)
Farmer	130	(32.0)
House wife	113	(27.8)
Others***	126	(31.0)
Family size		
≤4	236	(58.1)
>4	170	(41.9)

Others*: Gurage; others**: Muslim; Catholic; others***: merchant, daily labor, student, and unemployed classified by using mean score.

3.4. HIV Testing and Acceptance of Provider Initiated HIV Testing and Counseling Services. Of all the study participants 399 (98.2%) are initiated for HIV test by their TB treatment supervisor during TB treatment follow-up; of those, 369 (92.5%) TB patients accepted the initiation and 353 (95.7%) patients had undergone HIV test and received their test result. On the other hand, about 30 (7.5%) patients did not accept the initiation because of different reasons like waiting until TB treatment completion, unable to cope following positive result and the remaining 7 (1.8%) participants are not encouraged for PITC. 357 (87.9%) did not know their serostatus about HIV before the study period; of those 92 (25.5%) TB patients were willing to check their status for HIV in the past after advice was given. According to document review result the prevalence of HIV among TB patients who underwent HIV counseling and testing from October 8, 2009, to August 18, 2010, was 137 (33.7%).

Table 2: Knowledge related to TB/HIV/AIDS among tuberculosis patients in East Wollega administrative zone at selected health centers, August 2010, ($N = 406$).

TB/HIV/AID related questions	Frequency	(%)
Source of TB#		
From TB patients	402	(99.0)
Polluted air	381	(93.8)
Contaminated water	81	(20.0)
Lump of earth	93	(22.9)
Others*	8	(1.90)
Risk of acquiring TB#		
Poor people	328	(80.8)
Living with TB patient	380	(93.6)
Having HIV/AIDS	306	(75.4)
TB increased after the era of HIV/AIDS		
Increase	327	(88.4)
No difference	79	(11.6)
Controlling of HIV/AIDS is important in TB control		
Yes	359	(88.4)
No	47	(88.4)
Route of HIV transmission#		
Sexual contact	406	(100)
Mother to child	402	(99.0)
Transfusion of blood	404	(99.5)
Sharing of sharp materials with PLHIV	406	(100)
Blood contact	402	(99.0)
Mosquito bite	60	(14.8)
Share wearing clothes	29	(7.40)
Others**	3	(0.70)
Methods of HIV prevention#		
Limiting sex to one uninfected partner	404	(99.5)
Abstain from sexual intercourse	401	(98.8)
Use of condom during sexual intercourse	392	(96.6)
Comprehensive knowledge of HIV		
Knowledgeable	338	(83.3)
Not knowledgeable	68	(16.7)
Self-perceived risk of HIV infection		
No risk	48	(11.8)
Risk	358	(88.2)

#Multiple responses; others*: sexual intercourse, evil spirit; others**: shaking hand, sharing meal.

3.5. Analysis of Factors Associated with Acceptance of PITC among TB Patients. In bivariate logistic regression analysis,

TABLE 3: Bivariate and multiple logistic regression analysis of factors associated with acceptance of PITC (n = 369).

Variables	Accepter	Not accepter	OR (95% CI)	AOR (95% CI)	P value
Educational status					**0.03**
Not formal education[R]	200	26	1.0	1.0	
Formal education	169	4	5.49 (1.88–16.05)	3.51 (1.13–10.91)	
Controlling of HIV could help in control of TB					**0.04**
No[R]	36	10	1.0	1.0	
Yes	333	20	4.63 (2.01–10.64)	3.89 (1.54–9.83)	
Comprehensive knowledge on HIV/AIDS					**0.011**
Not knowledgeable[R]	49	13	1.0	1.0	
Knowledgeable	320	17	4.99 (2.84–10.92)	3.22 (1.3–7.97)	
Self-perceived risk of contracting HIV					**0.028**
No risk[R]	38	9	1.0	1.0	
Risk	331	21	3.73 (1.6–8.73)	2.93 (1.12–7.66)	
Knowledge of PITC					**0.017**
Not knowledgeable[R]	5	3	1.0	1.0	
Knowledgeable	364	27	8.09 (1.83–35.67)	7.56 (1.14–40.35)	

[R]Reference category.

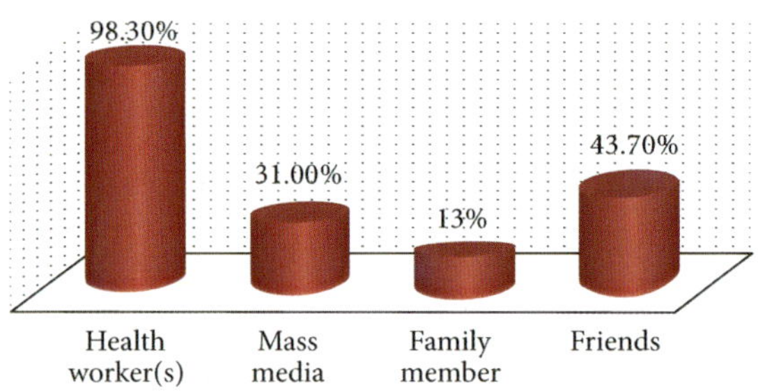

FIGURE 1: Source of information about PITC, among TB patients in East Wollega administrative zone at selected health centers, August 2010.

each explanatory variable with the outcome variable (acceptance of PITC) was assessed for its association. Variables with P value >0.3 were not imported to multiple logistic regression for further analysis. Participants with formal education were 3.51 times more likely to accept PITC following their TB treatment supervisor initiation, as compared with who had not formal education (AOR = 3.51, 95% CI: 1.13–10.91). Similarly, those who had comprehensive knowledge about HIV/AIDS way of transmission were 3.22 times more likely to accept PITC than who had not (AOR = 3.22, 95% CI: 1.3–7.97). Who understand the importance of controlling HIV/AIDS helps in controlling of TB were 3.89 times more likely to accept PITC than those who do not know (AOR = 3.89, 95% CI: 1.54–9.83) (Table 3).

4. Discussion

Most of the TB patients were initiated for HIV test by their TB treatment supervisors 399 (98.7%) during TB treatment follow-up. Among those initiated 369 (92.5%) accepted PITC and of those 353 (95.7%) were tested and received their test result. In this study there is a high acceptance of PITC (92.5%) among TB patients. The study results that were not comparable with the previous studies conducted in Addis Ababa (capital city of Ethiopia) and Arba Minch (south nation, nationality people) among TB patients showed 66.6% and 73%, respectively [13, 14]. This difference may relate to the recent introduction of free life-saving antiretroviral therapy at selected health centers throughout Ethiopia. Similarly, this finding was comparable with studies done in India, Kenya, Cameroon, and Congo which showed 97%, 91.5%, 94.5%, and 96.25%, respectively [15, 16]. The reason for increment number of acceptances was that those patients who refuse to undergo an HIV test at the beginning of TB treatment may accept PITC initiation during TB treatment follow-up.

According to documents reviewed result, the prevalence of HIV among TB patients who undergo HIV test was 33.7%. This result is comparable with studies done in North West Ethiopia and South Ethiopia [17–19]. However, this finding is not in line with the Federal HIV/AIDS prevention and a control office report in March 2010 which accounts for 20% [17]; the reason for this might be that the increment of awareness and knowledge on TB-HIV infection and PITC services during TB treatment follow-up may increase the chance of positivity.

Patients who had self-perceived risk of contracting HIV/AIDS accept PITC as compared to not self-perceived risk patients (OR = 3.73 95%, CI: 1.6–8.73). This result was in agreement with a study done in Arba Minch hospital among TB patients that showed self-perceived risk patients were five times more willing to accept the initiation than non-self-perceived risk patients [20]. The possible explanation for this may be those patients who considered themselves at risk of getting HIV in the past are more interested to know their serostatus in order to benefit from the available treatment options related to HIV including provision of ART as compared to not self-perceived risk individuals (Table 3). Similarly, patients who had knowledge about provider initiated HIV testing and counseling service were more likely to accept PITC than unknowledgeable patients (OR = 8.09, 95%, CI: 1.83–35.67). This finding is in agreement with study done in North West Ethiopia [17].

Generally, in this study there is a high acceptance of PITC among TB patients following the initiation of TB treatment supervisor. This is important for the control, prevention, and treatment of TB-HIV coinfection strategies. Despite the high knowledge of TB/HIV, still there is a misconception about TB/HIV means of transmission. Therefore, information or health education about TB and HIV, particularly on way of transmission, prevention, and control, should be provided intensively by health extension workers during home-to-home visiting and TB treatment supervisors provide counseling regularly for all forms of TB patients.

Authors' Contribution

Wakjira Kebede conceived the study, undertook statistical analysis, and drafted the paper. Fikru Keno, Gutu Mamo, and Temesgen Ewunetu were involved in data collection and data entry. All authors contributed to the writing of the paper and approved the submitted version of the paper.

Acknowledgments

The authors acknowledge the Zonal Health Bureau of East Wollega for providing important information. Their acknowledgment is also for all health center staff members for their technical assistance. Finally, their thanks also go to all the study participants for their trust and cooperation.

References

[1] WHO, "Joint newsletter of the TB/HIV and MDR-TB working groups of the stop TB partnership," 2012, http://www.stoptb.org/wg/tb_hiv/.

[2] WHO, *Tuberculosis Control, Epidemiology Strategy and Financing Report*, World Health Organization, Geneva, Switzerland, 2009.

[3] V. M. Vashishtha, "WHO Global Tuberculosis Control Report 2009: tuberculosis elimination is a distant dream," *Indian Pediatrics*, vol. 46, no. 5, pp. 401–402, 2009.

[4] WHO, *Networking for Policy Change*, TB/HIV Participant's Guide, 2007.

[5] WHO, "Stop TB partnership," Tuberculosis facts, 2009, http://www.who.int/tb/.

[6] Ministry of Health, *Health and Health Related Indicators*, Planning and Programming Department, FMOH, Addis Ababa, Ethiopia, 2004.

[7] E. L. Corbett, C. J. Watt, N. Walker et al., "The growing burden of tuberculosis: global trends and interactions with the HIV epidemic," *Archives of Internal Medicine*, vol. 163, no. 9, pp. 1009–1021, 2003.

[8] Federal Ministry of Health, *TB/HIV Implementation Guideline*, Federal Ministry of Health, Addis Ababa, Ethiopia, 2005.

[9] WHO/UNAIDS, *Guidance on Provider-Initiated HIV Testing and Counseling in Health Facilities*, World Health Organization, Geneva, Switzerland, 2007.

[10] Central Statistical Authority and ORC Macro, *Demographic and Health Survey of Ethiopia, Addis Ababa: CSA and ORC Macro, Calverton*, 2005.

[11] MOH, *AIDS in Ethiopia*, Ministry of Health, 5th edition, 2004.

[12] N. B. Njozing, "Assessing the accessibility of HIV care packages among tuberculosis patients in the Northwest Region, Cameroon," *BMC Public Health*, vol. 10, article 129, 2010.

[13] A. Van Rie, M. Sabue, N. Jarrett et al., "Counseling and testing TB patients for HIV: evaluation of three implementation models in Kinshasa, Congo," *International Journal of Tuberculosis and Lung Disease*, vol. 12, no. 3, pp. S73–S78, 2008.

[14] A. Aklilu, *Assessment of Willingness of TB Patients Towards VCT in Selected Health Centers*, North Gondar Administrative Zone, Addis Ababa, Ethiopia, 2005.

[15] H. Michael, C. Jira, K. Tushune, and B. Girma, "Health workers perspectives on incentive structure: the case of East wollega zone," *Ethiopian Journal of Health Sciences*, vol. 19, no. 3, 2009.

[16] B. E. Thomas, P. K. Dewan, S. Vijay et al., "Perceptions of tuberculosis patients on provider-initiated HIV testing and counseling—a study from south India," *PLoS ONE*, vol. 4, no. 12, article e8389, 2009.

[17] D. Jerene, A. Endale, and B. Lindtjørn, "Acceptability of HIV counselling and testing among tuberculosis patients in south Ethiopia," *BMC International Health and Human Rights*, vol. 7, article 4, 2007.

[18] A. Ayenew, A. Leykun, R. Colebunders, and A. Deribew, "Predictors of HIV testing among patients with tuberculosis in North West Ethiopia: a case-control study," *PloS ONE*, vol. 5, no. 3, article e9702, 2010.

[19] M. Melaku, "Assessment of VCT utilization and willingness to accept provider-initiated HIV counseling and testing among tuberculosis patients in Addis Ababa Ethiopia," *Ethio Journal*, p. 5, 2007.

[20] J. Odhiambo, W. Kizito, A. Njoroge et al., "Provider-initiated HIV testing and counselling for TB patients and suspects in Nairobi, Kenya," *International Journal of Tuberculosis and Lung Disease*, vol. 12, no. 3, pp. S63–S68, 2008.

27

Treatment Outcome of Tuberculosis Patients at Enfraz Health Center, Northwest Ethiopia: A Five-Year Retrospective Study

Mengistu Endris,[1] Feleke Moges,[1] Yeshambel Belyhun,[1,2] Eleni Woldehana,[3] Ahmed Esmael,[4] and Chandrashekhar Unakal[1]

[1] *School of Biomedical and Laboratory Sciences, University of Gondar, P.O. Box 196, Gondar, Ethiopia*
[2] *Institute of Virology, Faculty of Medicine, University of Leipzig, Leipzig, Germany*
[3] *Enfranz Health Center, Enfranz, Ethiopia*
[4] *Department of Microbiology, Immunology & Parasitology, Debre Markos University, Debre Marqos, Ethiopia*

Correspondence should be addressed to Mengistu Endris; mengistu06@gmail.com

Academic Editor: W. N. Rom

Objectives. The aim of this study was to assess treatment outcome and associated risk factors among TB patients registered for anti-TB treatment at Enfraz health center, northwest Ethiopia. *Methods.* A five-year retrospective data (2007–2011) of tuberculosis patients ($n = 417$) registered for anti-TB treatment at Enfraz health center, northwest Ethiopia, were reviewed. Tuberculosis outcomes were following the WHO guidelines. Data were entered and analyzed using SPSS version 20. *Results.* Among 417 study participants, 95 (22.8%), 141 (33.8%), and 181 (43.4%) were smear-positive, smear-negative, and extrapulmonary tuberculosis patients, respectively. Of the 417 study participants, 206 (49.4%) were tested for HIV. The TB-HIV coinfection was 24/206 (11.7%). Seventeen study participants (4.2%) were transferred to other health facilities. Among the 400 study participants, 379 (94.8%) had successful treatment outcome (302 treatment completed and 77 cured). The overall death, default, and failure rates were 3.4%, 0.5%, and 1.2%, respectively. There was no significant association between sex, age, residence, type of TB, HIV status, and successful TB treatment outcome. *Conclusion.* Treatment outcome of patients who attended their anti-TB treatment at Enfraz health center was successful. Therefore, this treatment success rate should be maintained and strengthened to achieve the millennium development goal.

1. Background

Tuberculosis (TB) is a major global health problem. It causes illness among millions of people each year and ranks as the second leading cause of death from an infectious disease worldwide, next to HIV infection. According to the World Health Organization (WHO) 2012 report, almost 9 million new cases and 1.4 million TB deaths occur worldwide by the year 2011 [1]. These deaths occurred in the presence of treatments that were able to cure most of the cases.

Geographically, the burden of TB is the highest in Asia and Africa. The African region has 24% of the world's cases and the highest rates of cases and deaths per capita [1]. Almost 80% of TB cases among people living with HIV reside in Africa [1]. Among 22 high burden countries (HBCs) of TB, Ethiopia ranks the 7th with an estimated prevalence of 394/100,000 population [1].

According to the Ethiopian Ministry of Health report, TB is the leading cause of morbidity, the third leading cause of hospital admission, and the second cause of death in Ethiopia [2]. Recording and reporting the number of cases detected by national TB control programmes (NTPs) and the outcomes of treatment are of the five component packages of the directly observed therapy short-course strategy (DOTS) [1]. In 1992 Ethiopia has started the implementation of DOTS within the standardized TB prevention and control program [2]. Currently DOTS coverage is estimated at 100% geographical and 95% health facility level [1].

Ethiopia is one of the seven HBCs that reported lower rates of treatment success rate (83%) [1]. The treatment outcome monitoring in order to evaluate the effectiveness of the DOTS program is essential [3]. Furthermore, understanding the specific reasons for unsuccessful outcomes is important in order to improve treatment strategy [4]. In this regard, studies in Ethiopia ranged from 26% to 93.7% [5–13]. Previous report of the TB defaulter, failure, and death rates in Ethiopia ranged from 0.6% to 18.3% [5–8, 12–15], 0.2% to 18.6% [5–8, 12], and 2.6% to 10.1% [5–7, 9, 12, 13, 16, 17], respectively. Some of the identified independent risk factors for poor treatment outcome were being on retreatment, age being more than 55 years, being male, distance from home to treatment centre, and the added burden of using public transport to get to a treatment centre.

Despite high DOTS coverage in northwest Ethiopia, the treatment outcome of TB patients in health centers has not been assessed so far. There is little information about factors responsible for unsuccessful treatment outcome in the region. In this study, we assessed the treatment outcomes of TB patients in DOTS program and associated risk factors with unsuccessful TB treatment outcome in Enfraz health center, northwest Ethiopia.

2. Methods

2.1. Study Area. Enfraz health center is located in the northwest part of Ethiopia. Enfraz is a historic town 678 Kilometers away from Addis Ababa, capital city of Ethiopia. The health center is the only facility that renders DOTS service for the people living in and around Enfraz. Patients were diagnosed, registered, treated, and referred to other DOTS clinics following the National Tuberculosis and Leprosy Control Program (NTLCP) guideline [2].

2.2. Study Design and Data Collection. A retrospective study was conducted among TB patients registered from 2007 to 2011 at DOTS clinic. The sociodemographic data (such as sex, age, and residence), category of TB at the start, and the treatment outcomes of the TB patients were collected from the DOTS registration book.

2.3. Definitions. The Ethiopian NTLCP guideline [2], adopted from WHO, was used for the following clinical case and treatment outcome definitions.

2.3.1. Smear-Positive Pulmonary TB Case. Smear-positive pulmonary TB is the case of a patient with one or more initial sputum smear examinations (direct smear microscopy) AFB-positive or one sputum examination AFB-positive plus radiographic abnormalities consistent with active pulmonary TB as determined by a clinician.

2.3.2. Smear-Negative Pulmonary TB Case. Smear-negative pulmonary TB is the case of a patient with pulmonary TB who does not meet the above criteria for smear-positive disease. Diagnostic criteria should include the following: at least two AFB-negative sputum smear examinations; radiographic abnormalities consistent with active pulmonary TB; no response to a course of broad-spectrum antibiotics (except in a patient for whom there is laboratory confirmation or strong clinical evidence of HIV infection); and a decision by a clinician to treat the patient with a full course of anti-TB chemotherapy. A patient with positive culture but AFB-negative sputum examinations is also a smear-negative case of pulmonary TB.

2.3.3. Extrapulmonary TB Case. Extrapulmonary TB is the case of a patient with TB of organs other than the lungs (e.g., pleura, lymph nodes, abdomen, genitourinary tract, skin, joints and bones, and meninges). Diagnosis should be based on one culture-positive specimen or histological or strong clinical evidence consistent with active extrapulmonary disease, followed by a decision by a clinician to treat a patient with a full course of anti-TB chemotherapy. A patient in whom both pulmonary and extrapulmonary TB has been diagnosed should be classified as a pulmonary case.

2.3.4. Treatment Outcome. *Cured*: a patient who was initially sputum smear-positive and who was sputum smear-negative in the last month of treatment and on at least one previous occasion. *Completedtreatment*: when a patient completed treatment but did not meet the criteria for cure or failure. This definition applies to sputum smear-positive and sputum smear-negative patients with pulmonary TB and to patients with extrapulmonary disease. *Died*: when a patient died from any cause during treatment. *Failed*: when a patient was initially sputum smear-positive and when a patient remained sputum smear-positive at month 5 or later during treatment. *Defaulted*: when a patient whose treatment was interrupted for 2 consecutive months or more. *Successfully treated*: when a patient was cured or completed treatment.

2.4. Statistical Analysis. Data were entered, cleaned, and analyzed using SPSS version 20 statistical software. Data were entered into a computer and analyzed twice by two independent investigators to ensure their quality. Bivariate and multivariate analysis were done to analyze whether there is association between the TB treatment outcomes and independent variables. Crude and adjusted odd ratio were computed and used to see the strength of association. P values less than 0.05 were considered statistically significant.

2.5. Ethical Considerations. Institutional ethical clearance was obtained from the college of Medicine and Health Sciences research ethical committee of University of Gondar.

3. Results

3.1. Characteristics of Study Participants. A total of 417 TB patients whose age ranged from 0.17 to 80 years, mean and standard deviation of 31.91 ± 1.69 years, were included in the study. Among 417 study participants 108 (52.3%) were females and 199 (47.7%) were males. Children ≤ 14 years accounted for 14.6% of the study participants. Majority of the patients were rural residents (270 (64.7%)) (Table 1).

Most of the TB patients 407/417 (97.6%) were new cases. At the start of TB treatment, the TB patients relapse, defaulter, and failure rates were 6 (1.4%), 3 (0.7%), and

TABLE 1: Characteristics of TB patients with types of TB at DOTS clinic of Enfraz health center, 2007–2011.

Characteristics	Total	Type of TB		
		Smear-positive	Smear-negative	EPTB
Sex				
Male	199 (47.7)*	41 (20.6)	74 (37.2)	84 (42.2)
Female	218 (52.3)	54 (24.8)	67 (30.7)	97 (44.5)
Residence				
Urban	147 (35.3)	33 (22.4)	55 (37.4)	59 (40.1)
Rural	270 (64.7)	62 (23.0)	86 (31.9)	122 (45.2)
Age (years)				
≤14	61 (14.6)	3 (4.9)	29 (47.5)	29 (47.5)
15–24	78 (18.7)	19 (24.4)	18 (23.1)	41 (52.6)
25–34	112 (26.9)	34 (30.4)	25 (22.3)	53 (47.3)
35–44	70 (16.8)	19 (27.1)	31 (44.3)	20 (28.6)
45–54	45 (10.8)	14 (31.1)	17 (37.8)	14 (31.1)
55–64	30 (7.2)	3 (10.0)	14 (46.7)	13 (43.3)
≥65	21 (5.0)	3 (14.3)	7 (33.3)	11 (52.4)
HIV test				
Negative	182 (43.6)	39 (21.4)	65 (35.7)	78 (42.9)
Positive	24 (5.8)	10 (41.7)	9 (37.5)	5 (20.8)
Unknown	200 (48.0)	45 (22.5)	62 (31.0)	93 (46.5)
Refused to test	11 (2.6)	1 (9.1)	5 (45.5)	5 (45.5)
Total	417 (100)	95 (22.8)	141 (33.8)	181 (43.4)

*Figures in parenthesis indicate percentage, EPTB: extrapulmonary tuberculosis.

1 (0.2%), respectively. The smear-positive, smear-negative, and extrapulmonary TB cases were 95 (22.8%), 141 (33.8%), and 181 (43.4%), respectively (Table 1).

Of 417 TB patients registered for anti-TB treatment 49.4% (n = 206) were tested for HIV. The TB-HIV co-infection was 11.7% (24/206). The smear positive, smear negative pulmonary TB and EPTB type of TB among TB-HIV co-infected patients was 41.7% (n = 10), 37.5% (n = 9), and 20.8% (n = 5), respectively (Table 1).

3.2. Treatment Outcome. The treatment outcome of most study participants was successful (302 completed their anti-TB treatment and 77 cured). The treatment failure, defaulter, and death rates were 0.5%, 1.2%, and 3.4%, respectively (Table 2).

Since the status of 17 TB patients (transferred out cases) is not known we excluded them from the treatment success rate analysis. The overall five-year treatment success rate of the TB patients was 94.8% (379/400).

The provider initiated HIV counseling and testing (PHICT) was not started in the health center up to 2008. Among the 50 in 2009, 78 in 2010, and 78 in 2011 TB patients tested for HIV, 5/50 (11.1%), 8/78 (11.4%), and 11/78 (16.4%) were positive for HIV, respectively.

In the bivariate analysis, age between 35 and 44 years and ≥65 years showed statistically significant association with unsuccessful treatment outcome as compared to patients aged between 15 and 24 years. The multiple logistic regression showed no significant association between unsuccessful treatment outcome and the different characteristics of the TB patients including age, sex, residence, and HIV status (P > 0.05 in all cases) (Table 3).

In this study, in the first three years (2007–2009) smear-positive pulmonary TB was the leading type of TB (ranged from 17.9% to 27.4%), while the last two years showed an increment in smear-negative pulmonary TB cases (ranged from 20.6% to 25.5%). The highest smear-positive rate recorded was 26/99 (27.4%) in the year 2009 (Table 4). The treatment success rate of TB patients showed increment from 2007 to 2009 with 88.7% and 100% rates, respectively. In the last two years of this study (2010 and 2010) the treatment success rate was 93.4% and 94.0%, respectively (Table 4).

4. Discussion

Among 417 TB patients registered in DOTS clinic of Enfraz health center only 17 (4.1%) were transferred to other health institutions. Almost one out of five patients (22.8%; 95/417) registered for anti-TB treatment in the health center had smear-positive pulmonary tuberculosis. Majority of the smear-positive pulmonary tuberculosis patients (81.1%; 77/95) were cured at the end of their anti-TB treatment. This smear-positive pulmonary cure rate was comparable with reports from Tigray region (85.5%) [8].

TABLE 2: Treatment outcomes of TB patients with their characteristics at DOTS clinic of Enfarz health center, 2007–2011.

Characteristics	Treatment outcomes					
	Cured	Treatment completed	Defaulter	Failure	Dead	Transferred out
Sex						
Male	32 (16.1)*	145 (72.9)	2 (1.0)	2 (1.0)	9 (4.5)	9 (4.5)
Female	45 (20.6)	157 (72.0)	3 (1.4)	0 (0.0)	5 (2.3)	8 (3.7)
Residence						
Urban	23 (15.6)	105 (71.4)	3 (2.0)	0 (0.0)	7 (4.8)	9 (6.1)
Rural	54 (20.0)	197 (73.0)	2 (0.7)	2 (0.7)	7 (2.6)	8 (3.0)
Age (years)						
0–14	2 (3.3)	55 (90.2)	0 (0.0)	0 (0.0)	0 (0.0)	4 (6.6)
15–24	17 (21.8)	57 (73.1)	0 (0.0)	0 (0.0)	1 (1.3)	3 (3.8)
25–34	27 (24.1)	74 (66.1)	1 (0.9)	1 (0.9)	5 (4.5)	4 (3.6)
35–44	13 (18.6)	47 (67.1)	2 (2.9)	1 (1.4)	4 (5.7)	3 (4.3)
45–54	12 (26.7)	31 (68.9)	0 (0.0)	0 (0.0)	1 (2.2)	1 (2.2)
55–64	3 (10.0)	24 (80.0)	2 (6.7)	0 (0.0)	1 (3.3)	0 (0.0)
≥65	3 (14.3)	14 (66.7)	0 (0.0)	0 (0.0)	2 (9.5)	2 (9.5)
TB type						
Smear-positive	77 (81.1)	13 (13.7)	1 (1.1)	1 (1.1)	2 (2.1)	1 (1.1)
Smear-negative	—	128 (90.8)	2 (1.4)	0 (0.0)	8 (5.7)	3 (2.1)
EPTB	—	161 (89.0)	2 (1.1)	1 (0.6)	4 (2.2)	13 (7.2)
HIV status						
Negative	35 (19.2)	133 (73.1)	1 (0.5)	0 (0.0)	7 (3.8)	6 (3.3)
Positive	7 (29.2)	13 (54.2)	1 (4.2)	0 (0.0)	1 (4.2)	2 (8.3)
Unknown	35 (17.5)	145 (72.5)	3 (1.5)	2 (1.0)	6 (3.0)	9 (4.5)
Refused to test	0 (0.0)	11 (100.0)	0 (0.0)	0 (0.0)	0 (0.0)	0 (0.0)

*Figures in parenthesis indicate percentage.

The majority of TB patients, 379/400 (94.8%), had successful treatment outcome (cured + treatment completed). Similar successful treatment outcomes were reported by Muñoz-Sellart et al. [9] from different health institutions, Leku health center and Yirgalem health center, 90.5% and 93.7%, respectively. The present study successful treatment outcome was higher than previous reports from different parts of Ethiopia, namely, Gondar University Hospital (29.5%) [5], Felege Hiwot Referral Hospital (26%) [12], Hadiya Treatment Centers (49%) [7], Gambo Rural Hospital (66.9%) [6], Kolladiba Health Center (85.6%) [13], and Mazandaran in Iran (87.8%). The present study showed successful treatment outcome (94.8%) which met the target (90%) set in the Global Plan to Stop TB by 2015 [1].

In the present study, the prevalence of HIV among TB patients was 11.7%. This was comparable from different parts of Ethiopia such as Nekemte 11.5% [11], West Arsi 13.6% [6], and Dembia with 10.9% [13]. However, the present study TB-HIV coinfection was lower than previous reports from different health centers at Addis Ababa, Gondar University Hospital, and Felege Hiwot Referral Hospital, 27.2% [18], 52.1% [19], and 25% [12], respectively. TB-HIV coinfection in present study (11.7%) was also lower than in the WHO estimate (39%) in Africa [1]. The lowered TB-HIV coinfection in this study might be due to the higher number of rural study participants than urban residents (64.7% versus 35.5%) (Table 1).

Fourteen (3.4%) study participants died during their course of their treatment. This report was consistent with reports from Kolladiba Health Center (3.3%) [13] and different health centers in Addis Ababa (3.7%) [16] and Tigray (3.9%) [8]. The death rate of this study was lower than reports from Gondar University Hospital [5], Felege Hiwot Referral Hospital [12], and Gambo Rural Hospital [6], 10.1%, 5.8%, and 5.3%, respectively. The lower death rates in the present study might be due to the difference in the study sites, by which the study was done in rural health center, while the higher death rates in hospitals might be due to hospitalization of more critical TB patients in hospitals than in health centers. Health professionals working in DOTS clinic of the health centers

Table 3: Treatment success rate among TB patients at DOTS clinic of Enfraz health center 2007–2011.

Characteristics	Treatment success		OR (95% CI)	*P* value	AOR (95 % CI)	*P* value
	Yes	No				
Sex						
Male	177 (93.2)*	13 (6.8)	1.00	—	1.00	—
Female	202 (96.2)	8 (3.8)	1.85 (0.70–5.02)	0.26	0.61 (0.23–1.57)	0.30
Residence						
Urban	128 (92.8)	10 (7.2)	1.00	—	1.00	—
Rural	251 (95.8)	11 (4.2)	1.78 (0.68–4.66)	0.28	0.51 (0.19–1.30)	0.16
Age (years)						
≤14	57 (100)	0 (0.0)	0.00 (0.00–23.10)	1.00	0.00 (0.00– —)	0.99
15–24	74 (98.7)	1 (1.3)	1.00	—	1.00	—
25–34	101 (93.5)	7 (6.5)	0.19 (0.01–1.63)	0.09	5.42 (0.63–46.56)	0.12
35–44	60 (89.6)	7 (10.4)	0.12 (0.01–0.98)	0.03	7.79 (0.89–68.25)	0.06
45–54	43 (97.7)	1 (2.3)	0.58 (0.02–21.91)	0.60	1.52 (0.08–26.20)	0.77
55–64	27 (90.0)	3 (10.0)	0.12 (0.00–1.41)	0.07	7.12 (0.68–73.71)	0.10
≥65	17 (89.5)	2 (10.5)	0.11 (0.00–1.76)	0.04	6.72 (0.56–80.83)	0.13
TB type						
Smear PTB	90 (95.7)	4 (4.3)	1.00	—	1.00	—
Smear NTB	128 (92.8)	10 (7.2)	0.57 (0.15–2.06)	0.51	2.05 (0.59–7.15)	0.26
EPTB	161 (95.8)	7 (4.2)	1.02 (0.24–4.02)	0.60	1.31 (0.34–4.90)	0.69
HIV status						
Negative	168 (95.5)	8 (4.5)	1.00	—	1.00	—
Positive	20 (90.9)	2 (9.1)	0.48 (0.08–3.50)	0.31	1.06 (0.18–6. 09)	0.95
Unknown	180 (94.2)	11 (5.8)	0.78 (0.28–2.15)	0.77	1.13 (0.42–3.05)	0.81
Refused to test	11 (100.0)	0 (0.0)	Undefined	0.61	0.00 (0.00– —)	0.99
Total	379 (94.8)	21 (5.2)				

*Figures in parenthesis indicate percentage.

Table 4: Trends of TB type and treatment outcomes of TB patients at Enfraz heath center 2007–2011.

Treatment outcomes and TB type	Year					Total
	2007	2008	2009	2010	2011	
Category at start						
New	62 (15.2)*	88 (21.6)	98 (24.1)	77 (18.9)	82 (20.1)	407 (97.6)
Relapse	1 (16.7)	1 (16.7)	1 (16.7)	2 (33.3)	1 (16.7)	6 (1.4)
Defaulter	0 (0.0)	1 (33.3)	0 (0.0)	0 (0.0)	2 (66.7)	3 (0.7)
Failure	0 (0.0)	0 (0.0)	0 (0.0)	0 (0.0)	1 (100.0)	1 (0.2)
Tuberculosis type						
Smear-positive PTB	17 (17.9)	20 (21.1)	26 (27.4)	16 (16.8)	16 (16.8)	95 (22.8)
Smear-negative PTB	20 (14.2)	30 (21.3)	26 (18.4)	29 (20.6)	36 (25.5)	141 (33.8)
EPTB	26 (14.4)	40 (22.1)	47 (26.0)	34 (18.8)	34 (18.8)	181 (43.4)
Treatment outcomes						
Treatment success	55 (88.7)	80 (95.2)	94 (100.0)	71 (93.4)	79 (94.0)	379 (94.8)
Dead	3 (4.8)	3 (3.3)	0 (0.0)	4 (5.1)	4 (4.7)	14 (3.4)
Failure	2 (3.2)	0 (0.0)	0 (0.0)	0 (0.0)	0 (0.0)	2 (0.5)
Default	2 (3.2)	1 (1.1)	0 (0.0)	1 (1.3)	1 (1.2)	5 (1.2)
Transferred out	1 (1.6)	6 (6.7)	5 (5.1)	3 (3.8)	2 (2.3)	17 (4.1)
Overall	63 (15.1)	90 (21.6)	99 (23.7)	79 (18.9)	86 (20.6)	417 (100.0)

*Figures in parenthesis indicate percentage.

might reach and advise TB patients who discontinue their anti-TB treatment than hospital workers due to their smaller catchment area and less work load. This work in turn might lead to a decrease in death rate. The other reason for low death rate in the present study might be due to the lower TB-HIV co-infection (11.7%) as compared to previous studies done at Felege Hiwot Referral Hospital (25%) [12] and Gambo Rural Hospital (13.6%) [6].

The TB treatment failure rate of this study was 0.5%, which was lower than the average TB treatment failure rate of the 22 HBCs [20]. Failure rates that ranged from 0.2% to 18.6% were reported from the different parts of Ethiopia [5–8, 12].

In this study, in the first three years (2007–2009) smear-positive pulmonary TB was the leading type of TB (ranged from 17.9% to 27.4%), while the last two years showed an increment in smear-negative pulmonary TB cases (ranged from 20.6% to 25.5%). This might be due to the increase in the HIV prevalence in the health center from year to year (11.1% in 2009 to 16.4% in 2011).

There was no significant association between unsuccessful treatment outcome and the different characteristics of the TB patients in the present study. Similar finding was reported by Datiko and Lindtjørn [17] in Southern part of Ethiopia. This result might be due to the poor characteristics of the retrospective study design to identify possible risk factors.

5. Conclusions

This study shows that treatment outcome of patients that attended their anti-TB treatment at Enfraz health center was successful. Enfraz health center has met the target success rate set by WHO. There was no associated risk factor identified for unsuccessful treatment outcome. Therefore, this treatment success rate should be maintained and strengthened to achieve the development goal. Further studies are needed to identify possible risk factors for unsuccessful treatment outcome.

Authors' Contribution

Mengistu Endris conceived the study, designed, participated in data collection, conducted data analysis, and drafted the paper for publication. Feleke Moges and Yeshambel Belyhun entered data, interpreted the results, and reviewed the initial and final drafts of the paper. Eleni Woldehana, Mengistu Endris, and Ahmed Esmael participated in data collection and reviewed the initial and final drafts of the paper. Chandrashekhar Unakal and Ahmed Esmael participated in the preparation of first draft of paper. All authors read and approved the final paper.

Acknowledgment

The authors would like to thank all the staff members of Enfraz Health center, DOTS clinic, for their kind cooperation during data collection.

References

[1] World Health Organization, *G Global Tuberculosis Report 2012*, WHO, Geneva, Switzerland, 2012.

[2] Ministry of Health of Ethiopia, *Tuberculosis, Leprosy and TB/HIV Prevention and Control Program Manual*, MOH, Addis Ababa, Ethiopia, 4th edition, 2008.

[3] J. Veen, M. Raviglione, H. L. Rieder et al., "Standardized tuberculosis treatment outcome monitoring in Europe," *European Respiratory Journal*, vol. 12, no. 2, pp. 505–510, 1998.

[4] T. Vasankari, P. Holmström, J. Ollgren, K. Liippo, M. Kokki, and P. Ruutu, "Risk factors for poor tuberculosis treatment outcome in Finland: a cohort study," *BMC Public Health*, vol. 7, article 291, 2007.

[5] B. Tessema, A. Muche, A. Bekele, D. Reissig, F. Emmrich, and U. Sack, "Treatment outcome of tuberculosis patients at Gondar University Teaching Hospital, Northwest Ethiopia. A five—year retrospective study," *BMC Public Health*, vol. 9, article 371, 2009.

[6] J. M. Ramos, F. Reyes, and A. Tesfamariam, "Childhood and adult tuberculosis in a rural hospital in Southeast Ethiopia: a ten-year retrospective study," *BMC Public Health*, vol. 10, article 215, 2010.

[7] E. B. Shargie and B. Lindtjørn, "DOTS improves treatment outcomes and service coverage for tuberculosis in South Ethiopia: a retrospective trend analysis," *BMC Public Health*, vol. 5, 2005.

[8] G. Berhe, F. Enquselassie, and A. Aseffa, "Treatment outcome of smear-positive pulmonary tuberculosis patients in Tigray Region, Northern Ethiopia," *BMC Public Health*, vol. 12, p. 537, 2012.

[9] M. Muñoz-Sellart, L. E. Cuevas, M. Tumato, Y. Merid, and M. A. Yassin, "Factors associated with poor tuberculosis treatment outcome in the Southern Region of Ethiopia," *International Journal of Tuberculosis and Lung Disease*, vol. 14, no. 8, pp. 973–979, 2010.

[10] M. Muoňz-Sellart, M. A. Yassin, M. Tumato, Y. Merid, and L. E. Cuevas, "Treatment outcome in children with tuberculosis in southern Ethiopia," *Scandinavian Journal of Infectious Diseases*, vol. 41, no. 6-7, pp. 450–455, 2009.

[11] E. Eyasu, L. Mengistu, and A. Gobena, "Preliminary study on the epidemiology of tuberculosis in Nekemte and its surroundings -Western Ethiopia," *STAR*, vol. 1, no. 1, pp. 18–25, 2012.

[12] F. Biadglegne, B. Anagaw, T. Debebe et al., "A retrospective study on the outcomes of tuberculosis treatment in Felege Hiwot Referral Hospital, Northwest Ethiopia," *International Journal of Medical Sciences*, vol. 5, no. 2, pp. 85–91, 2013.

[13] M. G. Beza, M. T. Wubie, M. D. Teferi, Y. S. Getahun, S. M. Bogale, and S. B. Tefera, "A five years tuberculosis treatment outcome at Kolla Diba Health Center, Dembia District, Northwest Ethiopia: a retrospective crosssectional analysis," *Journal of Infectious Diseases and Therapy*, vol. 1, no. 1, pp. 1–6, 2013.

[14] B. Tekle, D. H. Mariam, and A. Ali, "Defaulting from DOTS and its determinants in three districts of Arsi Zone in Ethiopia," *International Journal of Tuberculosis and Lung Disease*, vol. 6, no. 7, pp. 573–579, 2002.

[15] K. W. Michael, T. Belachew, and C. Jira, "Tuberculosis defaulters from the "DOTS" regimen in Jimma zone, southwest Ethiopia," *Ethiopian Medical Journal*, vol. 42, no. 4, pp. 247–253, 2004.

[16] B. Getahun, G. Ameni, S. Biadgilign, and G. Medhin, "Mortality and associated risk factors in a cohort of tuberculosis patients treated under DOTS programme in Addis Ababa, Ethiopia," *BMC Infectious Diseases*, vol. 11, article 127, 2011.

[17] D. G. Datiko and B. Lindtjørn, "Mortality in successfully treated tuberculosis patients in southern Ethiopia: retrospective follow-up study," *International Journal of Tuberculosis and Lung Disease*, vol. 14, no. 7, pp. 866–871, 2010.

[18] A. Deribew, N. Negussu, Z. Melaku, and K. Deribe, "Investigation outcomes of tuberculosis suspects in the health centers of addis ababa, ethiopia," *PLoS ONE*, vol. 6, no. 4, Article ID e18614, 2011.

[19] A. Kassu, G. Mengistu, B. Ayele et al., "Coinfection and clinical manifestations of tuberculosis in human immunodeficiency virus-infected and -uninfected adults at a teaching hospital, northwest Ethiopia," *Journal of Microbiology, Immunology and Infection*, vol. 40, no. 2, pp. 116–122, 2007.

[20] WHO, *Global Tuberculosis Control: Surveillance,Planning, Financing. WHO Report 2005*, WHO/HTM/TB/2005/49, WHO, Geneva, Switzerland, 2005.

TB Risk Perceptions among Medical Residents at a Tertiary Care Center in India

Geeta S. Pardeshi,[1] Dileep Kadam,[2] Ajay Chandanwale,[2] Andrea Deluca,[3] Pranali Khobragade,[2] Malan Parande,[2] Nishi Suryavanshi,[4] Aarti Kinikar,[2] Anita Basavaraj,[2] Sunita Girish,[2] Sangita Shelke,[2] Nikhil Gupte,[3,4] Jason Farley,[5] and Robert Bollinger[6]

[1] *Department of Community Medicine, Vardhman Mahavir Medical College and Safdarjung Hospital, New Delhi, India*
[2] *Byramjee Jeejeebhoy Government Medical College/Sassoon General Hospital, Pune, Maharashtra, India*
[3] *Department of International Health, Johns Hopkins Bloomberg School of Public Health, Baltimore, MD, USA*
[4] *Byramjee Jeejeebhoy Government Medical College/Johns Hopkins Clinical Trials Unit, Pune, Maharashtra, India*
[5] *School of Nursing, Johns Hopkins University, Baltimore, MD, USA*
[6] *Division of Infectious Diseases and International Health, Johns Hopkins University School of Medicine, Baltimore, MD, USA*

Correspondence should be addressed to Geeta S. Pardeshi; kanugeet@gmail.com

Academic Editor: David C. Perlman

Setting. Government tertiary health care center in India. *Objective*. To understand the perceptions of medical residents about their risk of developing TB in the workplace. *Design*. Cross-sectional study in which a semistructured questionnaire which included an open-ended question to assess their main concerns regarding TB in workplace was used to collect data. *Results*. Out of 305 resident doctors approached, 263 (94%) completed a structured questionnaire and 200 of these responded to an open-ended question. Daily exposure to TB was reported by 141 (64%) residents, 13 (5%) reported a prior history of TB, and 175 (69%) respondents were aware of TB infection control guidelines. A majority reported concerns about acquiring TB (78%) and drug-resistant TB (88%). The key themes identified were concerns about developing drug-resistant TB (n = 100; 50%); disease and its clinical consequences (n = 39; 20%); social and professional consequences (n = 37; 19%); exposure to TB patients (n = 32; 16%); poor infection control measures (n = 27; 14%); and high workload and its health consequences (n = 16; 8%). *Conclusion*. Though many resident doctors were aware of TB infection control guidelines, only few expressed concern about lack of TB infection control measures. Doctors need to be convinced of the importance of these measures which should be implemented urgently.

1. Introduction

Health Care Workers (HCWs) are known to be at risk of acquiring tuberculosis in the workplace [1]. In response to this risk, the World Health Organization published guidelines for prevention of TB in health care facilities and policy on TB infection control [2, 3]. In India, studies have also reported an increased risk of TB among HCWs [4–8]. The government has issued airborne infection control recommendations for health care settings [9]. However, due to structural, administrative, and behavioral factors [10–13], implementation of these guidelines has been poor [14–17].

Recently a study estimated TB incidence of 3,279 per 100,000 person years among resident doctors in a tertiary care center in India [18]. In our study at the same institute which was conducted to assess the resident doctors' attitudes toward TB patients, only 49% reported feeling compassion for and desire to help TB patients. The remaining 51% reported either feeling compassion yet avoiding TB pateints, having a fear and thinking that they may cause infection, or having no particular feeling [19].

These results raise concerns about the ability of the residents to follow the TB prevention guidelines and its impact on their attitudes towards TB patients. Health care workers are key stakeholders for interventions to prevent occupationally acquired TB. Understanding the resident doctors TB risk perceptions will aid in implementing effective interventions for prevention of occupationally acquired TB at institutional level.

2. Methods

2.1. Study Design and Setting. A cross-sectional study was conducted at B.J. Government Medical College and Sassoon General Hospital, a large, public tertiary health care center in Pune, India. Sassoon General Hospital is a government medical college hospital which has total bed strength of 1,296 and an average OPD (Out-Patient Department) attendance of 45,000 per month.

2.2. Study Population. The study participants were postgraduate medical resident doctors, assigned to clinical and laboratory departments. A total of 325 residents were eligible for study participation in September 2014, when the data were collected.

2.3. Tool. A semiquantitative questionnaire was administered to consenting residents. The questionnaire was finalized after pretesting in a pilot study. It included questions on sociodemographic variables, duration of work, exposure to TB patients/specimens, past history of TB, and knowing a resident who had TB. Two questions assessed whether the residents were concerned about TB and drug-resistant TB at workplace. The knowledge and awareness of the resident doctors about the administrative measures, environmental measures, and use of respiratory protective devices for prevention of occupationally acquired TB in health care settings was assessed using a Likert scale (strongly disagree, disagree, no opinion, agree, strongly agree). In addition, the questionnaire included one open-ended question asking residents to document their main concerns regarding development of TB at workplace. All questions and answers were in English, the same language as their medical training.

2.4. Recruitment. The study investigators attended regular departmental meetings, where they explained the research project to the residents and invited them to participate in the study. The consenting residents were given a self-administered anonymous questionnaire.

2.5. Ethical Review. The study protocol was approved by the ethics committees of B.J. Government Medical College and the Johns Hopkins University School of Medicine. Written informed consent was obtained from each respondent.

2.6. Analysis. Descriptive analysis was done using proportions, mean, and standard deviation. For analyzing the responses on the Likert scale, responses "strongly disagree, disagree, and no opinion" were combined into one group and "strongly agree and agree" were combined into another group. The responses to the open-ended question were analyzed manually in an excel sheet, using thematic content analysis [20]. Two investigators developed a coding scheme for all the responses and applied it to the dataset. An interrater reliability analysis for the two sets of codes was done using Kappa statistic. Codes were transformed into subthemes, which were sorted into key themes by identifying similar patterns and commonalities. Exemplary quotations were identified for each theme. The frequency of respondents reporting each key theme was calculated.

3. Results

Out of the 325 residents registered for postgraduate courses at the institute, 305 (94%) could be contacted. Of them 263 (86%) responded to questions assessing knowledge and 200 (76%) responded to the open-ended question about their concerns for contracting TB in the workplace. The characteristics of residents who responded only to the structured questions and to both the structured and open-ended questions are described in Table 1. Overall, majority of the respondents were male (60%) and had daily exposure to a known TB patient or specimen (64%).

Thirteen (5%) residents reported that they were previously diagnosed and treated for TB and 40 (16%) had been assessed for TB based on symptoms during their period of medical education. Most residents were concerned about being infected with TB at the workplace (78%) and an even greater proportion of residents (88%) expressed specific concern about acquiring drug-resistant TB in the workplace.

Table 2 describes the knowledge of the resident medical doctors regarding measures for prevention of occupationally acquired TB. A majority of the respondents had knowledge about administrative measures like early detection and separation of patients and cough etiquette in patients as well as environmental measures like good ventilation. Only 175 (69%) of resident doctors were aware of any guidelines for prevention of transmission of TB in health care settings. Many residents, that is, 145 (56%), were not aware of the use of ultraviolet (UV) gamma radiation for reducing the risk of transmission of TB in health care setting. While 166 (64%) respondents knew that N 95 masks reduce the risk of acquiring TB only 96 (37%) were aware about the need for fit testing.

To further understand the residents' main concerns about acquiring TB in the workplace, the 200 responses to the open-ended question were coded and analyzed. The level of agreement between the coders was high, with a Kappa of 0.85 ($p < 0.001$, 95% CI: 0.83–0.92). Six key themes were identified. Developing drug-resistant TB was the most common concern reported by 100 (50%) residents. The second most common concern, expressed by 39 (20%) residents, was about developing TB disease and its clinical consequences. Concerns about social and professional consequences of developing TB were reported by 37 (19%) residents. Other concerns expressed included exposure to TB patients at the workplace ($n = 32$; 16%); poor TB infection control measures ($n = 27$; 14%); and high workload and its health consequences ($n = 16$; 13%).

The six key themes, their subthemes, and representative comments from the responses to open-ended question are as follows.

Table 1: Characteristics of medical residents responding to TB risk questionnaire.

Variables	Responded to only structured questions	Responded to structured and open-ended questions*
Study participants: *N*	263	200
Mean age: years (SD)	27.2 (3.6)	27.3 (3.6)
Male gender: *N*/responses (%)	147/263 (60)	111/200 (56)
Year of residency: *N*/responses (%)		
First year	97/263 (37)	73/200 (36)
Second year	87/263 (33)	66/200 (33)
Third year	79/263 (30)	61/200 (31)
Working ≥12 hours/day: *N*/responses (%)	115/251 (46)	94/194 (49)
Daily exposure to known TB patients or specimens: *N*/responses (%)	141/222 (64)	104/168 (62)
Assessed for TB in the past: *N*/responses (%)	40/254 (16)	35/193 (18)
Past history of TB: *N*/responses (%)	13/253 (5)	12/193 (6)
Know a resident colleague with TB: *N*/responses (%)	115/251 (46)	94/194 (49)
Concerned about being infected with TB at workplace: *N*/responses (%)	205/263 (78)	161/200 (81)
Concerned about being infected with drug-resistant TB at workplace: *N*/responses (%)	232/263 (88)	183/200 (92)

*Subset of residents who responded to the open-ended question about TB risk concerns.

Table 2: Knowledge about measures to prevent occupationally acquired tuberculosis amongst medical resident doctors.

Measures	Responses *N* (%)	
	Agree	Disagree/ No opinion
Administrative measures		
Early detection and separation of patients with TB will reduce the risk of TB for HCWs ($N = 261$)	229 (88)	32 (12)
Cough etiquette in patients will reduce the risk of TB in HCWs ($N = 257$)	230 (89)	27 (11)
There are guidelines for prevention of transmission of TB in Health Care Set Up ($N = 252$)	175 (69)	77 (31)
Environmental measures		
Good ventilation at workplace will reduce the risk of TB in HCWs ($N = 261$)	238 (91)	23 (9)
Ultraviolet gamma irradiation can be used to reduce risk of transmission of TB at workplace ($N = 257$)	112 (44)	145 (56)
Respiratory protective devices		
HCWs can reduce their risk of acquiring TB by wearing N 95 masks ($N = 259$)	166 (64)	93 (36)
Fit testing is needed before using N 95 masks ($N = 259$)	96 (37)	163 (63)

3.1. Concern about Developing Drug-Resistant TB (DR-TB) in the Workplace. Concern about developing drug-resistant TB in the workplace was the most common key theme reported by 100 residents who responded to the open-ended question. Subthemes from these responses included concerns about side effects of DR-TB treatment, delayed diagnosis of DR-TB, and poor treatment outcomes due to DR-TB.

Representative responses about this theme and subthemes included the following:

> *"I am worried about the risk of MDR/XDR TB, as the treatment is very difficult to follow because of side effects."* (Age 27, Female, Ophthalmology)

> *"...worried about getting diagnosed with MDR/XDR TB. I would prefer to be screened directly for MDR TB and start treatment accordingly to prevent delays."* (Age 26, Male, Surgery)

> *"About MDR TB, there will be no definitive line of management; because I have seen Category IV patients go in relapse/failure."* (Age 27, Male, Orthopedics)

3.2. Concern about Developing TB Disease and Clinical Consequences of TB. Concern about developing TB in the workplace and its clinical consequences was the second most common key theme reported by the residents in response to the open-ended question. Subthemes from these responses included concerns about type of TB, clinical complications of TB, adverse effects of treatment, the long duration of treatment, and potential for hospitalization.

The following quotes represent this theme and subthemes:

> *"It can affect body system in the form of extra-pulmonary tuberculosis which remains undiagnosed for much time."* (Age 26, Female, Medicine)

> *"It could affect fertility."* (Age 26, Female, Pediatrics)

> *"The duration of treatment is lengthy."* (Age 27, Male, Medicine)

> *"I am worried about the adverse effects of drugs."* (Age 26, Female, Ophthalmology)

> *"Worried about the stay in TB ward."* (Age 30, Male, Psychiatry)

3.3. Concern about the Social and Professional Consequences of Developing TB. The residents expressed concern about a number of social and professional consequences of developing TB. The subthemes included academic loss, transmitting the infection to family members, and social stigma attached to the disease.

Responses representing this theme were as follows:

> *"I am worried about absenteeism from work, gap in residency."* (Age 26, Female, Medicine)

> *"Worried about transmitting TB to others."* (Age 26, Male, Preventive and Social Medicine)

> *"My colleagues will avoid staying with me if I develop TB."* (Age 28, Female, Medicine)

3.4. Concern about Exposure to TB Patients in the Workplace. This key theme included subthemes such as concerns about frequent encounters with TB patients, with undiagnosed and undisclosed TB patients, and patients with poor cough etiquettes. The residents from different departments expressed concern about specific types of exposures. For example, the resident doctors from the ophthalmology department perceived certain procedures, which they performed from close quarters, to increase the risk of infection.

Representative responses about this theme and subthemes included the following:

> *"There are many Koch's patients in the hospital campus. There is significant direct exposure to TB patients in OPD."* (Age 28, Male, Community Medicine)

> *"Many patients in the OPD have undiagnosed TB. Hence there is more risk."* (Age 26, Male, Surgery)

> *"Some patients hide their TB status from doctors."* (Age 25, Female, Otorhinolaryngology)

> *"Some patients cough right in front of our face in OPDs."* (Age 25, Female, Dermatology)

> *"When patients with TB and co-morbidity such as hypertension, diabetes mellitus are admitted in the wards a call is sent to ophthalmology department. We have to examine such patients with direct ophthalmoscope from close quarters. Other procedures like sac syringing, slit lamp examination also pose a risk of TB transmission."* (Age 28, Female, Ophthalmology)

3.5. Concern about Poor Infection Control Measures. There were multiple concerns expressed about poor infection control measures. The subthemes included inadequate patient screening for TB, lack of room ventilation, nonfunctional mechanical ventilation, and lack of N-95 masks. The resident doctors were concerned with both the natural and mechanical ventilation in general and specifically in the laboratories and enclosed rooms of radiology department. Only ten residents reported concern about lack of N-95 masks at workplace. Residents highlighted the importance of ventilation in enclosed rooms as well as practical difficulties and even a negligent attitude towards the use of protective equipment.

A few responses under this theme were as follows:

> *"...inadequate testing and screening for TB."* (Age 25, Male, Anesthesia)

> *"Being doctors we are exposed to burden of diverse (MDR) flora and still we have to work without necessary equipment (N 95 masks)"* (Age 28, Male, Pulmonary Medicine)

> *"We have a risk during certain procedures like USG. All our investigations are conducted in enclosed dark rooms with mechanical ventilation. If this fails and is not repaired, our risk increases."* (Age 26, Male, Radiology)

> *"...it is hardly possible for me to use the mask (N95) all the time. It causes suffocation and problems in communication."* (Age 26, Male, Ophthalmology)

> *"We do not use N 95 masks every time we do bronchoscopy. Use it only if we suspect the patient has TB...This is mere negligence."* (Age 29, Male, Pulmonary Medicine)

3.6. Concern about High Workload and Its Health Consequences. The subthemes under this key theme were concerns about excessive workload, long working hours, improper nutrition, and inadequate rest among the residents.

The following responses represent this theme:

> *"With odd working hours, sleep and food schedule we are at risk of developing TB"* (Age 26, Male, Anesthesia)

> *"Because of excessive physical strain and mental fatigue residents with heavy postings are not able to follow standard practices even if they know about them and then they fall for infection".* (Age 25, Male, Medicine)

TABLE 3: TB risk perceptions among resident doctors, key themes and subthemes.

Key themes	Subthemes
Developing drug-resistant TB ($n = 100$)	Side effects of DR-TB treatment; delayed diagnosis of DR-TB; poor treatment outcomes
Disease and its clinical consequences ($n = 39$)	Type of TB; clinical complications of TB; adverse effects of treatment; long duration of treatment; potential for hospitalization
Social and professional consequences ($n = 37$)	Academic loss; transmitting the infection to family members; social stigma attached to the disease
Exposure to TB patients/specimens ($n = 32$)	Frequent encounters with TB patients; encounters with undiagnosed cases; encounters with undisclosed TB patients; patients with poor cough etiquettes
Poor infection control measures ($n = 27$)	Inadequate patient screening for TB; Lack of room ventilation; Nonfunctional mechanical ventilation; Nonavailability and nonuse of N-95 masks
High workload and its health consequences ($n = 16$)	Workload; working hours; improper nutrition; inadequate rest

"There is excessive workload, especially in the first year. Need to redistribute the work among all residents..." (Age 28, Male, Pediatrics)

The key themes and subthemes which emerged from the study are summarized in Table 3.

4. Discussion

The study was conducted in a medical college hospital without a separate institutional TB infection control policy, in which residents have a heavy workload and frequent encounters with TB patients. The results of our study show that most medical residents in this public teaching hospital in India perceive TB as an occupational hazard, and many expressed concern about the consequences of developing TB disease. The incidence of TB among colleagues and the fact that many of the interventions for prevention of TB in health care settings need to be initiated at the institutional level rather than at an individual level could have contributed to these risk perceptions. There is a need to train the resident doctors as well as generate and highlight evidence demonstrating feasibility and effectiveness of the interventions for prevention of TB within health care settings in the Indian scenario. This may convince them of the need and also generate a demand for implementation of the TB infection control measures.

A majority of the resident doctors know about the role of administrative measures and ventilation in prevention of occupationally acquired TB. Less than 70% of them are aware of any guidelines for prevention of TB in health care settings, use of ultraviolet radiation and N 95 masks for prevention of occupationally acquired TB. Few were aware about the need of fit testing prior to using N 95 masks. In addition, only 39% of the residents reported to have been adequately trained in TB infection control measures. These gaps in knowledge indicate the need to incorporate the topic of prevention of occupationally acquired TB in their training program. The lack of knowledge about use of N 95 masks could also be due to either nonavailability or nonuse of the masks at workplace.

Responses to the open-ended questions indicate that their concerns go beyond the concerns about measures for preventing TB infection at workplace. These include concerns related to clinical, social, and professional implications of getting the disease and excessive workload.

A major concern is getting TB disease, including acquiring drug-resistant TB. Many of the resident doctors know of a colleague who has been diagnosed with TB. Having come across patients with TB and knowing another resident with TB reinforces this perception. A study conducted in this institute has reported that medical trainees in India are at risk of TB, including MDR TB [18]. Fear of death, duration, and side effects of the treatment regimens and hospitalization have been reported in this study. A study has reported similar fears among HCWs working in MDR/XDR TB wards in South Africa [21]. The perceptions of stigma about the disease may be influenced by the sociocultural milieu in the community. Being students, the resident doctors are also concerned about the anticipated extension of academic period resulting from the disease.

The resident doctors mention workload and its impact on their diet and resting hours. Concerns related to excessive workload and inadequate sleep and rest time leading to stress, especially in the first year of residency have been described in other studies too [22–25]. The hospital has a hierarchy system in which the major burden of work falls on the junior residents. Redistributing duties so that work hours are more evenly distributed among the health care workers will address some of the issues related to excessive workload. In certain procedures, the doctors examine the patients from close quarters, which is perceived to increase risk of TB transmission. Respondents in this study have mentioned some of these procedures, direct ophthalmoscopy, sac syringing, and slit lamp examination. Standard operating procedures should be established for trainees who perform them. TB wards, ART centers, bronchoscopy rooms, Intensive Care Units, radiology department, autopsy suites, and TB laboratories are designated high risk areas [9]. Good ventilation, masks for patients, and appropriate personal protective equipment for the doctors should be ensured for high risk procedures and areas. Using N-95 masks has been shown to lower the risk of incident LTBI [26]. However, the study respondents have reported practical problems in wearing masks for prolonged periods of time, as needed in high prevalence settings. Other studies have reported association of discomfort and headache with prolonged use of masks [27, 28]. The institute should formulate a policy for using N-95 masks and motivate and monitor its use among the residents. Addressing the resident doctors' concerns will not only facilitate prioritization of the implementation of interventions for prevention of TB transmission but also ensure compliance to the measures when they are implemented.

A majority of the medical resident doctors were concerned about TB disease, especially drug-resistant TB. Though many of the resident doctors were aware of TB infection control guidelines only few of them expressed concern about exposure to TB patients and lack of TB infection control measures at the institutional level. There is a need to train the resident doctors and highlight specific evidence demonstrating the feasibility and efficacy of these guidelines in prevention of TB in Indian scenario. Simultaneously, the health care system has to fulfill the reciprocal obligation of implementing these guidelines.

Disclosure

The content is solely the responsibility of the authors and does not necessarily represent the official views of the National Institutes of Health. An earlier version of this work was presented as an abstract at the "46th Union World Conference on Lung Health," 2015, in Cape Town, South Africa.

Authors' Contributions

Geeta Pardeshi contributed to conception and design, acquisition of data, analysis and interpretation of data, and drafting the manuscript; Dileep Kadam and Ajay Chandanwale contributed to design and final approval of the version to be published; Andrea Deluca contributed to study design, data analysis, and drafting the manuscript; Pranali Khobragde, Malan Parande, Aarti Kinikar, Anita Basavaraj, Sunita Girish, Sangita Shelke, Nishi Suryawanshi, and Nikhil Gupte contributed to study design and data collection; Jason Farley contributed to study design and development of study tool; and Robert Bollinger contributed to conception and design, revising it critically for important intellectual content, and final approval of the version to be published.

Acknowledgments

The authors acknowledge the valuable time spared by the residents for filling up the questionnaire. This work was supported by the BJGMC JHU HIV Program funded by the Fogarty International Center, NIH (Grant no. 1D43TW009574). The authors thank members of the CTU and BJGMC for their support and guidance.

References

[1] R. Joshi, A. L. Reingold, D. Menzies, and M. Pai, "Tuberculosis among health-care workers in low- and middle-income countries: a systematic review," *PLoS Medicine*, vol. 3, no. 12, pp. 2376–2391, 2006.

[2] World Health Organization (WHO), *Guidelines for Prevention of Tuberculosis in Health Care Facilities in Resource Limited Settings*, World Health Organization, Geneva, Switzerland, 1999, http://www.who.int/tb/publications/who_tb_99_269.pdf?ua=1.

[3] World Health Organization (WHO), *WHO Policy on TB Infection Control in Health-Care Facilities, Congregate Settings and Households*, World Health Organization, Geneva, Switzerland, 2009, http://apps.who.int/iris/bitstream/10665/44148/1/9789241598323_eng.pdf.

[4] D. Menzies, R. Joshi, and M. Pai, "Risk of tuberculosis infection and disease associated with work in health care settings," *The International Journal of Tuberculosis and Lung Disease*, vol. 11, no. 6, pp. 593–605, 2007.

[5] D. J. Christopher, P. Daley, L. Armstrong et al., "Tuberculosis infection among young nursing trainees in South India," *PLoS ONE*, vol. 5, no. 4, Article ID e10408, 2010.

[6] K. G. Rao, A. M. Aggarwal, and D. Behera, "Tuberculosis among physicians in training," *The International Journal of Tuberculosis and Lung Disease*, vol. 8, no. 11, pp. 1392–1394, 2004.

[7] M. Pai, K. Gokhale, R. Joshi et al., "Mycobacterium tuberculosis infection in health care workers in rural India: Comparison of a whole-blood interferon γ assay with tuberculin skin testing," *Journal of the American Medical Association*, vol. 293, no. 22, pp. 2746–2755, 2005.

[8] M. Pai, R. Joshi, S. Dogra et al., "Serial testing of health care workers for tuberculosis using interferon-γ assay," *American Journal of Respiratory and Critical Care Medicine*, vol. 174, no. 3, pp. 349–355, 2006.

[9] Directorate General of Health Services, *Guidelines on Airborne Infection Control in Healthcare and Other Settings in the Context of Tuberculosis and Other Airborne Infections*, Ministry of Health & Family Welfare, New Delhi, India, 2010, http://upsacs.in/pdf/Guidelines_on_Airborne_Infection_Control_April2010Provisional.pdf.

[10] J. E. Farley, C. Tudor, M. Mphahlele et al., "A national infection control evaluation of drug-resistant tuberculosis hospitals in South Africa," *The International Journal of Tuberculosis and Lung Disease*, vol. 16, no. 1, pp. 82–89, 2012.

[11] G. X. He, S. V. D. Hof, M. J. V. D. Werf et al., "Infection control and the burden of tuberculosis infection and disease in health care workers in China: a cross-sectional study," *BMC Infectious Diseases*, vol. 10, article 313, 2010.

[12] J. Robert, D. Affolabi, F. Awokou et al., "Assessment of organizational measures to prevent nosocomial tuberculosis in health facilities of 4 sub-saharan countries in 2010," *Infection Control and Hospital Epidemiology*, vol. 34, no. 2, pp. 190–194, 2013.

[13] S. Naidoo, K. Seevnarain, and D. L. Nordstrom, "Tuberculosis infection control in primary health clinics in eThekwini, KwaZulu-Natal, South Africa," *The International Journal of Tuberculosis and Lung Disease*, vol. 16, no. 12, pp. 1600–1604, 2012.

[14] B.-E. Ider, J. Adams, A. Morton, M. Whitby, and A. Clements, "Perceptions of healthcare professionals regarding the main challenges and barriers to effective hospital infection control in Mongolia: a qualitative study," *BMC Infectious Diseases*, vol. 12, article 170, 2012.

[15] H. A. Joseph, R. Shrestha-Kuwahara, D. Lowry et al., "Factors influencing health care workers' adherence to work site tuberculosis screening and treatment policies," *American Journal of Infection Control*, vol. 32, no. 8, pp. 456–461, 2004.

[16] D. Sissolak, F. Marais, and S. Mehtar, "TB infection prevention and control experiences of South African nurses—a phenomenological study," *BMC Public Health*, vol. 11, article 262, 2011.

[17] W. M. Woith, G. Volchenkov, and J. L. Larson, "Barriers and motivators affecting tuberculosis infection control practices of Russian health care workers," *The International Journal of Tuberculosis and Lung Disease*, vol. 16, no. 8, pp. 1092–1096, 2012.

[18] A. Basavaraj, A. Chandanwale, A. Patil et al., "High tuberculosis risk among medical trainees, Pune, India," *Emerging Infectious Diseases*, vol. 22, no. 3, pp. 541–543, 2016.

[19] G. S. Pardeshi, D. Kadam, A. Chandanwale, R. Bollinger, and A. Deluca, "Resident doctors' attitudes toward tuberculosis patients," *Indian Journal of Tuberculosis*, vol. 64, no. 2, pp. 89–92, 2017.

[20] B. L. Berg, *Qualitative Research Methods for the Social Sciences*, Pearson, Boston, Mass, USA, 5th edition, 2004.

[21] C. Tudor, M. Mphahlele, M. Van der Walt, and J. E. Farley, "Health care workers' fears associated with working in multidrug- and or extensively-resistant tuberculosis wards in South Africa," *The International Journal of Tuberculosis and Lung Disease*, vol. 17, no. 10, pp. 22–29, 2013.

[22] J. D. Deshpande, D. B. Phalke, P. Kalakoti, D. Qutub, and V. Agrawal, "Stress levels and depression amongst interns and resident doctors working in a tertiary care teaching hospital in rural area," *International Journal of Health and Rehabilitation Sciences*, vol. 2, no. 1, pp. 44–49, 2013.

[23] J. Stebbing and T. Powles, "Stress in the workplace amongst medical professionals," *Journal of Postgraduate Medicine*, vol. 53, no. 2, pp. 83-84, 2007.

[24] G. S. Azhar, A. Z. Azhar, and A. S. Azhar, "Overwork among residents in India: a medical resident's perspective," *Journal of Family Medicine and Primary Care*, vol. 1, no. 2, pp. 141–143, 2012.

[25] R. K. Bansal, P. Bharodiya, K. Jain et al., "Stress profile of post graduate medical residents in western India," *National Journal of Community Medicine*, vol. 1, no. 1, pp. 55-56, 2010.

[26] E. L. Maciel, M. C. Viana, R. C. Zeitoune, I. Ferreira, G. Fregona, and R. Dietze, "Prevalence and incidence of Mycobacterium tuberculosis infection in nursing students in Vitória, Espírito Santo," *Revista da Socieda de Brasileira de Medicina Tropical*, vol. 38, no. 6, pp. 469–472, 2005.

[27] J. H. Zhu, S. J. Lee, D. Y. Wang, and H. P. Lee, "Effects of long duration wearing of N 95 respirator and surgical facemask: a pilot study," *Journal of Lung, Pulmonary and Respiratory Research*, vol. 1, no. 4, 2014, http://medcraveonline.com/JLPRR/JLPRR-01-00021.pdf.

[28] E. C. H. Lim, R. C. S. Seet, K.-H. Lee, E. P. V. Wilder-Smith, B. Y. S. Chuah, and B. K. C. Ong, "Headaches and the N95 face-mask amongst healthcare providers," *Acta Neurologica Scandinavica*, vol. 113, no. 3, pp. 199–202, 2006.

29

Evolution of *M. bovis* BCG Vaccine: Is Niacin Production Still a Valid Biomarker?

Sarman Singh,[1] Manoj Kumar,[1] and Pragati Singh[2]

[1]*Division of Clinical Microbiology & Molecular Medicine, Department of Laboratory Medicine, All India Institute of Medical Sciences, New Delhi 110029, India*
[2]*National Polio Surveillance Project, Country Office for India, World Health Organization, Mathura 281001, India*

Correspondence should be addressed to Sarman Singh; sarman_singh@yahoo.com

Academic Editor: Vincent Jarlier

BCG vaccine is usually considered to be safe though rarely serious complications have also been reported, often incriminating contamination of the seed strain with pathogenic *Mycobacterium tuberculosis*. In such circumstances, it becomes prudent to rule out the contamination of the vaccine seed. *M. bovis* BCG can be confirmed by the absence of nitrate reductase, negative niacin test, and resistance to pyrazinamide and cycloserine. Recently in India, some stocks were found to be niacin positive which led to a national controversy and closer of a vaccine production plant. This prompted us to write this review and the comparative biochemical and genotypic studies were carried out on the these contentious vaccine stocks at the Indian vaccine plant and other seeds and it was found that some BCG vaccine strains and even some strains of *M. bovis* with eugenic-growth characteristics mainly old laboratory strains may give a positive niacin reaction. Most probably, the repeated subcultures lead to undefined changes at the genetic level in these seed strains. These changing biological characteristics envisage reevaluation of biochemical characters of existing BCG vaccine seeds and framing of newer guidelines for manufacturing, production, safety, and effectiveness of BCG vaccine.

1. Introduction

BCG, an attenuated strain of *Mycobacterium bovis* (*M. bovis*), has been used in more than 182 countries or territories as a prophylactic vaccine against tuberculosis (TB), for more than 90 years, albeit amidst a considerable controversy related to its efficacy. The true efficacy of BCG has been difficult to understand due to many experimental variables [1]. *M. bovis* is the etiological agent of bovine tuberculosis and is closely related to *Mycobacterium tuberculosis* (*M. tuberculosis*) in the *M. tuberculosis* complex (MTBC), which consists of *M. tuberculosis, M. bovis, M. bovis* BCG, *M. africanum, M. canettii, M. microti, M. caprae,* and *M. pinnipedii*. The *M. bovis* mainly infects cattle (*Bos taurus*), but it can infect other mammalians including humans [2, 3]. The BCG vaccine undoubtedly provides protection against childhood disseminated form of TB including TB meningitis. However its efficacy against pulmonary TB in adults has been reported to give variable results [4]. In 2011, World Health Organization (WHO) monitored study revealed that protection levels ranged from 53% in Equatorial Guinea and 54% in Ethiopia to more than 99.5% in India and China [5]. Its efficacy in programmed mode is reported to be more than 80% [6]. So far more than 3 billion doses of BCG vaccine have been given since 1948, and by and large it is considered safe [7]. However localized abscess formation, disseminated disease, and regional lymphadenopathy, especially in immunocompromised hosts are rare but well-recognized complications [8].

An estimated 8.6 million new cases and 1.3 million deaths due to tuberculosis occur every year [9]. Almost all cases of tuberculosis are caused by *M. tuberculosis*, and share of *M. bovis* is less than 1.4 percent of all pulmonary tuberculosis cases outside of Africa. Though, in Africa, *M. bovis* accounts for approximately 2.8 percent of cases of pulmonary tuberculosis, for a crude incidence of 7 cases per 100,000 populations [10], the global proportion of *M. bovis* is higher among patients with extrapulmonary tuberculosis, since the pathogen is frequently acquired via oral ingestion and gastrointestinal disease is an important clinical manifestation [11].

2. Historical Aspect of BCG

The original BCG vaccine "strain" was derived from an isolate of *M. bovis*. Since 1900, Albert Calmette (1863–1933) began his research on the *M. bovis* strain, which had been isolated from the milk of an infected cow by veterinarian Jean-Marie Camille Guérin (1872–1961) in 1904. In addition, the "strain" was named Bacillus of Calmette and Guérin. They cultivated these bacilli in a medium containing glycerin and potato, but they found that there was difficulty in the production of homogenous suspension of the bacilli. To make the bacteria homogenous they added ox bile to the medium and to their revelation, they found that the additive has lowered the virulence of bacteria. This unexpected observation became source of vaccine production from the attenuated tubercle bacilli [12]. Benjamin Weill-Hall (1875–1958), a French pediatrician and bacteriologist, was the first to feed the vaccine to infants in Paris who were at a risk for the disease. However, in 1908, Camille Guérin and Benjamin Weill-Hall, both at the Institute Pasteur in Lille, France, began attenuating the *M. bovis* by passing it through a growth medium they had developed specifically for this purpose and an actual BCG vaccine was thus developed at the Pasteur Institute in Lille and was first given to humans in 1921. The first formal trial of BCG outside France was organized among the North American Indians in the 1930s [13]. By the late 1940s, several studies provided evidence favouring its utility in protection against tuberculosis. For this, the original culture was subcultured and distributed to several laboratories throughout the world, where the vaccine strain was called BCG and was maintained by continuous subcultures. After many years, the various strains maintained in different laboratories were found to be no longer identical to each other. In fact, it was likely that various strains maintained by continuous subculture continued to undergo undefined genetic changes. Indeed, even the "original" strain of BCG maintained at Paris also continued to change its characteristic during the subcultures. To limit the genetic changes the procedures needed to maintain the strain were modified time to time. Currently, the *M. bovis* BCG is maintained by using a "seed-lot" production technique to limit further genetic variations.

Presently, five main strains or seed-lots, accounting for more than 90% of the vaccine produced, are used worldwide with each strain possessing different biological characteristics. These strains are Pasteur 1173 P2, the DANISH 1331, the Glaxo 1077 (derived from the DANISH strain), the Russian BCG-I, the Tokyo 172-1, and the Moreau RDJ strains [24]. Confusions are generated by the vague terminologies used by individual stakeholders (e.g. "American" strain), varying nomenclature (e.g., BCG Brazil is the synonym of BCG Moreau, although Moreau was from Uruguay), and unusual corporate events (e.g., Pasteur-MeÂrieux-Connaught produces BCG- Glaxo except in Canada where BCG-Connaught is used) [25]. Articles on BCG molecular biology reflect this confusion, with studies employing different strains, attributed to different historical periods [26]. In the extent of different vaccine efficacy and safety in humans, it is not clear at present; but some differences in the molecular and genetic characteristics are known and each BCG has been called by the location where it is produced; for example, BCG (Paris), BCG (Copenhagen), BCG (Tice), and BCG (Montreal).

In India, the BCG vaccination programme was started in 1948 and BCG vaccine laboratory was established in Madanpalle (Tamil Nadu, India). By 1960, the first round of mass BCG vaccination was completed in all states with about 254 million persons having been vaccinated by 1979. Yet BCG is one of the most controversial vaccines till today [27]. Since the 1950s, the reason for the failure of BCG in some populations has been a subject of debate, and to explain the observed variation, different hypotheses have been suggested [28]. The differences in the strain of BCG, the age at vaccination, or methodological differences are important factors [29]. One exception from this general rule is the consistent high efficacy when BCG is used to vaccinate newborns. Neonatal vaccination with BCG reports protection against the childhood manifestations of TB, especially the meningitis [30], but the efficacy decreases over a period of times, and therefore in the adult population the third world vaccine does not prevent against the later breakdown with pulmonary TB [28].

3. Biochemical and Genotypic Characteristics of BCG

Phenotypic characteristics have been a contentious issue and some strains are considered inferior over the others. Not only allegations of contamination with *M. tuberculosis* have been made occasionally, but also recently one batch of the Indian BCG vaccine was found to give niacin positive reaction and this led to the closure of vaccine plant in India. A high-level technical committee was formed by Government of India and one coauthor was part of this committee. As described in Table 1, the diagnostic features of BCG include growth in Lowenstein-Jensen and 7H11 media and in the modified Dubos liquid medium at 37°C; inhibition of growth in the presence of thiophene-2-carboxylic acid hydrazide; negative tests for niacin, catalase production at 68°C, nitrate reduction, Tween 80 hydrolysis; and a positive urease test [31]. On the basis of secreted proteins, MPB64 and MPB70 substrains of *M. bovis* BCG have been divided in two major groups: high and low producers of these proteins [16]. Polymerase chain reaction (PCR) and hybridization experiments indicate that the MPB64 gene is absent in the BCG substrains Pasteur, Glaxo, Copenhagen, and Tice. The species specificity of MPB64 and its occurrence in both *M. tuberculosis* and virulent strains of *M. bovis* may create further confusion [32]. Biochemical tests are currently used for the identification of bacterial species, including the genus *Mycobacterium* [33]. Several enzymes such as NAD and NADH quinone reductases, mycobacterial phospholipase A (MPLA) which catalyses the hydrolysis of lipids including Tween 80, and others appear to contribute to survival of the mycobacteria [34, 35]. An important virulence factor for *M. tuberculosis* and *M. bovis* is the nitrate reductase system. Chemically, BCG can be distinguished from *M. tuberculosis* by its weakly positive nitrate reduction ability. While the amidase test gives a strongly positive reaction to carbamide, whereas other amidases give negative results in Bônicke series [36].

TABLE 1: Characterization and comparison of different conventional biochemical and molecular tests to identify different *Mycobacterium bovis* (BCG) and *Mycobacterium tuberculosis* species.

Tests strain	*M. bovis* BCG P3	*M. tuberculosis* H37Rv	*Remarks*
Nitrate reduction	Negative	Positive	
Niacin	Positive	Positive	
Catalase	Negative	Negative	
hsp65-PCR	Positive	Positive	
esat6-PCR	Negative	Positive	
Mac-PCR	Negative	Negative	¥
MPT64 antigen	Negative	Positive	
MPT63 antigen	Positive	Positive	
Binary spoligotyping	■■□■■■■■□■■■■■■□■■■■■■■■■■■■■■■■■■■■■■□□□□□	■■■■■■■■■■■■■■■■■■■□□■■■■■■■■■■■■□□□□■■■■■■	
Octal number	676773777777600	777777477760771	
Shared type	482	451	
Lineage/sublineages	Bovis1_BCG	H37Rv	
Guinea pig virulence	Non-virulent	Virulent	Ψ
	M. bovis BCG (Tokyo)	*M. tuberculosis* H37Ra	
Nitrate reduction	Positive	Positive	
Niacin	Positive**	Positive	[14]
Catalase	Negative	Positive**	
	M. bovis BCG (ATCC 19274), *M. bovis BCG* (Biken)	*M. tuberculosis H37Rv* (TMC102), H37Rv (Biken), H37Ra (Biken)	
Niacin test	Weakly Positive	Pos	[15]
	BCG Copenhagen, BCG Glaxo, BCG Pasteur, BCG Tice	*M. tuberculosis* H37Rv, *M. tuberculosis* H37Ra	
MPB64	Negative	Positive	
MPB70	Positive	Positive	[15]
16SrRNA	Positive	Positive	
	BCG Tokyo, BCG Moreau, BCG Russia, BCG Sweden. *M. bovis* AN5	—	
MPB64	Positive	—	
MPB70	Positive	—	[16]
16SrRNA	Positive	—	
	M. bovis BCG (Glaxo, Pasteur, Tice)	*M. tuberculosis* (H37Rv)	
MPB64	Negative	Positive	[16]
IS6110 copy number	1	—	
	M. bovis BCG (Brazilian, Japanese, Russian, Swedish)		
MPB64	Positive		[16]
IS6110 copy number	2	—	
	M. bovis BCG	*M. tuberculosis (classical)*	
Nitrate reduction	Positive	Positive	[17]
Niacin	Negative	Positive	

Table 1: Continued.

	M. bovis BCG	*M. tuberculosis* (classical)	
Nitrate reduction	Negative	Positive	[18]
Niacin	Negative	Positive	
MPB70	Positive	Positive	
Mtp40	Negative	Positive* (very occasionally)	
	M. bovis BCG	*M. tuberculosis*	
Nitrate reduction	Negative	Positive	[19]
Niacin	Negative	Positive	
MPB70	Positive	Negative	
Mtp40	Negative	Positive	
Spoligotyping spacer 39–43	Negative	Positive	
	M. bovis	*M. tuberculosis*	
Nitrate reduction	Negative	Positive	[20]
Niacin accumulation	Negative	Positive	
Presence of mtp40	Negative	Positive	
Spoligotype (characteristic features)	At least one of spacers 39–43 present	Spacers 39–43 absent	
	M. bovis BCG	*M. tuberculosis* (H37Rv)	
Binary spoligotyping	■■□□□■■■□■■■■■■□■■■■□■■■■■■■■■■■■■■■■■□□□□□	■■■■■■■■■■■■■■■■■■■□□■■■■■■■■■■■□□□□■■■■■■■	[21]
Octal number	616773677777600	777777477760771	
Shared type	663	451	
	BOVIS1	H37Rv	
	M. bovis	*M. tuberculosis*	
Spacers 33 to 36 (derived from BCG)	—	*M. tuberculosis* does not hybridize to the spacers	[22]
Spacers 39 to 43 (derived from *M. tuberculosis*)	*M. bovis* and BCG do not hybridize to the spacers	—	
	M. bovis	*M. tuberculosis* (H37Rv)	
Capilia TB-Neo	Positive	Positive	[23]
SD MPT64	Positive	Positive	
TbcID	Positive	Positive	
	M. bovis BCG Tokyo	*M. bovis* BCG Connaught	
Capilia TB-Neo	Positive	Negative	[23]

¥Our analysis on the Indian seed-lot; Ψpersonal communication with the Director of the BCG vaccine producing laboratory; *very occasionally positive; **Weak Positive.

Niacin production during the adaptation to hosts of several strains of biovars 1 to 4 can more readily switch on and switch off the genes. It is reported that *M. bovis* strains of the "European" type (which possess a single IS*6110* fragment and which lack DR spacer sequences 39 to 43) branched off at an earlier stage than the other *M. bovis* strains. The *M. bovis* BCG has been reported as niacin test negative, nitrate reductase negative, and pyrazinamide and cycloserine resistance [37].

The elevated levels of nitrate reductase activity increase the virulence and consequently the success of some lineages of *M. tuberculosis* [38]. However, nitrite production has also been reported in some strains of *M. bovis* under different conditions such as longer incubation period and anaerobic conditions [39]. Both *M. tuberculosis* and *M. bovis* BCG express an anaerobic nitrate reductase (NarGHJI) activity and a *narG* *M. bovis* BCG mutant lacks the ability to reduce nitrate under anaerobic conditions [40]. A *narG* knockout mutant of BCG showed reduced virulence and reduced lung damage in severe combined immunodeficiency (SCID) mice. Thus *M. bovis* BCG, like *M. tuberculosis*, can form granulomas in different body sites and abscesses in various human tissues [41]. In MTB granuloma formation hypoxia plays an important role and this pathology is mediated by several enzymes including nitrate reductase [42, 43]. However, the role of hypoxia is not well defined in vaccine strain *M. bovis* BCG [44].

The human tubercle bacilli (*M. tuberculosis*) produce more niacin than other mycobacteria, and the detection of niacin production has been widely used for differentiating MTBC species from *M. bovis* which are usually niacin negative [45–47]. Recently, this biomarker created a huge crisis in Indian Government system, because the in-use lots of BCG vaccine were found to be niacin positive. Other manufacturers of the BCG vaccine alleged that the Indian seed-lot was contaminated with *M. tuberculosis*. Besides closing the vaccine production plant, the Government of India set up a technical committee to examine the controversy. Several seed-lots along with the alleged Indian lots were analyzed in Table 1. These results indicated that besides Indian seed-lot (BCG-P3) several other strains have also become niacin positive, without any evidence. The strain BCG-P3 has been found to lack genes normally present in *M. tuberculosis* but absent in BCG and was nonvirulent for Guinea pigs, ruling out contamination by *M. tuberculosis*, important fact. All vaccine producers are required to follow standard vaccine virulence testing guidelines as per WHO guidelines [45]. The literature also indicates that some bovine strains with eugenic-growth characteristic, mainly old laboratory strains, and some BCG vaccine strains may give a positive niacin reaction; on the other hand, certain *M. tuberculosis* strains with dysgenic-growth characteristics, such as isoniazid-resistant strains, may give a niacin negative reaction [48, 49].

4. *M. bovis* Genome and Biological Lifestyle

At genetic level also heterogeneity of niacin accumulation has been observed among BCG substrains. The *M. bovis* cell wall contains phenolic glycolipids that are absent in *M. tuberculosis*. A family of membrane-spanning proteins involved in the export of the phenolic cell wall glycolipids in the *M. bovis* genome (TbD1 locus) consists of the *mmp* genes [50]. A group of antigens of ESAT-6 family such as CPF-7 and CPF-10 which were originally described as T-cell antigens are secreted by *M. tuberculosis* [51], but these are also encoded by the genome of *M. bovis*. Other members of the family act in match-up; possibly in a mix-and-match array the interaction between ESAT-6 and CPF-10 is exhibited, whereas in *M. tuberculosis* the six members of the ESAT-6 familyare absent from the genome of *M. bovis* [52, 53].

5. *M. bovis* BCG Infection

BCG infections are infrequent, but rarely some children can develop localized or disseminated BCG infections. To differentiate these manifestations from other conditions recovery of the BCG strain of *M. bovis* from the pretentious focus is mandatory. The identification process of *M. bovis* is not simple as it relies on the isolation of the bacteria from the site of localized infection, usually the injection site, or from other tissues including the blood such as in case of disseminated infection. In adults, when BCG vaccine is used in bladder cancer therapy, dissemination can lead to fatal infection. Recently, molecular techniques have been frequently used to identify the true pathogens even when it is not culturable. The commonest molecular methods used to identify and confirm the diagnosis of BCG vaccine infections are PCR followed by single stranded conformation polymorphism (SSCP). The *pncA* gene is the most specific target due to the fact that polymorphic site at the 169 position of this gene, *M. bovis* BCG vaccine can be differentiated from *M. tuberculosis* using PCR-RFLP [54]. The standard mycobacterial culture techniques currently used in clinical microbiology laboratories are capable of identifying mycobacteria to the level of the *M. tuberculosis* complex. On the basis of morphology and biochemical criteria, it is difficult to differentiate between virulent *M. bovis* and *M. bovis* BCG. More sophisticated methods are probably needed to confirm a diagnosis of *M. bovis* BCG. Complications after BCG vaccination and the intrinsic resistance of *M. bovis* BCG to pyrazinamide, as well as knowledge on BCG infection, would be of particular interest to the clinician responsible for guiding therapy. After PCR-based diagnosis, therapy is based on drug susceptibility with BCG sensitive regimens, that is, isoniazid, rifampin, and ethambutol. However, the prevalence of BCG infection is not known, mainly because most laboratories cannot quickly differentiate between BCG and other members of the *M. tuberculosis* complex. Utilization of an allele-specific PCR combined with a multiplex PCR was found to be a sensitive and rapid test for the detection of *M. bovis* BCG in clinical specimens [37].

6. Complications of BCG Vaccination

BCG vaccine has been given to more than a billion people, but the protective efficacy is reported to vary in various human trials and the utility is further limited by their propensity to induce tuberculin reactivity [55, 56]. The current global threat of tuberculosis and the emergence of drug-resistant strains are compelling the scientific community to improve BCG vaccine or develop an entirely new vaccine against tuberculosis [57]. BCG vaccine has been considered to be safe, and although complications are rare after vaccination and the outcome is usually favourable, serious BCG infections can occur. Localized abscesses, regional lymphadenopathy, and disseminated disease in immunocompromised hosts are uncommon but well-recognized complications [58]. The retrospective review identified 60 cases of dissemination for which the mortality rate was 50%. BCG vaccine has been administered per cutaneous in Brazil since 1968 using the multiple puncture method. More than 1,000 publications made between 1921 and 1982 reported approximately 10,000 complications of BCG vaccination [58]. Recent molecular work has demonstrated differences between BCG and *M. tuberculosis* as well as within the BCG strains [59, 60]. Since BCG strains vary in protein expression [61], lipid composition [62], pathobiology in laboratory animals [63, 64] and humans, an understanding of genetic differences may provide insights into the determinants of protective immunity and vaccine associated complications [65–67].

The mild adverse reaction is characterized by a papule at an injection site, which may progress to become ulcerated. This may heal after 2–5 months leaving a superficial scar, and swelling of the epilateral regional lymph nodes may also occur. Multiple cutaneous lesions may signal disseminated BCG disease usually in an immunocompromised host [24]. Severe adverse events include subcutaneous abscess and keloids at the injection site and occurrence of a number of cutaneous lesions (such as TB chancre, lupus vulgaris, scrofuloderma, papulonecrotic, and disseminated tuberculosis) at the sites distinct from the vaccination site [68]. The incidence of local complications depends on the age of the recipient and the dose of vaccine. In newborn, BCG administration as an intradermal injection at any age is not easy; the commonest error is to inject the vaccine too deep. This deep injection can cause injection abscesses (2% cases). In more serious injection related complications, deep ulcers, osteomyelitis (0.04%), and lymphadenopathy (1%), especially in younger infants under one year, may occur. The immune dysfunction is directly related to disseminated disease, in the order of 1/1,000,000 doses, but is thought to be rare [69].

7. BCG Complications in HIV Infected Hosts

Following *M. bovis* BCG vaccination, development of disseminated disease in immune-compromised individuals has been reported which can be fatal in several cases [70]. The significantly high risk of disseminated BCG (dBCG) disease is reported in HIV-positive infants, with rates approaching 1% in South Africa [71]. Immune reconstitution inflammatory syndrome (IRIS) has recently been identified as a BCG vaccine-related adverse event in immunocompromised individuals after antiretroviral therapy (ART) [72]. The cellular primary immunodeficiency predisposes to the condition [73, 74]. The place of BCG vaccination in TB control programs is being carefully assessed as of the considerable risk of human to human transmission in immune-compromised patients, particularly in TB nonendemic countries [75–77].

8. BCG Vaccine and Tuberculin Skin Test (TST)

BCG-induced tuberculin reactivity is identical with reactivity induced by *M. tuberculosis* infection and the increased degree has been found in BCG revaccination in school children. The influence of BCG vaccination in past has been reported on tuberculin skin test (TST) surveys used as an auxiliary tool to estimate latent or active tuberculosis [78, 79].

9. Current Understanding of BCG Vaccination

The production of *M. bovis* BCG from different strains and by different manufacturers resulted in variable quality of vaccine and viabilities per dose of vaccine, as discussed in the previous paragraphs [80, 81]. Therefore, the World Health Organization is contemplating the revision in vaccine production guidelines, scope, terminology, and requirement of BCG vaccines. To discuss issues regarding the standardization, characterization of live and attenuated BCG vaccines, and evaluation of these vaccines, a consultative meeting of regulators, BCG vaccine manufacturers, researchers, and program managers was organized in 2010. The development of live attenuated TB vaccines, new recombinant BCG, and the characterization of different BCG sub-strains were also reviewed using state-of-the-art technologies to revise and update the various important issues related to current recommendations focused on the scope, terminology, manufacturing issues, and the incorporation of new reference reagents and new quality control test [82]. Interestingly, recent studies have shown that the combination of priming with recombinant BCG such as Δ*ureC* *hly*$^{+}$ rBCG and boosting it with most efficacious subunit vaccine would provide more powerful intervention measure against tuberculosis [83, 84]. The results of a long-term controlled trial of a BCG vaccine provides supports to investigators aspiring to produce vaccine with similar or improved characteristics as trial of a BCG vaccine found to have good protective efficacy against TB that extended up to 60 years after vaccination except some cases of pulmonary and extrapulmonary TB [85, 86].

10. Guidelines on Administration of BCG Vaccine

Tuberculosis emerged as a major concern in the aftermath of World War II, and subsequently, the use of BCG was encouraged in many countries, particularly by UNICEF and by Scandinavian Red Cross Societies and then by the WHO. Major trials were set up by the British Medical Research Council (BMRC) and by the United States Public Health Service (USPHS) in the early 1950s. The procedure employed by the BMRC provided high efficacy against tuberculosis [86, 87]. In contrast, BCG used by the USPHS (Park or Tice strains given to tuberculin-negatives of various ages) provided very little protection [55]. Respective public health agencies reported that BCG was recommended as a routine for tuberculin-negative adolescents in the UK, whereas in USA, BCG was restricted to certain high-risk populations but was not recommended for routine use [88]. Following major policy changes in the field of infectious disease control and immunization programs, and the amendment of the Immunization Law in 2001 BCG vaccination campaign was introduced [83, 89] according to various schedules (e.g., at birth, school entry, or school leaving) in the majority of countries [82].

11. Molecular Biology of BCG

11.1. Genetic Evolution. BCG is a derivative of *M. bovis* after the loss of the region of deletion 1 (RD1) that encodes the ESX-1 secretion system [90]. During the first half of the 20th century BCG was maintained by serial passage throughout the world, as mentioned in the history section. Over the decades, multiple BCG daughter strains were produced which resulted in several regions of genomic deletions as well as regions of genomic duplication and other mutations [83–86]. A tremendous opportunity is provided by the complete genome sequence of *M. tuberculosis* for investigating molecular mechanisms of overlapping disease manifestations produced by *M. bovis* BCG and *M. tuberculosis* and it is now evident that both share 99.9% of their DNA. It also shows that the BCG strain retained at least some of its original virulence characters [91–93]. The attenuation of BCG due to the loss of RD1 region from *M. bovis* and reintroduction of RD1 into BCG increased virulence significantly. Because of complementation neither BCG Pasteur nor the least passaged strain, BCG Russia, with RD1 resulted in the restoration of virulence to levels characteristic of *M. tuberculosis* or *M. bovis*. The reported genetic studies weaken the theory that the RD3, RD4, RD5, RD7, and RD9 loci are responsible for virulence among the tubercle bacilli [90]. The immune suppressive capacity of BCG is perhaps the most apparent feature in-vivo [87–91].

Some of the *M. bovis* BCG isolates that are reported to be sensitive to ethambutol, streptomycin, and p-nitrobenzoic acid reacted positively to cycloserine, but they are found to be resistant to isoniazid, rifampicin, pyrazinamide, and thiophen-2-carbonic acid hydrazide. However, lately, the cloning of pyrazinamidase gene (*pncA*) shows a single point mutation in the gene which is unique to *M. bovis* [94–98]. Therefore, to differentiate *M. tuberculosis* and *M. bovis* polymorphism, this gene could be a good option for diagnosis methods.

The standard mycobacterial culture techniques currently used in clinical microbiology laboratories are capable of identifying mycobacteria to the level of the *M. tuberculosis* complex.

It has been reported that most of *M. bovis* strainscontainspacers 40 to 43, whereas they lacks spacer 39 [36]. In 1993, Hoffner studied a high degree of biochemical heterogeneity within strains of the *M. tuberculosis* complex isolated [98], when subtyped by DNA fingerprinting using the insertion element IS*6110* and spoligotyping [92]. Variable-number tandem repeats (VNTRs) occur throughout the chromosome of *M. tuberculosis*. Mycobacterial interspersed repetitive units (MIRUs) are polymorphic VNTRs and also have proved to be useful tools in molecular epidemiology; their biological significance is less well understood. The copy number of VNTR 3690 varies among Indian clinical isolates of *M. tuberculosis* (one to twelve copies), *M. tuberculosis* H37Rv TMC102 (four copies), *M. tuberculosis* H37Ra (two to four copies), and *M. bovis* BCG (one copy) [99]. A detailed comparison among virulent *M. tuberculosis*, *M. bovis*, and *M. bovis* BCG based on published literature [14, 15, 17–23] and on our own work is summarized in Table 1.

12. Conclusion

M. bovis strains are more virulent for cattle, while classical *M. tuberculosis* strains are thought to be more virulent for humans. The benefit of BCG immunization against *M. tuberculosis* infection has been the subject of much controversy. It is of uncertain efficacy and is associated with significant safety concerns in untreated HIV-infected infants and in those on ART.

The diagnosis and management of BCG disease are complex, leading to under recognition and suboptimal care in resource-limited settings often due to misdiagnosis. Better safety and efficacy profiles under investigations are highly needed for the new BCG vaccines. Vaccination policy attempt to balance risk and benefit needs to be revived. Various biochemical tests currently being used are useful methods for identifying *M. bovis* BCG virulence pathology, especially niacin positivity, which differs in the results of these tests among BCG substrains. The differences observed in different parts of the world could be attributed to the long passages of the BCG strains that have been subcultured in different laboratories leading to the divergence of *M. bovis* BCG strains in due course of time.

Acknowledgments

The authors acknowledge the Indian BCG Special Investigation Committee Members Dr. Kiran Katoch and Dr. DS Chauhan of National Jalma Institute of Leprosy and other Mycobacterial Diseases, Agra; Dr. Vanaja Kumar and Dr. Aleyamma Thomas of National Institute of Research in Tuberculosis, Chennai, for the experiments carried out on the Indian seed-lot of BCG vaccine under question; and Dr. Surinder Singh, Drug Controller General of India and Dr. RK Srivastava, Director General of Health Services, India, for their regulatory and administrative comments. The authors specially thank Dr. VM Katoch, Director General of Indian Council of Medical Research and Secretary to Government of India, Ministry of Health & Family welfare and Chairman of this committee for his technical inputs and encouragement to write this review.

References

[1] J. F. T. Griffin, D. N. Chinn, C. R. Rodgers, and C. G. Mackintosh, "Optimal models to evaluate the protective efficacy of tuberculosis vaccines," *Tuberculosis*, vol. 81, no. 1-2, pp. 133–139, 2001.

[2] P. H. Lagrange, B. Hurtrel, and J. L. Stach, "Vaccines against mycobacteria and other intracellular multiplying bacteria," *Annales de l'Institut Pasteur D—Immunology*, vol. 136, no. 2, pp. 151–162, 1985.

[3] B. M. Buddle, N. A. Parlane, D. L. Keen et al., "Differentiation between *Mycobacterium bovis* BCG-vaccinated and *M. bovis*-infected cattle by using recombinant mycobacterial antigens," *Clinical and Diagnostic Laboratory Immunology*, vol. 6, no. 1, pp. 1–5, 1999.

[4] World Health Organization, "Tuberculosis," WHO, Geneva, Switzerland, 2014, http://www.who.int/topics/tuberculosis/en/.

[5] World Health Organization, "BCG Vaccines," WHO, Geneva, Switzerland, 2014, http://www.who.int/biologicals/areas/vaccines/en/.

[6] World Health Organization, *BCG Vaccine: Safety*, WHO, Geneva, Switzerland, 2014, http://www.who.int/vaccine_safety/committee/topics/bcg/en/.

[7] E. A. Talbot, M. D. Perkins, S. F. M. Suva, and R. Frothingham, "Disseminated bacille Calmette-Guerin disease after vaccination: case report and review," *Clinical Infectious Diseases*, vol. 24, no. 6, pp. 1139–1146, 1997.

[8] I. S. Aljada, J. K. Crane, N. Corriere, D. G. Wagle, and D. Amsterdam, "*Mycobacterium bovis* BCG causing vertebral osteomyelitis (Pott's disease) following intravesical BCG therapy," *Journal of Clinical Microbiology*, vol. 37, no. 6, pp. 2106–2108, 1999.

[9] WHO, *WHO Global Tuberculosis Report 2013*, WHO, 2014, http://www.who.int/tb/publications/global_report/en/.

[10] B. Müller, S. Dürr, S. Alonso et al., "Zoonotic *Mycobacterium bovis*-induced tuberculosis in humans," *Emerging Infectious Diseases*, vol. 19, no. 6, pp. 899–908, 2013.

[11] L. M. O'Reilly and C. J. Daborn, "The epidemiology of *Mycobacterium bovis* infections in animals and man: a review," *Tubercle and Lung Disease*, vol. 76, supplement 1, pp. 1–46, 1995.

[12] M. Gheorghiu, J. Augier, and P. H. Lagrange, "Maintenance and control of the French BCG strain 1173p2 (primary and secondary seed-lots)," *Bulletin de l'Institut Pasteur*, vol. 81, pp. 281–288, 1983.

[13] J. D. Aronson, "Protective vaccination against tuberculosis with special reference to BCG vaccination," *The American Review of Tuberculosis*, vol. 58, pp. 255–281, 1948.

[14] T. Udou, "Adaptation of mycobacteria on solid, egg-based media to anaerobic conditions and characterization of their diagnostic phenotypes," *Journal of UOEH*, vol. 35, no. 2, pp. 109–117, 2013.

[15] T. Hirai, "Distribution of η precipitinogen in mycobacteria," *International Journal of Systematic Bacteriology*, vol. 34, no. 4, pp. 401–404, 1984.

[16] H. Li, J. C. Ulstrup, T. O. Jonassen, K. Melby, S. Nagai, and M. Harboe, "Evidence for absence of the MPB64 gene in some substrains of *Mycobacterium bovis* BCG," *Infection and Immunity*, vol. 61, no. 5, pp. 1730–1734, 1993.

[17] L. M. Parsons, R. Brosch, S. T. Cole et al., "Rapid and simple approach for identification of *Mycobacterium tuberculosis* complex isolates by PCR-based genomic deletion analysis," *Journal of Clinical Microbiology*, vol. 40, no. 7, pp. 2339–2345, 2002.

[18] A. Aranaz, E. Liébana, E. Gómez-Mampaso et al., "*Mycobacterium tuberculosis* subsp. *caprae* subsp. nov.: a taxonomic study of a new member of the *Mycobacterium tuberculosis* complex isolated from goats in Spain," *International Journal of Systematic Bacteriology*, vol. 49, no. 3, pp. 1263–1273, 1999.

[19] R. K. Tenguria, F. N. Khan, S. Quereshi, and A. Pandey, "Epidemiological study of zoonotic tuberculosis complex (Ztbc)," *World Journal of Science and Technology*, vol. 1, pp. 31–56, 2011.

[20] S. Niemann, E. Richter, and S. Rüsch-Gerdes, "Biochemical and genetic evidence for the transfer of *Mycobacterium tuberculosis* subsp. caprae Aranaz et al. 1999 to the species *Mycobacterium bovis* Karlson and Lessel 1970 (approved list 1980) as *Mycobacterium bovis* subsp. caprae comb. nov.," *International Journal of Systematic and Evolutionary Microbiology*, vol. 52, no. 2, pp. 433–436, 2002.

[21] P. Brodin, K. Eiglmeier, M. Marmiesse et al., "Bacterial artificial chromosome-based comparative genomic analysis identifies *Mycobacterium microti* as a natural ESAT-6 deletion mutant," *Infection and Immunity*, vol. 70, no. 10, pp. 5568–5578, 2002.

[22] J. Kamerbeek, L. Schouls, A. Kolk et al., "Simultaneous detection and strain differentiation of *Mycobacterium tuberculosis* for diagnosis and epidemiology," *Journal of Clinical Microbiology*, vol. 35, no. 4, pp. 907–914, 1997.

[23] K. Chikamatsu, A. Aono, H. Yamada et al., "Comparative evaluation of three immunochromatographic identification tests for culture confirmation of *Mycobacterium tuberculosis* complex," *BMC Infectious Diseases*, vol. 14, article 54, 2014.

[24] World Health Organization, *Information Sheet-Observed Rate of Vaccine Reactions Bacille Calmette-Guérin (Bcg) Vaccine Global Vaccine Safety, Immunization, Vaccines and Biologicals*, World Health Organization, Geneva, Switzerland, 2012, http://www.who.int/vaccine_safety/initiative/tools/BCG_Vaccine_rates_information_sheet.pdf.

[25] F. T. Perkins, *Analysis of the Replies to a Questionnaire*, vol. 17 of *Series in Immunobiology Stand*, 1971.

[26] E. A. Talbot, D. L. Williams, and R. Frothingham, "PCR identification of *Mycobacterium bovis* BCG," *Journal of Clinical Microbiology*, vol. 35, no. 3, pp. 566–569, 1997.

[27] V. Seth, S. Kabra, Y. Jain, and O. P. Semwal, "BCG revisited," *Indian Pediatrics*, vol. 31, no. 12, pp. 1585–1593, 1994.

[28] L. Brandt, J. F. Cunha, A. W. Olsen et al., "Failure of the *Mycobacterium bovis* BCG vaccine: some species of environmental mycobacteria block multiplication of BCG and induction of protective immunity to tuberculosis," *Infection and Immunity*, vol. 70, no. 2, pp. 672–678, 2002.

[29] J. D. Clemens, J. J. H. Chuong, and A. R. Feinstein, "The BCG controversy. A methodological and statistical reappraisal," *The Journal of the American Medical Association*, vol. 249, no. 17, pp. 2362–2369, 1983.

[30] G. A. Colditz, C. S. Berkey, F. Mosteller et al., "The efficacy of bacillus Calmette-Guerin vaccination of newborns and infants in the prevention of tuberculosis: meta-analyses of the published literature," *Pediatrics*, vol. 96, no. 1, pp. 29–35, 1995.

[31] H. C. Engbaek, B. Vergmann, and K. Bunch-Christensen, "Pulmonary tuberculosis due to BCG in a technician employed in a BCG laboratory," *Bulletin of the World Health Organization*, vol. 55, no. 4, pp. 517–520, 1977.

[32] D. Thierry, A. Brisson-Noel, V. Vincent-Lévy-Frébault, S. Nguyen, J.-L. Guesdon, and B. Gicquel, "Characterization of a *Mycobacterium tuberculosis* insertion sequence, IS6110, and its application in diagnosis," *Journal of Clinical Microbiology*, vol. 28, no. 12, pp. 2668–2673, 1990.

[33] D. Hayashi, T. Takii, T. Mukai et al., "Biochemical characteristics among *Mycobacterium bovis* BCG substrains," *FEMS Microbiology Letters*, vol. 306, no. 2, pp. 103–109, 2010.

[34] H. I. M. Boshoff, X. Xu, K. Tahlan et al., "Biosynthesis and recycling of nicotinamide cofactors in *Mycobacterium tuberculosis*:

an essential role for NAD in nonreplicating bacilli," *Journal of Biological Chemistry*, vol. 283, no. 28, pp. 19329–19341, 2008.

[35] C. D. Sohaskey and L. Modesti, "Differences in nitrate reduction between *Mycobacterium tuberculosis* and *Mycobacterium bovis* are due to differential expression of both *narGHJI* and *narK2*," *FEMS Microbiology Letters*, vol. 290, no. 2, pp. 129–134, 2009.

[36] G. Källenius, T. Koivula, S. Ghebremichael et al., "Evolution and clonal traits of *Mycobacterium tuberculosis* complex in Guinea-Bissau," *Journal of Clinical Microbiology*, vol. 37, no. 12, pp. 3872–3878, 1999.

[37] W.-J. Su, C.-Y. Huang, and R.-P. Perng, "Utility of PCR assays for rapid diagnosis of BCG infection in children," *International Journal of Tuberculosis and Lung Disease*, vol. 5, no. 4, pp. 380–384, 2001.

[38] K. S. Goh, N. Rastogi, M. Berchel, R. C. Huard, and C. Sola, "Molecular evolutionary history of tubercle bacilli assessed by study of the polymorphic nucleotide within the nitrate reductase (narghji) operon promoter," *Journal of Clinical Microbiology*, vol. 43, no. 8, pp. 4010–4014, 2005.

[39] M. Stermann, A. Bohrssen, C. Diephaus, S. Maass, and F.-C. Bange, "Polymorphic nucleotide within the promoter of nitrate reductase (NarGHJI) is specific for *Mycobacterium tuberculosis*," *Journal of Clinical Microbiology*, vol. 41, no. 7, pp. 3252–3259, 2003.

[40] R. J. North and A. A. Izzo, "Mycobacterial virulence. Virulent strains of *Mycobacteria tuberculosis* have faster in vivo doubling times and are better equipped to resist growth-inhibiting functions of macrophages in the presence and absence of specific immunity," *The Journal of Experimental Medicine*, vol. 177, no. 6, pp. 1723–1733, 1993.

[41] C. Fritz, S. Maass, A. Kreft, and F.-C. Bange, "Dependence of *Mycobacterium bovis* BCG on anaerobic nitrate reductase for persistence is tissue specific," *Infection and Immunity*, vol. 70, no. 1, pp. 286–291, 2002.

[42] D. R. Sherman, M. Voskuil, D. Schnappinger, R. Liao, M. I. Harrell, and G. K. Schoolnik, "Regulation of the Mycobacterium tuberculosis hypoxic response gene encoding alpha-crystallin," *Proceedings of the National Academy of Sciences of the United States of America*, vol. 98, no. 13, pp. 7534–7539, 2001.

[43] C. D. Sohaskey and L. G. Wayne, "Role of narK2X and narGHJI in hypoxic upregulation of nitrate reduction by *Mycobacterium tuberculosis*," *Journal of Bacteriology*, vol. 185, no. 24, pp. 7247–7256, 2003.

[44] S. Virtanen, "A study of nitrate reduction by mycobacteria," *Acta Tuberculosea Scandinavica*, vol. 48, pp. 1–119, 1960.

[45] World Health Organization, *Recommendations to Assure the Quality, Safety and Efficacy of BCG Vaccines Replacement of: WHO Technical Report Series, no. 745, Annex 2 and Amendment to WHO Technical Report Series, no. 771, Annex 12*, World Health Organization, Geneva, Switzerland, 2012, http://www.who.int/biologicals/BCG_DB_HK_23_April_2012.pdf.

[46] T. P. Kent and G. P. Kubica, *Public Health Mycobacteriology. A Guide for Level III Laboratory*, vol. 30, United States Department of Health and Human Services, Centre for Disease Control, Atlanta, Ga, USA, 1985.

[47] K. S. Goh and N. Rastogi, "Simple and rapid method for detection of nitrate reductase activity of *Mycobacterium tuberculosis* and *Mycobacterium canettii* grown in the Bactec MGIT960 system," *Journal of Microbiological Methods*, vol. 81, no. 2, pp. 208–210, 2010.

[48] L. Sula and M. Langerova, "Drug sensitivity-resistance determination and simple enzymatic tests for the differentiation of Mycobacteria," *Bulletin of the World Health Organization*, vol. 29, pp. 579–588, 1963.

[49] G. P. Kubica, P. P. Gontijo Filho, and T. Kim, "Preservation of mycobacteria at −70°C: persistence of key differential features," *Journal of Clinical Microbiology*, vol. 6, no. 2, pp. 149–153, 1977.

[50] M. Ventura, C. Canchaya, A. Tauch et al., "Genomics of *Actinobacteria*: tracing the evolutionary history of an ancient phylum," *Microbiology and Molecular Biology Reviews*, vol. 71, no. 3, pp. 495–548, 2007.

[51] A. L. Sørensen, S. Nagai, G. Houen, P. Andersen, and A. B. Andersen, "Purification and characterization of a low-molecular-mass T-Cell antigen secreted by *Mycobacterium tuberculosis*," *Infection and Immunity*, vol. 63, no. 5, pp. 1710–1717, 1995.

[52] P. S. Renshaw, P. Panagiotidou, A. Whelan et al., "Conclusive evidence that the major T-cell antigens of the *Mycobacterium tuberculosis* complex ESAT-6 and CFP-10 form a tight, 1:1 complex and characterization of the structural properties of ESAT-6, CFP-10, and the ESAT-6·CFP-10 complex. Implications for pathogenesis and virulence," *The Journal of Biological Chemistry*, vol. 277, no. 24, pp. 21598–21603, 2002.

[53] P. Akhtar, S. Srivastava, A. Srivastava, M. Srivastava, B. S. Srivastava, and R. Srivastava, "Rv3303c of *Mycobacterium tuberculosis* protects tubercle bacilli against oxidative stress *in vivo* and contributes to virulence in mice," *Microbes and Infection*, vol. 8, no. 14-15, pp. 2855–2862, 2006.

[54] A. S. Barouni, C. Augusto, M. V. N. P. Queiroz, M. T. P. Lopes, M. S. Zanini, and C. E. Salas, "BCG lymphadenopathy detected in a BCG-vaccinated infant," *Brazilian Journal of Medical and Biological Research*, vol. 37, no. 5, pp. 697–700, 2004.

[55] G. W. Comstock and C. E. Palmer, "Long-term results of BCG vaccination in the Southern United States," *The American Review of Respiratory Disease*, vol. 93, no. 2, pp. 171–183, 1966.

[56] P. E. M. Fine, "Bacille Calmette-Guérin vaccines: a rough guide," *Clinical Infectious Diseases*, vol. 20, no. 1, pp. 11–14, 1995.

[57] A. S. Malin and D. B. Young, "Designing a vaccine for tuberculosis," *British Medical Journal*, vol. 312, no. 7045, p. 1495, 1996.

[58] A. Lotte, O. Wasz-Höckert, N. Poisson, N. Dumitrescu, M. Verron, and E. Couvet, "BCG complications. Estimates of the risks among vaccinated subjects and statistical analysis of their main characteristics," *Advances in Tuberculosis Research. Fortschritte der Tuberkuloseforschung. Progres de la exploration de la tuberculose*, vol. 21, pp. 107–193, 1984.

[59] G. G. Mahairas, P. J. Sabo, M. J. Hickey, D. C. Singh, and C. K. Stover, "Molecular analysis of genetic differences between *Mycobacterium bovis* BCG and virulent *M. bovis*," *Journal of Bacteriology*, vol. 178, no. 5, pp. 1274–1282, 1996.

[60] N. G. Fomukong, J. W. Dale, T. W. Osborn, and J. M. Grange, "Use of gene probes based on the insertion sequence IS986 to differentiate between BCG vaccine strains," *Journal of Applied Bacteriology*, vol. 72, no. 2, pp. 126–133, 1992.

[61] M. Harboe and S. Nagai, "MPB70, a unique antigen of *Mycobacterium bovis* BCG," *The American Review of Respiratory Disease*, vol. 129, no. 3, pp. 444–452, 1984.

[62] D. E. Minnikin, J. H. Parlett, M. Magnusson, M. Ridell, and A. Lind, "Mycolic acid patterns of representatives of *Mycobacterium bovis* BCG," *Journal of General Microbiology*, vol. 130, no. 10, pp. 2733–2736, 1984.

[63] J. Bøe, "Variations in the virulence of BCG," *Acta Tuberculosea Scandinavica*, vol. 22, no. 1, pp. 125–133, 1948.

[64] M. R. R. Lagranderie, A.-M. Balazuc, E. Deriaud, C. D. Leclerc, and M. Gheorghiu, "Comparison of immune responses of mice immunized with five different *Mycobacterium bovis* BCG vaccine strains," *Infection and Immunity*, vol. 64, no. 1, pp. 1–9, 1996.

[65] K. M. Edwards, M. H. Cynamon, R. K. Voladri et al., "Iron-co-factored superoxide dismutase inhibits host responses to *Mycobacterium tuberculosis*," *The American Journal of Respiratory and Critical Care Medicine*, vol. 164, pp. 2213–2219, 2001.

[66] J. A. Tree, A. Williams, S. Clark, G. Hall, P. D. Marsh, and J. Ivanyi, "Intranasal bacille Calmette-Guérin (BCG) vaccine dosage needs balancing between protection and lung pathology," *Clinical and Experimental Immunology*, vol. 138, no. 3, pp. 405–409, 2004.

[67] K. Bunch-Christensen, A. Ladefoged, and J. Guld, "The virulence of some strains of BCG for golden hamsters. Further studies," *Bulletin of the World Health Organization*, vol. 43, no. 1, pp. 65–70, 1970.

[68] J. S. Bellet and N. S. Prose, "Skin complications of Bacillus Calmette-Guérin immunization," *Current Opinion in Infectious Diseases*, vol. 18, no. 2, pp. 97–100, 2005.

[69] F. M. Turnbull, P. B. McIntyre, H. M. Achat et al., "National study of adverse reactions after vaccination with bacille Calmette-Guérin," *Clinical Infectious Diseases*, vol. 34, no. 4, pp. 447–453, 2002.

[70] F. Altare, D. Lammas, P. Revy et al., "Inherited interleukin 12 deficiency in a child with bacille Calmette-Guérin and *Salmonella enteritidis* disseminated infection," *The Journal of Clinical Investigation*, vol. 102, no. 12, pp. 2035–2040, 1998.

[71] J. J. C. Nuttall and B. S. Eley, "BCG vaccination in HIV-infected children," *Tuberculosis Research and Treatment*, vol. 2011, Article ID 712736, pp. 1–6, 2011.

[72] J. A. DeSimone, R. J. Pomerantz, and T. J. Babinchak, "Inflammatory reactions in HIV-1-infected persons after initiation of highly active antiretroviral therapy," *Annals of Internal Medicine*, vol. 133, no. 6, pp. 447–454, 2000.

[73] G. Aslan, N. Kuyucu, E. Aydin, S. Günal, and G. Emekdaş, "A case of fatal disseminated infection caused by *Mycobacterium bovis* BCG strain and the identification of the isolate by spoligotyping," *Mikrobiyoloji Bulteni*, vol. 44, no. 2, pp. 297–302, 2010.

[74] A. Lotte, O. Wasz-Hockert, N. Poisson et al., "Second IUATLD study on complications induced by intradermal BCG-vaccination," *Bulletin of the International Union Against Tuberculosis and Lung Disease*, vol. 63, no. 2, pp. 47–59, 1988.

[75] M. J. Cayabyab, L. Macovei, and A. Campos-Neto, "Current and novel approaches to vaccine development against tuberculosis," *Frontiers in Cellular and Infection Microbiology*, vol. 2, no. 154, pp. 1–16, 2012.

[76] P. E. Fine, "BCG vaccines and vaccination," in *Tuberculosis: A Comprehensive International Approach*, L. B. Reichman and E. S. Hershfield, Eds., pp. 503–522, Marcel Dekker, New York, NY, USA, 2nd edition, 2001.

[77] V. Romanus, H. O. Hallander, P. Wåhlén, A. M. Olinder-Nielsen, P. H. W. Magnusson, and I. Juhlin, "Atypical mycobacteria in extrapulmonary disease among children. Incidence in Sweden from 1969 to 1990, related to changing BCG-vaccination coverage," *Tubercle and Lung Disease*, vol. 76, no. 4, pp. 300–310, 1995.

[78] J. Singh, M. M. Sankar, S. Kumar et al., "Incidence and prevalence of tuberculosis among household contacts of pulmonary tuberculosis patients in a peri-urban population of South Delhi, India," *PLoS ONE*, vol. 8, no. 7, Article ID e69730, 2013.

[79] M. O. C. Ota, R. H. Brookes, P. C. Hill et al., "The effect of tuberculin skin test and BCG vaccination on the expansion of PPD-specific IFN-γ producing cells ex vivo," *Vaccine*, vol. 25, no. 52, pp. 8861–8867, 2007.

[80] J. B. Milstien and J. J. Gibson, "Quality control of BCG vaccine by WHO: a review of factors that may influence vaccine effectiveness and safety," *Bulletin of the World Health Organization*, vol. 68, no. 1, pp. 93–108, 1990.

[81] S. Luca and T. Mihaescu, "History of BCG vaccine," *Mædica*, vol. 8, no. 1, pp. 53–58, 2013.

[82] M. M. Ho, J. Southern, H.-N. Kang, and I. Knezevic, "WHO Informal Consultation on standardization and evaluation of BCG vaccines Geneva, Switzerland 22-23 September 2009," *Vaccine*, vol. 28, no. 43, pp. 6945–6950, 2010.

[83] A. L. Bierrenbach, S. S. Cunha, M. L. Barreto et al., "Tuberculin reactivity in a population of schoolchildren with high BCG vaccination coverage," *Pan American Journal of Public Health*, vol. 13, no. 3, pp. 285–286, 2003.

[84] L. Grode, P. Seiler, S. Baumann et al., "Increased vaccine efficacy against tuberculosis of recombinant *Mycobacterium bovis* bacille Calmette-Guérin mutants that secrete listeriolysin," *The Journal of Clinical Investigation*, vol. 115, no. 9, pp. 2472–2479, 2005.

[85] N. E. Aronson, M. Santosham, G. W. Comstock et al., "Long-term efficacy of BCG vaccine in American Indians and Alaska natives: a 60-year follow-up study," *The Journal of the American Medical Association*, vol. 291, no. 17, pp. 2086–2091, 2004.

[86] P. D. Hart and I. Sutherland, "BCG and vole bacillus vaccines in the prevention of tuberculosis in adolescence and early adult life. Final report to the Medical Research Council," *British Medical Journal*, vol. 2, no. 6082, pp. 293–295, 1977.

[87] C. E. Palmer, L. W. Shaw, and G. W. Comstock, "Community trials of BCG vaccination," *American Review of Tuberculosis*, vol. 77, no. 6, pp. 877–907, 1958.

[88] P. E. M. Fine, I. A. M. Carneiro, and C. J. Clements, *Issues Relating to the Use of BCG in Immunization Programmes*, World Health Organization, Geneva, Switzerland, 1999.

[89] H. Nakatani, T. Sano, and T. Iuchi, "Development of vaccination policy in Japan: current issues and policy directions," *Japanese Journal of Infectious Diseases*, vol. 55, no. 4, pp. 101–111, 2002.

[90] A. S. Pym, P. Brodin, R. Brosch, M. Huerre, and S. T. Cole, "Loss of RD1 contributed to the attenuation of the live tuberculosis vaccines *Mycobacterium bovis* BCG and *Mycobacterium microti*," *Molecular Microbiology*, vol. 46, no. 3, pp. 709–717, 2002.

[91] R. Brosch, S. V. Gordon, C. Buchrieser, A. S. Pym, T. Gamier, and S. T. Cole, "Comparative genomics uncovers large tandem chromosomal duplications in *Mycobacterium bovis* BCG Pasteur," *Yeast*, vol. 17, no. 2, pp. 111–123, 2000.

[92] R. Brosch, S. V. Gordon, T. Garnier et al., "Genome plasticity of BCG and impact on vaccine efficacy," *Proceedings of the National Academy of Sciences of the United States of America*, vol. 104, no. 13, pp. 5596–5601, 2007.

[93] M. A. Behr, M. A. Wilson, W. P. Gill et al., "Comparative genomics of BCG vaccines by whole-genome DNA microarray," *Science*, vol. 284, no. 5419, pp. 1520–1523, 1999.

[94] D. M. Collins, R. P. Kawakami, G. W. de Lisle, L. Pascopella, B. R. Bloom, and W. R. Jacobs Jr., "Mutation of the principal sigma factor causes loss of virulence in a strain of the *Mycobacterium*

tuberculosis complex," *Proceedings of the National Academy of Sciences of the United States of America*, vol. 92, no. 17, pp. 8036–8040, 1995.

[95] I. Weber, C. Fritz, S. Ruttkowski, A. Kreft, and F.-C. Bange, "Anaerobic nitrate reductase (*narGHJI*) activity of *Mycobacterium bovis* BCG in vitro and its contribution to virulence in immunodeficient mice," *Molecular Microbiology*, vol. 35, no. 5, pp. 1017–1025, 2000.

[96] S. Sadagopal, M. Braunstein, C. C. Hager et al., "Reducing the activity and secretion of microbial antioxidants enhances the immunogenicity of BCG," *PLoS ONE*, vol. 4, no. 5, Article ID e5531, 2009.

[97] A. Scorpio and Y. Zhang, "Mutations in *pncA*, a gene encoding pyrazinamidase/nicotinamidase, cause resistance to the antituberculous drug pyrazinamide in tubercle bacillus," *Nature Medicine*, vol. 2, no. 6, pp. 662–667, 1996.

[98] S. E. Hoffner, S. B. Svenson, R. Norberg, F. Dias, S. Ghebremichael, and G. Kallenius, "Biochemical heterogeneity of *Mycobacterium tuberculosis* complex isolates in Guinea-Bissau," *Journal of Clinical Microbiology*, vol. 31, no. 8, pp. 2215–2217, 1993.

[99] P. Akhtar, S. Singh, P. Bifani, S. Kaur, B. S. Srivastava, and R. Srivastava, "Variable-number tandem repeat 3690 polymorphism in Indian clinical isolates of *Mycobacterium tuberculosis* and its influence on transcription," *Journal of Medical Microbiology*, vol. 58, no. 6, pp. 798–805, 2009.

30

The Use of Interferon Gamma Release Assays in the Diagnosis of Active Tuberculosis

Silvan M. Vesenbeckh,[1] Nicolas Schönfeld,[1] Harald Mauch,[2] Thorsten Bergmann,[2] Sonja Wagner,[2] Torsten T. Bauer,[1] and Holger Rüssmann[2]

[1] *Department of Pneumology, Lungenklinik Heckeshorn, HELIOS Klinikum Emil von Behring, 14165 Berlin, Germany*
[2] *Institute of Microbiology, Immunology and Laboratory Medicine, HELIOS Klinikum Emil von Behring, 14165 Berlin, Germany*

Correspondence should be addressed to Silvan M. Vesenbeckh, vesenbeckh@gmail.com

Academic Editor: Soumitesh Chakravorty

Interferon gamma release assays (IGRAs) are *in vitro* immunologic diagnostic tests used to identify *Mycobacterium tuberculosis* infection. They cannot differentiate between latent and active infections. The cutoff suggested by the manufacturer is 0.35 IU/mL for latent tuberculosis. As IGRA tests were recently approved for the differential diagnosis of active tuberculosis, we assessed the diagnostic accuracy of the latest generation IGRA for detection of active tuberculosis in a low-incidence area in Germany. Our consecutive case series includes 61 HIV negative, *Mycobacterium tuberculosis* culture positive patients, as well as 234 control patients. The retrospective analysis was performed over a period of two years. In 11/61 patients with active tuberculosis (18.0%) the test result was <0.35 IU/mL, resulting in a sensitivity of 0.82. We recommend establishing a new cut-off value for the differential diagnosis of active tuberculosis assessed by prospective clinical studies and in various regions with high and low prevalence of tuberculosis.

1. Introduction

Tuberculosis (TB) remains a major public health problem affecting one-third of the world's population [1, 2]. Diagnosis of TB is usually based on a combination of anamnestic symptoms, clinical presentation, radiological and pathological changes, bacteriological findings of acid/alcohol-fast bacilli, and molecular tests [3]. Definitive TB diagnosis is based on the detection of *Mycobacterium tuberculosis* (MTB) in the culture, which usually takes four to six weeks. For decades, tuberculin skin test (TST) has been used as diagnostic tool to support the physician's decision process. With the introduction of interferon gamma release assays (IGRAs), a more specific method became available. Although primarily developed for the diagnosis of latent TB, clinicians have also been searching for improved diagnostic tools and explored IGRAs for the immunodiagnosis of active TB. In 2010, the Centers for Disease Control and Prevention (CDC) updated their guidelines for testing for TB infection, concluding that IGRAs "may be used instead of a tuberculin skin test in all situations in which the CDC recommends the tuberculin skin test as an aid in diagnosing *M. tuberculosis* infection" [4, 5].

Nevertheless, with the cutoff for the diagnosis of latent TB as given by the producers, pooled sensitivity for the diagnosis of culture positive TB did not exceed 80% in the most recent meta-analyses [6, 7]. The present case series constitutes one of the largest reports of latest generation IGRA used in culturally proven HIV-negative TB cases in a low-prevalence country. Our study is meant to help evaluate the cutoff for the IGRA in the differential diagnosis of TB.

2. Study Population and Methods

This is a retrospective study performed on inpatients of a regional hospital specialized in lung diseases (Lungenklinik Heckeshorn, Berlin). At least one IGRA is routinely performed on a blood sample of each TB-suspect patient, and every suspicious sample (smear, lymph node biopsy, pleural effusion, or biopsy) is routinely cultured for TB. All

Table 1: (a) Median and range for patient age and IGRA test result for all culture positive cases of active tuberculosis, by organ manifestation. (b) Median and range for age and IGRA test result for all controls, by diagnosis. "Others" includes other lung diseases such as asbestosis, aspergillosis, asthma, bronchiectasis, pleural effusion, haemoptysis, fibrosis, and sarcoidosis. (c) Study results for TB cases and controls. (*n*: sample size, CI: confidence interval).

(a)

MTB infection	Male	Female	Total	Median age, years (range)	Median QFT, IU/mL (range)
Lung	28	25	53	45 (4–83)	2.40 (0,00–103,4)
Pleura	2	3	5	26 (17–76)	2,45 (0,96–300)
Lymph node	2	1	3	65 (25–69)	21,32 (3,78–86,8)
Total	32	29	61	46 (5–84)	3.46 (0,00–300)

(b)

Diagnosis	Male	Female	Total	Median age, years (range)	Median QFT, IU/mL (range)
Malignancy	22	23	45	69 (39–90)	0,01 (0,00–23,9)
Bronchitis	27	13	40	64 (1–90)	0,00 (0,00–1,84)
Pneumonia	30	17	47	67 (1–99)	0,00 (0,00–75)
Others	53	49	102	62,5 (5–99)	0,02 (0,00–103,4)
Total	132	102	234	66 (1–99)	0,00 (0,00–103,4)

(c)

	n	QFT			Age		
		Mean	95% CI	*P*	Mean	95% CI	*P*
TB	61	14.13	3.44–24.82	<0.05	47.8	41.88–53.79	<0.05
Control	234	1.33	0.24–2.43		63	60.56–65.39	

samples of patients included in this study were taken prior to initiation of antibiotic therapy. Over a two-year period (1/2008–1/2010), IGRA results of all MTB culture positive cases of active TB were analyzed. Patients with other lung diseases than TB, including negative history for MTB infection and without radiological findings suggestive of MTB infection in the past and with no signs of active disease, were chosen as control group. All HIV-positive patients were excluded from the database.

2.1. IGRA. We used the latest generation IGRA (QuantiFERON-TB Gold in-Tube, Cellestis, Carnegie, Australia), later referred to as QFT-GIT, on all samples. Peripheral blood samples were obtained by trained personnel in specific blood collection tubes following the manufacturer's instructions. All blood samples were processed within 4 h of phlebotomy. Otherwise, the test was performed as previously described [8].

2.2. TB Culture. Specimens were stained, processed, and cultured by standard procedures in mycobacteriology [9]. The isolates were cultured for 4 weeks on Löwenstein-Jensen (L-J) medium at 37°C and tested for growth rate, pigment production, and by biochemical testing using standard methods [10, 11].

2.3. Statistical Analysis. Data were analyzed using STATA 12.0 (StataCorp, College Station, Texas, USA). The *t*-test for independent samples (two-tailed) was carried out to assess significance level of detected differences in both groups (IGRA test results, age).

3. Results

A total of 61 patients with active TB as ascertained through positive MTB culture were examined using QFT-GIT between 1/2008 and 1/2010 (see Table 1(a)). 53 patients presented with pulmonary TB, three patients with lymph node TB, and five patients with tuberculous pleurisy. The median QFT-GIT value for all TB patients was 3.46 IU/mL, ranging from 0.00 to 300 IU/mL. In 11 patients, the test result was <0.35 IU/mL (see Figure 1). Assuming the cutoff for latent TB suggested by the producer, these are false-negative (FN) test results (11/61 = 0.18; 18% FN). We calculated the sensitivity (the proportion of patients with active TB who are correctly identified as such) as 1-FN (=82%). Only in one patient four months after therapy with adalimumab, the result was 0.00 IU/mL, and in one other patient with lung cancer under concomitant chemotherapy, it was 0.02 IU/mL. All other patients showed values of 0.07 IU/mL or above. The median age of our patients was 46 years (range: 5–84 years), in the group with a test result ≥0.07 and <0.35 IU/mL, the median age was 80 years (range: 44–84 years), and, in the group testing ≥0.35 IU/mL, it was 36 years (range: 5–84 years).

Within the control group (see Table 1(b)), QFT-GIT values ranged from 0.00 to 103.4 IU/mL in one patient with pneumonia. The median was 0.00 IU/mL. In 50% of all cases (116/234), no Interferon gamma (IFN-γ) release was measured (0.00 IU/mL). In 51/234 patients (21%), test results

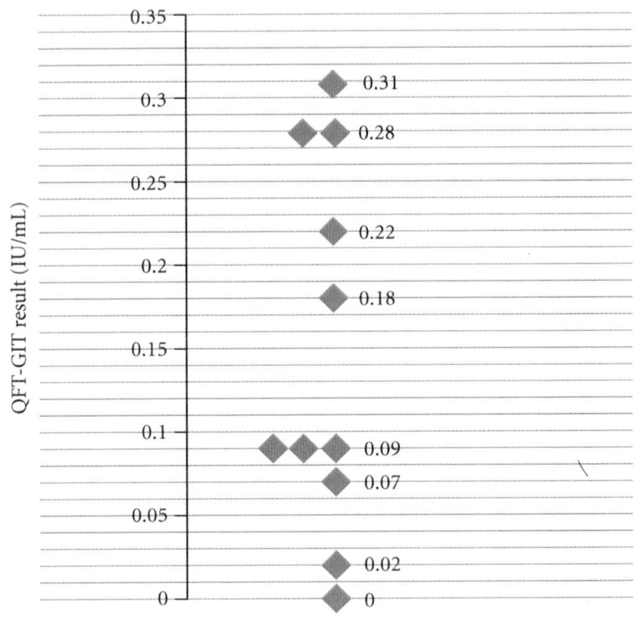

FIGURE 1: Range of QFT-GIT values below the cutoff of 0.35 IU/mL for patients with active tuberculosis.

were above 0.35 IU/mL. The median age in the control group was 66 years with a range from 1 to 99 years.

Patients in the study group were significantly younger than in the control group and had significantly higher QFT-GIT test results ($P < 0.05$ for both, see Table 1(c)).

4. Discussion

IGRAs are *in vitro* immunologic diagnostic tests to identify MTB infection. Latent and active infections are not differentiated. Several test systems are commercially available: QuantiFERON-TB Gold (QFT), QuantiFERON-TB Gold in-Tube (QFT-GIT), both Cellestis Limited, Chadstone, Australia, and T-SPOT.TB (Oxford Immunotec, Abingdon, UK). The QFT-GIT measures IFN-γ responses to the MTB specific antigens early secretory antigenic target 6 (ESAT-6), culture filtrate protein 10 (CFP-10), and Rv2654 (TB 7.7). Their use in clinical practice is more and more widespread. Whereas the test was initially conceived to support diagnosis of latent infection, an increasing body of evidence is published on its use in detection of active TB infection [12–14]. More and more guidelines now include recommendations for or against the use of IGRAs in the differential diagnosis of active TB [15].

Several systematic reviews and meta-analyses have recently been published specifically on the diagnostic accuracy of IGRAs in active TB [6, 16, 17]. Strong heterogeneity between study populations is a major limitation of these meta-analyses, and most studies had small sample sizes. Overall, few studies were done with the latest generation QFT-GIT in areas of low endemicity such as Germany (2 studies in [17], 13 studies in [16]). Among those, even fewer restricted sensitivity analysis to patients with culturally proven MTB infection and confirmed HIV-negative status [12, 18].

Specificity depends highly on the definition of the control group. Pai et al. reported a pooled specificity of 99% among non-BCG vaccinated and 96% among BCG-vaccinated low-risk groups [17]. According to a recent meta-analysis that did not restrict studies on specificity to low-risk groups [6], a situation more compatible to our clinical setting, the specificity of QFT-GIT was only 0.79 (95% CI 0.75–0.82). In our study, 51 out of 234 control patients (21%) showed test results above 0.35 IU/mL, indicative of latent TB according to the producer. However, this finding is also consistent with the expected number of false positives assuming a specificity of around 0.8 according to Sester et al. [6]. The retrospective design of our study does not allow any conclusion about the test specificity in our study population.

Sensitivity in these studies was also found to be highly dependent on the study population, notably local TB prevalence, and ranged from 0.58 in a high-prevalence country [19] to 1.00 in a low-prevalence country [20], when QFT-GIT was assessed. Diel et al. found a pooled sensitivity of 0.84 (95% CI 0.81–0.87) when including only developed countries [16], consistent with the results published by Sester et al. (0.77, 95% CI 0.75–0.80) [6].

In our consecutive case series of 61 TB culture positive, HIV-negative patients in a low-prevalence setting in Germany, we found a sensitivity of 82.0% (95% CI: 0.696, 0.902) for the QFT-GIT, when the cutoff recommended for the diagnosis of latent TB was used (<0.35 IU/mL). In a low-prevalence country such as Germany with a TB prevalence of 5.4/100,000 inhabitants [21], case finding is an outstanding priority in the management of this disease. Therefore, highly sensitive test systems are needed for screening purposes. If the use of IGRA in the differential diagnosis of active TB is recommended, at least under certain conditions, then the cut-off point for active TB should be lower compared to latent TB, as previously discussed by Davidow [22]. Prospective clinical studies in different defined regions, with high- and low-prevalence of active TB, should be performed to evaluate the use of IGRAs in the diagnostic workup of TB patients. The cutoff for the detection of latent TB does not seem applicable for that purpose.

5. Conclusions

We suggest that the cutoff for the use of IGRA in the differential diagnosis of active TB in low incidence settings be reevaluated. Further prospective studies including clinical criteria for TB are needed to determine a new cutoff for active TB.

Authors' Contribution

H. Mauch, N. Schönfeld, and S. M. Vesenbeckh designed the study, T. Bergmann and S. Wagner managed data acquisition and compilation, N. Schönfeld and S. M. Vesenbeckh analysed the data, T. T. Bauer and S. M. Vesenbeckh did statistical analysis, S. M. Vesenbeckh wrote the paper, and T. T. Bauer, H. Mauch, H. Rüssmann, and N. Schönfeld reviewed and edited the manuscript.

Funding

This work was funded by HELIOS Klinikum Emil von Behring and received support by DZK (Deutsches Zentralkomitee zur Bekämpfung der Tuberkulose) and OHH (Stiftung Oskar-Helene-Heim).

References

[1] C. Dye et al., "Consensus statement. Global burden of tuberculosis: estimated incidence, prevalence, and mortality by country. WHO Global Surveillance and Monitoring Project," *the Journal of the American Medical Association*, vol. 282, no. 7, pp. 677–686, 1999.

[2] World Health Organization, "Tuberculosis," 2011, http://www.who.int/mediacentre/factsheets/fs104/en/.

[3] World Health Organization, "Treatment of tuberculosis: guidelines for national programmes," WHO/CDS/TB/2003.313, Geneva, Switzerland, 2003.

[4] G. H. Mazurek, J. Jereb, A. Vernon, P. LoBue, S. Goldberg, and K. Castros, "Updated guidelines for using interferon gamma release assays to detect Mycobacterium tuberculosis infection—United States, 2010," *Morbidity and Mortality Weekly Report*, vol. 59, no. RR-5, pp. 1–25, 2010.

[5] L. Barclay, "CDC issues updated guidelines for testing for tuberculosis infection," http://www.medscape.com/viewarticle/724390.

[6] M. Sester, G. Sotgiu, C. Lange et al., "Interferon-γ release assays for the diagnosis of active tuberculosis: a systematic review and meta-analysis," *European Respiratory Journal*, vol. 37, no. 1, pp. 100–111, 2011.

[7] J. Z. Metcalfe, C. K. Everett, K. R. Steingart et al., "Interferon-γ release assays for active pulmonary tuberculosis diagnosis in adults in low-and middle-income countries: systematic review and meta-analysis," *Journal of Infectious Diseases*, vol. 204, supplement 4, pp. S1120–S1129, 2011.

[8] B. Kampmann, E. Whittaker, A. Williams et al., "Interferon-γ release assays do not identify more children with active tuberculosis than the tuberculin skin test," *European Respiratory Journal*, vol. 33, no. 6, pp. 1374–1382, 2009.

[9] E. D. Roberts, E. W. Koneman, and Y. K. Kim, "Mycobacterium," in *Manual of Clinical Microbiology*, H. W. J. J. Balows, K. L. Herrmann, H. D. Isenberg, and H. J. Shadomy, Eds., pp. 304–339, Washington, DC, USA, 1991.

[10] P. T. Kent and G. P. Kubica, *Public Health Mycobacteriology—A Guide for the Level III Laboratory*, vol. 86, U. S. Department of Health and Human Services Publication (CDC), 1985.

[11] V. V. Levy-Frebault and F. Portaels, "Proposed minimal standards for the genus Mycobacterium and for description of new slowly growing Mycobacterium species," *International Journal of Systematic Bacteriology*, vol. 42, no. 2, pp. 315–323, 1992.

[12] A. K. Detjen, T. Keil, S. Roll et al., "Interferon-γ release assays improve the diagnosis of tuberculosis and nontuberculous mycobacterial disease in children in a country with a low incidence of tuberculosis," *Clinical Infectious Diseases*, vol. 45, no. 3, pp. 322–328, 2007.

[13] L. Bianchi, L. Galli, M. Moriondo et al., "Interferon-gamma release assay improves the diagnosis of tuberculosis in children," *Pediatric Infectious Disease Journal*, vol. 28, no. 6, pp. 510–514, 2009.

[14] V. Bartu, M. Havelkova, and E. Kopecka, "QuantiFERON-TB gold in the diagnosis of active tuberculosis," *Journal of International Medical Research*, vol. 36, no. 3, pp. 434–437, 2008.

[15] C. M. Denkinger, K. Dheda, and M. Pai, "Guidelines on interferon-γ release assays for tuberculosis infection: concordance, discordance or confusion?" *Clinical Microbiology and Infection*, vol. 17, no. 6, pp. 806–814, 2011.

[16] R. Diel, R. Loaddenkemper, and A. Nienhaus, "Evidence-based comparison of commercial Interferon-γ Release assays for detecting active TB a metaanalysis," *Chest*, vol. 137, no. 4, pp. 952–968, 2010.

[17] M. Pai, A. Zwerling, and D. Menzies, "Systematic review: T-cell-based assays for the diagnosis of latent tuberculosis infection: an update," *Annals of Internal Medicine*, vol. 149, no. 3, pp. 177–184, 2008.

[18] R. Palazzo, F. Spensieri, M. Massari et al., "Use of whole-blood samples in in-house bulk and single-cell antigen-specific gamma interferon assays for surveillance of Mycobacterium tuberculosis infections," *Clinical and Vaccine Immunology*, vol. 15, no. 2, pp. 327–337, 2008.

[19] K. Baba, S. Sørnes, A. A. Hoosen et al., "Evaluation of immune responses in HIV infected patients with pleural tuberculosis by the QuantiFERON TB-Gold interferon-gamma assay," *BMC Infectious Diseases*, vol. 8, article no. 35, 2008.

[20] I. Sauzullo, F. Mengoni, M. Lichtner et al., "In vivo and in vitro effects of antituberculosis treatment on mycobacterial interferon-γ T cell response," *PLoS One*, vol. 4, no. 4, Article ID e5187, 2009.

[21] Robert Koch Institut, "RKI-Bericht zur epidemiologie der tuberkulose in deutschland für 2009," 2011; http://www.rki.de/cln_178/nn_274324/DE/Content/InfAZ/T/Tuberkulose/Download/TB2009.html.

[22] A. L. Davidow, "Interferon-gamma release assay test characteristics depend upon the prevalence of active tuberculosis," *International Journal of Tuberculosis and Lung Disease*, vol. 13, no. 11, pp. 1411–1415, 2009.

31

Is Chemoprophylaxis for Child Contacts of Drug-Resistant TB Patients Beneficial?

C. Padmapriyadarsini,[1] Mrinalini Das,[2] Sharath Burugina Nagaraja,[3] Mahalakshmi Rajendran,[1] Richard Kirubakaran,[4] Sarabjit Chadha,[5] and Prathap Tharyan[4]

[1]*National Institute for Research and Tuberculosis, Chennai, India*
[2]*Médecins Sans Frontières, New Delhi, India*
[3]*ESIC Medical College and PGIMSR, Bangalore, India*
[4]*Christian Medical College, Vellore, India*
[5]*The International Union Against TB and Lung Disease, New Delhi, India*

Correspondence should be addressed to C. Padmapriyadarsini; darsini69@hotmail.com

Academic Editor: Brian Eley

Background. Preventive therapy for child contacts of multidrug-resistant tuberculosis (MDR-TB) patients is poorly studied, and no consensus about the role and the rationale of chemoprophylaxis has been reached. *Objective.* To conduct systematic review with an aim to determine the effectiveness of TB preventive therapy in reducing the incidence of TB disease in pediatric contacts of MDR-TB patients. *Methods.* We conducted a literature search for randomized control trials, cohort studies, and case reports of chemoprophylaxis for pediatric contacts of MDR-TB patients in PubMed, EMBASE, Cochrane Databases of Systematic Reviews, metaRegister of Controlled Trials, and other clinical registries through March 2017, using appropriate search strategy. In addition we searched abstracts from international conferences and references of published articles and reviews. *Results.* Of the 153 references assessed from various databases, seven studies were identified as relevant after adaption of eligibility criteria and assessed for systematic review. Of these, only two studies contributed data for the pooled meta-analysis. *Conclusions.* Though the available evidences suggest that the chemoprophylaxis for child contacts of MDR-TB patients is beneficial, data to support or reject preventive therapy is very limited. Further clinical research, in Tb endemic settings like India, needs to be performed to prove the beneficial effect of chemoprophylaxis for pediatric contacts of MDR-TB.

1. Introduction

The World Health Organization (WHO) estimates that, globally in 2016, there were around 600,000 incident cases of rifampicin-resistant tuberculosis (TB) of which 490,000 had multidrug-resistant tuberculosis (MDR-TB) with India, China, and Russian federation accounting for almost 47% of these cases [1]. The burden of childhood TB is estimated to be 10–15% of the total TB burden with an annual risk of TB infection at 2–5% [2]. About 5% of those infected are likely to develop the disease in the first year after acquiring the infection and another 5% during rest of their lifetime. In children MDR-TB is mainly due to primary transmission from the index case, rather than acquired from prior exposure to TB treatment. Thirty-five countries have reported at least one pediatric MDR-TB case between 1994 and 2011, with increased morbidity and mortality compared to drug-sensitive disease [3]. Early diagnosis and effective treatment of adult MDR-TB case remain the main strategy to reduce TB transmission. However, given the poor success rate of currently used treatment regimens, it is wiser to adapt other modalities to prevent the occurrence of MDR-TB among the countries who pledge to achieve End TB goal by 2035 [4]. One such strategy is to target the latent TB reservoir, with either drugs or vaccines, and prevent the progression of latent TB infection to active TB disease. But optimal chemoprophylaxis for pediatric contacts of MDR-TB patients is poorly studied, and no consensus about the role and the rationale of different preventive treatments has been reached. A systematic review in 2006 by Fraser et al. concluded that there is lack of studies from randomized controlled trials to confirm or refute the need for chemoprophylaxis for childhood contacts of DR-TB patients [5]. A recent systematic review by Marks et al. further added that though preventive therapy showed effectiveness in prevention of MDR-TB among contacts, they often resulted in treatment discontinuation due to the adverse effects from the drugs in the regimen [6].

Frequent monitoring of these children was emphasized as much as the need for more clinical trials to determine the drugs that will be effective for pediatric contacts of these patients. Therefore, to address the gaps in evidence and look for newer studies for chemoprophylaxis for child contacts of MDR-TB patients, a systematic review was carried out with the following objectives: (i) to determine the effectiveness of chemoprophylaxis or TB preventive therapy in reducing the incidence of tuberculosis disease in childhood contacts of drug-resistant pulmonary tuberculosis patients and (ii) to determine the occurrence of any adverse events during the course of chemoprophylaxis or TB preventive therapy.

2. Methods

A protocol for the systematic review was registered with PROSPERO and is available online. The search is up to date as on 31 June 2017: https://www.crd.york.ac.uk/PROSPERO/display_record.php?RecordID=39330.

2.1. Eligibility and Inclusion Criteria

2.1.1. Types of Studies. We intended to include all randomized and quasi-randomized controlled trials (RCT): prospective and retrospective cohort studies and case reports of chemoprophylaxis for children of MDR-TB patients. Studies performed among children of MDR-TB patients without active disease, HIV infected or uninfected, and studies performed in any country and published in any language were included. Systematic reviews, policy papers/briefs, case reports, letters to the editors, programme reports, correspondence, and non-human studies were not included in the review.

2.1.2. Types of Participants. All childhood contacts of MDR-TB patients between the age of 0 and 14 years were included. Definition of "contacts" was retained as they were defined in the original study. For example, Seddon et al. 2013 defined "contacts" as children < 5 years of age with significant exposure to an infectious (sputum smear of culture positive) pulmonary MDR-TB source patient [7].

2.1.3. Types of Interventions. Interventions with chemoprophylaxis for MDR-TB of any duration were considered. Comparison in RCT was the control or comparator arm while the comparison in the cohort study was the standard of care.

2.1.4. Types of Outcome Measures. The primary outcome measures were occurrence of TB disease or serious adverse events among childhood contacts of MDR-TB patients on chemoprophylaxis. The secondary outcomes were occurrence of adverse events and occurrence of MDR-TB among children on chemoprophylaxis.

2.1.5. Search Strategy. We searched separately for randomized control trials, cohort studies, and case reports regardless of publication status (published and in press) in PubMed, EMBASE, Cochrane Databases of Systematic Reviews, and other clinical registries (WHO, United States, South Africa, and Australia-New Zealand clinical registry). The search was also extended to metaRegister of Controlled Trials (mRCT): ClinicalTrials.gov website to identify progressive trials and abstracts from international conferences: (i) The Union World Conference on Lung Health from 2000 to 2017 and (ii) the American Thoracic Society Conference from 2000 to 2017.

2.2. Data Collection and Analysis

2.2.1. Selection of Studies. The systematic review was carried out in accordance with the Preferred Reporting Items for Systematic Reviews and Meta-Analyses guidelines. The search strategy was developed considering the population, intervention, comparator, and outcome of the systematic review. The following terms in PubMed were used for search: ((((((((Tuberculosis [MeSH Terms]) OR Latent tuberculosis [MeSH Terms]) OR Extensively Drug-Resistant Tuberculosis [MeSH Terms]) OR Tuberculosis, Multidrug-Resistant [MeSH Terms]) OR Tuberculosis, Pulmonary [MeSH Terms]) OR Mycobacterium tuberculosis [MeSH Terms])) AND ((((((Child [MeSH Terms]) OR child)) OR ((Pediatrics [MeSH Terms]) OR pediatric*)) OR children)) AND (("Family Characteristics"[Mesh]) OR contact tracing [MeSH Terms]))) AND (((chemotherapy) OR chemoprevention [MeSH Terms]) OR prophylaxis). Similar searches were carried out in all relevant electronic sources and stored as online bibliography in open access web-based application: Rayan (https://rayyan.qcri.org/). We also contacted the authors of ongoing clinical trials, journal editors of International Journal of TB and Lung Diseases, Public Health Action for manuscript in press, and experts in the field for details on the study.

The titles and abstracts of screened studies in bibliography were evaluated by PP, MD, and SBN independently for relevance according to the prespecified criteria.

2.2.2. Data Extraction and Management. Data were extracted individually by two authors (PP and MD) using standardized data extraction forms (Figure 1). Separate forms for randomized trials and prospective and retrospective cohort studies were used. We attempted to contact the trial authors for clarification when methodological details are unclear. Any disagreement was resolved by discussion with third author SBN.

2.2.3. Data Synthesis. We assessed the similarity across the included studies on the characteristics of population intervention and the outcomes to provide a meaningful result to perform meta-analysis. Studies which did not describe

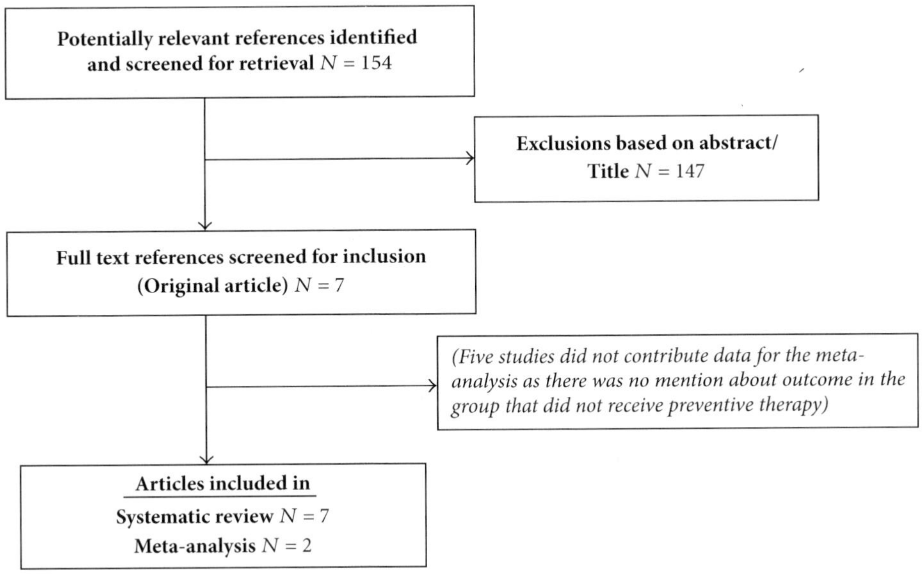

FIGURE 1: Search result of the topic.

the event or outcome in one of the groups—either the intervention group or the comparator group—were excluded from meta-analysis, though they will be included in the systematic review. We used Revman 5.3 software for meta-analysis. Mantel Hanzel method was used for dichotomous outcome reporting the relative risk along with 95% CI with fixed effect model. Inverse variance method was used for continuous data using fixed effect model presented with the mean difference with 95% CI [14]. We created subgroup according to type of intervention and age categories (0–5, 6–9, 10–14) and drug resistance profile and sensitivity analysis by excluding the high risk of bias studies. However, due to the limited data available, we did not undertake the subgroup and sensitivity analysis.

2.2.4. Assessment of Heterogeneity. We assessed the heterogeneity with *i*2 statistics which describes the percentage of variation across the included studies rather than due to random error.

2.2.5. Assessment of Risk of Bias. For randomized controlled trials Cochrane risk of bias tool was used for assessment following the standards given in the Cochrane handbook [15]. Downs and Black checklist was used for observational studies [16]. All the risk of bias figure was created in Revman 5.3 by modifying the domains depending upon the tool.

2.2.6. Summary of Findings. Gradepro software was used for creating the summary of findings table. There are five domains for assessing certainty of evidence for randomized controlled trials (risk of bias, inconsistency, indirectness, imprecision, and publication bias). However for observational studies in addition to these existing domains the following domains were also considered (large effect, plausible confounding, and dosage response gradient).

Two authors (PP and MD) independently assessed the risk of bias of the selected studies using the Cochrane tool to assess the risk of bias and the quality of the evidence of the included studies was assessed using GRADE Pro software. Any disagreements were discussed with third author (SBN).

3. Findings and Results

The search strategy extracted 154 studies from the various databases published during January 2000 to June 2017; of these seven studies were considered potentially relevant (Figure 1). Three systematic reviews were identified and these were assessed for relevant references. Of these studies, after adaption of eligibility criteria, seven studies were included for the systematic review while only two studies were included for the pooled meta-analysis.

3.1. Characteristics of Included Studies. The relevant characteristics of studies included are shown in Table 1. A study by Seddon et al. (2013) described the tolerability and toxicity of a standard MDR-TB preventive therapy regimen given to childhood contacts of adults with ofloxacin-susceptible MDR-TB and described the treatment outcomes [7]. This study included children below 5 years of age and children living with human immunodeficiency virus (HIV) infection below 15 years at the time of screening between May 2010 and April 2011. Children were initiated on preventive therapy with ofloxacin, ethambutol, and high dose isoniazid for a period of six months. A total of 186 childhood contacts were identified, given preventive therapy, and followed up for a period of at least 12 months.

Another study by Schaaf et al. (2002) described the long-term prevalence of tuberculous infection and disease in young children in household contact of adults with drug-resistant (DR) pulmonary TB in an area with high incidence of TB [8]. This study included 41 children below 5 years of

Table 1: Summary of the seven studies showing their relevant details of included parameters.

Number	Author	Study design	Treatment regimen	Study subjects	Number of children	Treatment completion rate	Adverse event	Incidence TB	Mortality	Follow-up months	Remark
(1)	Seddon et al. [7] (2013)	Prospective cohort South Africa	Ofloxacin, ethambutol, and high dose isoniazid*	Children < 5 years, CLHIV < 15 years	186	75.8% (141/186)	7/186 (3.7%)	6/141 on PT 4/45 not on PT	1 (0.5%)	219 p-y (12–24 months)	-
(2)	Schaaf et al. [8] (2002)	Prospective cohort S. Africa	High dose isoniazid, pyrazinamide, ethionamide, ethambutol/ofloxacin*	Children < 5 years old	41 + 64		30/61 Eth 1/15 OFX	2/41 on PT 13/64 not on PT	No deaths	30	-
(3)	Adler-Shohet et al. [9] (2014)	Prospective cohort California	9 mon levofloxacin and pyrazinamide	Children	31	8/26 (31%) (7 changed Rx 11 did not complete)	All children	0	No deaths	24	*No separate mention on outcome in those who refused PT*
(4)	Gracia-Prats et al. [10] (2014)	Retrospective community cohort S. Africa	Ofloxacin, ethambutol, and high dose isoniazid*	<15 years	38	24/34 (71%)	No	No TB	No deaths	12	*PT offered only to HHC < 5 years of age*
(5)	Bamrah et al. [11] (2014)	Prospective cohort Micronesia	12 mon levofloxacin and ethambutol	Children < 12 years	119 *(only 26 children)*	25/26 (95%)	Not clear	0/104 on PT 3/15 not on PT	No deaths	36	*Not mentioned who developed TB—adult or child*
(6)	Feja et al. [12] (2008)	Retrospective chart review NYC	9 mon quinolones, cycloserine, ethionamide, pyrazinamide, ethambutol	Children < 15 years	51	36/41 (88%) at DOHMH; 2/9 (22%)	8/22 (24%)	No TB	No deaths	24	*No comparator group without PT*
(7)	Attamna et al. [13] (2009)	Retrospective chart review Israel	Ciprofloxacin and pyrazinamide*		476 (387 no Rx versus 89 PT)	Not clear	Not clear	No TB in any group	Not clear	72	*Low TB prevalence area*

Study or subgroup	FQ combination Events	FQ combination Total	No treatment Events	No treatment Total	Weight	Risk ratio M-H, fixed, 95% CI
Schaaf et al. 2002	2	41	13	64	62.6%	0.24 [0.06, 1.01]
Seddon et al. 2013	2	141	4	45	37.4%	0.16 [0.03, 0.84]
Total (95% CI)		*182*		*109*	*100.0%*	*0.21 [0.07, 0.63]*
Total events	4		17			

Heterogeneity: $\chi^2 = 0.14$, df = 1 ($P = 0.71$); $I^2 = 0\%$

Test for overall effect: $Z = 2.77$ ($P = 0.006$)

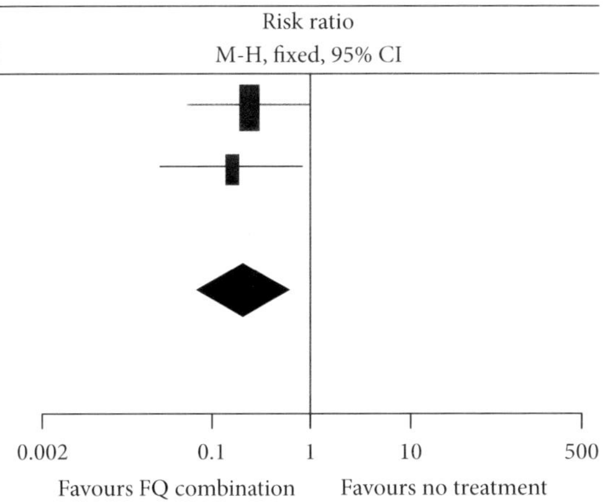

Figure 2: Forest plot of comparison of effect of preventive therapy versus no therapy for pediatric contacts of MDR-TB patients.

age who were initiated on chemoprophylaxis according to the index's strain susceptibility and included high dose isoniazid, pyrazinamide, ethionamide, and ethambutol or high dose isoniazid, pyrazinamide, ethionamide, and ofloxacin daily for a period of six months. All children were followed up to thirty months.

Other studies on TB prevention for MDR-TB contacts included both adults and a small number of children and do not specify the outcome in children on preventive therapy or on placebo. For example, Adler-Shohet et al. (2014) described 31 children who developed latent infection after exposure to an index MDR-TB patient. Twenty-six were treated with levofloxacin and pyrazinamide; none developed TB but twelve required a change in therapy secondary to adverse effects [9]. However, there is no mention of any outcome in the five children who did not receive preventive therapy. Hence though this study was included for the systematic review, data from this study was not included for the meta-analysis. Similarly in the Garcia-Prats study, of the 38 who received preventive therapy, only 23 were children <5 years of age. Of them none developed TB. However among the comparator group (total = 4) who received no preventive therapy all seemed to be adults and no children [10]. Hence though these studies were included in the systematic review, they did not contribute data to the meta-analysis.

3.2. Effect of Intervention. Between the two studies combined, there were four cases of TB in the contacts group that received chemoprophylaxis to prevent MDR-TB as compared to 17 cases of TB in the contacts group that did not receive any chemoprophylaxis (Figure 2). The relative risk for developing TB was 0.21 (95% CI 0.07–0.63). As the number of events were low, the confidence interval was wide. The other predefined outcomes were treatment completion rate, adverse events, and mortality rate. The pooled estimate of treatment completion rate was 0.74 (95% CI 0.64–0.82) among the included studies. Though adverse events were observed in all the studies, due to heterogeneity in the reporting of adverse events between the studies, a pooled estimate could not be calculated. There was only one reported death in the abovementioned studies.

3.3. Risk of Bias Assessment. Figure 3 shows the summary of the risk of bias assessment using the Black and Downs tool to assess the risk of bias for cohort studies. The tool assessed three domains, namely, (1) selection bias, (2) outcome ascertain bias, and (3) performance bias. A study could be awarded a maximum of "definitely yes," showing a low risk of bias to a "definitely no" indicating high risk of bias for the three different domains. These studies do not mention any adjustments for confounders; hence, all have risk of bias.

3.4. Certainty of Evidence. The certainty of the evidence of the included studies was assessed using GRADE Pro software. As there were not any serious inconsistencies, imprecision, or indirectness in the results of the two studies, the quality of evidence could be upgraded. The quality of evidence for the effectiveness of chemoprophylaxis for child contacts of MDR-TB patients was thus assessed to be moderate (Table 2).

4. Discussions

This systematic review adds up to the evidences available on this topic in the scientific domain. Globally, the National Health Programmes have laid lot of emphasis on diagnosing and treating drug-resistant tuberculosis which is in line with the End TB strategy; however, the components of chemoprophylaxis for contacts of TB patients remain under prioritized or in primitive stage due to lack of standardized chemoprophylaxis regimens with respect to the drugs, dosages, and duration of therapy. The same has been opined in the recent systematic review by Fox et al. in 2017 [17].

We found that preventive therapy with second-line drugs, in line with the susceptibility profile of index case isolate or with fluoroquinolone, should be considered for chemoprophylaxis of contacts of MDR-TB patients. Our finding is supported by another retrospective review on pediatric contacts of MDR-TB patients in South Africa, where the authors

TABLE 2: Quality of evidence and results from included studies.

Quality assessment							Number of patients		Effect		Quality	Importance
Number of studies	Study design	Risk of bias	Inconsistency	Indirectness	Imprecision	Other considerations	Preventive therapy	No preventive therapy	Relative (95% CI)	Absolute (95% CI)		
Incidence of TB												
2	Observational studies	Not serious	Not serious	Not serious	Not serious	Strong association	4/182 (2.2%)	17/109 (15.6%)	RR 0.21 (0.07 to 0.63)	123 fewer per 1,000 (from 58 fewer to 145 fewer)	⊕⊕⊕○ Moderate	

	Exposed and nonexposed cohorts drawn from same population	Assessment of exposure	Outcome of interest not present at start of study	Study match exposed and unexposed	Presence or absence of prognostic factors	Assessment of outcome	Follow-up adequate	Cointervention similar between groups
Adler-Shohet et al. 2014	+	+	+	?	?	+	+	?
Attamna et al. 2009	?	+	+	?	?	?	+	?
Bamrah et al. 2014	+	+	?	?	?	+	+	?
Feja et al. 2008	?	+	+	?	?	+	+	?
Garcia-Prats et al. 2014	+	+	+	?	?	?	?	?
Schaaf et al. 2002	+	+	+	?	?	+	+	?
Seddon et al. 2013	+	+	+	?	?	+	+	?

FIGURE 3: Summary of risk of bias assessment of the seven included studies.

concluded that children developed MDR-TB if they received chemoprophylaxis with either isoniazid or a combination of isoniazid, rifampin, and pyrazinamide and at least 2 second-line drugs should be considered for chemoprophylaxis of 6–12 months [18]. Other studies have reported varied results and the evidences are not sufficient to support or reject chemoprophylaxis for contacts of MDR-TB patients [19].

Currently, very few studies are conducted and published in this thematic area. Even the rigorous search in various databases of last two decades revealed only few studies. The quality of evidence provided by these studies is low to moderate and given the heterogeneity of these studies, one needs to be cautious while interpreting the results of these studies. However, there is evidence to support the reduction of risk of developing TB among contacts who receive chemoprophylaxis and the protection ranges from 37 to 90%.

All the studies reported adverse events irrespective of the type of drugs used. However, higher adverse events were recorded with ethionamide and pyrazinamide while fluoroquinolones had minimal toxicity. Discontinuation of treatment was noted among the contacts on ethionamide containing regimens predominantly due to gastrointestinal side effects.

To conclude, available evidences suggest that the chemoprophylaxis for child contacts of MDR-TB patient is beneficial, though the available evidence is of moderate quality. Further researches under controlled conditions in *TB endemic settings* are required to prove the beneficial or no effect of chemoprophylaxis for pediatric contacts of MDR-TB patients.

Authors' Contributions

The titles and abstracts of screened studies in bibliography were evaluated by C. Padmapriyadarsini, Mrinalini Das, and Sharath Burugina Nagaraja independently for relevance according to the prespecified criteria.

References

[1] WHO, *Global Tuberculosis Report 2017. World Health Organisation*, 2017, http://www.who.int/tb/publications/childtb_guidelines/en/.

[2] WHO, *Guidance for national tuberculosis programmes on the management of tuberculosis in children*, 2014, http://www.who.int/tb/publications/childtb_guidelines/en/.

[3] M. Zignol, C. Sismanidis, D. Falzon, P. Glaziou, M. Dara, and K. Floyd, "Multidrug-resistant tuberculosis in children: Evidence from global surveillance," *European Respiratory Journal*, vol. 42, no. 3, pp. 701–707, 2013.

[4] WHO, *WHO End TB Strategy*, World Health Organization, 2015, http://www.who.int/tb/post2015_strategy/en/.

[5] A. Fraser, M. Paul, A. Attamna, and L. Leibovici, "Drugs for preventing tuberculosis in people at risk of multiple-drug-resistant pulmonary tuberculosis.," *Cochrane Database of Systematic Reviews (Online)*, no. 2, p. CD005435, 2006.

[6] S. M. Marks, S. R. Mase, and S. B. Morris, "Systematic review, meta-analysis, and cost-effectiveness of treatment of latent tuberculosis to reduce progression to multidrug-resistant tuberculosis," *Clinical Infectious Diseases*, vol. 64, no. 12, pp. 1670–1677, 2017.

[7] J. A. Seddon, A. C. Hesseling, H. Finlayson et al., "Preventive therapy for child contacts of multidrug-resistant tuberculosis: A prospective cohort study," *Clinical Infectious Diseases*, vol. 57, no. 12, pp. 1676–1684, 2013.

[8] H. S. Schaaf, R. P. Gie, M. Kennedy, N. Beyers, P. B. Hesseling, and P. R. Donald, "Evaluation of young children in contact with adult multidrug-resistant pulmonary tuberculosis: A 30-month follow-up," *Pediatrics*, vol. 109, no. 5, pp. 765–771, 2002.

[9] F. C. Adler-Shohet, J. Low, M. Carson, H. Girma, and J. Singh, "Management of latent tuberculosis infection in child contacts of multidrug-resistant tuberculosis," *The Pediatric Infectious Disease Journal*, vol. 33, no. 6, pp. 664–666, 2014.

[10] A. J. Garcia-Prats, K. Zimri, Z. Mramba, H. S. Schaaf, and A. C. Hesseling, "Children exposed to multidrug-resistant tuberculosis at a homebased day care centre: A contact investigation," *The International Journal of Tuberculosis and Lung Disease*, vol. 18, no. 11, pp. 1292–1298, 2014.

[11] S. Bamrah, R. Brostrom, F. Dorina et al., "Treatment for LTBI in contacts of MDR-TB patients, Federated States of Micronesia, 2009-2012," *The International Journal of Tuberculosis and Lung Disease*, vol. 18, no. 8, pp. 912–918, 2014.

[12] K. Feja, E. McNelley, C. S. Tran, J. Burzynski, and L. Saiman, "Management of pediatric multidrug-resistant tuberculosis and latent tuberculosis infections in New York City from 1995 to 2003," *The Pediatric Infectious Disease Journal*, vol. 27, no. 10, pp. 907–912, 2008.

[13] A. Attamna, D. Chemtob, S. Attamna et al., "Risk of tuberculosis in close contacts of patients with multidrug resistant tuberculosis: A nationwide cohort," *Thorax*, vol. 64, no. 3, p. 271, 2009.

[14] "RevMan 5 Download," http://community.cochrane.org/tools/review-production-tools/revman-5/revman-5-download.

[15] "Cochrane Methods, Bias," http://methods.cochrane.org/bias/assessing-risk-bias-included-studies.

[16] S. H. Downs and N. Black, "The feasibility of creating a checklist for the assessment of the methodological quality both of randomized and non-randomized studies of health care interventions," *Journal of Epidemiology Community Health*, vol. 52, pp. 377–384, 1998.

[17] G. Fox, C. Dobler, B. Marais, and J. Denholm, "Preventive therapy for latent tuberculosis infection—the promise and the challenges," *International Journal of Infectious Diseases*, vol. 56, pp. 68–76, 2017.

[18] D. B. Sneag, H. S. Schaaf, M. F. Cotton, and H. J. Zar, "Failure of chemoprophylaxis with standard antituberculosis agents in child contacts of multidrug-resistant tuberculosis cases," *The Pediatric Infectious Disease Journal*, vol. 26, no. 12, pp. 1142–1146, 2007.

[19] M. J. Van Der Werf, M. W. Langendam, A. Sandgren, and D. Manissero, "Lack of evidence to support policy development for management of contacts of multidrug-resistant tuberculosis patients: Two systematic reviews," *The International Journal of Tuberculosis and Lung Disease*, vol. 16, no. 3, pp. 288–296, 2012.

32

Roles of Mucosal Immunity against *Mycobacterium tuberculosis* Infection

Wu Li,[1,2] Guangcun Deng,[1,2] Min Li,[1,2] Xiaoming Liu,[1,2] and Yujiong Wang[1,2]

[1] *Key Laboratory of Ministry of Education for Conservation and Utilization of Special Biological Resources in the Western, Ningxia University, Yinchuan, Ningxia 750021, China*
[2] *College of Life Science, Ningxia University, 539 W. Helanshan Road, Xixia District, Yinchuan, Ningxia 750021, China*

Correspondence should be addressed to Yujiong Wang, yujiongw@gmail.com

Academic Editor: Euzenir N. Sarno

Mycobacterium tuberculosis (Mtb), the causative agent of tuberculosis (TB), is one of the world's leading infectious causes of morbidity and mortality. As a mucosal-transmitted pathogen, Mtb infects humans and animals mainly through the mucosal tissue of the respiratory tract. Apart from providing a physical barrier against the invasion of pathogen, the major function of the respiratory mucosa may be to serve as the inductive sites to initiate mucosal immune responses and sequentially provide the first line of defense for the host to defend against this pathogen. A large body of studies in the animals and humans have demonstrated that the mucosal immune system, rather than the systemic immune system, plays fundamental roles in the host's defense against Mtb infection. Therefore, the development of new vaccines and novel delivery routes capable of directly inducing respiratory mucosal immunity is emphasized for achieving enhanced protection from Mtb infection. In this paper, we outline the current state of knowledge regarding the mucosal immunity against Mtb infection, including the development of TB vaccines, and respiratory delivery routes to enhance mucosal immunity are discussed.

1. Introduction

Tuberculosis (TB) is one of the world's leading infectious disease with approximately two million deaths and eight million new cases annually. It is also a severe pulmonary disease and a public health burden caused by the infection of *Mycobacterium tuberculosis* (Mtb) [1]. Mtb is a facultative intracellular bacterium capable of surviving and persisting in host mononuclear cells where it is able to escape the elimination through numerous mechanisms [2]. The capacity of Mtb to survive within a host cell for decades without replicating may be partially due to the fact that it is a metabolically, fastidious, acid-fast bacillus that grows very slowly, as well as its ability to inhibit phagosomal maturation by preventing phagosome-lysosome fusion and acidification of the phagosome [3]. Transcriptomic analysis has revealed that Mtb was able to gain its abilities to evade the host immune surveillance, adopted its specialized intracellular niche, and resisted various agents and antibiotic drugs, by expressing various genes against the host immune responses [4]. The ability of Mtb to evade the host immune surveillance and establish a latent metabolic state in the host causes the difficulty to eradicate tuberculosis, even though most of patients infected with Mtb could be cured with appropriate therapy. In addition, the reactivation of Mtb at a latent state in immunocompromised patients and the emergency of the multidrug-resistant Mtb strains and a coinfection with HIV have also increased the difficulty to prevent this disease [5]. To date, vaccination remains one of the most effective approaches for controlling TB worldwide.

It is well known that the mucosa is the largest immune organ in the body, and it is generally believed that almost all infectious diseases are initiated at mucosal surface [6]. The respiratory tract is the natural route for Mtb infection, where Mtb infects the individual mainly through the mucosal tissue of the respiratory tract after inhalation of mycobacteria-containing droplets from the external environment. Normally, the pathogen (Mtb) infection could be eliminated by the host's immune system, but it is desirable to induce immunity prior to the infection by means of vaccination in most of the cases. In order to effectively prevent Mtb infection, the approach of mucosal immunization has recently received increasing attention in the field of tuberculosis vaccination owing to its potency in inducing mucosa-associated protection from mucosal infectious diseases [7–9]. Several lines of evidence have suggested that mucosal immunity can provide unique advantages for protection against mycobacterial infection, by which the immune cells, such as macrophages, dendritic cells, and leukocytes recognize the pathogen associated molecular patterns (PAMPs), and sequentially activate the antimycobacterial immune responses including the activation of specific T-cell and antibody synthesis [10–13].

In general, the mucosal protection includes the physical and chemical mucosal barriers, and a wide range of immune components for the recognition of invading pathogen by different cell types, the secretions of antimicrobial peptides, and factors of immune mediator/effector. This paper aims to summarize our current understanding of the mucosal immunity against Mtb infection, and some ongoing approaches of developing mucosal TB vaccines to enhance the mucosal immunity.

2. The Mucosal System in the Respiratory Tract

The immune system is composed of two primary compartments: the mucosal immune system and the systemic immune system. The mucosal immune system functions as the first line of defense against pathogens and is composed of inductive sites and effector sites. The inductive sites are responsible for antigen uptake and priming of naïve T and B cells that then migrate to other mucosal effector sites, while the effector sites are the mucosa where secretory IgA (sIgA) is produced and mucosal immunity is initiated [14]. In the mucosal surface, the epithelial cells line to establish a barrier and perform its "barrier functions," and the immune cells play vital roles in host defense against infection of pathogens by migrating to the lamina propria of respiratory tract and other sites after they are primed.

Mucosal surfaces are classically defined as the body's mucus-covered surfaces and include surfaces of the respiratory, gastrointestinal, and urogenital tracts as well as the exposed cornea/conjunctiva [15]. They are constantly in contact with external environments to perform physiological functions including nutrient transport, ion and water homeostasis, and respiration. The surface area of human adult mucosa is about $400\,m^2$, and almost 80% of the total immune cell population is present at mucosal sites, with over 90% of human infections at the body's mucosal borders. Additionally, most of mucosal surfaces contain specialized mucosa-associated lymphoid tissues (MALT); the MALT consisted of gastrointestinal-associated lymphoid tissue, bronchial and nasal-associated lymphoid tissue (B/NALT), and conjunctiva- and urogenital-associated lymphoid tissue [15], all of which are necessary for antigen sampling and induction of mucosal immune responses [16]. The attachment of bacteria to mucosal surfaces is the first step in the pathogenesis of most infectious diseases; equally important, it is the first-line defense of mucosa against invading microbial pathogens. Thus, the mucosal immune system has been suggested to be the port of entry for many pathogens and is one of the most important immune organs against Mtb infection in the body.

2.1. The Role of Mucosal Epithelial Cells in Mucosal Immunity against Mtb. In humans and animals, the mucosal surface is lined by epithelial cells and mucus-secreting cells that form tight barriers separating the external environments from the internal compartments. It is an important interface bridging the host cells with the environments. Since mucosal epithelial cells are constantly exposed to external environments, they are vulnerable to microbial attacks and play active roles in regulating mucosal immune responses by locally adapting of microbial recognition, maintaining of immune homeostasis, and modulating of antigen-presenting cells and adaptive immune responses, during the interaction of host and external pathogens (see review [17]). In addition, the interaction of epithelial cells with Mtb is an important step for Mtb to entry into the host body. Teitelbaum et al. found that epithelial M cells play important roles in this process [18]. Furthermore, a microbial attack may damage the mucosal layer; the mucosal epithelial cells, however, are able to rapidly restore the integrity of mucosal epithelium by initiating a programmed series of interdependent responses after the injury [19].

The mucosal epithelial cells play a prominent role in protecting the host from the invasion of pathogens through secreting many kinds of antimicrobial substances into the mucosal fluid (e.g., mucins, defensins, lysozyme, nitric oxide, and others), among which the production of sIgA is one of the important activities of mucosal epithelial cells. These defensive compounds in the mucosal surfaces form a physical barrier and have direct antimicrobial activity. Mucin glycoproteins are secreted in large quantities by mucosal epithelia, and they play a central role in accommodating the resident commensal flora and limiting infectious disease [20]. Defensins have an activity against a broad range of pathogens, which are a family of evolutionarily related vertebrate antimicrobial peptides with characteristics of β-sheet-rich folds and frame work of six disulphide-linked cysteines [21]. Defensins can act on the mycobacterial cell envelope and disrupt the membrane architecture to directly kill bacillus [22]. Such an antimycobacterial activity has also been proved in both mouse models [23] and humans [24]. Nitric oxide and other reactive nitrogen intermediates (RNI) produced by alveolar macrophages also aid the host's defense against the infection of Mtb (see review [25]). Furthermore, the mucosal epithelial cells can also secrete a series of proinflammatory cytokines against Mtb (see Section 4). These proinflammatory factors can eradicate organisms and infected cells by recruiting and activating phagocytic cells [26–28]. The mucosal epithelial cells also produce other compounds important for host against the invasion of Mtb. For example, surfactant protein A and surfactant protein D, which are produced by pulmonary epithelial cells, play important roles in the innate immunity by influencing the ability of pathogens to be taken up by host cells and/or cleared by host defense mechanisms [29]. Together with the family of Toll-like receptors, the surfactant proteins also play a key role in the recognition and binding of the pathogen to epithelial cells during Mtb infection (see review [30]).

2.2. The Role of sIgA in Mucosal Immunity against Mtb. It is generally accepted that cell-mediated immunity (CMI) plays a pivotal role in the immune response against Mtb infection. However, the protective role of Mtb-specific humoral immunity remains controversial. Recently, several lines of evidence showed a protective role of antibodies against Mtb [31–33], where sIgA is the most abundantly produced natural antibody isotype in mucosal tissue. sIgA has been found to play important roles in the exclusion of different antigens from mucosal surfaces. It serves as a first line of defense against pathogens in mucosal areas by agglutinating potential invaders and facilitating their clearance by peristaltic and mucociliary movements [34]. In addition, sIgA is the most characteristic component of the mucosal immunity [35].

sIgA can serve as a carrier of antigens; it also has the potential functions in the inhibition of bacterial adherence, neutralization of toxin and virus, and prevention of antigen uptake by epithelial cells, in part through a mechanism of binding and intercepting the invasion of pathogens and/or neutralizing their toxic products, during the transcytosis or in the mucosal fluids [36–39]. These imply that sIgA in mucosal secretions may play an important role in the host's early defense against invading pathogens in respiratory tract [40]. The above notion is supported by a previous human study in which the mucosal BCG vaccination could induce significant increases of sIgA [41]. This finding was also attested in a recent study using a mouse model; mice vaccinated with Ag85A-Esat-6-IL-21 DNA vaccine showed an improved level of sIgA in the bronchoalveolar lavage (BAL) [42]. Moreover, the sIgA could prevent the adsorption of pathogens at the mucosal epithelium [37–39]; the initial infection of Mtb could therefore be blocked at the mucosal surface by sIgA. Such finding was supported by a study in a murine model in which the entrance of mycobacterial bacilli into the lungs was blocked by sIgA [43].

3. Mucosal Immune Effector Cells against Mtb Infection

The immune cell types in MALT include a variety of phenotypical and functional distinct T-cell, B-cell, and accessory cell subpopulations, by which the MALT plays a central role in regulating mucosal immunity. It has been well established that the cell-mediated immune responses (CMIRs) are the primary defense against intracellular pathogens such as Mtb infection. The functional "effectors" of these responses are various immune cells. In response to Mtb infection, the $CD4^+$ and $CD8^+$ subsets of T-cell population, as well as alveolar macrophages and dendritic cells (DCs), are the major immune effector cell types, which have been well documented by others; here we will only focus on the functions displayed by these immune cells in the mucosal microenvironment.

3.1. $CD4^+$, $CD8^+$, and Other T-Cell Subsets. As an intracellular pathogen, Mtb resides within the vacuole of host macrophages; the $CD4^+$ T cells and $CD8^+$ T cells are of primary importance in the host's protection against Mtb. $CD4^+$ T cells are involved in primary resistance to Mtb by producing IFN-γ and other cytokines to activate macrophages, of which it is critical in the controlling and eliminating of Mtb [25]. In response to Mtb infection, the host initiates the $CD4^+$ T-cell responses in the mediastinal lymph node (MLN) [44] and lung-draining lymph node (LN) [45, 46]. The critical role of $CD4^+$ T cells in defending Mtb infection became evident during epidemiological studies of HIV-1 infection [47]. When mice were challenged with Mtb via an aerosol method, the $CD4^+$ T cells in the lungs were highly activated during the acute phase of infection [48]. Recent study by Khader and coworkers also found that when mice were vaccinated, antigen-specific $CD4^+$ T cells can be induced in the lungs of vaccinated mice [49]. Additionally, mice vaccinated with a recombinant adenovirus-basis TB vaccine delivered by a mucosal route exhibited an increasing number of Ag-specific $CD4^+$ and $CD8^+$ T cells, while parenteral vaccination intramuscular injection (i.m.) failed to elicit airway luminal T cells and protect the lung from Mtb infection in mice [50]. These studies suggested the important roles of $CD4^+$ T cells in the mucosal immunity against Mtb. Interestingly, increasing evidence suggests that the effector $CD4^+$ T-cell responses to Mtb are apparently delayed [45, 46, 51]. Although the reason for the delay is not completely understood, the delay was suggested to be likely to allow the bacteria sufficient time to establish persistent infection [44].

Other $CD4^+$ T lineages cells, such as Th17 lineage cells, CD4 TEM cells, invariant T cells, and regulatory T cells, have also been demonstrated to be important for mucosal immunity against Mtb. For example, Th17 cells, which are distinct lineage of $CD4^+$ T cells [52], play crucial roles in mucosal immune responses to major respiratory pathogens, and they are capable of regulating the production of antimicrobial proteins in mucosal epithelium and clearing various pathogens [53, 54]. In addition, regulatory T cells are important to maintain peripheral tolerance and homeostasis at mucosal surface [55].

$CD8^+$ T cells are another subset of T cells necessary for the clearance of intracellular pathogens at mucosal sites. There seem to be three primary effector functions for $CD8^+$ T cells in tuberculosis as compared to $CD4^+$ T cells; these include lysis of infected cells in the mucosal surfaces (e.g., macrophages and DCs), direct killing of the intracellular bacteria, and production of IFN-γ cytokines. Similar to $CD4^+$ cells, $CD8^+$ cells are also important sources of IFN-γ against Mtb infection, even if the production is less relative to $CD4^+$ T cells. The importance of $CD8^+$ cells was also evidenced by the appearance of Mtb antigen (Ag)-specific $CD8^+$ cells in the airway lumen at the time of Mtb infection [50, 56, 57]. Murine study suggested that intranasal (i.n.)

delivery of low dose of soluble Mtb Ags was able to recruit and retain Ag-specific $CD8^+$ cells in the airway lumen over time, while the Ags delivered via an i.m. route failed to induce the Ag-specific $CD8^+$ cells [58]. Intranasal vaccination of recombinant adenoviral TB vaccines showed the accumulation and retention of antigen-specific $CD8^+$ and $CD4^+$ T cells in the airway lumen of mice [59]. Recent study by Mu and coworkers also found that $CD4^+$ T-cell-depleted mice intranasally vaccinated with adenovirus vector expressing Mtb antigen Ag85A led to suboptimal generation of Ag-specific $CD8^+$ T cells in the lung and spleen at the early time following the immunization [60].

Except $CD4^+$ T cells and $CD8^+$ T cells, other subsets of T cells such as $\alpha\beta$ T cells and $\gamma\delta$ T cells also have been found to play important roles in the mucosal immunity against Mtb. For instance, $\gamma\delta$ T cells are abundant on mucosal and epithelial surfaces; they are capable of lysing infected macrophages and containing mycobacterial growth [61, 62]. By using a pulmonary murine model of Mtb, Lockhart and coworkers found that the major producers of IL-17 in T cells isolated from the lungs of infected mice were $\gamma\delta$ T cells; this suggested that $\gamma\delta$ T cells are more potent producers of IL-17 during the early immune response at mucosal sites following the infections [63].

3.2. Mucosal Dendritic Cells. There are two types of dendritic cells (DCs), tissue DCs (refer to those that reside in the peripheral tissues such as mucosa, skin, and internal organs) and blood DCs [64]. Mucosal DCs, especially the airway mucosal DCs, are key effectors in response to Mtb infection. In tuberculosis, DCs are involved in the induction of antimycobacterial T-cell immune response; Mtb-infected DCs have the ability to produce interferon [65] and phagocytose the Mtb in murine model [66, 67]. In the airway mucosa, DCs are present in the epithelium and underlying lamina propria, as well as in the lung parenchyma and alveolar spaces of the lower respiratory tract [68]. They are the first responders to infection at epithelial surfaces of mucosal tissues, in which DCs are distributed throughout intra and subepithelial sites. Mucosal DCs are able to recognize pathogens through engagement of pattern recognition receptors (PRRs) [69]. Upon an appropriate stimulation, DCs undergo further maturation and migrate to secondary lymphoid tissues where they present Ags to T cell. The activated effector T cells then migrate back to the infection sites to produce cytokines, activate macrophages, and lyse target cells for eliminating the pathogens. Thus, DCs are unique antigen-presenting cells (APCs) with a capacity to stimulate naïve T cells. In response to Mtb, the invasion of this pathogen may stimulate DCs to initiate immune responses, but they also may impair the function of DCs function to provide a mean of immune evasion for Mtb [70]. The constituents of mycobacteria possess a capacity to induce the activation and maturation of DCs [71–73]. However, exposure of attenuated or virulent Mtb could cause the death of human DCs [74].

3.3. Alveolar Macrophages. Macrophages, especially alveolar macrophages, are important immune cells against Mtb infection. It is generally accepted that alveolar macrophages are one of the first cell types that encounter Mtb in the lungs. They are a primary host cell type for Mtb to live in and the first-line of defense in the lung against infection of these bacilli. Mtb could survive and grow in the activated macrophages [75, 76] or be killed by the host cells through a mechanism of producing reactive nitrogen intermediates [77, 78]. As a successful pathogen, virulent Mtb is capable of escaping the host's immune surveillance and living and replicating in the resting macrophages, partially by a mechanism of impairing macrophage plasma membrane repair [79, 80].

A large body of study has shown that autophagy plays a role in innate immune responses to intracellular bacterial infections. Murine studies have shown that the autophagy participated in the process of mycobacterial destruction in infected macrophage, although a rapid macrophage apoptosis could be induced after the infection [81]. These results suggested that the autophagy might contribute an important part for the host to defend against Mtb invasion [82–85].

Phagolysosome fusion is another antimycobacterial mechanism of macrophages, which is an evident mechanism for the mononuclear phagocyte lineage to inhibit and kill intracellular pathogens within cells [86]. Fusion of the lysosome with a phagosome-containing ingested bacterium is a primary mechanism by which macrophages kill a pathogen. In an activated macrophage, phagosomes in which the pathogens are enclosed fuse with lysosomes to form phagosomes and kill the pathogens. However, mycobacteria have evolved mechanisms to inhibit phagosome maturation, prevent it fusion with lysosomes, acidify, and expose bacteria to lysosomal hydrolases [87, 88]. Hence, the inhibition of autophagosome formation may be one of the most important mechanisms for Mtb to escape from host immune surveillance [89].

4. Cytokines in Mucosal Immunity against Mtb

Mtb infection usually results in the induction of large number of cytokines. These cytokines are key effectors in the host defense against Mtb (see review [25]), among which IFN-γ, TNF-α, IL-12, and granulocyte-macrophage colony-stimulating factor (GM-CSF) are of most importance in the mucosal immunity to Mtb. IFN-γ is a critical cytokine in protective immunity against Mtb. Except for $CD4^+$, $CD8^+$ T cells, and NK cells [90], pulmonary mucosal epithelial cells are another source of IFN-γ in response to Mtb infection [91]. IFN-γ can activate infected macrophages to directly inhibit the intracellular replication and growth of Mtb in the macrophages. IFN-γ-deficient mice challenged with a sublethal dose of Mtb showed a loss of cohesive structure of multiple foci of bacterial growth in the lung, suggesting a key role of IFN-γ in primary Mtb infection [92]. Another murine study demonstrated that mice immunized with Ag85A DNA vaccine through an oral route showed the expression of targeted antigen in the mucosal epithelial cells of the small intestine, striking increased levels of IFN-γ in the intraepithelial lymphocytes (IELs), as well as relevantly decreased bacterial loads, in the lungs in comparison with the control group [93]. Furthermore, the depletion of IFN-γ by antibodies could lead to increased number of Mtb in the lungs of mice, which strongly implied that IFN-γ might play critical roles in governing the outcome of latent infection [94]. Similar function of IFN-γ was found in human studies; individuals deficient in functional IFN-γ or IFN-γ-receptor exhibited an enhanced susceptibility to Mtb [95, 96]. *In vitro* study using human lung epithelial cells also showed an increased production of IFN-γ and IFN-γ receptors in A549 cell infected with Mtb, indicating that IFN-γ might play important roles in innate immunity against tuberculosis [91]. In addition, a direct evidence of defective macrophage activation in IFN-γ knockout mice showed that IFN-γ was responsible for activation of infected macrophages following Mtb challenge [97]. Apart from its function in activating macrophages to inhibit intracellular growth of Mtb, IFN-γ is also a critical regulator for APC by increasing MHC and costimulatory molecular expression [98]. Moreover, IFN-γ can be used as an index for the diagnosis of tuberculosis infection, which is able to avoid cross-reactivity with BCG immunization and nontuberculous mycobacterial infections [99].

TNF-α is another important immune mediator secreted by the activated macrophages and lung epithelial cells, which is capable of stimulating an acute phase reaction in response to Mtb infections. This mediator is able to play multiple roles in the host's immune response and pathogenesis of tuberculosis. By eliciting the production of TNF-α, Mtb may gain a capability to penetrate alveolar epithelium after infection. On the other hand, TNF-α is essential for the initiation of immune response against Mtb infection [114, 115], and for an effective granuloma formation. The formation of granuloma is important in mediating prolonged containment of mycobacteria, and it has been suggested to be the hallmark of containment of Mtb bacterial growth in the lung [116, 117]. Like IFN-γ, TNF-α is another important component for macrophage activation [117] and induction of apoptosis and necrosis of infected macrophages [118, 119]. In spite of its essential roles in the host's immunity to Mtb infection, overproduction of TNF-α in pulmonary TB may cause fevers, weakness, night sweats, necrosis, and progressive weight loss [120]. Experiments with recombinant BCG-expressing TNF-α demonstrated that high levels of TNF-α could cause destructive inflammation; the relative amount of TNF-α at the site of infection determined whether the cytokine acts as a protective or a destructive mediator [121].

In addition to IFN-γ and TNF-α, IL-12 is another cytokine with an immunoregulatory function that bridges the innate and adaptive immunities [122]. IL-12 is mainly produced by macrophages, which is essential for immunity against of Mtb infection. IL-12 p40$^{-/-}$ mice, genetic modified mice lacking the gene for the IL-12 p40 subunit, have been found to be extremely susceptible to Mtb infection as compared with the C57BL/6 WT mice. It is thought that exogenous administration of IL-12 to mice was able to increase resistance to the infection and improve the granuloma formation, while a depletion of IL-12 with specific antibodies altered granuloma formation [115, 123, 124]. These studies indicated an important role of IL-12 in the formation of protective granulomas. However, IL-12 could not induce a protection against Mtb in the absence of IFN-γ in mice [115]. Other biological functions of IL-12 include its ability to increase the production of IFN-γ and activate naïve NK and T cells [123, 125].

GM-CSF is another important cytokine that contributes to the control of Mtb infection and the containment of Mtb growth, which is produced by many cell types including airway epithelial cells, macrophages, and type II alveolar epithelial cells [126]. The production of GM-CSF induced by rBCG is enabled to enhance antimycobacterial T-cell responses and could improve immune protection [127]. Mice with GM-CSF gene disruption were unable to contain the bacterial growth in the lungs, while the GM^{+} mice were able to limit bacterial growth to an extent. Unlike those seen in their wild-type littermates, GM-CSF disrupted mice and GM^{+} mice did not exhibit a detectable granuloma formation in the lungs where the GM-CSF was overexpressed; this indicated that GM-CSF might play a role in the granuloma formation [128]. In addition to its immunoregulatory function, GM-CSF is also an effective adjuvant and immune regulatory molecule for vaccine development against TB [129, 130].

5. Mucosal Adjuvants and Vaccine Candidates against Mtb

The mucosal immunity has been suggested to play central roles in TB. However, most conventional vaccines are designed for delivery via systemic routes, which augment systemic immunity, but induce a lesser immune response at the mucosal site of pathogen entry. Increasing numbers of studies have documented that the respiratory mucosa provides a valuable target site for immunization against respiratory pathogens including Mtb. The Bacillus Calmette Guerin (BCG), the only licensed vaccine against TB, has been used for almost a century. However, BCG does not protect all age groups, and its protective efficacy in adults is highly varied from different trials with complications (0–80%) [131–133]. Additionally, the BCG-induced protection lasts no longer than fifteen years [134], and it neither prevents the establishment of latent tuberculosis infection, nor is suitable for use with immunocompromised patients. Therefore, novel and more effective vaccines and vaccination strategies are needed.

Despite the great efforts that have been focused on producing an effective vaccine capable of inducing a cell-mediated immune response to kill the intracellular bacilli, such vaccine candidates and approaches have not induced a significantly better protection than BCG. It has been extensively demonstrated that mucosal immune response and mucosal antibodies (in particular the sIgA) are important in protecting the host from Mtb infection [36, 135]. The vaccines, adjuvants, and delivery strategies attempted to enhance respiratory mucosal immunity will help gain further attention in the research of TB vaccine (Table 1).

A range of subunit antigens of Mtb have been tested as antimycobacterial vaccine candidates, such as the 6-kDa early secretory antigenic target (ESAT-6), 10-kDa culture

TABLE 1: Respiratory delivery of vaccine candidates against mycobacteria infection⁺.

Antigen	Delivery route and/or adjuvant	Tested species	Results or immune responses	Reference
Live rBCG	Delivered by intranasal (i.n.) route	Mice	Induce strong antibody responses	[100]
Live BCG	Delivered aerosol inhalation	Possum	Protection from *M. bovis* infection	[101, 102]
Live BCG	Delivered by i.n. route	Mice	Protection from H37Rv challenge	[103]
Live BCG	Delivered by i.n. route	Mice	Increase protective effect of BCG vaccine	[11]
Mtb cell wall MDP	Delivered by aerosol inhalation	Guinea pig	Activate alveolar macrophages	[104]
Killed BCG	Delivered in Eurocine L3 adjuvant *via* i.n. route	Mice	Induce high immune responses	[105]
ESAT-6 protein	Delivered by PLA microsphere *via* i.n. route	Mice	Induce specific immune responses	[106]
FbpA, HtpX	Intranasally delivered by an *E. coli* vector	Mice	Induce specific T-cell response and protection from Mtb challenge	[107]
Ag85A	Delivered with adenoviral and VSV vectors *via* i.n. route	Mice	Induce mucosal T-cell response	[108]
HSP65 (DNA)	Delivered by liposome *via* i.n. route	Mice	Induce strong cellular immune response	[109]
Ag85A, CFB10	Adenoviral vector *via* i.n. route	Mice	Induce specific immune response and protection from Mtb challenge	[33, 110, 111]
Ag85A	Delivered with Adenoviral and VSV vectors *via* i.n. route	Mice	Induce mucosal T-cell response	[108]
HSP65 (DNA)	Delivered by liposome *via* i.n. route	Mice	Induce strong cellular immune response	[109]
Ag85A, CFB10	Adenoviral vector *via* i.n. route	Mice	Induce specific immune response and protection from Mtb challenge	[33, 110, 111]
Ag85B, ESAT-6	Delivered by LTK63 vehicle *via* i.n. route	Mice	Increase anti-Mtb-specific CD4 T cells	[12]
Soluble mycobacterial antigens	Directly delivered by i.n. route	Mice	Restore antigen specific immune responses	[57]
ulticomponent subunits recombinant proteins of Mtb	Delivered with DDA-MPL vehicle *via* i.n. route	Mice	Induce strong antigen-specific T-cell responses	[112]
MPT51	Delivered by Lentiviral vector *via* intratracheal route	Mice	Induce MTP51-specific CD8 T cells and decrease the number of Mtb in lung following challenge	[113]

⁺MDP: muramyl dipeptide; PLA: poly(lactide); VSV: vesicular stomatitis virus.

filtrate protein (CFP-10), a 30 to 32 kDa family of three proteins (Ag85A, Ag85B, and Ag85C), MPT64, MPT83, Hsp65, and KATG of the bacilli; these subunit antigens were used either alone or in combination (Table 1). As a mucosal pathogen, a vaccine capable of efficiently inducing mucosal responses may offer a desirable protection against Mtb. Indeed, increasing evidence does suggest that vaccination via a mucosal route produce better protective effects relative to a conventional intramuscular or subcutaneous injection against mucosal infectious diseases [136]. Currently, great efforts have been devoted to improve the protective efficacy of TB vaccines. These efforts include genetical modification of BCG (rBCG), defining and producing protective subunit antigens or epitopes, and development of adjuvant, vehicles, and/or vectors for targeting mucosal surfaces, as well as delivery strategies for enhancing mucosal immunity. For instance, Ballester and coworkers recently developed a synthetic vaccine delivery platform with nanoparticles (NPs) loaded with the tuberculosis antigen Ag85B; such a formulated vaccine candidate was capable of inducing mucosal and systemic Th17 responses in mice [137]. A strategy of multistage vaccination, in which the Mtb antigens Ag85B and ESAT-6 were combined with the latency-associated protein Rv2660c, was able to control reactivation of Mtb and significantly lower the bacterial load [138].

Three criteria may be essential for determining a successful mucosal immunization strategy: effective delivery of antigen to the mucosal immune inductive site, the enhancement of mucosal immune responses by the use of mucosal immunomodulators (adjuvant), and the route of immunization [139]. It has long been recognized that most vaccines require the addition of adjuvant to enhance their immunogenicity, particularly in the mucosal immunization with soluble proteins or peptides, of which vaccination with such soluble immunogens without mucosal adjuvant may induce a state of antigen-specific immunological tolerances [140]. BCG itself is an effective adjuvant and has been used for the active immunotherapy of various cancers for many years [141]. Recently, whole cell lysate of Mtb was also used as a potent mucosal adjuvant [142]. In addition to conventional aluminum salts, oil-in-water emulsions [143], components of microbial origin (DNA motifs, lipid A, cholera enterotoxin (CT), and *Escherichia coli* heat-labile enterotoxin (LT)) [144, 145], emulsions and particles (immunostimulating complexes (ISCOMs), liposomes, PLGA, and saponins) [146, 147], Eurocine L3 [148], and cytokines are in use or under development for adjuvant and/or vaccine delivery vehicles. Notably, ISCOMs, CT, LT, Eurocine L3, and saponins are the most available mucosal adjuvants. For example, antigen encapsulated in biodegradable poly-L-lactide microspheres was capable of conferring an adjuvants effect [149], and the mucosal delivery of Mtb in microspheres enabled to induce robust cell-mediated responses in the lungs [106].

Apart from the immunogenicity and adjuvanticity, an appropriate antigen delivery route and system for vaccination is also critical for an effective immunization. Since the primary targeting site of Mtb is in respiratory mucosa, the respiratory mucosal immunization has received increasing attention recently. Mucosal vaccination via the respiratory tract such as intranasal delivery, displays many advantages over other routes including the subcutaneous immunization. The intranasal delivery approach is much easier and more flexible, and more importantly, mucosal delivery exhibited a capacity to trigger both mucosal and systemic immune responses [150]. Vaccination through an intranasal route was also superior to the subcutaneous route in the protection against pulmonary TB [151]. Additionally, it has been demonstrated that intranasal immunization of antigens with mucosal adjuvant could effectively induce the production of sIgA. The sIgA was thought to play an important role in the host's defense against mucosal pathogens including the Mtb [152, 153].

6. Concluding Remarks

Mtb is an airborne transmitted pathogen, and the immune responses, especially the mucosal immune response, play fundamental roles for the host to defend the primary and the containment of Mtb infection. Despite the fact that BCG has made a tremendous contribution to the control of Mtb infection, particularly in child population and newborns, there is not a consistent effective vaccine available for TB. Therefore, the development of novel, safer, and more effective vaccines and vaccination strategy capable of conferring a broad protection at the respiratory mucosa is required. Given the fact that more than one-third of the population is infected with Mtb, but only 10% of them develop active disease while >90% of all who contained infections remain dormant, suggests that the variability of immune responses may be attributed to the outcome of Mtb infection. There is growing evidence demonstrating that the mucosal immunity plays a central role in the host against Mtb infection; thus, a better understanding of the mucosal immunity will aid us to improve the diagnostic procedures and the development of efficient vaccines against TB. Nevertheless, there are surprising gaps in the knowledge of mucosal immunity against Mtb, which highlight the need for additional research to fully understand the mechanisms of mucosal immunity, especially mechanisms of immune evasion by Mtb and molecular pathogenesis of Mtb.

Acknowledgments

This work was supported by a Grant from the National key Basic Research Program of China (973 Program) (nos. 2012CB126301, 2012CB518801) and a Grant from the National Natural Science Foundation of China (nos. 31160515, 30960289).

References

[1] C. Dye, S. Scheele, P. Dolin, V. Pathania, and M. C. Raviglione, "Global burden of tuberculosis: estimated incidence, prevalence, and mortality by country," *Journal of the American Medical Association*, vol. 282, no. 7, pp. 677–686, 1999.

[2] M. S. Gomes, S. Paul, A. L. Moreira, R. Appelberg, M. Rabinovitch, and G. Kaplan, "Survival of Mycobacterium avium and *Mycobacterium tuberculosis* in acidified vacuoles of murine macrophages," *Infection and Immunity*, vol. 67, no. 7, pp. 3199–3206, 1999.

[3] B. B. Finlay and S. Falkow, "Common themes in microbial pathogenicity revisited," *Microbiology and Molecular Biology Reviews*, vol. 61, no. 2, pp. 136–169, 1997.

[4] S. Mukhopadhyay, S. Nair, and S. Ghosh, "Pathogenesis in tuberculosis: transcriptomic approaches to unraveling virulence mechanisms and finding new drug targets," *FEMS Microbiology Reviews*, vol. 36, no. 2, pp. 463–485, 2012.

[5] R. Hershberg, M. Lipatov, P. M. Small et al., "High functional diversity in *Mycobacterium tuberculosis* driven by genetic drift and human demography," *PLoS Biology*, vol. 6, no. 12, pp. 2658–2671, 2008.

[6] L. Ye, R. Zeng, Y. Bai, D. C. Roopenian, and X. Zhu, "Efficient mucosal vaccination mediated by the neonatal Fc receptor," *Nature Biotechnology*, vol. 29, no. 2, pp. 158–163, 2011.

[7] P. L. Ogra, H. Faden, and R. C. Welliver, "Vaccination strategies for mucosal immune responses," *Clinical Microbiology Reviews*, vol. 14, no. 2, pp. 430–445, 2001.

[8] L. Stevceva, A. G. Abimiku, and G. Franchini, "Targeting the mucosa: genetically engineered vaccines and mucosal immune responses," *Genes and Immunity*, vol. 1, no. 5, pp. 308–315, 2000.

[9] J. M. Kyd, A. R. Foxwell, and A. W. Cripps, "Mucosal immunity in the lung and upper airway," *Vaccine*, vol. 19, no. 17–19, pp. 2527–2533, 2001.

[10] N. P. Goonetilleke, H. McShane, C. M. Hannan, R. J. Anderson, R. H. Brookes, and A. V. S. Hill, "Enhanced immunogenicity and protective efficacy against *Mycobacterium tuberculosis* of bacille Calmette-Guérin vaccine using mucosal administration and boosting with a recombinant modified vaccinia virus Ankara," *The Journal of Immunology*, vol. 171, no. 3, pp. 1602–1609, 2003.

[11] L. Chen, J. Wang, A. Zganiacz, and Z. Xing, "Single intranasal mucosal *Mycobacterium bovis* BCG vaccination confers improved protection compared to subcutaneous vaccination against pulmonary tuberculosis," *Infection and Immunity*, vol. 72, no. 1, pp. 238–246, 2004.

[12] J. Dietrich, C. Andersen, R. Rappuoli, T. M. Doherty, C. G. Jensen, and P. Andersen, "Mucosal administration of Ag85B-ESAT-6 protects against infection with *Mycobacterium tuberculosis* and boosts prior bacillus Calmette-Guérin immunity," *The Journal of Immunology*, vol. 177, no. 9, pp. 6353–6360, 2006.

[13] T. H. Mogensen, "Pathogen recognition and inflammatory signaling in innate immune defenses," *Clinical Microbiology Reviews*, vol. 22, no. 2, pp. 240–273, 2009.

[14] S. I. Tamura and T. Kurata, "Defense mechanisms against influenza virus infection in the respiratory tract mucosa," *Japanese Journal of Infectious Diseases*, vol. 57, no. 6, pp. 236–247, 2004.

[15] B. S. McKenzie, J. L. Brady, and A. M. Lew, "Mucosal immunity: overcoming the barrier for induction of proximal responses," *Immunologic Research*, vol. 30, no. 1, pp. 35–71, 2004.

[16] I. W. Lugton, "Mucosa-associated lymphoid tissues as sites for uptake, carriage and excretion of tubercle bacilli and other pathogenic mycobacteria," *Immunology and Cell Biology*, vol. 77, no. 4, pp. 364–372, 1999.

[17] A. K. Mayer and A. H. Dalpke, "Regulation of local immunity by airway epithelial cells," *Archivum Immunologiae et Therapiae Experimentalis*, vol. 55, no. 6, pp. 353–362, 2007.

[18] R. Teitelbaum, W. Schubert, L. Gunther et al., "The M cell as a portal of entry to the lung for the bacterial pathogen *Mycobacterium tuberculosis*," *Immunity*, vol. 10, no. 6, pp. 641–650, 1999.

[19] Y. S. López-Boado, C. L. Wilson, L. V. Hooper, J. I. Gordon, S. J. Hultgren, and W. C. Parks, "Bacterial exposure induces and activates matrilysin in mucosal epithelial cells," *The Journal of Cell Biology*, vol. 148, no. 6, pp. 1305–1315, 2000.

[20] S. K. Linden, P. Sutton, N. G. Karlsson, V. Korolik, and M. A. McGuckin, "Mucins in the mucosal barrier to infection," *Mucosal Immunology*, vol. 1, no. 3, pp. 183–197, 2008.

[21] M. E. Selsted, S. S. L. Harwig, and T. Ganz, "Primary structures of three human neutrophil defensins," *Journal of Clinical Investigation*, vol. 76, no. 4, pp. 1436–1439, 1985.

[22] S. Sharma, I. Verma, and G. K. Khuller, "Biochemical interaction of human neutrophil peptide-1 with *Mycobacterium tuberculosis* H37Ra," *Archives of Microbiology*, vol. 171, no. 5, pp. 338–342, 1999.

[23] B. Rivas-Santiago, E. Sada, V. Tsutsumi, D. Aguilar-Léon, J. L. Contreras, and R. Hernández-Pando, "β-defensin gene expression during the course of experimental tuberculosis infection," *Journal of Infectious Diseases*, vol. 194, no. 5, pp. 697–701, 2006.

[24] B. Rivas-Santiago, S. K. Schwander, C. Sarabia et al., "Human β-defensin 2 is expressed and associated with *Mycobacterium tuberculosis* during infection of human alveolar epithelial cells," *Infection and Immunity*, vol. 73, no. 8, pp. 4505–4511, 2005.

[25] J. A. L. Flynn and J. Chan, "Immunology of tuberculosis," *Annual Review of Immunology*, vol. 19, no. 1, pp. 93–129, 2001.

[26] M. I. Gómez and A. Prince, "Airway epithelial cell signaling in response to bacterial pathogens," *Pediatric Pulmonology*, vol. 43, no. 1, pp. 11–19, 2008.

[27] A. M. Cooper and S. A. Khader, "The role of cytokines in the initiation, expansion, and control of cellular immunity to tuberculosis," *Immunological Reviews*, vol. 226, no. 1, pp. 191–204, 2008.

[28] W. Peters and J. D. Ernst, "Mechanisms of cell recruitment in the immune response to *Mycobacterium tuberculosis*," *Microbes and Infection*, vol. 5, no. 2, pp. 151–158, 2003.

[29] L. Hall-Stoodley, G. Watts, J. E. Crowther et al., "Mycobactenum tuberculosis binding to human surfactant proteins A and D, fibronectin, and small airway epithelial cells under shear conditions," *Infection and Immunity*, vol. 74, no. 6, pp. 3587–3596, 2006.

[30] Y. Li, Y. Wang, and X. Liu, "The role of airway epithelial cells in response to mycobacteria infection," *Clinical and Developmental Immunology*, vol. 2012, Article ID 791392, 11 pages, 2012.

[31] Y. López, D. Yero, G. Falero-Diaz et al., "Induction of a protective response with an IgA monoclonal antibody against *Mycobacterium tuberculosis* 16 kDa protein in a model of progressive pulmonary infection," *International Journal of Medical Microbiology*, vol. 299, no. 6, pp. 447–452, 2009.

[32] A. Williams, R. Reljic, I. Naylor et al., "Passive protection with immunoglobulin A antibodies against tuberculous early infection of the lungs," *Immunology*, vol. 111, no. 3, pp. 328–333, 2004.

[33] F. Abebe and G. Bjune, "The protective role of antibody responses during *Mycobacterium tuberculosis* infection," *Clinical and Experimental Immunology*, vol. 157, no. 2, pp. 235–243, 2009.

[34] J. Mestecky, M. W. Russell, and C. O. Elson, "Intestinal IgA: novel views on its function in the defence of the largest mucosal surface," *Gut*, vol. 44, no. 1, pp. 2–5, 1999.

[35] P. C. McNabb and T. B. Tomasi, "Host defense mechanisms at mucosal surfaces," *Annual Review of Microbiology*, vol. 35, no. 1, pp. 477–496, 1981.

[36] R. Reljic, A. Williams, and J. Ivanyi, "Mucosal immunotherapy of tuberculosis: Is there a value in passive IgA?" *Tuberculosis*, vol. 86, no. 3, pp. 179–190, 2006.

[37] M. B. Mazanec, J. G. Nedrud, C. S. Kaetzel, and M. E. Lamm, "A three-tiered view of the role of IgA in mucosal defense," *Immunology Today*, vol. 14, no. 9, pp. 430–435, 1993.

[38] R. C. Williams and R. J. Gibbons, "Inhibition of bacterial adherence by secretory immunoglobulin A: a mechanism of antigen disposal," *Science*, vol. 177, no. 4050, pp. 697–699, 1972.

[39] Y. Kurono, K. Shimamura, H. Shigemi, and G. Mogi, "Inhibition of bacterial adherence by nasopharyngeal secretions," *The Annals of Otology, Rhinology and Laryngology*, vol. 100, no. 6, pp. 455–458, 1991.

[40] M. E. Lamm, "Interaction of antigens and antibodies at mucosal surfaces," *Annual Review of Microbiology*, vol. 51, pp. 311–340, 1997.

[41] R. M. Brown, O. Cruz, M. Brennan et al., "Lipoarabinomannan-reactive human secretory immunoglobulin A responses induced by mucosal bacille Calmette-Guérin vaccination," *Journal of Infectious Diseases*, vol. 187, no. 3, pp. 513–517, 2003.

[42] B. Ten berge, M. S. Paats, I. M. Bergen et al., "Increased IL-17A expression in granulomas and in circulating memory T cells in sarcoidosis," *Rheumatology*, vol. 51, no. 1, pp. 37–46, 2012.

[43] A. Tjärnlund, A. Rodríguez, P. J. Cardona et al., "Polymeric IgR knockout mice are more susceptible to mycobacterial infections in the respiratory tract than wild-type mice," *International Immunology*, vol. 18, no. 5, pp. 807–816, 2006.

[44] W. W. Reiley, M. D. Calayag, S. T. Wittmer et al., "ESAT-6-specific CD4 T cell responses to aerosol *Mycobacterium tuberculosis* infection are initiated in the mediastinal lymph

nodes," *Proceedings of the National Academy of Sciences of the United States of America*, vol. 105, no. 31, pp. 10961–10966, 2008.

[45] A. A. Chackerian, J. M. Alt, T. V. Perera, C. C. Dascher, and S. M. Behar, "Dissemination of *Mycobacterium tuberculosis* is influenced by host factors and precedes the initiation of T-cell immunity," *Infection and Immunity*, vol. 70, no. 8, pp. 4501–4509, 2002.

[46] A. J. Wolf, L. Desvignes, B. Linas et al., "Initiation of the adaptive immune response to *Mycobacterium tuberculosis* depends on antigen production in the local lymph node, not the lungs," *The Journal of Experimental Medicine*, vol. 205, no. 1, pp. 105–115, 2008.

[47] E. L. Corbett, R. W. Steketee, F. O. Ter Kuile, A. S. Latif, A. Kamali, and R. J. Hayes, "HIV-1/AIDS and the control of other infectious diseases in Africa," *The Lancet*, vol. 359, no. 9324, pp. 2177–2187, 2002.

[48] L. A. H. van Pinxteren, J. P. Cassidy, B. H. C. Smedegaard, E. M. Agger, and P. Andersen, "Control of latent *Mycobacterium tuberculosis* infection is dependent on CD8 T cells," *European The Journal of Immunology*, vol. 30, no. 12, pp. 3689–3698, 2000.

[49] S. A. Khader, G. K. Bell, J. E. Pearl et al., "IL-23 and IL-17 in the establishment of protective pulmonary $CD4^+$ T cell responses after vaccination and during *Mycobacterium tuberculosis* challenge," *Nature Immunology*, vol. 8, no. 4, pp. 369–377, 2007.

[50] M. Santosuosso, X. Zhang, S. McCormick, J. Wang, M. Hitt, and Z. Xing, "Mechanisms of mucosal and parenteral tuberculosis vaccinations: adenoviral-based mucosal immunization preferentially elicits sustained accumulation of immune protective CD4 and CD8 T cells within the airway lumen," *The Journal of Immunology*, vol. 174, no. 12, pp. 7986–7994, 2005.

[51] A. M. Cooper, J. E. Callahan, M. Keen, J. T. Belisle, and I. M. Orme, "Expression of memory immunity in the lung following re-exposure to *Mycobacterium tuberculosis*," *Tubercle and Lung Disease*, vol. 78, no. 1, pp. 67–73, 1997.

[52] H. Park, Z. Li, X. O. Yang et al., "A distinct lineage of CD4 T cells regulates tissue inflammation by producing interleukin 17," *Nature Immunology*, vol. 6, no. 11, pp. 1133–1141, 2005.

[53] C. T. Weaver, L. E. Harrington, P. R. Mangan, M. Gavrieli, and K. M. Murphy, "Th17: an effector CD4 T cell lineage with regulatory T cell ties," *Immunity*, vol. 24, no. 6, pp. 677–688, 2006.

[54] S. J. Aujla, P. J. Dubin, and J. K. Kolls, "Th17 cells and mucosal host defense," *Seminars in Immunology*, vol. 19, no. 6, pp. 377–382, 2007.

[55] S. Sakaguchi, "Regulatory T cells: key controllers of immunologic self-tolerance," *Cell*, vol. 101, no. 5, pp. 455–458, 2000.

[56] A. B. Kamath, J. Woodworth, X. Xiong, C. Taylor, Y. Weng, and S. M. Behar, "Cytolytic $CD8^+$ T cells recognizing CFP10 are recruited to the lung after *Mycobacterium tuberculosis* infection," *The Journal of Experimental Medicine*, vol. 200, no. 11, pp. 1479–1489, 2004.

[57] M. Jeyanathan, J. Mu, K. Kugathasan et al., "Airway delivery of soluble mycobacterial antigens restores protective mucosal immunity by single intramuscular plasmid DNA tuberculosis vaccination: role of proinflammatory signals in the lung," *The Journal of Immunology*, vol. 181, no. 8, pp. 5618–5626, 2008.

[58] M. Santosuosso, S. McCormick, E. Roediger et al., "Mucosal luminal manipulation of T cell geography switches on protective efficacy by otherwise ineffective parenteral genetic immunization," *The Journal of Immunology*, vol. 178, no. 4, pp. 2387–2395, 2007.

[59] Z. Xing and B. D. Lichty, "Use of recombinant virus-vectored tuberculosis vaccines for respiratory mucosal immunization," *Tuberculosis*, vol. 86, no. 3-4, pp. 211–217, 2006.

[60] J. Mu, M. Jeyanathan, C. R. Shaler et al., "Respiratory mucosal immunization with adenovirus gene transfer vector induces helper CD4 T cell-independent protective immunity," *Journal of Gene Medicine*, vol. 12, no. 8, pp. 693–704, 2010.

[61] K. Tsukaguchi, K. N. Balaji, and W. H. Boom, "$CD4^+ \alpha\beta$ T cell and $\gamma\delta$ T cell responses to *Mycobacterium tuberculosis*: similarities and differences in Ag recognition, cytotoxic effector function, and cytokine production," *The Journal of Immunology*, vol. 154, no. 4, pp. 1786–1796, 1995.

[62] F. Dieli, M. Troye-Blomberg, J. Ivanyi et al., "Granulysin-dependent killing of intracellular and extracellular *Mycobacterium tuberculosis* by V-γ9/Vδ2 T lymphocytes," *Journal of Infectious Diseases*, vol. 184, no. 8, pp. 1082–1085, 2001.

[63] E. Lockhart, A. M. Green, and J. L. Flynn, "IL-17 production is dominated by $\gamma\delta$ T cells rather than CD4 T cells during *Mycobacterium tuberculosis* infection," *The Journal of Immunology*, vol. 177, no. 7, pp. 4662–4669, 2006.

[64] A. A. Itano and M. K. Jenkins, "Antigen presentation to naive CD4 T cells in the lymph node," *Nature Immunology*, vol. 4, no. 8, pp. 733–739, 2003.

[65] E. Giacomini, E. Iona, L. Ferroni et al., "Infection of human macrophages and dendritic cells with *Mycobacterium tuberculosis* induces a differential cytokine gene expression that modulates T cell response," *The Journal of Immunology*, vol. 166, no. 12, pp. 7033–7041, 2001.

[66] K. A. Bodnar, N. V. Serbina, and J. A. L. Flynn, "Fate of *Mycobacterium tuberculosis* within murine dendritic cells," *Infection and Immunity*, vol. 69, no. 2, pp. 800–809, 2001.

[67] M. Gonzalez-Juarrero and I. M. Orme, "Characterization of murine lung dendritic cells infected with *Mycobacterium tuberculosis*," *Infection and Immunity*, vol. 69, no. 2, pp. 1127–1133, 2001.

[68] C. von Garnier, L. Filgueira, M. Wikstrom et al., "Anatomical location determines the distribution and function of dendritic cells and other APCs in the respiratory tract," *The Journal of Immunology*, vol. 175, no. 3, pp. 1609–1618, 2005.

[69] A. C. Soloff and S. M. Barratt-Boyes, "Enemy at the gates: dendritic cells and immunity to mucosal pathogens," *Cell Research*, vol. 20, no. 8, pp. 872–885, 2010.

[70] A. J. Wolf, B. Linas, G. J. Trevejo-Nuñez et al., "*Mycobacterium tuberculosis* infects dendritic cells with high frequency and impairs their function in vivo," *The Journal of Immunology*, vol. 179, no. 4, pp. 2509–2519, 2007.

[71] I. D. Jung, S. K. Jeong, C. M. Lee et al., "Enhanced efficacy of therapeutic cancer vaccines produced by Co-treatment with *Mycobacterium tuberculosis* heparin-binding hemagglutinin, a novel TLR4 agonist," *Cancer Research*, vol. 71, no. 8, pp. 2858–2870, 2011.

[72] D. R. Heo, S. J. Shin, W. S. Kim et al., "*Mycobacterium tuberculosis* lpdC, Rv0462, induces dendritic cell maturation and Th1 polarization," *Biochemical and Biophysical Research Communications*, vol. 411, no. 3, pp. 642–647, 2011.

[73] A. Mihret, G. Mamo, M. Tafesse, A. Hailu, and S. Parida, "Dendritic cells activate and mature after infection with *Mycobacterium tuberculosis*," *BMC Research Notes*, vol. 4, article 247, 2011.

[74] R. C. M. Ryan, M. P. O'Sullivan, and J. Keane, "*Mycobacterium tuberculosis* infection induces non-apoptotic cell death

of human dendritic cells," *BMC Microbiology*, vol. 11, Article ID 237, 2011.

[75] G. A. W. Rook, J. Steele, M. Ainsworth, and B. R. Champion, "Activation of macrophages to inhibit proliferation of *Mycobacterium tuberculosis*: comparison of the effects of recombinant gamma-interferon on human monocytes and murine peritoneal macrophages," *Immunology*, vol. 59, no. 3, pp. 333–338, 1986.

[76] M. Denis, "Interferon-gamma-treated murine macrophages inhibit growth of tubercle bacilli via the generation of reactive nitrogen intermediates," *Cellular Immunology*, vol. 132, no. 1, pp. 150–157, 1991.

[77] J. Chan, Y. Xing, R. S. Magliozzo, and B. R. Bloom, "Killing of virulent *Mycobacterium tuberculosis* by reactive nitrogen intermediates produced by activated murine macrophages," *The Journal of Experimental Medicine*, vol. 175, no. 4, pp. 1111–1122, 1992.

[78] J. L. Flynn, "Immunology of tuberculosis and implications in vaccine development," *Tuberculosis*, vol. 84, no. 1, pp. 93–101, 2004.

[79] M. Divangahi, M. Chen, H. Gan et al., "*Mycobacterium tuberculosis* evades macrophage defenses by inhibiting plasma membrane repair," *Nature Immunology*, vol. 10, no. 8, pp. 899–906, 2009.

[80] L. S. Meena and T. Rajni, "Survival mechanisms of pathogenic *Mycobacterium tuberculosis* H 37Rv," *FEBS Journal*, vol. 277, no. 11, pp. 2416–2427, 2010.

[81] L. Zhang, H. Zhang, Y. Zhao et al., "Effects of *Mycobacterium tuberculosis* ESAT-6/CFP-10 fusion protein on the autophagy function of mouse macrophages," *DNA and Cell Biology*, vol. 31, no. 2, pp. 171–179, 2012.

[82] E. K. Jo, "Innate immunity to mycobacteria: vitamin D and autophagy," *Cellular Microbiology*, vol. 12, no. 8, pp. 1026–1035, 2010.

[83] C. L. Birmingham, A. C. Smith, M. A. Bakowski, T. Yoshimori, and J. H. Brumell, "Autophagy controls Salmonella infection in response to damage to the Salmonella-containing vacuole," *Journal of Biological Chemistry*, vol. 281, no. 16, pp. 11374–11383, 2006.

[84] V. Deretic, M. Delgado, I. Vergne et al., "Autophagy in immunity against *Mycobacterium tuberculosis*: a model system to dissect immunological roles of autophagy," *Current Topics in Microbiology and Immunology*, vol. 335, no. 1, pp. 169–188, 2009.

[85] S. J. Cherra III, S. M. Kulich, G. Uechi et al., "Regulation of the autophagy protein LC3 by phosphorylation," *The Journal of Cell Biology*, vol. 190, no. 4, pp. 533–539, 2010.

[86] J. W. Moulder, "Comparative biology of intracellular parasitism," *Microbiological Reviews*, vol. 49, no. 3, pp. 298–337, 1985.

[87] D. G. Russell, "*Mycobacterium tuberculosis*: here today, and here tomorrow," *Nature Reviews Molecular Cell Biology*, vol. 2, no. 8, pp. 569–586, 2001.

[88] V. Deretic, S. Singh, S. Master et al., "*Mycobacterium tuberculosis* inhibition of phagolysosome biogenesis and autophagy as a host defence mechanism," *Cellular Microbiology*, vol. 8, no. 5, pp. 719–727, 2006.

[89] M. G. Gutierrez, S. S. Master, S. B. Singh, G. A. Taylor, M. I. Colombo, and V. Deretic, "Autophagy is a defense mechanism inhibiting BCG and *Mycobacterium tuberculosis* survival in infected macrophages," *Cell*, vol. 119, no. 6, pp. 753–766, 2004.

[90] S. J. Szabo, B. M. Sullivan, C. Sternmann, A. R. Satoskar, B. P. Sleckman, and L. H. Glimcher, "Distinct effects of T-bet in Th1 lineage commitment and IFN-γ production in CD4 and CD8 T cells," *Science*, vol. 295, no. 5553, pp. 338–342, 2002.

[91] M. Sharma, S. Sharma, S. Roy, S. Varma, and M. Bose, "Pulmonary epithelial cells are a source of interferon-γ in response to *Mycobacterium tuberculosis* infection," *Immunology and Cell Biology*, vol. 85, no. 3, pp. 229–237, 2007.

[92] A. M. Cooper, D. K. Dalton, T. A. Stewart, J. P. Griffin, D. G. Russell, and I. M. Orme, "Disseminated tuberculosis in interferon γ gene-disrupted mice," *The Journal of Experimental Medicine*, vol. 178, no. 6, pp. 2243–2247, 1993.

[93] D. Wang, J. Xu, Y. Feng et al., "Liposomal oral DNA vaccine (mycobacterium DNA) elicits immune response," *Vaccine*, vol. 28, no. 18, pp. 3134–3142, 2010.

[94] C. A. Scanga, V. P. Mohan, H. Joseph, K. Yu, J. Chan, and J. L. Flynn, "Reactivation of latent tuberculosis: variations on the cornell murine model," *Infection and Immunity*, vol. 67, no. 9, pp. 4531–4538, 1999.

[95] T. H. M. Ottenhoff, D. Kumararatne, and J. L. Casanova, "Novel human immunodeficiencies reveal the essential role of type-I cytokines in immunity to intracellular bacteria," *Immunology Today*, vol. 19, no. 11, pp. 491–494, 1998.

[96] E. Jouanguy, F. Altare, S. Lamhamedi et al., "Interferon-γ-receptor deficiency in an infant with fatal bacille Calmette-Guérin infection," *New England Journal of Medicine*, vol. 335, no. 26, pp. 1956–1961, 1996.

[97] D. K. Dalton, S. Pitts-Meek, S. Keshav, I. S. Figari, A. Bradley, and T. A. Stewart, "Multiple defects of immune cell function in mice with disrupted interferon-γ genes," *Science*, vol. 259, no. 5102, pp. 1739–1742, 1993.

[98] W. H. Boom, D. H. Canaday, S. A. Fulton, A. J. Gehring, R. E. Rojas, and M. Torres, "Human immunity to *M. tuberculosis*: T cell subsets and antigen processing," *Tuberculosis*, vol. 83, no. 1, pp. 98–106, 2003.

[99] N. Altet-Gómez, M. de Souza-Galvao, I. Latorre et al., "Diagnosing TB infection in children: analysis of discordances using in vitro tests and the tuberculin skin test," *European Respiratory Journal*, vol. 37, no. 5, pp. 1166–1174, 2011.

[100] L. Kremer, L. Dupré, G. Riveau, A. Capron, and C. Locht, "Systemic and mucosal immune responses after intranasal administration of recombinant *Mycobacterium bovis* bacillus Calmette-Guerin expressing glutathione S-transferase from Schistosoma haematobium," *Infection and Immunity*, vol. 66, no. 12, pp. 5669–5676, 1998.

[101] L. A. L. Corner, B. M. Buddle, D. U. Pfeiffer, and R. S. Morris, "Aerosol vaccination of the brushtail possum (Trichosurus vulpecula) with bacille Calmette-Guérin: the duration of protection," *Veterinary Microbiology*, vol. 81, no. 2, pp. 181–191, 2001.

[102] F. E. Aldwell, D. L. Keen, V. C. Stent et al., "Route of BCG administration in possums affects protection against bovine tuberculosis," *New Zealand Veterinary Journal*, vol. 43, no. 7, pp. 356–359, 1995.

[103] G. Falero-Diaz, S. Challacombe, D. Banerjee, G. Douce, A. Boyd, and J. Ivanyi, "Intranasal vaccination of mice against infection with *Mycobacterium tuberculosis*," *Vaccine*, vol. 18, no. 28, pp. 3223–3229, 2000.

[104] R. J. Pettis, I. Hall, D. Costa, and A. J. Hickey, "Aerosol delivery of muramyl dipeptide to rodent lungs," *The American Association of Pharmaceutical Scientists*, vol. 2, no. 3, p. E25, 2000.

[105] M. Haile, U. Schröder, B. Hamasur et al., "Immunization with heat-killed *Mycobacterium bovis* bacille Calmette-Guerin (BCG) in Eurocine L3 adjuvant protects against tuberculosis," *Vaccine*, vol. 22, no. 11-12, pp. 1498–1508, 2004.

[106] Z. K. Carpenter, E. D. Williamson, and J. E. Eyles, "Mucosal delivery of microparticle encapsulated ESAT-6 induces robust cell-mediated responses in the lung milieu," *Journal of Controlled Release*, vol. 104, no. 1, pp. 67–77, 2005.

[107] P. Brun, A. Zumbo, I. Castagliuolo et al., "Intranasal delivery of DNA encoding antigens of *Mycobacterium tuberculosis* by non-pathogenic invasive *Escherichia coli*," *Vaccine*, vol. 26, no. 16, pp. 1934–1941, 2008.

[108] E. K. Roediger, K. Kugathasan, X. Zhang, B. D. Lichty, and Z. Xing, "Heterologous boosting of recombinant adenoviral prime immunization with a novel vesicular stomatitis virus-vectored tuberculosis vaccine," *Molecular Therapy*, vol. 16, no. 6, pp. 1161–1169, 2008.

[109] R. S. Rosada, L. G. de la Torre, F. G. Frantz et al., "Protection against tuberculosis by a single intranasal administration of DNA-hsp65 vaccine complexed with cationic liposomes," *BMC Immunology*, vol. 9, no. 1, article 38, 2008.

[110] J. Wang, L. Thorson, R. W. Stokes et al., "Single mucosal, but not parenteral, immunization with recombinant adenoviral-based vaccine provides potent protection from pulmonary tuberculosis," *The Journal of Immunology*, vol. 173, no. 10, pp. 6357–6365, 2004.

[111] E. O. Ronan, L. N. Lee, P. C. L. Beverley, and E. Z. Tchilian, "Immunization of mice with a recombinant adenovirus vaccine inhibits the early growth of *Mycobacterium tuberculosis* after infection," *PLoS One*, vol. 4, no..12, Article ID e8235, 2009.

[112] S. B. Sable, M. Cheruvu, S. Nandakumar et al., "Cellular immune responses to nine *Mycobacterium tuberculosis* vaccine candidates following intranasal vaccination," *PLoS One*, vol. 6, no. 7, Article ID e22718, 2011.

[113] D. Hashimoto, T. Nagata, M. Uchijima et al., "Intratracheal administration of third-generation lentivirus vector encoding MPT51 from *Mycobacterium tuberculosis* induces specific $CD8^+$ T-cell responses in the lung," *Vaccine*, vol. 26, no. 40, pp. 5095–5100, 2008.

[114] A. G. D. Bean, D. R. Roach, H. Briscoe et al., "Structural deficiencies in granuloma formation in TNF gene-targeted mice underlie the heightened susceptibility to aerosol *Mycobacterium tuberculosis* infection, which is not compensated for by lymphotoxin," *The Journal of Immunology*, vol. 162, no. 6, pp. 3504–3511, 1999.

[115] J. L. Flynn, M. M. Goldstein, K. J. Triebold, J. Sypek, S. Wolf, and B. R. Bloom, "IL-12 increases resistance of BALB/c mice to *Mycobacterium tuberculosis* infection," *The Journal of Immunology*, vol. 155, no. 5, pp. 2515–2524, 1995.

[116] O. C. Turner, R. J. Basaraba, A. A. Frank et al., "Granuloma formation in mouse and guinea pig models of experimental tuberculosis," in *Granulomatous Infections and Inflammations: Cellular and Molecular Mechanisms*, pp. 65–84, ASM Press, Washington, DC, USA, 2003.

[117] B. M. Saunders and A. M. Cooper, "Restraining mycobacteria: role of granulomas in mycobacterial infections," *Immunology and Cell Biology*, vol. 78, no. 4, pp. 334–341, 2000.

[118] S. Guo, R. Xue, Y. Li et al., "The CFP10/ESAT6 complex of *Mycobacterium tuberculosis* may function as a regulator of macrophage cell death at different stages of tuberculosis infection," *Medical Hypotheses*, vol. 78, no. 3, pp. 389–392, 2012.

[119] J. Keane, M. K. Balcewicz-Sablinska, H. G. Remold et al., "Infection by *Mycobacterium tuberculosis* promotes human alveolar macrophage apoptosis," *Infection and Immunity*, vol. 65, no. 1, pp. 298–304, 1997.

[120] J. M. Tramontana, U. Utaipat, A. Molloy et al., "Thalidomide treatment reduces tumor necrosis factor alpha production and enhances weight gain in patients with pulmonary tuberculosis," *Molecular Medicine*, vol. 1, no. 4, pp. 384–397, 1995.

[121] L. G. Bekker, A. L. Moreira, A. Bergtold, S. Freeman, B. Ryffel, and G. Kaplan, "Immunopathologic effects of tumor necrosis factor alpha in murine mycobacterial infection are dose dependent," *Infection and Immunity*, vol. 68, no. 12, pp. 6954–6961, 2000.

[122] G. Trinchieri, "Interleukin-12: a proinflammatory cytokine with immunoregulatory functions that bridge innate resistance and antigen-specific adaptive immunity," *Annual Review of Immunology*, vol. 13, pp. 251–276, 1995.

[123] A. M. Cooper, A. D. Roberts, E. R. Rhoades, J. E. Callahan, D. M. Getzy, and I. M. Orme, "The role of interleukin-12 in acquired immunity to *Mycobacterium tuberculosis* infection," *Immunology*, vol. 84, no. 3, pp. 423–432, 1995.

[124] D. Nolt and J. A. L. Flynn, "Interleukin-12 therapy reduces the number of immune cells and pathology in lungs of mice infected with *Mycobacterium tuberculosis*," *Infection and Immunity*, vol. 72, no. 5, pp. 2976–2988, 2004.

[125] C. Demangel and W. J. Britton, "Interaction of dendritic cells with mycobacteria: where the action starts," *Immunology and Cell Biology*, vol. 78, no. 4, pp. 318–324, 2000.

[126] Y. Shi, C. H. Liu, A. I. Roberts et al., "Granulocyte-macrophage colony-stimulating factor (GM-CSF) and T-cell responses: What we do and don't know," *Cell Research*, vol. 16, no. 2, pp. 126–133, 2006.

[127] A. A. Ryan, T. M. Wozniak, E. Shklovskaya et al., "Improved protection against disseminated tuberculosis by *Mycobacterium bovis* bacillus Calmette-Guérin secreting murine GM-CSF is associated with expansion and activation of APCs," *The Journal of Immunology*, vol. 179, no. 12, pp. 8418–8424, 2007.

[128] M. Gonzalez-Juarrero, J. M. Hattle, A. Izzo et al., "Disruption of granulocyte macrophage-colony stimulating factor production in the lungs severely affects the ability of mice to control *Mycobacterium tuberculosis* infection," *Journal of Leukocyte Biology*, vol. 77, no. 6, pp. 914–922, 2005.

[129] S. Yuan, C. Shi, W. Han, R. Ling, N. Li, and T. Wang, "Effective anti-tumor responses induced by recombinant bacillus Calmette-Guérin vaccines based on different tandem repeats of MUC1 and GM-CSF," *European Journal of Cancer Prevention*, vol. 18, no. 5, pp. 416–423, 2009.

[130] A. C. Maue, W. R. Waters, M. V. Palmer et al., "An ESAT-6:CFP10 DNA vaccine administered in conjunction with *Mycobacterium bovis* BCG confers protection to cattle challenged with virulent M. bovis," *Vaccine*, vol. 25, no. 24, pp. 4735–4746, 2007.

[131] A. A. Al-Hassan and A. M. Ahsanullah, "Bacillus Calmette-Guerins vaccination at birth causing tuberculous ranulomatous lymphadenitis," *Saudi Medical Journal*, vol. 32, no. 4, pp. 412–414, 2011.

[132] J. J. Nuttall, M. A. Davies, G. D. Hussey, and B. S. Eley, "Bacillus Calmette-Guérin (BCG) vaccine-induced complications in children treated with highly active antiretroviral therapy," *International Journal of Infectious Diseases*, vol. 12, no. 6, pp. e99–e105, 2008.

[133] T. Bolger, M. O'Connell, A. Menon, and K. Butler, "Complications associated with the bacille Calmette-Guérin vaccination in Ireland," *Archives of Disease in Childhood*, vol. 91, no. 7, pp. 594–597, 2006.

[134] P. E. M. Fine, "BCG: the challenge continues," *Scandinavian Journal of Infectious Diseases*, vol. 33, no. 4, pp. 243–245, 2001.

[135] G. Källenius, A. Pawlowski, P. Brandtzaeg, and S. Svenson, "Should a new tuberculosis vaccine be administered intranasally?" *Tuberculosis*, vol. 87, no. 4, pp. 257–266, 2007.

[136] J. McGhee, C. Czerkinsky, and J. Mestecky, "Mucosal vaccines: an overview," *Mucosal Immunology*, vol. 2, pp. 741–757, 1999.

[137] M. Ballester, C. Nembrini, N. Dhar et al., "Nanoparticle conjugation and pulmonary delivery enhance the protective efficacy of Ag85B and CpG against tuberculosis," *Vaccine*, vol. 29, no. 40, pp. 6959–6966, 2011.

[138] C. Aagaard, T. Hoang, J. Dietrich et al., "A multistage tuberculosis vaccine that confers efficient protection before and after exposure," *Nature Medicine*, vol. 17, no. 2, pp. 189–195, 2011.

[139] A. W. Cripps, J. M. Kyd, and A. R. Foxwell, "Vaccines and mucosal immunisation," *Vaccine*, vol. 19, no. 17–19, pp. 2513–2515, 2001.

[140] P. K. Giri and G. K. Khuller, "Is intranasal vaccination a feasible solution for tuberculosis?" *Expert Review of Vaccines*, vol. 7, no. 9, pp. 1341–1356, 2008.

[141] R. Reid, V. DeVita, S. Hellman, and S. A. Rosenberg, "Biologic therapy of cancer," *Histopathology*, vol. 20, no. 3, p. 278, 1992.

[142] V. Dwivedi, C. Manickam, R. Patterson et al., "Cross-protective immunity to porcine reproductive and respiratory syndrome virus by intranasal delivery of a live virus vaccine with a potent adjuvant," *Vaccine*, vol. 29, no. 23, pp. 4058–4066, 2011.

[143] M. L. Mbow, E. de Gregorio, N. M. Valiante, and R. Rappuoli, "New adjuvants for human vaccines," *Current Opinion in Immunology*, vol. 22, no. 3, pp. 411–416, 2010.

[144] T. Shimizu, K. Sasaki, M. Kato et al., "Induction of thymus-derived $\gamma\delta$ T cells by Escherichia coli enterotoxin B subunit in peritoneal cavities of mice," *Clinical and Diagnostic Laboratory Immunology*, vol. 12, no. 1, pp. 157–164, 2005.

[145] N. Lycke, T. Tsuji, and J. Holmgren, "The adjuvant effect of Vibrio cholerae and *Escherichia coli* heat-labile enterotoxins is linked to their ADP-ribosyltransferase activity," *European Journal of Immunology*, vol. 22, no. 9, pp. 2277–2281, 1992.

[146] A. Helgeby, N. C. Robson, A. M. Donachie et al., "The combined CTA1-DD/ISCOM adjuvant vector promotes priming of mucosal and systemic immunity to incorporated antigens by specific targeting of B cells," *The Journal of Immunology*, vol. 176, no. 6, pp. 3697–3706, 2006.

[147] C. R. Kensil, "Saponins as vaccine adjuvants," *Critical Reviews in Therapeutic Drug Carrier Systems*, vol. 13, no. 1-2, pp. 1–55, 1996.

[148] B. Hamasur, M. Haile, A. Pawlowski et al., "*Mycobacterium tuberculosis* arabinomannan-protein conjugates protect against tuberculosis," *Vaccine*, vol. 21, no. 25-26, pp. 4081–4093, 2003.

[149] J. E. Eyles, V. W. Bramwell, E. D. Williamson, and H. O. Alpar, "Microsphere translocation and immunopotentiation in systemic tissues following intranasal administration," *Vaccine*, vol. 19, no. 32, pp. 4732–4742, 2001.

[150] S. S. Davis, "Nasal vaccines," *Advanced Drug Delivery Reviews*, vol. 51, no. 1–3, pp. 21–42, 2001.

[151] P. K. Giri, S. B. Sable, I. Verma, and G. K. Khuller, "Comparative evaluation of intranasal and subcutaneous route of immunization for development of mucosal vaccine against experimental tuberculosis," *FEMS Immunology and Medical Microbiology*, vol. 45, no. 1, pp. 87–93, 2005.

[152] Y. Kurono, M. Yamamoto, K. Fujihashi et al., "Nasal immunization induces Haemophilus influenzae-specific Th1 and Th2 responses with mucosal IgA and systemic IgG antibodies for protective immunity," *Journal of Infectious Diseases*, vol. 180, no. 1, pp. 122–132, 1999.

[153] L. de Haan, W. R. Verweij, M. Holtrop et al., "Nasal or intramuscular immunization of mice with influenza subunit antigen and the B subunit of *Escherichia coli* heat-labile toxin induces IgA- or IgG-mediated protective mucosal immunity," *Vaccine*, vol. 19, no. 20–22, pp. 2898–2907, 2001.

33

Health Seeking Behaviour and Associated Factors among Pulmonary Tuberculosis Suspects in Lay Armachiho District, Northwest Ethiopia: A Community-Based Study

Eshetu Haileselassie Engeda,[1] Berihun Assefa Dachew,[2] Hiwot Kassa Woreta,[1] Mengistu Mekonnen Kelkay,[1] and Tesfaye Demeke Ashenafie[1]

[1]*Department of Nursing, College of Medicine and Health Sciences, University of Gondar, P.O. Box 196, Gondar, Ethiopia*
[2]*Department of Epidemiology and Biostatistics, Institute of Public Health, College of Medicine and Health Sciences, University of Gondar, P.O. Box 196, Gondar, Ethiopia*

Correspondence should be addressed to Eshetu Haileselassie Engeda; eshet143@gmail.com

Academic Editor: Isamu Sugawara

Studies in the northern part of Ethiopia showed high prevalence of undiagnosed cluster of tuberculosis cases within the community which demanded an investigation of the health care seeking behaviour of tuberculosis suspects. A community-based cross-sectional study was conducted in Lay Armachiho district, Northwest Ethiopia. Individuals who had cough for at least two weeks and aged greater than or equal to 15 years were included in the study. Data were collected by interview using pretested and structured questionnaire. Logistic regression was computed and adjusted odds ratio with 95% confidence interval was calculated. Out of the total population surveyed (29, 735), 663 (2.2%) individuals were found to be pulmonary tuberculosis suspects. Majority of the suspects reported that they had visited a modern health care facility. Those aged 15 to 34 and aged 35–54 had secondary educational level and above; those who were civil servants, those who were farmers, those who had previous history of tuberculosis treatment, and those who perceived that they were sick were more likely to visit a modern health care facility. The proportion of respondents who had taken traditional measures was found to be higher than some other districts. Improving the socioeconomic status of the community is recommended.

1. Background

According to the 2015 World Health Organization (WHO) global tuberculosis (TB) report, TB remains a major global health problem that killed 1.5 million people in 2014 alone. This report also showed that an estimated number of 9.6 million new tuberculosis cases are diagnosed in the same year [1].

Evidences showed that over 81% of TB related morbidity and mortality occurred in developing countries [2]. This enormous burden of TB was mainly because of high prevalence of human immune deficiency virus infection [3], emergence of multidrug resistant (MDR) TB, social inequalities, ineffective TB control efforts, and low TB case detection rates [2, 4]. Moreover, many studies indicated that reservoirs for the extensive transmission of TB found predominantly in the community are being undiagnosed [2, 4, 5].

In Ethiopia, TB is the major cause of hospital admission and mortality [6]. The country stands 7th among the 22 high TB burden countries and grouped among the 27 high MDR tuberculosis burden countries [1]. The estimated annual incidence and prevalence of TB in Ethiopia is 258 and 237 per 100,000 population, respectively [6]. A TB trend analysis study also indicated that the incidence rate of TB in Ethiopia was increasing at a rate of 5 new TB cases per 100,000 population per year [7].

Ethiopia adopted the internationally recommended TB control strategy, the Directly Observed Treatment Short (DOTS) course, by early 1900s. The major components of this strategy included case detection by sputum smear microscopy and standardized treatment with supervision [6]. However, despite the early introduction of such an important strategy, a recent national report showed a TB case detection rate of 58.9% which is below the national target of detecting 82.7% of infectious TB cases [8]. Low TB case detection rate may be related to individual or organizational factors. That is to say, either the patients fail to seek health care or the health care system fails to address TB case detection particularly at the community level [9]. In one or another way, this usually ends up with a delay in diagnosis of TB patients.

Health seeking behaviour is defined as any action taken by the individual TB suspect to get relief from his/her presenting symptoms [10]. This action may include any form of traditional illness management including self-treatments by taking or applying local remedies, visit to traditional healers, "Holy Water," local injectors, and/or buying medications from drug stores without prescription. On the other hand, people with TB symptoms may visit government or private modern health care facilities to get prescribed treatment [9, 10].

The health care seeking behaviour of TB suspects varies from country to country. In Ukraine, for instance, 88% of the respondents reported that they visited polyclinic or hospital as a primary choice [11]. In Northern India, 87% of the study participants reported that they had taken some kind of self-initiated action such as home remedies [10]. In another Indian study, 72% of respondents reported that they had consulted nonprofessional private healer [12]. In Vietnam, TB case suspects visits to pharmacy and private practitioner were the initial actions for alleviating TB symptoms [5]. In Gambia, majority of people from the study population seek help from modern health institutions early [13]. Respondents from Uganda reported that they used self-treatment as a primary choice and visited health institutions when they became bedridden in most cases [14]. A study done in Ethiopia demonstrated that 60% of the respondents visited modern health institutions while 22% and 18% of the respondents sought traditional healers and took no action, respectively [9].

There are several factors which can affect the health seeking behaviour of TB suspects. According to the literature, health seeking behaviour is a dynamic process which is influenced by cultural, religious, sociodemographic, environmental, political, and other issues [9]. These factors shape the behaviour of individual patients by influencing their perception about symptoms. Moreover, their decision on the choice of a particular health care action is largely influenced by those factors [15].

In relation to the health seeking behaviour of TB suspects, a considerable degree of diagnosis and treatment delay had been observed in some studies. For instance, the median time between the start of symptoms and first visit to health care provider in Ukraine and Ethiopian studies was 30 days [9, 11]. A delay in visiting modern health care facilities results in a delay in detecting infectious tuberculosis [16]. This in turn results in a more complicated disease process, increased patient suffering, extensive transmission of the infection within the community, and higher risk of TB associated mortality [17].

Various strategies had been tried in the past to bring the health seeking behaviour of TB suspects on the right track and to overcome diagnostic delays. Among these, public health education, identifying target groups for health education, and targeting vulnerable and difficult to reach groups were the major ones [5, 10, 11].

In Ethiopia a significant number of facility-based studies had been conducted on the health seeking behaviour of newly diagnosed TB patients. However, community-based studies are rarely available at national level in general and no information is found at the current study area in particular. Nevertheless, the health seeking behaviour of TB suspects who preferred to stay within the community may be different as compared to those who visited modern health care facilities. Therefore, this study will be immensely important to describe the level of modern health care seeking practice in the rural community and factors associated with it.

2. Materials and Methods

A community-based cross-sectional study was conducted from January 17 to February 24, 2014, in the rural kebeles (the lowest administrative units) of Lay Armachiho district. The district is found in North Gondar administrative zone, Amhara Regional State, 768 km far from Addis Ababa to the Northwest of Ethiopia. The total population of the district was estimated to be 175,114. Within the district there are 33 rural kebeles and one urban kebele. With regard to health facilities, there were 34 health posts (one per each kebele) and 7 health centres. According to the health care delivery system of Ethiopia, health posts are the lowest units and do not have sputum diagnostic facility for tuberculosis. On the other hand a health centre, serving as a referral centre for five satellite health posts in its catchment area, is supposed to have a sputum diagnostic facility for pulmonary tuberculosis. However, only two out of the seven health centres had sputum diagnostic facility during the study period.

All individuals aged above 15 who had experienced cough for two or more weeks during the time of the survey were included in the study.

The outcome variable of this study is "modern heath care facility visit." The independent variables include sociodemographic characteristics (age, sex, religion, marital status, occupation, and educational level) and illness related factors (history of hemoptysis, previous history of TB treatment, and perceived health status).

Sample size was determined by using single population proportion formula by considering the following assumptions: 95% confidence interval (CI), 0.22% proportion (prevalence of TB in rural Northern Ethiopia [18]), 0.1% margin of error, a design effect of 2, and a 10% nonresponse rate, and the minimum sample size was 18,553 individuals.

Cluster sampling technique was utilized in this study. From the 33 rural kebeles (clusters) under the administration of Lay Armachiho district, 9 kebeles (27.3%) were selected by simple random sampling. Then all individuals (within the target age group) found within the randomly selected nine kebeles were surveyed house to house.

Data were collected by pretested and structured Amharic version questionnaire (Amharic is the local language of the district spoken by all people in the study kebeles) using interview technique. Eighteen health extension workers and nine BSc nurses were recruited for data collection and supervision, respectively. Before data collection, two data collectors were assigned to each kebele. Then each data collector conducted a house-to-house survey among the randomly selected households. During the survey, the head of the household was asked about whether or not any family member had cough for a duration more than or equal to two weeks. When such a case was found, the data collectors interviewed suspects using the questionnaire about TB symptoms, sociodemographic variables, and the different health care actions taken. Repeat visits were conducted for those individuals who were not available during the first visit. At each data collection spot, sufficient explanation about the aim of the research was given to the study participants before the interview.

The quality of data was assured by applying the following methods. First, the questionnaires were carefully designed based on the literature. Second, pretest was conducted at one of the rural kebeles of the nearby district equivalent to 5% of the sample size. Third, appropriate modifications were made on the questionnaires after viewing the pretest result. Fourth, a two-day training was given for data collectors and supervisors just before the actual data collection time. Every day after data collection, questionnaires were reviewed and checked for completeness, accuracy, and clarity by the supervisors and principal investigator and the necessary feedback was offered to data collectors in the next morning.

The collected data were coded, entered into Epi Info 7, and exported to SPSS version 20 software for analysis. Descriptive statistics was used to illustrate the means, standard deviations, medians, and frequencies of the study variables. Bivariate analysis was computed and those variables whose P values were less than or equal to 0.2 were fitted into backward multivariate logistic regression model. Odds ratios with 95% confidence interval were used to determine the strength of association between dependent and independent variables. P values less than or equal to 0.05 were considered statistically significant.

In this study, when respondents reported that they visited a health post, a health centre, a private clinic, or a hospital, it had been taken as they visited a modern health care facility. On the contrary, when they reported that they had taken actions such as self-treatment with home remedies, bought medicines without prescription, took traditional medicine (herbs), went to "Holy Water," and took no action, it was considered as if they had taken traditional measures.

Ethical clearance was obtained from institutional ethical review board of College of Medicine and Health Sciences, University of Gondar. Moreover, letter of support was secured from the woreda health office and each kebele administration. In addition to that, following an explanation of the purpose, the benefits, and the possible risks of the study, consent was obtained from all study subjects who assured that participation was on voluntarily basis. On top of that, to keep the anonymity of study participants, code numbers rather than personal identifiers were used and all questionnaires were sealed with post following data collection at each kebele every day. When TB suspects were identified during the survey, they were counseled in order to go to the nearby health centre (for those health centres which have sputum examination facility) or hospital for sputum examination. Finally, the questionnaires were kept locked all the time except during data entry.

3. Results

3.1. Sample Characteristics and Prevalence of PTBC Suspects. A total of 29,735 illegible individuals participated in the study of whom the majority were male, 15,833 (53.2%). Out of those study participants, 663 (2.2%) individuals were fund to be pulmonary tuberculosis suspects. The prevalence of PTBC suspects among male and female participants was 1.3 and 3.3, respectively. The median age (IQR) of PTBC suspects was 37 (32–45 years). Majority of PTBC suspects were females (68.8%), married (71.9%), and Orthodox Christian followers (74.1%). Approximately 58% of PTBC suspects attended elementary school education and 48% of them were unemployed (Table 1).

3.2. Duration of Cough and Past History of TB Treatment. In this study, the median duration of cough (IQR) was 3 weeks (2–4 weeks). Four hundred ninety-nine (75.3%), 125 (18.9%), 17 (2.6%), and 22 (3.3%) of PTBC suspects had a cough that lasted 1–4 weeks, 2–5 weeks, 9–12 weeks, and greater than 12 weeks, respectively. One hundred fifty-two (22.9%) of the PTBC suspects had previous history of TB treatment.

3.3. Perception of Illness. Among the total PTBC suspects who had been asked about perception of their symptoms, 177 (26.7%) perceived their symptom as common cold. One hundred sixty-four (24.7%) reported that their symptoms were due to "bird" or "Nefas," a common local description of an illness believed to be resulting from exposure to cold weather or wind. Similarly, 130 (19.6%) of the PTBC suspects reported that their symptoms were due to "mitch" or "gerefta," another local description of illness given to an illness similar to pneumonia (usually treated traditionally by hot steam in which leaves will be boiled in water and the patient will inhale the steam). One hundred thirty-nine (21%), 30 (4.5%), and 15 (2.3%) of the respondents perceived that their symptoms were because of pneumonia, asthma, and pulmonary tuberculosis, respectively, whereas 8 (1.2%) reported that they had no disease.

3.4. Health Care Seeking Behaviour. All respondents were asked about the first action they had taken to alleviate their symptoms. The majority of PTBC suspects (60.9%) visited modern health care facilities first whereas the rest of PTBC suspects took some other kind of individual action which included but not limited to home treatment and traditional medicine (Table 2). The median time (IQR) elapsed to take first action after the onset of symptoms was 13 days (10–17).

TABLE 1: Sociodemographic characteristics of pulmonary tuberculosis suspects in Lay Armachiho district, Northwest Ethiopia, 2014.

Characteristics	Number	Percent ($n = 663$)
Age		
15–34	183	27.6
35–54	375	53.8
55 and above	123	18.6
Sex		
Male	207	31.2
Female	456	68.8
Marital status		
Unmarried[a]	186	28.1
Married	477	71.9
Religion		
Orthodox Christian	491	74.1
Muslim	107	16.1
Protestant	65	9.8
Educational level		
Illiterate	193	29.1
Elementary	382	57.6
Secondary and above	88	13.3
Occupation		
Unemployed[b]	318	48
Farmer	300	45.2
Civil servant	45	6.8

[a]Unmarried includes single (never married), widowed, separated, and divorced.
[b]Unemployed includes those who have no job and students.

TABLE 2: First action taken by pulmonary tuberculosis suspects in Lay Armachiho district, Northwest Ethiopia, 2014 ($n = 663$).

Action taken	Number	Percent
Visited health post	152	22.9
Visited health centre	190	28.7
Visited hospital	16	2.4
Visited private clinic	46	6.9
Self-treatment with safe home remedies (tea, honey, etc.)	53	8
Bought drugs without prescription	7	1.1
Taken traditional medicine (herbs)	70	10.6
Went to "Holy Water"	92	13.9
No action taken	37	5.6
Total	663	100

3.5. Bivariate and Multivariate Findings: Factors Associated with Health Care Seeking Behaviour. In the bivariate analysis, age (those younger than 55 years), occupation (farmers and civil servants), having history of hemoptysis, perceived health status (perceived wellness), and having previous history of TB treatment showed statistical significance with visiting modern health care facility. However, in the multivariate model, age (15–34 years and 35–54 years), educational level (secondary and above), occupation (farmers and civil servants), perceived health status (perceived wellness), and having previous history of TB treatment are yielded as factors associated with visiting modern health care facility among PTBC suspects.

Age was significantly associated with visiting modern health care facility. Pulmonary tuberculosis suspects aged 15 to 34 and aged 35–54 were more likely to visit a modern health care facility than PTBC suspects aged 55 and above (AOR (95% CI) 4.59 (2.71–7.76) and 2.45 (1.54–3.88), resp.). The other significant factor was level of education with respondents who had secondary educational level and above and were more likely to visit a modern health care facility than those who were illiterate (AOR (95% CI) 2.61 (1.35–5.04)). Occupation was also among the significant factors as PTBC suspects who were civil servants or farmers were more likely to report that they visited a modern health care facility than PTBC suspects who were unemployed (AOR (95% CI) 3.02 (1.26–5.58) and 1.43 (1.01–2.05), resp.). History of TB treatment was also significantly associated with visiting a modern health care facility. Pulmonary tuberculosis suspects who had previous history of TB treatment were more likely to visit a modern health care facility than PTBC suspects who had no previous history of TB treatment (AOR (95% CI) 3.47 (2.16–5.58)). Perceived health status was also among the significant factors as PTBC suspects who perceived they were sick were more likely to visit a modern health care facility than who perceived they were well (AOR (95% CI) 3.19 (1.98–5.13)) (Table 3).

4. Discussion

In developing countries like Ethiopia where TB case detection rate is below the WHO set value and majority of the population live in rural areas in which TB diagnostic facilities are not fulfilled, understanding the health care seeking behaviour of PTBC suspects could be very crucial in order to design appropriate behaviour modification mechanisms.

In this study 39.1% of PTBC suspects had not visited modern health care facilities during the study period. This might imply that the respondents either did not consider their symptoms as a serious health problem or they had used other traditional methods to alleviate their symptoms. Although this finding is lower than a West Gojjam (Northwest Ethiopia) study [9], it is higher than a study done in Dabat district (Northwest Ethiopia) [19] in which the proportions of PTBC suspects who had not visited modern health care facility were 40% and 20%, respectively. Despite a relatively similar geographic location, significant variations have been observed between the Dabat and the current studies. One possible explanation for these discrepancies might be due to the fact that strategies to increase community awareness about tuberculosis might not be implemented uniformly and effectively across districts. On the other hand, a variation in socioeconomic and sociocultural variables which affect

TABLE 3: Bivariate and multivariate logistic regression analysis of factors associated with visiting modern health care facility among pulmonary tuberculosis suspects in Lay Armachiho district, Northwest Ethiopia, 2014.

Variable	Visited modern health care facility first		Crude odds ratio with 95% CI	Adjusted odds ratio with 95% CI
	Yes	No		
Age				
15–34	135	48	4.87 (2.97–7.98)	4.59 (2.71–7.76)***
35–54	224	133	2.91 (1.90–4.46)	2.45 (1.54–3.88)***
55 and above	45	78	1.00	
Sex				
Male	134	73	1.00	
Female	270	186	0.791 (0.56–1.11)	1.14 (0.72–1.80)
Marital status				
Unmarried[a]	120	66	1.00	
Married	284	193	0.80 (0.56–1.15)	0.84 (0.57–1.26)
Religion				
Orthodox Christian	290	201	1.00	
Muslim	74	33	1.55 (0.99–2.43)	0.76 (0.41–1.14)
Protestant	40	25	1.10 (0.65–1.88)	0.98 (0.46–2.08)
Educational level				
Illiterate	125	68	1.00	1.00
Elementary	219	163	0.73 (0.5–1.04)	1.10 (0.72–1.67)
Secondary and above	60	28	1.16 (0.68–1.99)[a]	2.61 (1.35–5.04)**
Occupation				
Unemployed[b]	172	146	1.00	1.00
Farmer	195	105	1.57 (1.14–2.17)	1.43 (1.004–2.05)*
Civil servant	37	8	3.92 (1.7–8.69)	3.02 (1.26–7.25)*
History of TB treatment				
Yes	120	32	2.99 (1.95–4.59)	3.47 (2.16–5.58)***
No	284	227	1.00	1.00
Hemoptysis				
Yes	28	8	2.33 (1.04–5.20)	2.57 (0.99–6.63)
No	376	251	1.00	
Perceived health status				
Well	50	67	1.00	1.00
Sick	354	192	2.47 (1.4–3.70)	3.16 (1.98–5.13)***

[a]* P value < 0.05; ** P value < 0.001; *** P value < 0.0001.

[b]Unemployed includes those who do not have any kind of job and students.

medical health care seeking behaviour among districts could partly explain the situation.

In our study, more than 50% of PTBC suspects described their symptoms as "bird" or "gerefta." This finding is in line with another Ethiopian study in that 46% of respondents reported their symptoms as "bird" [9]. This implies that knowledge about TB symptoms and when to visit a medical care provider is low among the majority of the population in the study area. As acknowledged by other studies [6, 19, 20], this in turn will lead to misconception about TB within the community, delay in modern health care seeking, and as a result increased period of communicability.

In this study, PTBC suspects aged 55 years and older were less likely to visit a modern health care facility than those who were younger than 55 years. In most parts of Ethiopia in general and in the Northern part of the country in particular, it is not uncommon to see traditional treatment of illness among the elderly community by either traditional healers or "Holy Water." On the other hand, unlike the younger age groups, the elderly people hardly get access to information about TB symptoms through modern education and peer education and, therefore, misconceptions are common in this age group. Literature also showed a downward trend of knowledge about health related matters as age increases [21]. Moreover, the fact that elderly people are economically dependent on others and may refrain from visiting modern health care facilities could also be one possible explanation for the finding.

Consistent with other local and international studies [22, 23], the current study also showed that respondents who had secondary educational level and above were more likely to visit modern health care facility than those who were illiterate. This is due to the fact that people at this educational level usually have higher chance of accessing health related information easily from various media and through their formal education. Moreover, the more the educational level of people is, the better their understanding of diseases processes, availability of diagnosis, treatment options, and the risk of delay in medical care seeking will be [21].

In this study, those who had some kind of occupation (civil servants or farmers) were more likely to visit a modern health care facility than those who were unemployed. The possible explanation for this finding might be attributed to the fact that when people have some kind of job which generates income, they could be motivated to visit a modern health care facility. This is usually because of direct (e.g., cost of medicine) and indirect (e.g., transport) costs associated with modern health care facility. Moreover, apart from relatively affording medical health care service associated costs, those people who had job and were able to generate better income may have television or radio or both to access appropriate information about TB [19].

In line with another Ethiopian community-based survey [9], our study also showed that PTBC suspects who had previous history of TB treatment were more likely to visit a modern health care facility than PTBC suspects who had no previous history of TB treatment. One possible reason for this finding could be the fact that preexisting knowledge regarding the seriousness of TB infection, its causative agent, and the availability of services (e.g., free of charge diagnosis and treatment in Ethiopian context) shaped their health seeking behaviour and influenced their decision to visit a modern health care facility [24].

In this study, respondents who had perceived that they were sick were more likely to visit a modern health care facility than those who perceived that they were well. The possible explanation for this finding might be that the high risk perception of PTBC suspects could ultimately lead them to visit a modern health care facility as supported by a study conducted in Bangladesh [24].

One of the possible limitations of this study could be its cross-sectional nature in which it does not confirm definitive cause and effect relationship. Moreover, since the major of the study participants had no formal (modern) education and we used self-reported data, the reliability and validity of the results might be influenced to some extent.

5. Conclusion

This study revealed that the majority of pulmonary tuberculosis suspects had visited modern health care facility; however, the proportion of respondents who had taken traditional measures was still higher as compared with some other districts. Younger age, educational level (secondary and above), occupation (farmers and civil servants), perceived health status (perceived wellness), and having previous history of TB treatment were factors significantly associated with visiting modern health care facilities. Interventions aimed at reducing unemployment rate, increasing literacy rate, and improving the socioeconomic status of communities in the district are recommended for the sustainable modification of health care seeking behaviour of TB suspects.

Authors' Contribution

Eshetu Haileselassie Engeda was involved in all steps of the study from its commencement to write-up as a principal investigator; Berihun Assefa Dachew, Hiwot Kassa Woreta, Mengistu Mekonnen Kelkay, and Tesfaye Demeke Ashenafie were coinvestigators and involved in proposal write-up and data analysis. All authors have reviewed and approved the submission of the paper.

Acknowledgments

The authors would like to acknowledge the University of Gondar for financial support. Their deepest gratitude also goes to those who participated in this study.

References

[1] World Health Organization (WHO), "Global Tuberculosis Report 2015," 2015, http://apps.who.int/iris/bitstream/10665/191102/1/9789241565059_eng.pdf?ua=1.

[2] T. Tadesse, M. Demissie, Y. Berhane, Y. Kebede, and M. Abebe, "Two-thirds of smear-positive tuberculosis cases in the community were undiagnosed in Northwest Ethiopia: population based cross-sectional study," *PLoS ONE*, vol. 6, no. 12, Article ID e28258, 2011.

[3] A. Cambanis, A. Ramsay, M. A. Yassin, and L. E. Cuevas, "Duration and associated factors of patient delay during tuberculosis screening in rural Cameroon," *Tropical Medicine and International Health*, vol. 12, no. 11, pp. 1309–1314, 2007.

[4] T. Tadesse, M. Demissie, Y. Berhane, Y. Kebede, and M. Abebe, "The clustering of smear-positive tuberculosis in dabat, ethiopia: a population based cross sectional study," *PLoS ONE*, vol. 8, no. 5, Article ID e65022, 2013.

[5] N. T. Huong, M. Vree, B. D. Duong et al., "Delays in the diagnosis and treatment of tuberculosis patients in Vietnam: a cross-sectional study," *BMC Public Health*, vol. 7, article 110, 2007.

[6] G. Abebe, A. Deribew, L. Apers et al., "Knowledge, health seeking behavior and perceived stigma towards tuberculosis among tuberculosis suspects in a rural community in southwest Ethiopia," *PLoS ONE*, vol. 5, no. 10, Article ID e13339, 2010.

[7] T. Nigatu and M. Abraha, "Epidemiological analysis of tuberculosis trends in Ethiopia: 2000–2009," *Tüberküloz ve Toraks Dergisi*, vol. 58, no. 4, pp. 375–384, 2010.

[8] Federal Democratic Republic of Ethiopia Ministry of Health, "Policy and practice information for action," *Quarterly Health Bulletin*, vol. 6, no. 1, pp. 1–51, 2014.

[9] S. Yimer, C. Holm-Hansen, T. Yimaldu, and G. Bjune, "Health care seeking among pulmonary tuberculosis suspects and patients in rural Ethiopia: a community-based study," *BMC Public Health*, vol. 9, article 454, 2009.

[10] A. Grover, R. Kumar, and S. K. Jindal, "Socio-demographic determinants of treatment-seeking behavior among chest symptomatics," *Indian Journal of Community Medicine*, vol. 31, no. 3, pp. 145–149, 2006.

[11] M. J. van der Werf, Y. Chechulin, O. B. Yegorova et al., "Health care seeking behaviour for tuberculosis symptoms in Kiev City, Ukraine," *The International Journal of Tuberculosis and Lung Disease*, vol. 10, no. 4, pp. 390–395, 2006.

[12] G. Fochsen, K. Deshpande, V. Diwan, A. Mishra, V. K. Diwan, and A. Thorson, "Health care seeking among individuals with cough and tuberculosis: a population-based study from rural India," *International Journal of Tuberculosis and Lung Disease*, vol. 10, no. 9, pp. 995–1000, 2006.

[13] Y. Kasse, M. Jasseh, T. Corrah et al., "Health seeking behaviour, health system experience and tuberculosis case finding in Gambians with cough," *BMC Public Health*, vol. 6, article 143, 2006.

[14] E. Buregyeya, A. Kulane, R. Colebunders et al., "Tuberculosis knowledge, attitudes and health-seeking behaviour in rural Uganda," *International Journal of Tuberculosis and Lung Disease*, vol. 15, no. 7, pp. 938–942, 2011.

[15] B. T. Shaikh and J. Hatcher, "Health seeking behaviour and health service utilization in Pakistan: challenging the policy makers," *Journal of Public Health*, vol. 27, no. 1, pp. 49–54, 2005.

[16] E. Zerbini, M. C. Chirico, B. Salvadores, B. Amigot, S. Estrada, and G. Algorry, "Delay in tuberculosis diagnosis and treatment in four provinces of Argentina," *International Journal of Tuberculosis and Lung Disease*, vol. 12, no. 1, pp. 63–68, 2008.

[17] R. Basnet, S. G. Hinderaker, D. Enarson, P. Malla, and O. Mørkve, "Delay in the diagnosis of tuberculosis in Nepal," *BMC Public Health*, vol. 9, article 236, 2009.

[18] G. Berhe, F. Enqueselassie, E. Hailu et al., "Population-based prevalence survey of tuberculosis in the Tigray region of Ethiopia," *BMC Infectious Diseases*, vol. 13, no. 1, article 448, 2013.

[19] M. Senbeto, S. Tadesse, T. Tadesse, and T. Melesse, "Appropriate health-seeking behavior and associated factors among people who had cough for at least two weeks in northwest Ethiopia: a population-based cross-sectional study," *BMC Public Health*, vol. 13, article 1222, 2013.

[20] A. Esmael, I. Ali, M. Agonafir, A. Desale, Z. Yaregal, and K. Desta, "Assessment of patients' knowledge, attitude, and practice regarding pulmonary tuberculosis in Eastern Amhara Regional State, Ethiopia: cross-sectional study," *The American Journal of Tropical Medicine and Hygiene*, vol. 88, no. 4, pp. 785–788, 2013.

[21] X. Sun, Y. Shi, Q. Zeng et al., "Determinants of health literacy and health behavior regarding infectious respiratory diseases: a pathway model," *BMC Public Health*, vol. 13, article 261, 2013.

[22] C. M. Ford, A. M. Bayer, R. H. Gilman et al., "Factors associated with delayed tuberculosis test-seeking behavior in the Peruvian Amazon," *American Journal of Tropical Medicine and Hygiene*, vol. 81, no. 6, pp. 1097–1102, 2009.

[23] E. Gebeyehu, M. Azage, and G. Abeje, "Factors associated with patient's delay in tuberculosis treatment in Bahir Dar City Administration, Northwest Ethiopia," *BioMed Research International*, vol. 2014, Article ID 701429, 6 pages, 2014.

[24] K. Bam, L. P. Bhatt, R. Thapa, H. K. Dossajee, and M. R. Angdembe, "Illness perception of tuberculosis (TB) and health seeking practice among urban slum residents of Bangladesh: a qualitative study," *BMC Research Notes*, vol. 7, article 572, 2014.

34

Immigrant Arrival and Tuberculosis among Large Immigrant- and Refugee-Receiving Countries, 2005–2009

Zachary White,[1] John Painter,[1] Paul Douglas,[2] Ibrahim Abubakar,[3] Howard Njoo,[4] Chris Archibald,[4] Jessica Halverson,[4] John Robson,[5] and Drew L. Posey[1]

[1] *Division of Global Migration and Quarantine, National Center for Emerging and Zoonotic Infectious Diseases, Centers for Disease Control and Prevention, Atlanta, GA, USA*
[2] *Department of Immigration and Border Protection, Sydney, NSW, Australia*
[3] *Public Health England and University College London, London, UK*
[4] *Centre for Communicable Diseases and Infection Control, Public Health Agency of Canada, Ottawa, ON, Canada*
[5] *Immigration New Zealand, Wellington, New Zealand*

Correspondence should be addressed to Zachary White; zwhite@cdc.gov

Academic Editor: Alexander S. Apt

Objective. Tuberculosis control in foreign-born populations is a major public health concern for Australia, Canada, New Zealand, United Kingdom, and the United States, large immigrant- and refugee-receiving countries that comprise the Immigration and Refugee Health Working Group (IRHWG). Identifying and comparing immigration and distribution of foreign-born tuberculosis cases are important for developing targeted and collaborative interventions. *Methods.* Data stratified by year and country of birth from 2005 to 2009 were received from these five countries. Immigration totals, tuberculosis case totals, and multidrug-resistant tuberculosis (MDR TB) case totals from source countries were analyzed and compared to reveal similarities and differences for each member of the group. *Results.* Between 2005 and 2009, there were a combined 31,785,002 arrivals, 77,905 tuberculosis cases, and 888 MDR TB cases notified at the federal level in the IRHWG countries. India, China, Vietnam, and the Philippines accounted for 41.4% of the total foreign-born tuberculosis cases and 42.7% of the foreign-born MDR tuberculosis cases to IRHWG. *Interpretation.* Collaborative efforts across a small number of countries have the potential to yield sizeable gains in tuberculosis control for these large immigrant- and refugee-receiving countries.

1. Introduction

Tuberculosis is one of the world's largest public health challenges. Approximately one-third of the world's population is infected with tuberculosis (TB), and an estimated 1.5 million people die from the disease each year [1]. The World Health Organization (WHO) established targets for TB control by 2035 [2]. These goals include targets for rates of diagnosis and treatment completion rates for persons inside a country [2]. However, migration is a factor that provides challenges for meeting targets as well as opportunities for control, particularly for countries with low incidence for TB [3].

Worldwide, there are approximately 232 million international migrants, or 3.2% of the world's population [4]. Although western, industrialized countries receive a large percentage of international migrants, other parts of the world also receive a large number of international migrants. Parts of the world in which >10% of the population comprises international migrants include the Gulf countries, Eastern Europe, and even a few countries in Africa. Pertaining to TB, many of the top source countries for international migrants are also countries with a high burden of TB. For example, the top source country for international migrants in 2013 was India, a country with the highest burden of TB [1]. Other top countries for both international migrants and tuberculosis cases include the Russian Federation, China, Bangladesh, Pakistan, the Philippines, Afghanistan, and Indonesia.

Several of the world's largest immigrant- and refugee-receiving countries (Australia, Canada, New Zealand, the United States, and the United Kingdom) participate in the Immigration and Refugee Health Working Group (IRHWG), which aims to develop collaborative approaches for immigration and refugee resettlements, including TB. A majority of the TB cases in these countries are individuals who were born abroad, and the threat of multidrug-resistant (MDR) and extensively drug-resistant (XDR) TB is of significant concern [5–9]. Each participating country currently conducts TB screening overseas for immigrants (persons applying for permanent residency) and refugees; all members, except the United States, also perform TB screening overseas for persons who will live in the receiving country > 6 months, also known as long-term visitors [10–14].

To address modern TB threats, each IRHWG country is in the process of improving TB prevention-control efforts, especially as it relates to immigrant and refugee populations with high burden of TB. To better identify the primary source countries that contribute the largest migrating populations and most TB cases to the group as a whole, we conducted an analysis of arrivals and TB case diagnoses.

2. Methods

We analyzed data on TB cases and arrivals to Australia, Canada, New Zealand, the United Kingdom, and the United States. The arrival data from each IRHWG country include long-term visitors, immigrant arrivals, and refugee arrivals; the arrival data were obtained through the immigration bureau for each country. The TB data are comprised of an in-country diagnosis of foreign-born TB cases; the TB case reporting came from the National Reporting Agencies in each IRHWG country. The authors acknowledge that the TB cases in this analysis are not directly linked to the immigration data presented.

All TB case data were stratified by year, birth country, and type of TB (treatment-sensitive or MDR). For analysis purposes, cumulative totals from 2005 to 2009 were utilized to determine the total volume of immigrants and diagnosed tuberculosis for each IRHWG country. Microsoft Excel and JMP 9 were used to construct tables in order to compare relationships among immigration totals, TB cases, and MDR TB cases. The top 20 source countries for total immigrants, TB cases, and MDR TB cases were determined using Microsoft Excel. Bar graphs were constructed using Microsoft Excel and R statistical software and tables made from Microsoft Excel and JMP.

Because a goal of this analysis is to develop a perspective as to which source countries are the largest ones for the IRHWG members as a whole, irrespective of the numbers of arrivals or cases, we calculated the average of the percentages for each source country. This was calculated for arrivals, foreign-born TB cases, and foreign-MDR TB cases. The calculations in the bar graphs display the burden (immigration volume, TB case volume, and MDR TB case volume) for each member country, as well as the burden to the group as a whole. For example, the average of each country's proportion of TB cases born in specific countries is shown in Figure 2 as a bar graph. Each country's proportion to the total TB burden is also represented in the graph.

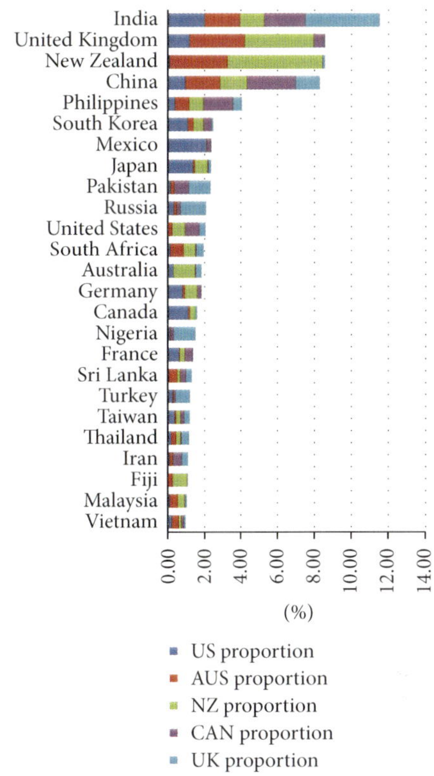

Figure 1: Combined averages of arrivals, 2005–2009.

Ethical Considerations. Ethical approval and informed consent were not required for this analysis.

3. Results

Between 2005 and 2009, there were 31,785,002 arrivals, 77,905 TB cases, and 888 MDR TB cases notified in these five countries. The data in Figures 1–3 represent the averages of each source country in respect to total arrivals, total TB cases, and total MDR TB cases from 2005 to 2009. The top five source countries for combined adjusted total arrivals (Figure 1) included India (11.5%), United Kingdom (8.6%), New Zealand (8.6%), China (8.3%), and the Philippines (4.1%), while the top five source countries for combined adjusted total tuberculosis cases (Figure 2) were India (19.0%), the Philippines (8.5%), China (8.3%), Vietnam (5.5%), and Mexico (5.0%). Similarly, the top five source countries for combined adjusted total MDR TB cases (Figure 3) were India (15.6%), China (14.7%), Papua New Guinea (8.5%), the Philippines (6.8%), and Vietnam (5.6%).

Data from the analysis reveal that India, China, Vietnam, and the Philippines supplied the majority of diagnosed TB counts. These four countries accounted for combined adjusted 41.4% of the total foreign-born TB cases (Figure 2) and 42.7% of the foreign-born MDR tuberculosis cases (Figure 3). Of these, India was the leading source country for arrivals (11.5% (Figure 1)), TB cases (19.0% (Figure 2)), and MDR TB cases from 2005 to 2009 (15.6% (Figure 3)).

Primary source countries for total immigrant arrivals, total TB cases, and total MDR TB cases varied for each of

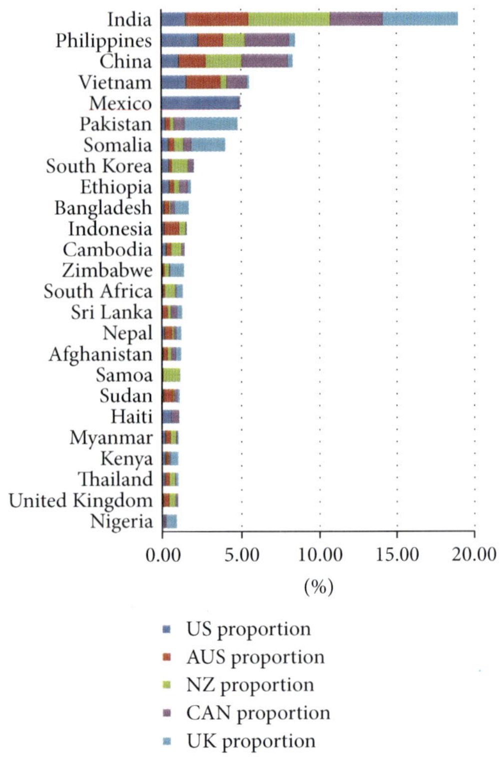

Figure 2: Combined averages of foreign-born TB cases, 2005–2009.

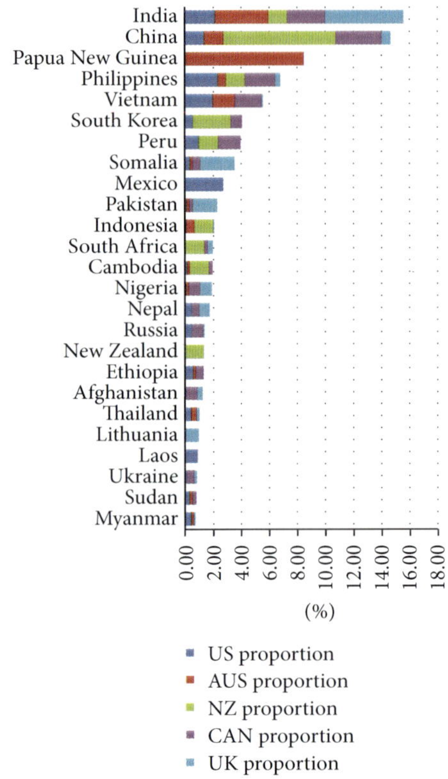

Figure 3: Combined averages of MDR TB cases, 2005–2009.

the five countries (Tables 1–3). Although multiple similarities were observed, the data reveal that four of the IRHWG countries have a specific source country/countries that contributes a significant amount of TB cases without affecting the group as a whole. Examples of specific source contributors include Papua New Guinea (3.4% of foreign-born TB cases and 42.4% of MDR TB cases) for Australia; Samoa (5.3% TB cases) for New Zealand; Somalia (10.6% TB cases and 12.3% MDR TB cases) and Pakistan (16.7% TB cases, 8.7% MDR TB cases) for the United Kingdom; and Mexico (24.1% TB cases and 13.7% MDR TB cases) for the United States (Tables 1, 2, and 3). Canada received the majority of cases from the four largest source countries (India, the Philippines, China, and Vietnam) but did not have a unique source country that was uncommon to the other members. In this analysis, instead of grouping countries by regions, we examined data for the individual source country to understand their specific impact on our immigration and TB programs.

4. Discussion

In this analysis, India, China, Vietnam, and the Philippines contributed the largest proportion of foreign-born TB cases to Australia, Canada, New Zealand, United Kingdom, and the United States as a whole during 2005–2009. The data used in this analysis is a couple of years old, but the immigration and TB trends are similar to the results of this analysis. The four countries accounted for 41.4% of combined adjusted foreign-born TB cases and 42.7% of the combined adjusted foreign-born MDR TB cases during this period of time. Each of these four countries is also included in the 2015 WHO list of high-burden countries with respect to TB [1].

However, these data also highlight the unique source countries for each of these countries, which illustrate differences in migration patterns. These unique situations may reflect factors related to geography, such as Mexico as a source country for the United States, or issues related to long-standing historical ties, such as Pakistan for the United Kingdom.

Although each country publishes immigration and TB surveillance figures, and the importance of foreign-born TB cases in industrialized countries has been described [15], this is the first comparison of immigration and TB data among large immigrant- and refugee-receiving countries to our knowledge.

The results of this analysis also mirror global comparisons over time. Just as the global trends in international migration have increased over time, so the volumes of arrivals have increased too during the study period. The growing importance of Asian arrivals, in particular, is also reflected in this analysis. In the United States, for example, the highest proportion of immigrants to the United States transitioned from Hispanics to Asians in 2009 [16].

The results also reflect global trends in TB, as many of the top birth countries for TB cases are also WHO high-burden countries. Although only five receiving countries are included in this analysis, the similarities (Figures 1–3) underscore the need to develop collaborative strategies to address the burden of TB in migrating populations [17].

Table 1: Top source countries for arrivals, 2005–2009.

Australia			Canada			New Zealand			United Kingdom			United States		
Country	Number	%	Country	Number	%	Country*	Number	%	Country	Number	%	Country	Number	%
New Zealand	114496	16.1	China	167658	13.4	United Kingdom	69316	18.6	India	2044222	20.1	Mexico	2021541	10.5
United Kingdom	109492	15.1	India	140599	11.3	China	26787	7.2	Russia	713690	7.0	India	1913293	9.9
China	70356	9.0	Philippines	105314	8.4	India	24180	6.5	China	656664	6.5	Japan	1294620	6.7
India	70173	9.9	United States	51594	4.1	Australia	21224	5.7	Pakistan	616792	6.1	United Kingdom	1096613	5.7
Philippines	28053	4.0	Pakistan	49713	4.0	Fiji	14361	3.9	Nigeria	605557	6.0	Canada	1027787	5.3
South Africa	26175	3.7	United Kingdom	39677	3.2	Philippines	14292	3.8	Turkey	390127	3.8	South Korea	1000637	5.2
Sri Lanka	16363	2.3	Iran	31312	2.5	Japan	12599	3.4	Saudi Arabia	266320	2.6	China	866419	4.5
Malaysia	15838	2.2	South Korea	30973	2.5	United States	12360	3.3	Philippines	239269	2.4	Germany	736608	3.8
Vietnam	14195	2.0	France	29700	2.4	Germany	12266	3.3	Thailand	208180	2.1	France	560047	2.9
Iraq	13587	1.9	Colombia	25912	2.1	South Africa	11600	3.1	Kuwait	202960	2.0	Brazil	401382	2.1
South Korea	11816	1.7	Sri Lanka	21892	1.8	South Korea	9788	2.6	South Africa	196602	1.9	Philippines	339139	1.8
Sudan	11147	1.6	United Arab Emirates	20856	1.7	Samoa	8402	2.3	United States	170199	1.7	Taiwan	321358	1.7
Thailand	10306	1.5	Algeria	18829	1.5	Malaysia	6506	1.7	Iran	166623	1.6	Australia	284135.5	1.5
Singapore	9792	1.4	Morocco	18717	1.5	Ireland	5526	1.5	Ukraine	163909	1.6	Russia	278332	1.4
Afghanistan	9774	1.4	Romania	17875	1.4	Canada	5425	1.5	Bangladesh	162765	1.6	Colombia	268298	1.4
Indonesia	8720	1.2	Germany	16358	1.3	France	4436	1.2	Sri Lanka	159197	1.6	Italy	258892	1.3
Fiji	8515	1.2	Bangladesh	15083	1.2	Taiwan	3875	1.0	Australia	154676	1.5	Spain	227517	1.2
Myanmar	7860	1.1	Mexico	14843	1.2	Tonga	3770	1.0	Taiwan	152157	1.5	Venezuela	213125	1.1
United States	7710	1.1	Lebanon	14788	1.2	Thailand	3722	1.0	Egypt	143768	1.4	Israel	212934	1.1
Pakistan	7301	1.0	Russia	14656	1.2	Sri Lanka	2441	0.7	Ghana	121162	1.2	Turkey	212565	1.1
Total	710627		Total	1250055		Total	373299		Total	10173350		Total	19277671	

*Reports list New Zealand as the top source for New Zealand.

TABLE 2: Top source countries for foreign-born TB cases, 2005–2009.

Australia			Canada			New Zealand			United Kingdom			United States		
Country	Number	%	Country	Number	%	Country	Number	%	Country	Number	%	Country	Number	%
India	1004	19.9	India	912	17.1	India	285	26.0	India	7009	24.4	Mexico	9098	24.1
Vietnam	551	10.9	China	795	14.9	China	124	11.3	Pakistan	4811	16.7	Philippines	4302	11.4
China	433	8.6	Philippines	759	14.3	Philippines	75	6.8	Somalia	3056	10.6	Vietnam	2885	7.7
Philippines	406	8.1	Vietnam	352	6.6	Samoa	58	5.3	Bangladesh	1229	4.3	India	2869	7.6
Indonesia	246	4.9	Pakistan	190	3.6	South Korea	55	5.0	Zimbabwe	1222	4.3	China	2019	5.4
Papua New Guinea	170	3.4	Ethiopia	149	2.8	South Africa	35	3.2	Nigeria	905	3.2	Guatemala	1154	3.1
Sudan	159	3.2	Somalia	144	2.7	Cambodia	35	3.2	Kenya	653	2.3	Haiti	1067	2.8
Nepal	123	2.4	Haiti	131	2.5	New Zealand*	33	3.0	South Africa	560	2.0	Ethiopia	887	2.4
United Kingdom	97	1.9	Sri Lanka	110	2.1	Somalia	30	2.7	Philippines	543	1.9	Honduras	853	2.3
Somalia	96	1.9	Unknown	106	2.0	Tonga	30	2.7	Afghanistan	457	1.6	South Korea	832	2.2
Sri Lanka	88	1.8	South Korea	103	1.9	Malaysia	25	2.3	Uganda	446	1.6	Somalia	786	2.1
Bangladesh	88	1.8	Afghanistan	85	1.6	United Kingdom	21	1.9	Sri Lanka	440	1.5	El Salvador	713	1.9
Myanmar	85	1.7	Bangladesh	79	1.5	Indonesia	21	1.9	China	421	1.5	Peru	692	1.8
Cambodia	84	1.7	Republic of Congo	73	1.4	Vietnam	20	1.8	Nepal	414	1.4	Ecuador	601	1.6
Pakistan	79	1.6	Sudan	60	1.1	Fiji	20	1.8	Eritrea	390	1.4	Cambodia	475	1.3
Afghanistan	78	1.6	Italy	53	1.0	Thailand	19	1.7	Ethiopia	274	0.95	Dominican Republic	434	1.2
Thailand	75	1.5	Cambodia	52	1.0	Myanmar	18	1.6	Republic of Congo	272	0.95	Pakistan	407	1.1
Ethiopia	74	1.5	Nepal	51	1.0	Ethiopia	18	1.6	Jamaica	246	0.86	Kenya	366	0.97
Malaysia	57	1.1	Kenya	45	0.8	Zimbabwe	15	1.4	Ghana	246	0.86	Myanmar	349	0.93
New Zealand	54	1.1	Eritrea	44	0.8	Kiribati	13	1.2	Zambia	223	0.78	Laos	344	0.91
Total	5036		Total	5327		Total	1098		Total	28760		Total	37684	

*New Zealand categorizes TB cases among non-New Zealand citizens as foreign-born. Thus, any persons born in New Zealand who are not New Zealand citizens but are diagnosed with TB will be included in the surveillance system among the foreign-born cases.

Table 3: Top source countries for foreign-born MDR TB cases, 2005–2009.

Australia			Canada			New Zealand			United Kingdom			United States		
Country	Number	%	Country	Number	%	Country	Number	%	Country	Number	%	Country	Number	%
Papua New Guinea	42	42.4	China	12	16.4	China	6	40.0	India	61	27.9	Mexico	66	13.7
India	19	19.2	India	10	13.7	South Korea	2	13.3	Somalia	27	12.3	Philippines	56	11.6
Vietnam	8	8.1	Philippines	8	11.0	New Zealand	1	6.7	Pakistan	19	8.7	India	51	10.6
China	7	7.1	Vietnam	7	9.6	Cambodia	1	6.7	Lithuania	10	4.6	Vietnam	47	9.8
Indonesia	3	3.0	Peru	6	8.2	South Africa	1	6.7	Nigeria	9	4.1	China	32	6.6
Philippines	3	3.0	Afghanistan	3	4.1	Indonesia	1	6.7	Nepal	8	3.7	Peru	24	5.0
United Kingdom	3	3.0	Russia	3	4.1	Peru	1	6.7	China	7	3.2	Laos	21	4.4
Thailand	2	2.0	Nigeria	3	4.1	Philippines	1	6.7	Zimbabwe	7	3.2	South Korea	14	2.9
Uzbekistan	2	2.0	South Korea	3	4.1	India	1	6.7	Bangladesh	6	2.7	Guatemala	14	2.9
Myanmar	1	1.0	Ukraine	2	2.7				Afghanistan	4	1.8	Ethiopia	13	2.7
Sudan	1	1.0	Ethiopia	2	2.7				South Africa	4	1.8	Dominican Republic	12	2.5
Ethiopia	1	1.0	Nepal	2	2.7				Philippines	4	1.8	Russia	11	2.3
Nigeria	1	1.0	Somalia	2	2.7				Kenya	3	1.4	Nepal	11	2.3
Cambodia	1	1.0	Guyana	2	2.7				Kazakhstan	3	1.4	Myanmar	10	2.1
Pakistan	1	1.0	Sudan	1	1.4				Cote d'Ivoire	3	1.4	Thailand	10	2.1
Somalia	1	1.0	Cambodia	1	1.4				Zambia	3	1.4	Haiti	10	2.1
East Timor	1	1.0	South Africa	1	1.4				Angola	3	1.4	Somalia	8	1.7
Sierra Leone	1	1.0	Pakistan	1	1.4				Latvia	3	1.4	Sudan	7	1.5
Lebanon	1	1.0	Kenya	1	1.4				Ukraine	2	0.91	Ecuador	7	1.5
Ukraine	0	0.0	Malaysia	1	1.4				Thailand	2	0.91	Moldova	4	0.83
Total	99		Total	73		Total	15		Total	219		Total	482	

During the period of this analysis, an average of 6 million persons were admitted annually to the five participating countries. Currently, approximately 2 million applicants for migration status to these five countries are screened for TB annually; the foreign-born TB cases which occur may or may not be discovered through the screening process. These examinations are performed by >2,000 panel physicians worldwide. Panel physicians are medical doctors who have agreements with each country to conduct the migrant medical exam overseas. Each of the IRHWG countries require overseas TB screening for all immigrants and refugees and each except for the United States routinely requires screening for long-term visitors. Moreover, all but the United Kingdom have historically required this screening [18]; following a successful pilot program in a limited number of countries, the United Kingdom began a targeted overseas screening program in 2012 for applicants from high-incidence countries [19]. Screening applicants for TB is very effective at preventing importation of active TB cases into the receiving countries [20, 21].

Managing a modern overseas TB screening program for migration and refugee resettlements results in development of laboratory and treatment capacity. The TB screening algorithms of IRHWG countries are similar in that they either require (United States) or use (Australia, Canada, New Zealand, and United Kingdom), where available, TB cultures for those suspected of having active pulmonary TB, drug susceptibility testing (DST) on positive isolates, and treatment delivered as directly observed therapy (DOT) prior to entry [10–14]. Since 2007, implementation of the US program's culture and DOT requirement has resulted in additional culture and DST laboratories as well as increased training for personnel involved with TB control [21, 22].

While each of these country's efforts in managing TB screening programs is invaluable for reducing importation of TB, they should also be leveraged to assist with control efforts within source countries. TB elimination in receiving countries is difficult without addressing TB in foreign-born populations [23]. For this reason, it is hoped that improved linkages between panel physician activities and TB control efforts within their countries would benefit the migrants and others in their source populations. This analysis helps demonstrate the fact that because panel physician volumes are large in key source countries, these countries are uniquely positioned to have their investments in the screening program also contribute to local control efforts [24]. And this analysis helps determine for which countries that contribution could be most needed. Additional benefits to screening programs could possibly be achieved by having panel physicians develop relationships with their TB controllers, share information on their experiences, share laboratory capacity, and comanage TB cases where DOT capacity is scarce.

The authors expected India to be a common source country but were surprised that the average number of cases was more than twice as high as that for the next two countries, the Philippines and China. The participating countries have collaborated closely with India, and this country was the first country for implementation of the United Kingdom screening program. However, the results of this analysis highlight the importance of collaborations with India for migrants, as well as for helping with overall TB control in India, since it is the highest-burden country for TB worldwide.

In many instances, TB treatment for those who travel to the US may not occur until years after they have arrived. While the data in this analysis shares source country of the migrants, it does not automatically imply importation. Individuals may acquire TB infection during travel or in the United States upon arrival.

Although this analysis yields important findings regarding migration and TB, there are some limitations. First, data for this analysis were only requested from 2005 to 2009, which is a short period of time. If additional years were observed for the analysis, additional trends for each country and the group as a whole might have been exposed. However, the data from these five countries for subsequent years suggest similar burdens of arrivals and diagnoses. Second, the analysis only included data for five countries. While these are some of the largest immigrant-receiving countries, additional future analyses should include countries outside the group. The analysis could have used data to separate the arrivals and TB cases by visa types for each receiving country. This would allow stratification of the arrivals and cases by populations to see which had the highest TB rates within each country. It is also important to note that the TB data were not stratified by time since arrival. Thus, the potential exists that trends among this subset may be slightly different. Finally, while this analysis can be used to help participating countries in the management of their screening programs by indicating which resources could be targeted, a cost-effectiveness review of screening programs on potential collaborations was beyond the scope of this analysis.

Australia, Canada, New Zealand, the United Kingdom, and the United States are the largest immigrant- and refugee-receiving countries in the world and are currently collaborating on preventing importation of TB into each of their countries. Joint efforts in a small number of high-burden countries can help prevent importation of TB cases and also contribute to control efforts within source countries.

Disclosure

The findings and conclusions of this article are those of the authors and do not necessarily represent the official position of the Centers for Disease Control and Prevention.

Authors' Contributions

Zachary White, John Painter, and Drew L. Posey were involved in the conception and design and performed the analysis. Paul Douglas, Ibrahim Abubakar, Howard Njoo, Chris Archibald, Jessica Halverson, and John Robson were involved in the study implementation, interpreted the data, and provided important intellectual input. Zachary White and Drew L. Posey wrote the first draft.

Acknowledgments

The authors thank Mr. Terry Comans for assistance garnering support for the analysis among participating countries; Mr. David Watt for assistance with data from Australia; Dr. Tom Navin for US TB case data; Mr. Yecai Liu for identifying long-term visitors in US arrival data; the panel physicians for performing overseas TB screening; and Ms. Courtney Chappelle for mapping activities. The authors acknowledge the support from Centers for Disease Control and Prevention, Public Health England, Department of Immigration and Border Protection Australia, Public Health Agency of Canada, and Immigration New Zealand.

References

[1] World Health Organization, *Global Tuberculosis Report 2015*, WHO, Geneva, Switzerland, 2015, http://www.who.int/tb/publications/global_report/en/.

[2] Global Strategy and Targets for Tuberculosis Prevention, Care and Control After 2015, May 2014, http://www.who.int/tb/post2015_strategy/en/.

[3] K. Lonnroith, G. B. Migliori, I. Abubakar et al., "Towards tuberculosis elimination: an action framework for low-incidence countries," *European Respiratory Journal*, vol. 45, no. 4, pp. 928–952, 2015.

[4] Department of Economic Affairs Population Division, *International Migration Report 2013*, United Nations Doc ST/ESA/SER.A/346, 2013.

[5] CDC, *Reported Tuberculosis in the United States, 2012*, U.S. Department of Health and Human Services, CDC, Atlanta, Ga, USA, 2013.

[6] C. Barry, J. Waring, R. Stapledon et al., "Tuberculosis notifications in Australia, 2008 and 2009," *Communicable Disease Intelligence*, vol. 36, no. 1, pp. 82–94, 2012, http://www.health.gov.au/internet/main/publishing.nsf/Content/cda-cdi3601c.htm#refs.

[7] Tuberculosis Prevention and Control in Canada, Centre for Communicable Disease and Infection Control, Public Health Agency of Canada, 2014, http://www.phac-aspc.gc.ca/.

[8] E. Lim and H. Heffernan, *Tuberculosis in New Zealand: Annual Report 2012*, Institute of Environmental Science and Research (ESR), Porirua, New Zealand, 2013.

[9] *Tuberculosis in the UK: Annual Report on Tuberculosis Surveillance in the UK*, Public Health England, London, UK, 2013.

[10] Department of Immigration and Citizenship, Global Health, Sydney, Australia, Instructions for medical and radiological examination of Australian visa applicants, Australian Government, March 2012.

[11] Government of Canada, *Citizenship and Immigration Canada: Immigration and Medical Examination Instructions*, 2013, http://www.cic.gc.ca/english/department/partner/pp/pdf/IMEI_Tuberculosis.pdf.

[12] Ministry of Health, *Guidelines for Tuberculosis Control in New Zealand 2010*, Ministry of Health, Wellington, New Zealand, 2010, http://www.moh.govt.nz.

[13] UK Visas & Immigration: UK Tuberculosis Technical Instructions (UKTBTI), Public Health England, September 2013 Version 6, https://www.gov.uk/government/uploads/system/uploads/attachment_data/file/245009/UK_tuberculosis_technical_instructions.pdf.

[14] CDC, *CDC Immigration Requirements: Technical Instructions for Tuberculosis Screening and Treatment*, U.S. Department of Health and Human Services, Atlanta, Ga, USA, 2007, http://www.cdc.gov/immigrantrefugeehealth/pdf/tuberculosis-ti-2009.pdf.

[15] K. P. Cain, S. R. Benoit, C. A. Winston, and W. R. Mac Kenzie, "Tuberculosis among foreign-born persons in the United States," *The Journal of the American Medical Association*, vol. 300, no. 4, pp. 405–412, 2008.

[16] Pew Research Center, *The Rise of Asian Americans*, 2013, http://www.pewsocialtrends.org/files/2013/04/Asian-Americans-new-full-report-04-2013.pdf.

[17] B. K. Moore, D. L. Posey, S. A. Maloney, M. Cetron, and K. Castro, *Tackling Tuberculosis Abroad—The Key to TB Elimination in the United States. June 2014. A Report of the CSIS Global Health Policy Center*, Center for Strategic and International Studies, 2014, https://csis.org/files/publication/140604_Moore_TacklingTBAbroad_Web.pdf.

[18] M. Dara, B. D. Gushulak, D. L. Posey, J.-P. Zellweger, and G. B. Migliori, "The history and evolution of immigration medical screening for tuberculosis," *Expert Review of Anti-Infective Therapy*, vol. 11, no. 2, pp. 137–146, 2013.

[19] UK Border Agency, "New screening to tackle tuberculosis in the UK," http://www.ukba.homeoffice.gov.uk/sitecontent/newsarticles/2012/may/42-tb-test.

[20] Y. Liu, M. S. Weinberg, L. S. Ortega, J. A. Painter, and S. A. Maloney, "Overseas screening for tuberculosis in U.S.-bound immigrants and refugees," *New England Journal of Medicine*, vol. 360, no. 23, pp. 2406–2415, 2009.

[21] D. L. Posey, M. P. Naughton, E. A. Willacy et al., "Implementation of new TB screening requirements for U.S.-bound immigrants and refugees—2007–2014," *Morbidity and Mortality Weekly Report*, vol. 63, pp. 234–236, 2014.

[22] Y. Liu, D. L. Posey, M. S. Cetron, and J. A. Painter, "Effect of a culture-based screening algorithm on tuberculosis incidence in immigrants and refugees bound for the United States a population-based cross-sectional study," *Annals of Internal Medicine*, vol. 162, no. 6, pp. 420–428, 2015.

[23] A. N. Hill, J. E. Becerra, and K. G. Castro, "Modelling tuberculosis trends in the USA," *Epidemiology and Infection*, vol. 140, no. 10, pp. 1862–1872, 2012.

[24] K. Schwartzman, O. Oxlade, R. Graham Barr et al., "Domestic returns from investment in the control of tuberculosis in other countries," *The New England Journal of Medicine*, vol. 353, no. 10, pp. 1008–1020, 2005.

35

Phenotypic and Genotypic Analysis of Multidrug-Resistant *Mycobacterium tuberculosis* Isolates from Sudanese Patients

Solima M. A. Sabeel,[1,2] Mohamed Ahmed Salih,[3] Manasik Ali,[4] Salah-Eldin EL-Zaki,[5] Nadir Abuzeid,[6] Zeinab Abubaker Mohammed Elgadi,[7] Hisham N. Altayb,[8] Asrar M. A. Elegail,[9] Nuha Y. Ibrahim,[9] and Bahaeldin K. Elamin[1,10]

[1] *Department of Microbiology, Faculty of Medical Laboratory Sciences, University of Khartoum, Khartoum, Sudan*
[2] *Microbiology Department, Faculty of Medical Laboratory Sciences, Ibn Sina University, Khartoum, Sudan*
[3] *Department of Bioinformatics, Africa City of Technology, Khartoum, Sudan*
[4] *Sudan Academy of Sciences, Khartoum, Sudan*
[5] *Department of Epidemiology, Tropical Medicine Research Institute, National Center for Research, Khartoum, Sudan*
[6] *Department of Microbiology, Faculty of Medical Laboratory Sciences, Omdurman Islamic University, Khartoum, Sudan*
[7] *Veterinary Research Institute, Khartoum, Sudan*
[8] *Microbiology Department, College of Medical Laboratory Sciences, Sudan University of Science and Technology, Khartoum, Sudan*
[9] *National Reference Laboratory-Tuberculosis (NRL-TB), National Public Health Laboratory, Khartoum, Sudan*
[10] *Department of Microbiology and Parasitology, College of Medicine, University of Bisha, Bisha, Saudi Arabia*

Correspondence should be addressed to Solima M. A. Sabeel; solima89@gmail.com

Academic Editor: Vincent Jarlier

Background. Currently, mutations in *rpoB*, *KatG*, and *rrs* genes and *inhA* promoter were considered to be involved in conferring resistance to rifampicin, isoniazid, and streptomycin in *Mycobacterium tuberculosis* (MTB). *Objective.* The aims of this study were to detect the prevalence of first-line tuberculosis (TB) drug resistance among a group of previously treated and newly detected TB patients, to determine the association between prevalence of multidrug resistance (MDR) and demographic information (age and sex), to explain genes correlated with MDR *Mycobacterium tuberculosis*, and to characterize MTB via 16S ribosomal RNA (16S rRNA) analysis. *Methods.* A hundred MTB isolates from Sudanese pulmonary TB patients were included in the study. The proportional method of drug susceptibility test was carried out on Löwenstein-Jensen media. Multiplex PCR of *rpoB* and *KatG* genes and *inhA* promoter was conducted; then *rrs* genes were amplified by conventional PCR and were sequenced. The sequences of the PCR product were compared with known *rrs* gene sequences in the GenBank database by multiple sequence alignment tools. *Result.* The prevalence of MDR was 14.7% among old cases and 5.3% among newly diagnosed cases. *Conclusion.* Mutations in *rrs* could be considered as a diagnostic marker.

1. Introduction

Monitoring of tuberculosis (TB) caused by drug-resistant *Mycobacterium tuberculosis* (MTB) has become one of the major problems throughout the world [1]. However, the detection of drug-resistant phenotypes of MTB takes at least 3–6 weeks by direct and indirect methods, respectively. Thus, treatment was prescribed empirically. Patients who fail to respond to drugs remain infectious [2]. They may be a source of transmission of infections [3].

Sudan is surrounded by high burden countries [4] and it harbors a high TB incidence among the East Mediterranean countries. The prevalence of TB infection in Sudan is probably variable in different regions [5]. The country has been severely affected by war, famine, and flood in recent decades and has a large population of internally displaced persons, which is considered risk factor of spreading TB. Cases among men exceeded those found in women by a ratio of 2 : 1 [6].

Multidrug-resistant TB (MDR-TB) is defined as MTB that is resistant to first-line anti-TB drugs such as rifampicin (RIF) and isoniazid (INH) [7]. RIF is a broad spectrum antimicrobial agent, which remains the most effective drug against *M. tuberculosis*. Resistance of rifampicin occurs via mutation in *rpoB* gene that encodes the β-subunit of RNA polymerase [8]. INH has the most powerful bactericidal activity against TB and has good tolerance and low price [7]. It is a prodrug, requiring activation through oxidation by a mycobacterial catalase-peroxidase enzyme encoded by *katG* gene [9]. Activated isoniazid interferes with the biosynthesis of essential mycolic acids through inhibition of nicotinamide adenine dinucleotide hydrogen (NADH) dependent enoyl-acyl carrier protein reductase, which is encoded by *inhA* promoter. Alterations in *katG* gene and *inhA* promoter were strongly associated with isoniazid resistance [10, 11]. Streptomycin (SM) was the foremost antibiotic successfully used against TB. Resistance to SM emerged as a result of monotherapy administration [12]. SM is an aminocyclitol glycoside that acts against actively growing bacilli by inhibiting the initiation of translation in protein synthesis at the level of the 30S subunit of the ribosome, specifically at the ribosomal protein S12 and the 16S rRNA coded by *rpsL* and *rrs* genes, respectively [13, 14]. Consequently, mutations in *rpsL* and *rrs* are the major mechanisms of resistance [10]. The aims of the current study were to detect the prevalence of monoresistance and multidrug-resistant *Mycobacterium tuberculosis* (MDR), to determine the association between prevalence of MDR and demographic information (age and sex), to explain the molecular characterization of *M. tuberculosis* through 16S rRNA, and to illustrate the frequency of *rrs* mutations among streptomycin-resistant *M. tuberculosis* isolates.

2. Materials and Methods

This study was approved by the Ethics Committee of the Africa City of Technology and the University of Khartoum, Sudan.

2.1. Mycobacterium tuberculosis Growth Properties. A hundred sputum samples were collected from pulmonary TB patients as a cross-sectional descriptive study conducted at the National Reference Laboratory-Tuberculosis (NRL-TB), Khartoum, Sudan. Samples were processed under biosafety cabinet level II via adding twice the volume of 4% NaOH to sputum in 50 mL centrifuge tube for decontamination and homogenization. Samples were neutralized by buffer, followed by centrifugation at 3000 RCF (Relative Centrifuge Force) for 20 min. Inoculation was adjusted by pipetting 3–5 drops of deposit in three Löwenstein-Jensen media (two containing glycerol and one containing pyruvate) which are egg based media. Then, cultured media were incubated at 37°C in slant position. Subsequently, weekly observation was made to check the growth of bacteria [15–17].

2.2. Drugs Susceptibility Test. Drugs susceptibility test was done through the conventional proportional method on Löwenstein-Jensen (LJ) media containing drugs according to CDC standard procedures [16, 18]. The grown colonies were picked up from the media and emulsified in a thick wall glass tube, containing DW + glass beads, by shaking the tubes well; furthermore, turbidity was adjusted with McFarland standard (number 0.5). The diluted suspension 10^{-4} was cultured on LJ drug-free media as a control and drug containing 0.2 μg/mL isoniazid (INH), 40.0 μg/mL rifampicin (RIF), 4.0 μg/mL streptomycin (SM), and 2.0 μg/mL ethambutol (EMB). The cultured media were incubated at 37°C and were observed after 4 weeks. If there are no colonies or if the ratio between the number of colonies in the media containing drug and the number of colonies in drug-free media is less than 1%, it will be considered sensitive, while if the ratio between the number of colonies in media including drug and the number of colonies in drug-free media is more than 1%, it will be interpreted as resistant to all four drugs. Species identification of *Mycobacterium* was carried out via testing the ability to grow on *p*-nitrobenzoic acid (PNB). All isolates were tested twice in media to confirm the accuracy of the results [19, 20].

2.3. Guanidine Chloride DNA Extraction Method. All scraped colonies were washed with phosphate buffer saline (PBS), followed by the addition of 2 mL lysis buffer, 5 μL proteinase K, 1 mL guanidine chloride, and 300 μL ammonium acetate. Suspensions were incubated overnight at 37°C; on the next day, 2 mL of chilled chloroform was added. After centrifugation, the clear upper layer was collected in a new tube and cold absolute ethanol was added to enhance precipitation of DNA. The pellet was washed with 70% ethanol and then decanted by 70% ethanol and allowed to dry. The pellet was then resuspended with nuclease-free water and qualified using NanoDrop ND-1000 spectrophotometer (NanoDrop Technologies, USA). The DNA samples were stored at −20°C until used for conventional PCR [21, 22].

2.4. GenoLyse Extraction Method. DNA extraction was performed as recommended by the manufacturer (Hain Lifescience). Firstly, collected bacterial colonies were heated for 20 minutes at 100°C in a water bath and then suspended in 100 μL of kit lysis buffer, followed by incubation at 95°C for 5 min; finally, 100 μL of neutralization buffer was added. The mixture was spun at full speed in a tabletop centrifuge with an aerosol tight rotor and then stored at −20°C and then used for multiplex PCR in Line Probe Assay [23].

2.5. Conventional PCR. Fifteen genomic DNA were used as templates for PCR amplification of complete *rrs* gene (16S rRNA). The two primers used were forward primer, namely, 27F (5′-AGAGTTTGATCCTGGCTCAG-3′), and reverse primer, namely, 1495R (5′-CTACGGCTACCTTGTTACGA-3′). The 25 μL reaction mixture contained 1 μL DNA, 1x reaction buffer (10x) with 3 mM $MgCl_2$, 2.5 U i-Taq™ DNA polymerase (5 U/μL), 2.5 mM dNTPs, 1 μL of 10 pmol of each primer, and 1x of gel loading buffer, followed by completing the volume to 25 μL by DW. PCR amplifying procedure was as follows: 5 min at 94°C, 30 cycles of 1 min at 94°C, 1 min at 58°C, 2 min at 72°C, and then 10 min at 72°C, which was performed on a Bio-Rad (DNA engine/Dyad Peltier) automatic thermal cycler. Duplicate PCR of every sample were carried out for more confirmation. The products of amplification were checked through running on 0.6% agarose gel electrophoresis [24, 25].

2.6. Multiplex PCR. Hybridization and detection were performed using the hybridization kits. Seventy-five isolated DNA were used by taking 5 μL of each DNA and mixing it with 10 μL Amplification Mix A and 35 μL Amplification Mix B containing biotinylated primers. The PCR amplifying procedure was as follows: 15 min at 95°C, 10 cycles of 30 seconds at 95°C, 20 cycles of 40 seconds at 50°C, and 8 min at 70°C, which was performed on a Hain Lifescience thermal cycler. The amplification product was visualized through reverse hybridization probes complementary to amplified nucleic acids on membrane strips. [26].

2.7. Sequencing of 16S rRNA. Isolates were packaged according to the International Air Transport Association guidelines and shipped with authorized permission to Macrogen Company (Seoul, South Korea). Purification and standard forward sequencing of 16S rRNA were done by ABI Genetic Analyser (Applied Biosystems).

2.8. Statistical and Bioinformatic Analysis. The result was analysed statistically using IBM SPSS Statistics version 21 (Statistical Package for the Social Sciences) which is a software package for statistical analysis; the chi-square test was used to check the statistical significance [27]. The chromatogram sequences were visualized through Finch TV program version 1.4.0 [28]. The nucleotides sequences of the *rrs* gene were searched for sequences similarity using nucleotide BLAST [29]. Highly similar sequences have accession numbers HM007576, KF796661, JX303293, and GU142936 and sequences of the reference *M. tuberculosis* H37Rv strain [X55588.1] were retrieved from NCBI (https://www.ncbi.nlm.nih.gov/) and subjected to multiple sequence alignment using BioEdit software version 7.2.5 [30]. Newick format was withdrawn from ClustalW (http://www.ebi.ac.uk/Tools/msa/clustalw2) [31] to create a phylogenetic tree in Phylogeny.fr software [32].

2.9. Nucleotide Sequence Accession Numbers. The nucleotide sequences of the *rrs* genes containing novel mutations were deposited in the GenBank database (National Center for Biotechnology Information; https://www.ncbi.nlm.nih.gov/) under the following accession numbers: KU372152, KU372153, KU372154, KU372155, KU372156, and KU372157.

3. Results

Among 100 sputum samples, twenty of them revealed no growth, two were contaminated, one was lysed, and two had grown in PNB indicating *Mycobacterium* other than tuberculosis (MOTT). The growth rate on LJ media is as follows: 39% (29/75) showed +3 (200–500 colonies), 33% (25/75) showed +2 (100–200 colonies), 26.7% (20/75) showed +1 (10–99 colonies), and 1.3% (1/75) showed 4 colonies.

TABLE 1: Percentage of MDR in different age groups.

Age group	MDR %	Account (number)
≤30	60%	9
31–40	13.3%	2
41–50	13.3%	2
51–60	13.3%	2
>60	0%	0

Most of the MDR growth appeared as +1 and probably had grown at 2–4 weeks (*P* value 0.426), showing a statistically insignificant association between growth rate and MDR. The prevalence of MDR was 20% (15/75) and 14.7% (11/15) among previously treated and old cases and 5.3% (4/15) among newly diagnosed cases (*P* value 0.003), which means drug resistance was associated with previous treatment. 73.3% of MDR cases were males, while 26.7% were females (*P* value 0.536). Sixty percent (9/15) of MDR cases were found in the age group ≤ 30 years (*P* value 0.652) (Table 1). Among seventy-five *Mycobacterium tuberculosis* isolates, 56% (42/75) were streptomycin-resistant, 29% (22/75) were rifampicin-resistant, 20% (15/75) were ethambutol-resistant, and 28% (21/75) were isoniazid-resistant. 20% (15/75) were resistant to RIF and INH. 16% (12/75) were resistant to all four drugs. The run progression of the final separation of PCR products was visualized under UV transilluminator documentation machine. Most of them fluoresced sharply, but two of them fluoresced faintly and were excluded. The most common mutation detected by LPA in the *rpoB* gene was S531L (80%, 12/15), followed by H526D; in *KatG* gene, the most common mutation was S315T (67%, 10/15) and in *InhA* promoter it was C15T (33.3%, 7/21).

Sixty-two percent (8/13 isolates) of streptomycin-resistant isolates revealed mutations in *rrs* gene which were identified in seven groups: four isolates (31%) have G → A transition at nucleoside position 892; three isolates (23%) have C → A transversion at nucleoside position 222; two isolates (15%) have A → G transition at nucleoside position 904; one isolate (8%) has G → T transversion at nucleoside position 855; one isolate (8%) has A → G transition at nucleoside position 906; one isolate (8%) has T → A transversion at nucleoside position 1238; and two isolates have G → A/G → C at nucleoside position 1400, which are more explained in Table 2.

3.1. Phylogenetic Tree. A phylogenetic tree represents the relationships among a set of *Mycobacterium tuberculosis*. The tree is classified into two branches. All isolates have a common ancestor except for isolate-9 which was outgroup. Isolate-2 and isolate-4 were sister groups as shown in Figure 1.

4. Discussions

The study found novel transversion mutation of C → A at position 222. To our knowledge, the present study is the first study that demonstrated 16S rRNA analysis among multidrug-resistant *M. tuberculosis* isolates from Sudan, and thus the prevalence of MDR was 20% (15/75) and 14.7% (11/15) among old cases and 5.3% (4/15) among newly diagnosed

TABLE 2: Explaining the position and frequency of polymorphism with resistance pattern of isolates.

Mutation position	Polymorphism	Frequency (%)	Resistance pattern			
			RIF	INH	STM	EMB
222	C → A	23%	R	R	R	S
			S	S	R	S
			R	S	R	S
885	G → T	8%	S	S	R	S
892	G → A	31%	S	R	R	S
			S	S	R	S
			R	R	R	S
			R	R	R	R
904	A → G	15%	S	R	R	S
			R	R	R	R
906	A → G	8%	S	R	R	S
	T → A	8%	R	S	R	S
1400	G → A	8%	R	R	R	R
	G → C	8%	S	S	R	S

R: resistance; S: sensitive; RIF: rifampicin; INH: isoniazid; STM: streptomycin; EMB: ethambutol.

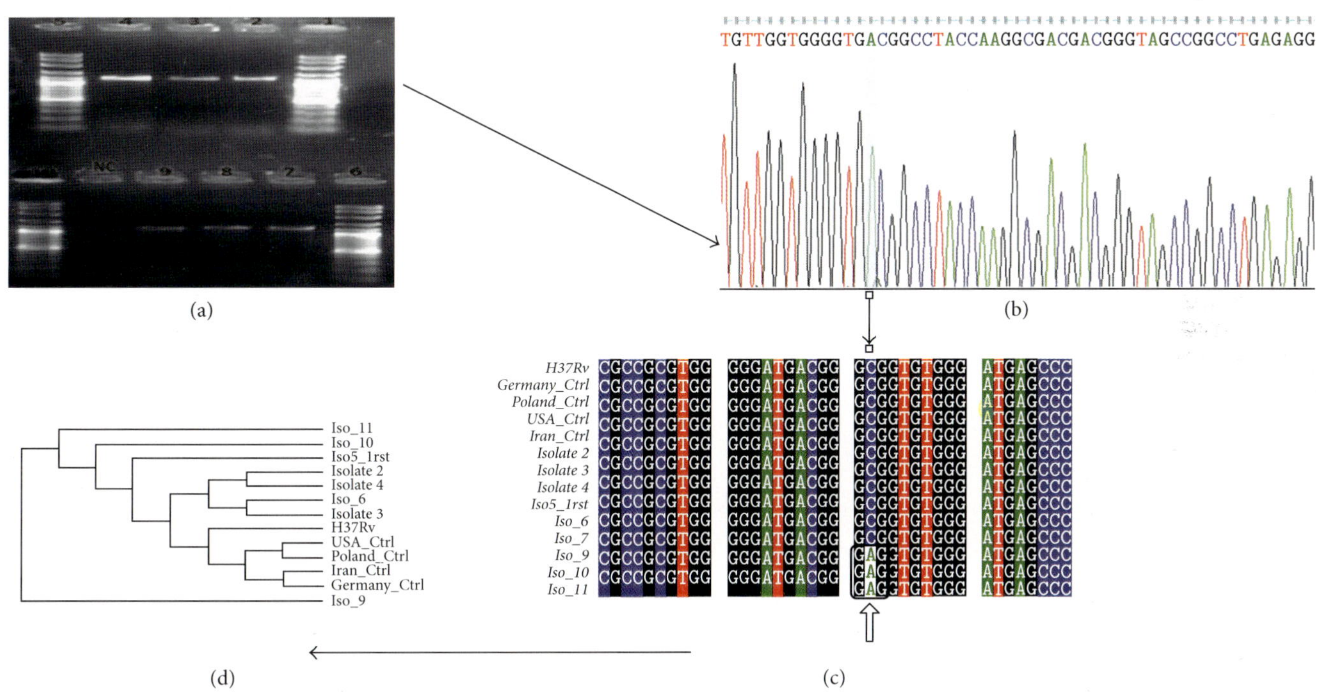

FIGURE 1: (a) Gel electrophoresis of PCR product. Lanes 1 and 5: DNA marker 1000+. Lanes 2, 3, and 4: amplified DNA products, 1500 bp. (b) Chromatogram sequence of 16S rRNA visualized via Finch TV software. (c) Alignment determining novel mutation at position 222, transversion of C to A in isolates 9, 10, and 11 via BioEdit software. (d) Phylogenetic tree using Phylogeny.fr software.

cases, which was lower than France's study with a prevalence of 23/323 (7.1%) in newly diagnosed patients and 33/105 (31.4%) in re-treated patients [33]; this difference could be due to the geographical variation. In the present study, 73.3% of MDR cases were males, while 26.7% were females, which agreed with Raizada et al.'s study where MDR-TB was predominant in males (72%, 230/320) [34] contrary to Melzer et al.'s study where 56.7% in males and 43.3% in females [35] may be due to the large numbers of males when compared with females included in this study. Most MDR cases were found in the age group ≤ 30 years (60%), corresponding with Melzer et al.'s study [35]. The genotype MTBDR*plus* test identified most frequent mutations involved in resistance to RIF and INH as follows: in *rpoB* gene, S531L was 54%

(12/22); this is similar to the findings of Barnard et al. [36]. The final result of mutation frequency in *rrs* gene is 62% which is approximately similar to Asho's study conducted in Pakistan that detected 35/50 (70%) strains [37]. Also, additional studies in China, Japan, and Latvia have reported the highest frequencies, 85.7%, 77.8%, and 85%, respectively [38–40], whereas, in North India, no mutation had been detected in streptomycin-resistant isolates [41]. Regarding mutation in the 912 region, 23% of the isolates have been revealed. A → G transition at position 904 corresponds to studies in Germany [42]. On the other hand, a study in Barcelona did not detect mutation in the rrs912 region [43]. The mutation at loop 530 of the *rrs* coding region had not been identified, which agreed with New York's study [44] and conflicted with Poland's study [45]. Novel mutation could be used as a diagnostic marker that represents a tool for rapid monitoring of streptomycin resistance and could be of value to the clinician.

Small sample size was one of the drawbacks that limited our study; therefore, a large sample size in further studies could be useful for the determination of other biomarkers that assist the diagnosis of streptomycin-resistant MTB.

5. Conclusion

Analysis of 16S rRNA sequences is considered the golden standard method for the identification and assessment of phylogenetic relationships among bacterial isolates.

Competing Interests

The authors declare that they have no competing interests.

Acknowledgments

The authors are grateful to Africa City of Technology, National Public Health Laboratory, Molecular Tuberculosis Laboratory, and all members of the National Reference Laboratory of Tuberculosis (NRL-TB), Sudan, Khartoum.

References

[1] World Health Organization, *Global Tuberculosis Report 2015*, chapter 4, WHO/HTM/TB/2015.22, Geneva, Switzerland, 20th edition, 2015.

[2] D. A. Mitchison and A. J. Nunn, "Influence of initial drug resistance on the response to short-course chemotherapy of pulmonary tuberculosis," *American Review of Respiratory Disease*, vol. 133, no. 3, pp. 423–430, 1986.

[3] A. L. Kritski, M. J. Ozorio Marques, M. F. Rabahi et al., "Transmission of tuberculosis to close contacts of patients with multidrug-resistant tuberculosis," *American Journal of Respiratory and Critical Care Medicine*, vol. 153, no. 1, pp. 331–335, 1996.

[4] WHO, *Global Tuberculosis Control 2014*, WHO, Geneva, Switzerland, 2014, http://www.who.int/tb/publications/global_report/.

[5] World Health Organization/IUATLD, "Global project on anti-tuberculosis drug resistance surveillance," Report 3, World Health Organization/IUATLD, Geneva, Switzerland, 2003.

[6] A. S. Rhines, "The role of sex differences in the prevalence and transmission of tuberculosis," *Tuberculosis*, vol. 93, no. 1, pp. 104–107, 2013.

[7] J. A. Caminero, Ed., *Guidelines for Clinical and Operational Management of Drug-Resistant Tuberculosis*, International Union Against Tuberculosis and Lung Disease, Paris, France, 2013.

[8] A. Somoskovi, L. M. Parsons, and M. Salfinger, "The molecular basis of resistance to isoniazid, rifampin, and pyrazinamide in *Mycobacterium tuberculosis*," *Respiratory Research*, vol. 2, no. 3, pp. 164–168, 2001.

[9] Y. Zhang, B. Heym, B. Allen, D. Young, and S. Cole, "The catalase—peroxidase gene and isoniazid resistance of *Mycobacterium tuberculosis*," *Nature*, vol. 358, no. 6387, pp. 591–593, 1992.

[10] S. H. Gillespie, "Evolution of drug resistance in *Mycobacterium tuberculosis*: clinical and molecular perspective," *Antimicrobial Agents and Chemotherapy*, vol. 46, no. 2, pp. 267–274, 2002.

[11] B. Heym, Y. Zhang, S. Poulet, D. Young, and S. T. Cole, "Characterization of the katG gene encoding a catalase-peroxidase required for the isoniazid susceptibility of *Mycobacterium tuberculosis*," *Journal of Bacteriology*, vol. 175, no. 13, pp. 4255–4259, 1993.

[12] J. Crofton and D. A. Mitchison, "Streptomycin resistance in pulmonary tuberculosis," *British Medical Journal*, vol. 2, pp. 1009–1015, 1948.

[13] D. Moazed and H. F. Noller, "Interaction of antibiotics with functional sites in 16S ribosomal RNA," *Nature*, vol. 327, no. 6121, pp. 389–394, 1987.

[14] M. Finken, P. Kirschner, A. Meier, A. Wrede, and E. C. Böttger, "Molecular basis of streptomycin resistance in Mycobacterium tuberculosis: alterations of the ribosomal protein S12 gene and point mutations within a functional 16S ribosomal RNA pseudoknot," *Molecular Microbiology*, vol. 9, no. 6, pp. 1239–1246, 1993.

[15] WHO, *Laboratory Services in Tuberculosis Control, Part II and III: Microscopy and Culture*, WHO, 1998.

[16] P. T. Kent and G. P. Kubica, *Public Health Mycobacteriology, Guides For Level III Laboratory*, US Department of Health and Human Services, Public Health Service, CDC, 1985.

[17] S.-J. Kim, G.-H. Bai, and H.-D. Hwang, "Efficiency of the direct and concentration methods in demonstrating tubercle bacilli in the sputum specimens," *Tuberculosis and Respiratory Diseases*, vol. 36, no. 4, pp. 354–361, 1989.

[18] V. Vincent and M. C. Gutiérrez, "*Mycobacterium*: laboratory characteristics of slowly growing mycobacteria," in *Manual of Clinical Microbiology*, pp. 573–588, American Society for Microbiology, Washington, DC, USA, 2007.

[19] C. Collins, J. Grange, and M. Yates, *Organization and Practice in Tuberculosis Bacteriology*, Butterworth, London, UK, 1985.

[20] G. Canetti, W. Fox, A. Khomenko et al., "Advances in techniques of testing mycobacterial drug sensitivity, and the use of sensitivity tests in tuberculosis control programmes," *Bulletin of the World Health Organization*, vol. 41, no. 1, pp. 21–43, 1969.

[21] DNA Extraction Guanidine Method, Modified from Black well Lab, Cambridge, UK.

[22] S. A. Miller, D. D. Dykes, and H. F. Polesky, "A simple salting out procedure for extracting DNA from human nucleated cells," *Nucleic Acids Research*, vol. 16, no. 3, p. 1215, 1988.

[23] Hain Life Science, Hardwiesenstraße, Nehren, Germany, http://www.hain-lifescience.de.

[24] W. Liu, Q. Bao, Jirimutu et al., "Isolation and identification of lactic acid bacteria from Tarag in Eastern Inner Mongolia of China by 16S rRNA sequences and DGGE analysis," *Microbiological Research*, vol. 167, no. 2, pp. 110–115, 2012.

[25] iNtRON BIOTECHNOLOGY, Maxime PCR PreMix Kit (i-Taq) for 20μl rxn, Cat. NO. 25025, http://www.intronbio.com/.

[26] "Genotype MTBDR*plus*™, version 1.0 [product insert]," Nehren, Germany: Hain Lifescience, GmbH. Hain lifescience website, http://www.hainlifescience.com/pdf/304xx_pbl.pdf.

[27] IBM SPSS Statistics for Windows, Version 21.0. Armonk, NY: IBM Corp, Released 2012, http://www.ibm.com/analytics/us/en/technology/spss/.

[28] http://www.geospiza.com/Products/finchtv.shtml.

[29] https://blast.ncbi.nlm.nih.gov/Blast.cgi.

[30] T. A. Hall, "BioEdit: a user-friendly biological sequence alignment editor and analysis program for Windows 95/98/NT," *Nucleic Acids Symposium Series*, vol. 41, pp. 95–98, 1999.

[31] H. McWilliam, W. Li, M. Uludag et al., "Analysis Tool Web Services from the EMBL-EBI," *Nucleic acids research*, vol. 41, pp. W597–W600, 2013.

[32] A. Dereeper, V. Guignon, G. Blanc et al., "Phylogeny.fr: robust phylogenetic analysis for the non-specialist," *Nucleic Acids Research*, vol. 36, pp. W465–W469, 2008.

[33] J. Lyu, M.-N. Kim, J. W. Song et al., "GenoType® MTBDR*plus* assay detection of drug-resistant tuberculosis in routine practice in Korea," *The International Journal of Tuberculosis and Lung Disease*, vol. 17, no. 1, pp. 120–124, 2013.

[34] N. Raizada, K. S. Sachdeva, D. S. Chauhan et al., "A Multi-site validation in India of the line probe assay for the rapid diagnosis of multi-drug resistant tuberculosis directly from sputum specimens," *PLoS ONE*, vol. 9, no. 2, Article ID e88626, 2014.

[35] M. Melzer, N. Gupta, I. Petersen, S. Cook, and B. Hall, "Previous treatment in predicting drug-resistant tuberculosis in an area bordering East London, UK," *International Journal of Infectious Diseases*, vol. 14, no. 8, pp. e717–e722, 2010.

[36] M. Barnard, H. Albert, G. Coetzee, R. O'Brien, and M. E. Bosman, "Rapid molecular screening for multidrug-resistant tuberculosis in a high-volume public health laboratory in South Africa," *American Journal of Respiratory and Critical Care Medicine*, vol. 177, no. 7, pp. 787–792, 2008.

[37] A. Ali, R. Hasan, K. Jabeen, N. Jabeen, E. Qadeer, and Z. Hasan, "Characterization of mutations conferring extensive drug resistance to *Mycobacterium tuberculosis* isolates in Pakistan," *Antimicrobial Agents and Chemotherapy*, vol. 55, no. 12, pp. 5654–5659, 2011.

[38] X.-Q. Wu, Y. Lu, J.-X. Zhang et al., "Detection of streptomycin resistance in *Mycobacterium tuberculosis* clinical isolates using four molecular methods in China," *Acta Genetica Sinica*, vol. 33, no. 7, pp. 655–663, 2006.

[39] C. Katsukawa, A. Tamaru, Y. Miyata, C. Abe, M. Makino, and Y. Suzuki, "Characterization of the *rpsL* and *rrs* genes of streptomycin-resistant clinical isolates of *Mycobacterium tuberculosis* in Japan," *Journal of Applied Microbiology*, vol. 83, no. 5, pp. 634–640, 1997.

[40] T. Tracevska, I. Jansone, A. Nodieva, O. Margab, G. Skendersc, and V. Baumanisa, "Characterization of *rpsl*, *rrs* and *embB* mutation associated Streptomycin and Euthambutol resistance in *Mycobacterium Tuberculosis*," *Microbiological Research*, vol. 155, pp. 830–834, 2007.

[41] N. Siddiqi, M. Shamim, S. Hussain et al., "Molecular characterization of multidrug-resistant isolates of *Mycobacterium Tuberculosis* from patients in North India," *Antimicrobial Agents and Chemotherapy*, vol. 46, no. 2, pp. 443–450, 2002.

[42] A. Meier, P. Kirschner, F.-C. Bange, U. Vogel, and E. C. Bottger, "Genetic alterations in streptomycin-resistant *Mycobacterium tuberculosis*: mapping of mutations conferring resistance," *Antimicrobial Agents and Chemotherapy*, vol. 38, no. 2, pp. 228–233, 1994.

[43] G. Tudó, E. Rey, S. Borrell et al., "Characterization of mutations in streptomycin-resistant *Mycobacterium tuberculosis* clinical isolates in the area of Barcelona," *Journal of Antimicrobial Chemotherapy*, vol. 65, no. 11, Article ID dkq322, pp. 2341–2346, 2010.

[44] R. C. Cooksey, G. P. Morlock, A. Mcqueen, S. E. Glickman, and J. T. Crawford, "Characterization of streptomycin resistance mechanisms among *Mycobacterium tuberculosis* isolates from patients in New York City," *Antimicrobial Agents and Chemotherapy*, vol. 40, no. 5, pp. 1186–1188, 1996.

[45] T. Jagielski, H. Ignatowska, Z. Bakuła et al., "Screening for streptomycin resistance-conferring mutations in *Mycobacterium tuberculosis* clinical isolates from Poland," *PLoS ONE*, vol. 9, no. 6, Article ID e100078, 2014.

36

Tuberculosis as an Etiological Factor in Liver Abscess in Adults

Jaideep Dey,[1] Hitender Gautam,[2] Shwetha Venugopal,[2] Chhavi Porwal,[2] Bijay Ranjan Mirdha,[2] Naresh Gupta,[3] and Urvashi B. Singh[2]

[1] *Department of Medicine, Lady Hardinge Medical College, New Delhi, India*
[2] *Department of Microbiology, All India Institute of Medical Sciences, New Delhi 110029, India*
[3] *Department of Medicine, Maulana Azad Medical College, New Delhi, India*

Correspondence should be addressed to Urvashi B. Singh; drurvashi@gmail.com

Academic Editor: Carlo Garzelli

Background. Tuberculosis of the liver without active pulmonary or miliary tuberculosis is considered as an uncommon diagnosis. The aim of the present study was to determine the etiological role of tuberculosis in adult patients presenting with features of liver abscess. *Methods.* A total of 40 patients with liver abscess were included in the study. The liver abscess aspirate was subjected to microscopy, culture, and polymerase chain reaction to determine the role of tuberculosis as an etiological factor in liver abscess. *Results.* Of the 40 patients enrolled, 25% (10/40) were diagnosed with having tubercular liver abscess. In a total of 40 specimens, 2.5% (1/40) were positive for acid fast bacilli by Ziehl-Neelsen method, while 10% (4/40) were positive for *M. tuberculosis* by culture using BACTEC 460 and the yield increased to 25% (10/40) by polymerase chain reaction for *M. tuberculosis*. *Conclusion.* 25% of the patients presenting with liver abscess had tubercular etiology without features of active pulmonary or miliary tuberculosis. Liver can act as the primary site of involvement in the absence of activity elsewhere in the body. Tuberculosis should be considered as an important differential diagnosis of liver abscess irrespective of evidence of active tuberculosis elsewhere in the body.

1. Introduction

Tuberculosis can involve possibly all organs in the human body [1]. Liver is an organ most susceptible to the development of abscesses, caused by numerous organisms, amoebic, bacterial, mycobacterial, or fungal in origin. Liver involvement in pulmonary and extrapulmonary TB is usually clinically silent [2].

Tubercular liver abscess in itself is a rare entity. The disease mimics liver abscess of other etiology, and the diagnosis is frequently missed due to lack of suspicion. Despite reports of involvement of liver in miliary TB, demonstrated in the form of tubercular granulomas in liver tissues [3, 4], local or primary hepatic TB without active pulmonary or miliary TB is considered an uncommon diagnosis [5].

Conventional methods for diagnosis of TB have been ineffective for peritoneal and liver TB; mean sensitivity of culture and AFB smear is 8.3–83% (depending on amount cultured and method utilized) and 3.2%, respectively [6]. In some studies, diagnosis was based on response to empirical antitubercular therapy (ATT) or laparotomy or even autopsy [5]. With increasing reports of resistance to ATT and the morbidity involved with its prolonged usage, response to empirical ATT is an inefficient diagnostic marker.

Liver abscess has traditionally been ascribed to etiologies other than TB [7–10]. The present study was designed to define the role of *Mycobacterium tuberculosis* (M. tb) as the etiological agent for liver abscess in adult patients with no evidence of active TB elsewhere in the body.

2. Materials and Methods

Forty consecutive subjects with clinical profile and radiological evidence of liver abscess from outpatient clinics, wards, and emergency departments of medicine at Lady Hardinge Medical College and Dr. Ram Manohar Lohia Hospital, New Delhi, were included in the study. Informed consent was obtained from each participant and clinical history collected.

Patients were excluded from this study if they were hemodynamically unstable, required monitoring in intensive care

TABLE 1: Presenting symptoms and history of patients in the study group.

Symptoms	Overall study group ($n = 40$)	Tubercular group ($n = 10$)	Nontubercular group ($n = 30$)	p value
Fever	92.5%	100%	90%	$p > 0.05\%$
Abdominal pain	92.5%	100%	90%	$p > 0.05\%$
Weight loss	44.5%	30%	53%	$p > 0.05\%$
Jaundice	17.5%	0%	23%	$p > 0.05\%$
Past h/o tuberculosis	20%	50%	10%	$p < 0.05$

TABLE 2: Laboratory profile of patients.

	Overall study group ($n = 40$)	Tubercular group ($n = 10$)	Nontubercular group ($n = 30$)	p value
Hb (<10 g/dL)	75%	88%	70%	$p > 0.05$
Leucocytosis	78%	80%	77%	$p > 0.05$
Raised ESR	85%	90%	83%	$p > 0.05$
Raised serum bilirubin	20%	10%	23%	$p > 0.05$
Raised serum liver enzymes	70%	80%	67%	$p > 0.05$
Raised alkaline phosphatase	95%	100%	93%	$p > 0.05$
Deranged coagulation profile	40%	40%	13%	$p > 0.05$
Mantoux test positive	23%	50%	13%	$p < 0.05$

units, were unable to undergo the requisite workup, and had uncontrolled coagulation defects. The clinical data obtained from each patient included (i) detailed medical history, (ii) clinical features, (iii) hematological laboratory profile like Hb%, leukocyte count, and erythrocyte sedimentation ratio, (iv) liver function test parameters, (v) Mantoux test reactivity, (vi) chest radiography, (vii) ultrasound examination of the abdomen, (viii) stool examination for ova/cyst, and (ix) serological tests for hepatitis B and hepatitis C and Human Immunodeficiency Virus (HIV).

Patients underwent diagnostic ultrasound guided aspiration for liver abscess. The aspirate was subjected to gram stain, bacterial culture, and microscopy for trophozoites and cysts of *Entamoeba histolytica.* The tubercular etiology of the liver abscess was diagnosed by Ziehl-Neelsen (ZN) staining for acid fast bacilli, culture by liquid culture (BACTEC 460), and detection of M. tb DNA using *Mpt64 gene* polymerase chain reaction performed on the liver aspirate.

Chi-square test was used to study the statistical significance of differences between patients with tubercular etiology and nontubercular etiology.

3. Results

Of 40 specimens, one (2.5%) was positive for acid fast bacilli by ZN method, while 4/40 (10%) were positive for M. tb by culture using BACTEC 460 (Becton Dickinson) and the yield increased to 10/40 (25%) by PCR for M. tb.

The mean age of the patients in the study was 40.35 ± 13.03 years (mean ± SD) and of the tubercular liver abscess patients was 41.9 ± 13.57 years. Male to female ratio in the study was 4.7 : 1 (82.5% male, 17.5% female) and in tubercular group was 4 : 1. The predominant symptoms in the study, in both tubercular and nontubercular liver abscess patients, were fever and abdominal pain (Table 1).

Twenty percent of the patients in the study but 50% of the patients in tubercular group had past history of TB and had taken ATT ($p < 0.05$) (Table 1). The family history of TB was given by 15% of the patients in the study, 20% in the tubercular group and 13% in nontubercular group. 20% each from the study group, tubercular and nontubercular group had past history of dysentery.

The mean body mass index (BMI) in the study group was 19.93 ± 2.47 kg/m^2, 20.46 ± 2.99 in tubercular group, and 19.27 ± 2.29 in nontubercular group. Hepatomegaly was present in all, mean 5.45 ± 2.75 cm in the study, 4.84 ± 1.55 in tubercular group and 5.66 ± 3.04 cm in nontubercular group. The liver span in the study group was 16.53 ± 3.42 cm, in tubercular group 16.35 ± 2.54 and in nontubercular group 16.6 ± 3.7.

The laboratory data including the hematological profile and liver function tests did not show statistically significant difference between the tubercular and nontubercular liver abscess patients (Table 2). The mantoux test gave 22.5% positives in the study group and 50% in the tubercular group ($p < 0.05$) (Table 2). Chest roentgenography was abnormal in 8 study patients (20%); only 2 (20%) were in tubercular group while the rest were in nontubercular group.

On ultrasonography of the abdomen, majority of patients (82.5%) had only right lobe liver abscess, 7.5% had only left lobe liver abscess and 10% had abscess involving both the lobes. Stool examination for cysts/trophozoites showed cysts of *Entamoeba histolytica* in one patient who belonged to the tubercular group. Acid fast bacilli were not detected in the stool of any patient.

The viral serological markers for hepatitis B were detected positive in 5% patients in the nontubercular group, while none of the patients were positive for hepatitis C and HIV. The aspirated pus of all the patients was negative using Gram stain, bacterial culture, and microscopy for trophozoites or cysts of *Entamoeba histolytica.*

4. Discussion

Smear examination for acid fast bacilli and conventional culture techniques are the widely used methods of TB diagnosis. Acid fast smears in hepatic TB have shown higher frequency among miliary TB patients [4, 11]. Yamaguchi and Braunstein have shown higher yield with fluorescent staining techniques [12]. In a recent study, sensitivity of conventional methods was 12% and that of PCR assay was 88% [13]. PCR assay increased the sensitivity of detection of M. tb among patients with hepatic granulomas. In the present study while the PCR detected 25% of liver abscess as tubercular, liquid culture and ZN staining could detect only 10% and 2.5%, respectively. More sensitive tests hence hold promise for increasing the yield of diagnosis.

Fever and abdominal pain were the predominant symptoms in the study and tubercular liver abscess group. The other symptoms were weight loss and jaundice, similar to previous studies in hepatic TB [3–5, 14, 15]. The past history of TB and history of previous treatment with ATT were statistically significant in the tubercular liver abscess group (Table 1). Careful history taking may provide a clue to the diagnosis of tubercular liver abscess.

On clinical examination, hepatomegaly was present in all the patients in the study; other studies [3–5, 14, 15] have shown hepatomegaly in 80–96% of patients with hepatic TB. The mean liver span was similar in the tubercular and nontubercular groups.

The liver function tests, though nonspecific, have been used to screen patients for hepatic TB. Some authors have shown raised serum-alkaline phosphatase (SAP) as suggestive of hepatic TB [4, 16], while others have shown presence of normal levels does not rule out hepatic TB [17]. In the present study, raised SAP was seen in 100% of tubercular group and 93% of the nontubercular group. This strengthens the view that abnormal SAP values should be considered with discretion. Serum levels of liver enzymes such as aspartate aminotransferase and alanine aminotransferase were raised in 80% in tubercular group; others have reported elevated levels in 70% [4]. Abnormalities in these enzyme levels in hepatic TB patients were present in 91–94% of jaundiced group and in only 5% of the nonjaundiced patients [18]. Other parameters like serum albumin, serum globulin, albumin/globulin ratio, and gamma-glutamyl transpeptidase were considered in some of the studies [4, 5, 15] but are nonspecific for hepatic TB. Thus abnormalities in liver function test parameters cannot be relied on for the diagnosis of hepatic TB.

In the present study, Mantoux test was positive in 22.5% and was statistically significant among tubercular group when compared with nontubercular group (Table 2). Oliva et al. in his review stated that out of 15 cases of isolated tuberculoma and tubercular liver abscess, 11 had positive reactions of tuberculin skin test whereas two patients were negative and two were anergic [14]. Guckian and Perry reported 41% patients were positive for tuberculin skin test [18].

Chest radiograph in the present study showed abnormalities in 20% study patients; only two belonged to the tubercular group; other studies have also reported normal chest X-rays in patients with local hepatic TB [19–23]. Some authors have shown abnormal chest X-ray in 65–78% in hepatic TB [4, 5, 15]. Essop et al. have published chest radiograph abnormality in 86% patients with acute (miliary) TB, while 25% of chest X-rays in chronic hepatic TB and all of the radiographs in local hepatic TB were normal [4]. Thus diagnosis cannot be excluded based on the normal chest radiograph.

The hypoechoic lesions and complex masses shown in ultrasound of the liver could not differentiate between liver abscess and carcinoma [24–28]. Though hypoechoic lesions are commonly seen in tubercular liver abscess, rarely hyperechoic lesions are also described in the literature [29]. In the present study, right lobe involvement was predominant and there was no statistically significant difference in the pattern of the abscess between tubercular and nontubercular group. Other imaging techniques like computed tomography of the abdomen, technetium colloid liver scans, and abdomen radiography are poorly suggestive of hepatic TB [4, 5, 15].

The study lent credence to the hypothesis that liver abscess can have etiologies other than *Entamoeba histolytica* causing amebiasis. One-quarter of the study patients were clearly shown to have TB as the only etiology of the liver abscess; the abscess probably develops from coalescing caseating nodules as described by Oliva et al. [14]. The study sums up that a patient presenting with symptoms of fever with abdominal pain in addition to an enlarged liver, with or without complaints of weight loss and usually without jaundice, along with a positive Mantoux test and a past history of TB should raise the suspicion of tubercular liver involvement even in the absence of chest/systemic involvement especially in a country with high prevalence of tuberculosis like India, which has one-fourth of the global incident TB cases, estimated annual incidence of 2.2 million TB cases, prevalence of 2.5 million, and annual mortality of 0.22 million, respectively [30]. It is important to keep the differential diagnosis of TB in order to reach the correct etiological diagnosis of liver abscess and instituting early treatment.

Competing Interests

The authors declare that they have no competing interests.

Acknowledgments

The authors acknowledge the cooperation of the patients and the support of the laboratory staff from Tuberculosis Division, Department of Microbiology, AIIMS, New Delhi.

References

[1] A. J. McAdam and A. H. Sharpe, "Infectious diseases: mycobacteria," in *Robbins and Cotran Pathologic Basis of Diseases*, pp. 381–386, Elsevier, Philadelphia, Pa, USA, 2004.

[2] T. B. Reynolds, J. L. Campra, and R. L. Peters, "Hepatic granuloma," in *Hepatology-A Textbook of Liver Disease*, D. Zakim and T. D. Boyer, Eds., p. 108, W.B. Saunders, Philadelphia, Pa, USA, 2nd edition, 1990.

[3] C. Hersch, "Tuberculosis of the liver. A study of 200 cases," *South African Medical Journal*, vol. 38, pp. 857–863, 1964.

[4] A. R. Essop, J. A. Posen, J. H. Hodkinson, and I. Segal, "Tuberculosis hepatitis: a clinical review of 96 cases," *Quarterly Journal of Medicine*, vol. 53, no. 212, pp. 465–477, 1984.

[5] S. Z. Alvarez and R. Carpio, "Hepatobiliary tuberculosis," *Digestive Diseases and Sciences*, vol. 28, no. 3, pp. 193–200, 1983.

[6] D. J. Hillebrand, B. A. Runyon, W. G. Yasmineh D, and G. P. Rynders, "Ascitic fluid adenosine deaminase insensitivity in detecting tuberculous peritonitis in the United States," *Hepatology*, vol. 24, no. 6, pp. 1408–1412, 1996.

[7] T. Tsunoda, T. Shiogama, M. Koga et al., "Tuberculous liver abscess with bronchobiliary and gastrobiliary fistulae-a case report," *The Japanese Journal of Surgery*, vol. 21, no. 1, pp. 100–104, 1991.

[8] A. R. Pottipati, P. B. Dave, V. Gumaste, and U. Vieux, "Tuberculous abscess of the liver in acquired immunodeficiency syndrome," *Journal of Clinical Gastroenterology*, vol. 13, no. 5, pp. 549–553, 1991.

[9] A. R. Essop, I. Segal, J. Posen, and N. Noormohamed, "Tuberculous abscess of the liver," *South African Medical Journal*, vol. 63, no. 21, pp. 825–826, 1983.

[10] D. Balsarkar and M. A. Joshi, "Isolated tuberculous hepatic abscess in a non-immunocompromised patient," *Journal of Postgraduate Medicine*, vol. 46, no. 2, pp. 108–109, 2000.

[11] P. T. Harrington, J. J. Gutiérrez, C. H. Ramirez-Ronda, R. Quiñones-Soto, R. H. Bermúdez, and J. Chaffey, "Granulomatous hepatitis.," *Reviews of Infectious Diseases*, vol. 4, no. 3, pp. 638–655, 1982.

[12] B. T. Yamaguchi and H. Braunstein, "Fluorescent stain for tubercle bacilli in histologic sections. II. Diagnostic efficiency in granulomatous lesions of the liver," *American Journal of Clinical Pathology*, vol. 43, pp. 184–187, 1965.

[13] D. E. Alcantara-Payawal, M. Matsumura, Y. Shiratori et al., "Direct detection of *Mycobacterium tuberculosis* using polymerase chain reaction assay among patients with hepatic granuloma," *Journal of Hepatology*, vol. 27, no. 4, pp. 620–627, 1997.

[14] A. Oliva, B. Duarte, O. Jonasson, and V. Nadimpalli, "The nodular form of local hepatic tuberculosis. A review," *Journal of Clinical Gastroenterology*, vol. 12, no. 2, pp. 166–173, 1990.

[15] B. Maharaj, W. P. Leary, and D. J. Pudifin, "A prospective study of hepatic tuberculosis in 41 black patients," *Quarterly Journal of Medicine*, vol. 63, no. 242, pp. 517–522, 1987.

[16] R. S. Ross, F. L. Iber, and A. M. Harvey, "The serum alkaline phosphatase in chronic infiltrative disease of the liver," *The American Journal of Medicine*, vol. 21, no. 6, pp. 850–856, 1956.

[17] B. B. Frank and E. C. Raffensperger, "Hepatic granulomata. Report of a case with jaundice improving on antituberculous therapy and review of the literature," *Archives of Internal Medicine*, vol. 115, pp. 223–234, 1965.

[18] J. C. Guckian and J. E. Perry, "Granulomatous hepatitis: an analysis of 63 cases and review of the literature," *Annals of Internal Medicine*, vol. 65, no. 5, pp. 1081–1100, 1966.

[19] B. S. Johri, M. P. Kane, and N. S. Mudbhatkal, "Isolated tuberculosis of the liver," *Indian Journal of Medical Sciences*, vol. 24, no. 1, pp. 15–21, 1970.

[20] A. Stevens and J. M. Little, "Isolated tuberculous hepatic abscess," *Australian and New Zealand Journal of Surgery*, vol. 57, no. 6, pp. 409–411, 1987.

[21] R. D. Zipser, J. E. Rau, R. R. Ricketts, and L. C. Bevans, "Tuberculous pseudotumors of the liver," *The American Journal of Medicine*, vol. 61, no. 6, pp. 946–951, 1976.

[22] J. Abascal, F. Martin, L. Abreu et al., "Atypical hepatic tuberculosis presenting as obstructive jaundice," *American Journal of Gastroenterology*, vol. 83, no. 10, pp. 1183–1186, 1988.

[23] R. B. Terry and R. M. Gunnar, "Primary miliary tuberculosis of the liver," *The Journal of the American Medical Association*, vol. 164, no. 2, pp. 150–157, 1957.

[24] R. A. Mustard, R. L. Mackenzie, and R. G. Gray, "Percutaneous drainage of a tuberculous liver abscess," *Canadian Journal of Surgery*, vol. 29, no. 6, pp. 449–450, 1986.

[25] S. Blangy, F. Cornud, A. Sibert, C. Vissuzaine, J. L. Saraux, and R. Benacerraf, "Hepatitis tuberculosis presenting as tumoral disease on ultrasonography," *Gastrointestinal Radiology*, vol. 13, no. 1, pp. 52–54, 1988.

[26] H. S. Chan and J. Pang, "Isolated giant tuberculomata of the liver detected by computed tomography," *Gastrointestinal Radiology*, vol. 14, no. 1, pp. 305–307, 1989.

[27] M. Brauner, M. D. Buffard, V. Jeantils, I. Legrand, and C. Gotheil, "Sonography and computed tomography of macroscopic tuberculosis of the liver," *Journal of Clinical Ultrasound*, vol. 17, no. 8, pp. 563–568, 1989.

[28] B. M. Epstein and C. B. Leibowitz, "Ultrasonographic and computed tomographic appearance of focal tuberculosis of the liver. A case report," *South African Medical Journal*, vol. 71, no. 7, pp. 461–462, 1987.

[29] H.-C. Chen, Y.-C. Chao, R.-Y. Shyu, and T.-Y. Hsieh, "Isolated tuberculous liver abscesses with multiple hyperechoic masses on ultrasound: a case report and review of the literature," *Liver International*, vol. 23, no. 5, pp. 346–350, 2003.

[30] TB, *Revised National Tuberculosis Control Programme Overview 2016*, Central TB Division, Directorate General of Health Services, Ministry of Health and Family Welfare, New Delhi, India, 2016.

Permissions

All chapters in this book were first published in TRT, by Hindawi Publishing Corporation; hereby published with permission under the Creative Commons Attribution License or equivalent. Every chapter published in this book has been scrutinized by our experts. Their significance has been extensively debated. The topics covered herein carry significant findings which will fuel the growth of the discipline. They may even be implemented as practical applications or may be referred to as a beginning point for another development.

The contributors of this book come from diverse backgrounds, making this book a truly international effort. This book will bring forth new frontiers with its revolutionizing research information and detailed analysis of the nascent developments around the world.

We would like to thank all the contributing authors for lending their expertise to make the book truly unique. They have played a crucial role in the development of this book. Without their invaluable contributions this book wouldn't have been possible. They have made vital efforts to compile up to date information on the varied aspects of this subject to make this book a valuable addition to the collection of many professionals and students.

This book was conceptualized with the vision of imparting up-to-date information and advanced data in this field. To ensure the same, a matchless editorial board was set up. Every individual on the board went through rigorous rounds of assessment to prove their worth. After which they invested a large part of their time researching and compiling the most relevant data for our readers.

The editorial board has been involved in producing this book since its inception. They have spent rigorous hours researching and exploring the diverse topics which have resulted in the successful publishing of this book. They have passed on their knowledge of decades through this book. To expedite this challenging task, the publisher supported the team at every step. A small team of assistant editors was also appointed to further simplify the editing procedure and attain best results for the readers.

Apart from the editorial board, the designing team has also invested a significant amount of their time in understanding the subject and creating the most relevant covers. They scrutinized every image to scout for the most suitable representation of the subject and create an appropriate cover for the book.

The publishing team has been an ardent support to the editorial, designing and production team. Their endless efforts to recruit the best for this project, has resulted in the accomplishment of this book. They are a veteran in the field of academics and their pool of knowledge is as vast as their experience in printing. Their expertise and guidance has proved useful at every step. Their uncompromising quality standards have made this book an exceptional effort. Their encouragement from time to time has been an inspiration for everyone.

The publisher and the editorial board hope that this book will prove to be a valuable piece of knowledge for researchers, students, practitioners and scholars across the globe.

List of Contributors

Poojan Shrestha, Amit Arjyal, Abhilasha Karkey, Sabina Dongol, Saruna Pathak, Shanti Prajapati and Buddha Basnyat
Oxford University Clinical Research Unit, Patan Hospital, Patan Academy of Health Sciences, Kathmandu, Nepal

Maxine Caws
Department of Clinical Sciences, Liverpool School of Tropical Medicine, Pembroke Place, Liverpool L3 5QA, UK
Oxford University Clinical Research Unit, Hospital for Tropical Diseases, Wellcome Trust Major Overseas Programme, 764 Vo Van Kiet, District 5, Ho Chi Minh City, Vietnam

Krishna Govinda Prajapati
Department of Microbiology and Immunology, Patan Hospital, Patan Academy of Health Sciences, Kathmandu, Nepal

Christopher Vinnard
Division of Infectious Diseases and HIV Medicine, College of Medicine, Drexel University, 245 N. 15th Street MS 461, New College Building 6314, Philadelphia, PA 19102, USA

Anand Gopal
College of Arts and Sciences, University of Pennsylvania, Philadelphia, PA 19104, USA

Darren R. Linkin
Division of Infectious Diseases, Department of Medicine, Perelman School of Medicine, University of Pennsylvania, Philadelphia, PA 19104, USA
Department of Medicine, Philadelphia VA Medical Center, Philadelphia, PA 19104, USA
Center for Clinical Epidemiology and Biostatistics, Perelman School of Medicine, University of Pennsylvania, Philadelphia, PA 19104, USA

Joel Maslow
Division of Infectious Diseases, Morristown Medical Center, Morristown, NJ 07962, USA

Gerardo Alvarez-Uria, Manoranjan Midde, Raghavakalyan Pakam and Praveen Kumar Naik
Department of Infectious Diseases, Bathalapalli Rural Development Trust Hospital, Kadiri Road, Anantapur District, Bathalapalli 515661, Andhra Pradesh, India

Olufemi O. Desalu, Alakija K. Salami and Ademola E. Fawibe
Department of Medicine, University of Ilorin Teaching Hospital, PMB 1459, Ilorin 240001, Nigeria

Adekunle O. Adeoti
Department of Medicine, Ekiti State University Teaching Hospital, PMB 5355, Ado-Ekiti, Nigeria

Abayomi Fadeyi
Department of Medical Microbiology, University of Ilorin Teaching Hospital, PMB 1459, Ilorin 240001, Nigeria

Olanrewaju O. Oyedepo
Department of Anaesthesia, University of Ilorin Teaching Hospital, PMB 1459, Ilorin 240001, Nigeria

Lilia Ponce Manangan, Cheryl Tryon, Elvin Magee and Roque Miramontes
Division of Tuberculosis Elimination, National Center for HIV/AIDS, Viral Hepatitis, STD, and Tuberculosis Prevention, Centers for Disease Control and Prevention (CDC), Mailstop E-10, 1600 Clifton Road, Atlanta, GA 30033, USA

Liberate J. Mleoh
Kibongóto National Tuberculosis Referral Hospital, Kilimanjaro, Tanzania

Stellah G. Mpagama
Kibongóto National Tuberculosis Referral Hospital, Kilimanjaro, Tanzania
Kilimanjaro Clinical Research Institute and Kilimanjaro Christian Medical College, Kilimanjaro Moshi, Tanzania

Charles Mtabho, Solomon Mwaigwisya, I Marion Sumari-de Boer and Gibson S. Kibiki
Kilimanjaro Clinical Research Institute and Kilimanjaro Christian Medical College, Kilimanjaro Moshi, Tanzania

Scott K. Heysell and Eric R. Houpt
Division of Infectious Diseases and International Health, University of Virginia, Charlotteville, VA 22908, USA

Fatemah Behnaz and Mahmoud Mohammadzadeh
Department of Infectious Diseases, Shahid Sadoughi University of Medical Sciences, Yazd, Iran

Golnaz Mohammadzade
Shahid Sadoughi University of Medical Sciences, Yazd, Iran

Michael Eisenhut
Paediatric Department, Luton and Dunstable University Hospital NHS Foundation Trust, Lewsey Road, Luton LU4 ODZ, UK

Katy Fidler
Department of Infection and Immunology, Brighton and Sussex Medical School, University of Sussex, Brighton, East Sussex BN1 9PX, UK

Luc Calvin Owono Owono
Laboratory for Simulations and Biomolecular Physics, Advanced Teachers Training College, University of Yaoundé I, Yaoundé, Cameroon
Centre for Atomic Molecular Physics and Quantum Optics (CEPAMOQ), University of Douala, Douala, Cameroon
International Centre for Science and High Technology, UNIDO, Area Science Park, Padriciano 99, 34012 Trieste, Italy

Melalie Keita and Eugene Megnassan
International Centre for Science and High Technology, UNIDO, Area Science Park, Padriciano 99, 34012 Trieste, Italy
Laboratoire de Physique Fondamentale et Appliquée, Université d'Abobo-Adjamé, 02 BP 801 Abidjan 02, Cote d'Ivoire

Vladimir Frecer
International Centre for Science and High Technology, UNIDO, Area Science Park, Padriciano 99, 34012 Trieste, Italy
Cancer Research Institute, Slovak Academy of Sciences, 83391 Bratislava, Slovakia
Department of Physical Chemistry of Drugs, Faculty of Pharmacy, Comenius University, 83232 Bratislava, Slovakia
International Centre for Applied Research and Sustainable Technology (ICARST), 81404 Bratislava, Slovakia

Stanislav Miertus
International Centre for Science and High Technology, UNIDO, Area Science Park, Padriciano 99, 34012 Trieste, Italy
International Centre for Applied Research and Sustainable Technology (ICARST), 81404 Bratislava, Slovakia
Faculty of Natural Sciences, University of Ss. Cyril and Methodius, 91701 Trnava, Slovakia

Oludotun Adebayo Phillips and Reny Varghese
Department of Pharmaceutical Chemistry, Faculty of Pharmacy, Kuwait University, Safat 13110, Kuwait

Edet Ekpenyong Udo
Department of Microbiology, Faculty of Medicine, Kuwait University, Safat 13110, Kuwait

Hyejin Kim, Young Kil Park and Sungweon Ryoo
Korean Institute of Tuberculosis, 168-5, Osong sangmyung 4 ro, Osong-eup, Cheongwon-gun, Chungbuk 363-954, Republic of Korea

Minji Seo
Novartis Korea LTD, CD&MA, Namdaemunro 5-ga, Joon-gu 100-753, Republic of Korea

Jae-Il Yoo, Yeong Seon Lee and Gyung Tae Chung
Centers for Infectious Diseases, National Institute of Health, Korea Centers for Disease Control and Prevention, 187 Osong sangmyung 2 ro, Osong-eup, Cheongwon-gun, Chungbuk 363-951, Republic of Korea

H. Ochoa-Díaz-López
Área Académica Sociedad, Cultura y Salud, El Colegio de la Frontera Sur (Ecosur), 29290 San Cristóbal de Las Casas, Chiapas, Mexico

J. C. Nájera-Ortiz and H. J. Sánchez-Pérez
Área Académica Sociedad, Cultura y Salud, El Colegio de la Frontera Sur (Ecosur), 29290 San Cristóbal de Las Casas, Chiapas, Mexico
Grups de Recerca d'Amèrica i Àfrica Latines, GRAAL-Ecosur, San Cristóbal de Las Casas, Chiapas, Mexico

G. Leal-Fernández
Departamento de Atención a la Salud, Universidad Autónoma Metropolitana-Xochimilco, 04960 México, DF, Mexico

A. Navarro-Giné
Grups de Recerca d'Amèrica i Àfrica Latines (GRAAL), Unitat de Bioestad´ıstica, Facultat de Medicina, Universitat Autónoma de Barcelona (UAB), 08193 Barcelona, Spain

Michael Eisenhut
Paediatric Department, Luton and Dunstable University Hospital, NHS Foundation Trust, Luton LU40DZ, UK

Detlef Thieme and Hans Sachs
Forensisch Toxikologisches Centrum, Munich 80335, Germany

Dagmar Schmid and Sybille Fieseler
Institut fur Rechtsmedizin, Ludwig-Maximilians Universität München, Munich 80336, Germany

Olarewaju Sunday, Folorunso Ebenezer, Babatunde Akintunde, Temitayo-Oboh Abiola and Abdulsalam Saliu
Department of Community Medicine, Ladoke Akintola University Teaching Hospital, Ogbomoso, Nigeria

Olanrewaju Oladimeji
Liverpool School of Tropical Medicine, Pembroke Place, Liverpool, UK

Oluwatoyin Abiodun
Department of Medical Microbiology, Ladoke Akintola University of Technology, Ogbomoso, Oyo State, Nigeria

Kabtamu Tolosie and M. K. Sharma
Addis Ababa University, Addis Ababa, Ethiopia

Lakshmi Krishnan, Katherine N. McIntire and Celine R. Gounder
Department of Medicine, Johns Hopkins University School of Medicine, Baltimore, MD 21287, USA

Tokunbo Akande, Anita V. Shankar and Wei-Teng Yang
Johns Hopkins Bloomberg School of Public Health, Baltimore, MD 21205, USA

Amita Gupta
Department of Medicine, Johns Hopkins University School of Medicine, Baltimore, MD 21287, USA
Johns Hopkins Bloomberg School of Public Health, Baltimore, MD 21205, USA
Center for Clinical Global Health Education, Johns Hopkins University, 600 North Wolfe Street, Phipps 540B, Baltimore, MD 21287, USA

Gezahegn Gebrekidan
Policy and Planning Directorate, Federal Ministry of Health (FMOH), Addis Ababa, Ethiopia

Gezahegn Tesfaye and Mitiku Teshome Hambisa
Department of Public Health, College of Health and Medical Sciences, Haramaya University, Harar, Ethiopia

Negussie Deyessa
School of Public Health, College of Medical Sciences, Addis Ababa University, Addis Ababa, Ethiopia

Ato Kwamena Tetteh
Laboratory Department, Metropolitan Hospital, Cape Coast, Ghana

Edward Agyarko
Department of Community Medicine and Health, Anglican University College of Technology, Nkoranza, Ghana

Joseph Otchere and Irene Ayi
Noguchi Memorial Institute for Medical Research, Department of Parasitology, College of Health Sciences, University of Ghana, Legon, Accra, Ghana

Langbong Bimi
Department of Animal Biology and Conservation Sciences, University of Ghana, Legon, Accra, Ghana

Shirin Karimi
Mycobacteriology Research Center, National Research Institute of Tuberculosis and Lung Diseases (NRITLD), Shahid Beheshti University of Medical Sciences, Tehran, Iran

Masoud Shamaei
Clinical Tuberculosis and Epidemiology Research Center, NRITLD, Shahid Beheshti University of Medical Sciences, Tehran, Iran

Mihan Pourabdollah and Mehrdad Karbasi
Pediatric Respiratory Diseases Research Center, National Research Institute of Tuberculosis and Lung Diseases (NRITLD), Shahid Beheshti University of Medical Sciences, Tehran, Iran

Makan Sadr and Arda Kiani
Tracheal Diseases Research Center, National Research Institute of Tuberculosis and Lung Diseases (NRITLD), Shahid Beheshti University of Medical Sciences, Tehran, Iran

Moslem Bahadori
Chronic Respiratory Diseases Research Center, National Research Institute of Tuberculosis and Lung Diseases (NRITLD), Shahid Beheshti University of Medical Sciences, Tehran, Iran

Tadesse Belayneh
Department of Medical Anesthesiology, CMHS, University of Gondar, Gondar, Ethiopia

Afework Kassu
Department of Microbiology Immunology and Parasitology, CMHS, University of Gondar, Gondar, Ethiopia

Desalgne Tigabu
Institute of Public Health, CMHS, University of Gondar, Gondar, Ethiopia

Gashaw Asmare and Sofanit Tilaye
University of Gondar Hospital, Gondar, Ethiopia

Eveline Klinkenberg
KNCV Tuberculosis Foundation, The Hague, Netherlands
Department of Global Health, Academic Medical Center, Amsterdam Institute for Global Health and Development, University of Amsterdam, Amsterdam, Netherlands

Senedu B. Gebreegziabher
Amhara Regional State Health Bureau, Bahir Dar, Ethiopia
Institute of Health and Society, University of Oslo, Blindern, 0318 Oslo, Norway

Gunnar A. Bjune
Institute of Health and Society, University of Oslo, Blindern, 0318 Oslo, Norway

Solomon A. Yimer
Amhara Regional State Health Bureau, Bahir Dar, Ethiopia
Institute of Health and Society, University of Oslo, Blindern, 0318 Oslo, Norway
Oslo University Hospital, 0424 Oslo, Norway
Norwegian Institute of Public Health, Nydalen, 0403 Oslo, Norway

Berhanu Seyoum
Haramaya University, College of Health and Medical Sciences, Harar, Ethiopia

Meaza Demissie and Alemayehu Worku
Addis Continental Institute of Public Health, Addis Ababa, Ethiopia

Shiferaw Bekele and Abraham Aseffa
Armauer Hansen Research Institute, Addis Ababa, Ethiopia

Sifrash Meseret Gelaw
Unit 12 A, Tuscany Condo, Ayala Avenue 6751, Makati City, 1226 Metro Manila, Philippines
24th Floor Citibank Tower, Paseo De Roxas 8741, Makati City, 1226 Metro Manila, Philippines

Omer Adjibodé, Prudence Wachinou, Narcisse Toundoh, Bérénice Awanou, Gildas Agodokpessi, Dissou Affolabi, Gabriel Adè and Séverin Anagonou
National Tuberculosis Programme, 01 BP 321 Cotonou, Benin

Anthony D. Harries
International Union against Tuberculosis and Lung Disease, Paris, France
London School of Hygiene and Tropical Medicine, London, UK

Serge Ade
National Tuberculosis Programme, 01 BP 321 Cotonou, Benin
Faculté de Médecine, Université de Parakou, Parakou, Benin
International Union against Tuberculosis and Lung Disease, Paris, France

Mahasweta Satpati
Population Services International (PSI), New Delhi, India

Sharath Burugina Nagaraja
ESIC Medical College and PGIMSR, Bangalore, India

Hemant Deepak Shewade and Sarabjit Chadha
International Union Against Tuberculosis and Lung Disease (The Union), South-East Asia Regional Office, New Delhi, India

Prabhakaran Ottapura Aslesh
Department of Community Medicine, Academy of Medical Sciences, Pariyaram, Kerala, India

Blesson Samuel
World Vision India, New Delhi, India

Ashwani Khanna
State TB Office, New Delhi, India

Wakjira Kebede and Temesgen Ewunetu
Department of Medical Laboratory Sciences and Pathology, College of Public Health and Medical Sciences, Jimma University, Jimma, Ethiopia

Fikru Keno
Oromia Regional Social and Labor Affairs Agency, Addis Ababa, Ethiopia

Gutu Mamo
Department of Pharmacy, College of Public Health and Medical Sciences, Nekemte Hospital, Jimma, Ethiopia

Mengistu Endris, Feleke Moges and Chandrashekhar Unakal
School of Biomedical and Laboratory Sciences, University of Gondar, Gondar, Ethiopia

Yeshambel Belyhun
School of Biomedical and Laboratory Sciences, University of Gondar, Gondar, Ethiopia Institute of Virology, Faculty of Medicine, University of Leipzig, Leipzig, Germany

Eleni Woldehana
Enfranz Health Center, Enfranz, Ethiopia

Ahmed Esmael
Department of Microbiology, Immunology and Parasitology, Debre Markos University, Debre Marqos, Ethiopia

Geeta S. Pardeshi
Department of Community Medicine, Vardhman Mahavir Medical College and Safdarjung Hospital, New Delhi, India

Dileep Kadam, Ajay Chandanwale, Pranali Khobragade, Malan Parande, Aarti Kinikar, Sunita Girish and Sangita Shelke
Byramjee Jeejeebhoy Government Medical College/ Sassoon General Hospital, Pune, Maharashtra, India

Andrea Deluca
Department of International Health, Johns Hopkins Bloomberg School of Public Health, Baltimore, MD, USA

Nikhil Gupte
Department of International Health, Johns Hopkins Bloomberg School of Public Health, Baltimore, MD, USA
Byramjee Jeejeebhoy Government Medical College/ Johns Hopkins Clinical Trials Unit, Pune, Maharashtra, India

Nishi Suryavanshi
Byramjee Jeejeebhoy Government Medical College/ Johns Hopkins Clinical Trials Unit, Pune, Maharashtra, India

Jason Farley
School of Nursing, Johns Hopkins University, Baltimore, MD, USA

Robert Bollinger
Division of Infectious Diseases and International Health, Johns Hopkins University School of Medicine, Baltimore, MD, USA

Sarman Singh and Manoj Kumar
Division of Clinical Microbiology and Molecular Medicine, Department of Laboratory Medicine,
All India Institute of Medical Sciences, New Delhi 110029, India

Pragati Singh
National Polio Surveillance Project, Country Office for India, World Health Organization, Mathura 281001, India

Silvan M. Vesenbeckh, Nicolas Schönfeld and Torsten T. Bauer
Department of Pneumology, Lungenklinik Heckeshorn, HELIOS Klinikum Emil von Behring, 14165 Berlin, Germany

Harald Mauch, Thorsten Bergmann, Sonja Wagner and Holger Rüssmann
Institute of Microbiology, Immunology and Laboratory Medicine, HELIOS Klinikum Emil von Behring, 14165 Berlin, Germany

C. Padmapriyadarsini and Mahalakshmi Rajendran
National Institute for Research and Tuberculosis, Chennai, India

Mrinalini Das
Médecins Sans Frontières, New Delhi, India

Sharath Burugina Nagaraja
ESIC Medical College and PGIMSR, Bangalore, India

Richard Kirubakaran and Prathap Tharyan
Christian Medical College, Vellore, India

Sarabjit Chadha
The International Union Against TB and Lung Disease, New Delhi, India

Wu Li, Guangcun Deng, Min Li, Xiaoming Liu and Yujiong Wang
Key Laboratory of Ministry of Education for Conservation and Utilization of Special Biological Resources in the Western, Ningxia University, Yinchuan, Ningxia 750021, China
College of Life Science, Ningxia University, 539 W. Helanshan Road, Xixia District, Yinchuan, Ningxia 750021, China

Eshetu Haileselassie Engeda, Hiwot Kassa Woreta, Mengistu Mekonnen Kelkay and Tesfaye Demeke Ashenafie
Department of Nursing, College of Medicine and Health Sciences, University of Gondar, Gondar, Ethiopia

Berihun Assefa Dachew
Department of Epidemiology and Biostatistics, Institute of Public Health, College of Medicine and Health Sciences, University of Gondar, Gondar, Ethiopia

Zachary White, John Painter and Drew L. Posey
Division of Global Migration and Quarantine, National Center for Emerging and Zoonotic Infectious Diseases, Centers for Disease Control and Prevention, Atlanta, GA, USA

Paul Douglas
Department of Immigration and Border Protection, Sydney, NSW, Australia

Ibrahim Abubakar
Public Health England and University College London, London, UK

Howard Njoo, Chris Archibald and Jessica Halverson
Centre for Communicable Diseases and Infection Control, Public Health Agency of Canada, Ottawa, ON, Canada

John Robson
Immigration New Zealand, Wellington, New Zealand

Solima M. A. Sabeel
Department of Microbiology, Faculty of Medical Laboratory Sciences, University of Khartoum, Khartoum, Sudan
Microbiology Department, Faculty of Medical Laboratory Sciences, Ibn Sina University, Khartoum, Sudan

Mohamed Ahmed Salih
Department of Bioinformatics, Africa City of Technology, Khartoum, Sudan

Manasik Ali
Sudan Academy of Sciences, Khartoum, Sudan

Salah-Eldin EL-Zaki
Department of Epidemiology, Tropical Medicine Research Institute, National Center for Research, Khartoum, Sudan

Nadir Abuzeid
Department of Microbiology, Faculty of Medical Laboratory Sciences, Omdurman Islamic University, Khartoum, Sudan

Zeinab Abubaker Mohammed Elgadi
Veterinary Research Institute, Khartoum, Sudan

Hisham N. Altayb
Microbiology Department, College of Medical Laboratory Sciences, Sudan University of Science and Technology, Khartoum, Sudan

Asrar M. A. Elegail and Nuha Y. Ibrahim
National Reference Laboratory-Tuberculosis (NRL-TB), National Public Health Laboratory, Khartoum, Sudan

Bahaeldin K. Elamin
Department of Microbiology, Faculty of Medical Laboratory Sciences, University of Khartoum, Khartoum, Sudan
Department of Microbiology and Parasitology, College of Medicine, University of Bisha, Bisha, Saudi Arabia

Jaideep Dey
Department of Medicine, Lady Hardinge Medical College, New Delhi, India

Hitender Gautam, Shwetha Venugopal, Chhavi Porwal, Bijay Ranjan Mirdha and Urvashi B. Singh
Department of Microbiology, All India Institute of Medical Sciences, New Delhi 110029, India

Naresh Gupta
Department of Medicine, Maulana Azad Medical College, New Delhi, India

Index